AF332967

NEXT GENERATION SEQUENCING - ADVANCES, APPLICATIONS AND CHALLENGES

Edited by **Jerzy K Kulski**

Next Generation Sequencing - Advances, Applications and Challenges

http://dx.doi.org/10.5772/60489
Edited by Jerzy K Kulski

Contributors

Manegold-Brauer Gwendolin, Olav Lapaire, Szilveszter Juhos, György Horváth, Krisztina Rigó, a Desai, Anamika Krishanpal, Vasco Azevedo, Mariana Santana, Flavia Aburjaile, Mariana Parise, Anne Cybelle Pinto, Sandeep Tiware, Artur Silva, Hiromasa Yamauchi, Shanrong Zhao, Yuan Lu, Ronald B. Walter, Yingjia Shen, Wesley Warren, David Rabbolini, Marie-Christine Morel-Kopp, Sara Gabrielli, Qiang Chen, Christopher Ward, William Stevenson, Urmila Dilip Kulkarni-Kale, Melaku Gedil, Andreas Gisel, Livia Stavolone, Ismail Rabbi, Gezahegn Girma, Morag Ferguson, Tatiana Tatusova, Leonid Zaslavsky, Stacy Ciufo, Igor Tolstoy, Boris Kiryutin, Boris Fedorov, Nirala Ramchiary, Rashmi Gaur, Ajay Kumar, Sushil Satish Chhapekar, Roger Dawkins, Ted Steele, Sally Lloyd, Takashi Shiina, Stephan Beck, Gareth A. Wilson, Jerzy Kazimierz Kulski

CBS, Edition **2017**

Published by InTech

Janeza Trdine 9, 51000 Rijeka, Croatia

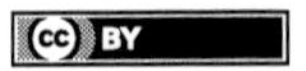

Notice

Statements and opinions expressed in the chapters are these of the individual contributors and not necessarily those of the editors or publisher. No responsibility is accepted for the accuracy of information contained in the published chapters. The publisher assumes no responsibility for any damage or injury to persons or property arising out of the use of any materials, instructions, methods or ideas contained in the book.

Publishing Process Manager Sandra Bakic

Technical Editor InTech DTP Team

Cover Designer InTech Design Team

Additional hard copies can be obtained from orders@intechopen.com

Next Generation Sequencing - Advances, Applications and Challenges, Edited by Jerzy K Kulski
p. cm.
ISBN 978-953-51-2240-1

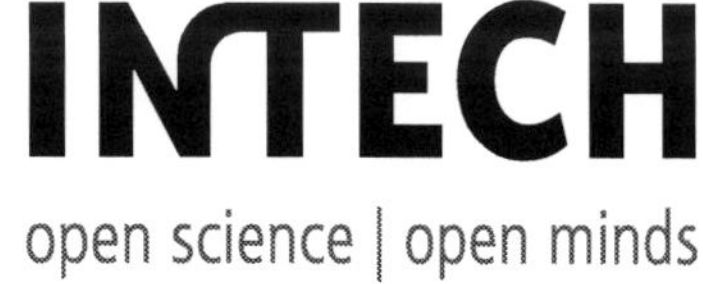

Contents

Preface

There is not a discovery in science, however revolutionary, however sparkling with insight that does not arise out of what went before.

Isaac Asimov, Adding a Dimension.

This year, 2015, marks the 150th anniversary of the Morovian monk Gregor Mendel's seminal paper on pea-plant genetics. He discovered the statistical patterns of inheritance from one generation to the next and deduced that the basic unit of inheritance was inherited in pairs, one unit from each parent that segregated and manifested in the offspring as dominant or recessive traits. Twenty-three years after Mendel's death in 1884, the English biologist William Bateson described the study of heredity as genetics, and a few years later the Danish botanist Wilhelm Johannsen named the gene as the physical and functional unit of inheritance. Soon after the rediscovery and understanding of Mendel's publication, his experimental observations became known in the biological sciences as Mendel's laws of heredity with (1) the law of segregation, (2) the law of independent assortment and (3) the law of dominance. Thus, by the early and mid-1900s, the science of genetics was well and truly born to evolve, amplify and spread far beyond the pea plants and impact on all the life sciences for the next 100 years, all the way across to the present age of next-generation genomics.

And what of the physical nature of the gene itself? It was only 62 years ago that Watson and Crick published their landmark paper 'Molecular structure of Nucleic Acids' in *Nature* on 25th April 1953. Their opening paragraph was *'We wish to suggest a structure for the salt of deoxyribose nucleic acid (D.N.A). This structure has novel feature which are of considerable biological interest.'* They put forward their hypothesis of the DNA structure as a sequence of four nucleotides as if these nucleotides were beads on two complementary helical strings or chains that coiled about each other in antiparallel and around the same axis. The nucleotides on the inside of the helix or strand always bound covalently to those on the opposite helix in a complimentary fashion, adenine to thymine and guanidine to cytosine. Thus, *'the two chains are held together by the purine and pyrimidine bases'* by hydrogen bonds. Further, *'It has not escaped our notice that the specific pairing we have postulated immediately suggests a possible copying mechanism for the genetic material.'* The history of how Watson and Crick surreptitiously established their DNA model as a double helix by using the unpublished X-ray diffraction data of Rosalind Franklin is well established and has been variously dramatized in print, theatre, film and on the TV screens. Two years prior to the Watson and Crick discovery, Erwin Chargaff and his colleagues had pointed out in a *Nature* paper that DNA was composed of equivalent amounts of nucleotides with A=T and G=C. Even earlier, in 1944, Oswald Avery and his colleagues, Colin MacLeod and Maclyn McCarty, already had identified DNA as the molecule of heredity in their published experimental work on bacterial transformation.

The impact of the Watson and Crick publication on the structure of DNA as a double helix was profound because it quickly led to the establishment of the Central Dogma that genetic information was transcribed from DNA to messenger RNA and translated to build a protein, and that it could not again flow in the reverse direction from protein to RNA. The proof that triplets or codons of the DNA sequence coded for amino acids that were the building blocks of peptides and proteins soon followed in the late 1950s and throughout the 1960s with the works of Marshall Nirenberg, Heinrich Matthaei, Sydney Brenner, Symour Benzer and others. Thus, DNA and RNA were strongly asserted to contain the genetic code and that the genetic information encoded within DNA was undoubtedly universal to all forms of life. It was not until 1970 that Crick's Central Dogma was jolted by Howard Temin and David Baltimore and their colleagues with the discovery that the reverse transcriptase enzyme allows the flow of genetic information from RNA to DNA by RNA retroviruses like human immunodeficiency virus and via certain cellular enzymes such as telomerase and a reverse transcriptase-like protein encoded by the RVT gene. Moreover, the sequencing of the human genome in 2001 revealed that at least half of our genome is made of fossils of past retrotransposon integrations, some of which have evolved to act as regulators and insulators in a complex, regulatory process of transcription and translation. Only 2–3 % of our genome consists of loci that we call genes and that code for proteins. The rest of the genome, once referred to as 'junk DNA', appears to be regulatory, although it remains mostly as *dark matter*, waiting to be fully deciphered. Nevertheless, Crick's fundamental insight that the sequence of the nucleotides in DNA is transcribed and translated into the synthesis of proteins via messenger RNA and amino acids carried by three-base coded (anticodons) transfer RNA molecules remains the basis of modern genetics and genomics.

The first published natural polynucleotide sequence was a yeast transfer RNA and not DNA. It was published in *Science* in 1965 by Robert W. Holley and his colleagues 12 years after the Watson and Crick paper proposed the structure of DNA, and it had taken them many years to obtain a gram of RNA by complicated purification procedures so that they had sufficient amounts to identify its sequence by spectrophotometry and chromatography. A number of different laborious DNA and RNA sequencing procedures were developed during the late 1960s and early 1970s mostly using two-dimensional chromatography and/or electrophoresis and hazardous chemicals and/or large doses of radioisotopes. The first genome to be sequenced was in 1976, a viral RNA genome from the bacteriophage MS2 by Walter Fiers' group at the University of Ghent in Belgium using an RNA sequencing technique based on RNA fragmentation and the separation of fragments by two-dimensional gel electrophoresis. The following year, Fred Sanger and his colleagues in the UK published the first DNA genome, the 5386 base-pair Phage Phi-X174. In the same year, they also published two technical papers on the rapid determination of DNA sequence that was safer, easier and more reliable than the other sequencing techniques such as the Maxam and Gilbert chemical method. The Sanger method was based on plasmid cloning of DNA fragments and DNA polymerase reactions using fluorescent-labelled or radiolabelled dideoxynucleotides to follow the sequencing reactions that were amendable more easily to automation. The coupling of the Sanger fluorescent DNA sequencing method with automated capillary electrophoresis led to the establishment of sequencing centres and factories with hundreds of DNA sequencing instruments operated in parallel by large numbers of personnel. This led to the domination of Sanger sequencing as the first-generation sequencing procedure and gold standard for 30 years since its inception, and it has had an enormous impact on our understanding of DNA and gene organization and what happens at the genomic level in humans and various plants and animals and microorganisms. By 2001, a mosaic version of the whole human genome was sequenced to 90 % completion with announcements of the accomplishment by the 42nd US President Bill Clinton at the White House, universal fanfare and two major papers published in *Science* and *Nature* at about the same time. In addition to the human genome, sequencing groups had already published the full genomes for eukaryotic and prokaryotic viruses, bacterial plasmids and partial genomes for a variety of different species.

Although the need for DNA sequencing and generating sequences for analytical consumption was great during the era of Sanger sequencing, the cost and effort of sequencing were still prohibitively expensive and far too slow for many laboratories to join in to work on the maturing field of genomics. This began to change dramatically by 2007 with the emergence of a number of different next-generation automated sequencing technologies such as those developed by 454 Life Sciences, Solexa, Applied Biosystems and Helicos that increased the number of sequencing reactions in miniaturized arrays, fibre-optic slides or flow cells and greatly reduced the cost of sequencing from millions to thousands of US dollars in only a few years. A single next-generation sequencing (NGS) run using any one of the new massively parallel-sequencing platforms could generate more sequencing data than simultaneously running a hundred Sanger sequencing machines. Although the short read lengths, sequencing errors and the large volumes of data generated by NGS were at first seen as a problem with the technology, the lower costs, large capacity, high coverage of reasonably accurate sequencing information and the versatility of NGS for a wide range of applications soon began to win over the scientific community and funding agents. The NGS market has grown exponentially over the last decade and promises to continue its enormous expansion with ongoing improvements and cost reductions provided by the manufacturers and service providers. It is envisaged that desktop sequencers for personal genomics and single investigators and small laboratory groups will be developed in the near future that will be no larger than portable hard drives stacked together and connected to laptop or desktop computers. However, with the sudden technical and economic ease to generate vast amounts of sequencing information comes the problem and burden of sequence data acquisition, storage, transmission and analysis. The bottleneck for genomics is no longer about generating sequences, the holdup is now at the level of bioinformatics, storing, processing, analysing and interpreting the sequencing information.

Unsurprisingly, the developments in DNA sequencing technology progressed almost hand in hand with those in computing and information systems technology. When Apple released the Macintosh 128K in 1984, its first Macintosh personal computer, the sequences available for analysis were from genes, genomic fragments, and genomes of plasmids and viruses. They were simple sequences that were analysed using the primitive, pioneering computer software such as DNA Inspector, DNAStrider and, later, GeneJockey, MacVector, Sequencher and others. With the arrival of the World Wide Web on the open Internet and personal computer web browsers in the early 1990s, the sequences available for analysis were increasing in number and complexity and they required more sophisticated algorithms, software and hardware with ever-increasing computation capacity and speed. The Human Genome Project was formally initiated in October of 1990 and it required a 13-year international effort to complete the sequence of most of the 3 billion DNA nucleotides and annotate the estimated 20,000–24,000 human genes for further study. Today, NGS and genomics are seen much more as a science of Biological Information Systems and 'Big Data'. There has been an inundation of DNA and RNA sequences that heavily taxes the limitations of the parallel development of computers to store and process the rapidly accumulating DNA and RNA data and to translate and manage the information systematically, efficiently and securely. For example, as of November 2014, half of the 7,597 prokaryote species in the NCBI Refseq dataset still were uncharacterized, and there are estimates that zetabases ($> 1 \times 10^{21}$) of sequence per year will need to be processed in a projected trillion dollar industry by 2025, including the personal data of a million or more human genome sequences. Thus, much attention is now drawn towards solving the problems of computational greed and how to integrate, process, filter and secure astronomical amounts of genomic data.

What is next-generation sequencing (NGS)? In brief, NGS is a sequencing technology that is faster, cheaper and more versatile than the first-generation sequencing methods that preceded it such as the Sanger sequencing method. NGS permits high-throughput sequencing of the whole genome (DNA-seq), exomes (exomic DNA-seq) or targeted genomic regions (targeted DNA-seq), genomic RNA or the transcriptome (RNA-seq), DNA methylation sites throughout the genome (Methyl-Seq) and the genomic regions involved in protein–DNA interactions (ChIP-seq) and three-dimensional genome structure (Hi-C) of any organism. However, NGS is not just a sequencing technology, it is also an information systems technology with enormous implications for man's future in various fields and aspects of life. It is the interrogation, collection and spread of biological information for our enlightenment and for the development of novel biological applications and innovations both good and bad in biotechnology, biodefense, the environment, ecosystems, agriculture, industry and human health.

Many of the advances, applications and challenges associated with NGS are dealt with comprehensively and insightfully in this book in the form of reviews and original studies by leading researchers providing expert and novel information and insights in their particular fields of interest. This is a book for scientists, clinicians, technicians, academics, specialists, graduate and postgraduate students and for all who are interested in DNA sequencing and bioinformatics across all fields of the life sciences. This book consists of 16 chapters presented in four sections. The first section, 'Genomics, Transcriptomics and Methylomics', contains five chapters starting with an overview of the basic tools and technological developments pertaining to NGS and 'omics', followed by examples of the application of NGS in the assembly of aquatic genomes, targeted NGS to genotype the polymorphisms of the MHC genomic region, NGS transcriptomic profiling and the computational analysis of methylome data. The three chapters in the second section, 'NGS of Microorganisms', cover the impact and progress of NGS techniques and the computational applications in the generation and analysis of NGS data for microorganisms, especially viruses and bacteria. The three chapters in the third section, 'NGS of Agricultural Plants', address the role of NGS in the study of plants that are part of the agricrops that sustain and feed humans and their livestock. The fourth and final section, 'NGS in Humanomics', consists of five chapters that focus on NGS in the analysis of ancestral haplotypes, ambiguities and quality measures using NGS for genotyping polymorphic HLA genes, NGS in the diagnosis of inherited macrothrombocytopenias as a Mendelian disease using signature sequence markers, NGS for the detection of non-invasive genetic diseases in the foetus using the pregnant mother's DNA, and it concludes with a chapter on the impact of RNA-seq data analysis on human gene annotation.

NGS is a vast and rapidly evolving area of science, and it is beyond the scope of this book to cover all the issues and topics related to this subject. The authors in this book are experts from various areas of NGS, structural and functional genomics, bioinformatics and complex data analysis who have devoted their time, despite their busy schedules, to write their valuable and thought-provoking chapters with tireless dedication in the few months allowed to them to meet the demanding deadlines. We thank them for their tireless dedication to overcome the challenges and to complete the book project on schedule. We welcome, savour and appreciate the information and knowledge imparted by these different authorities in their chapters presented in this book.

Last but not least, we thank the staff of InTech and the Publishing Process Manager Sandra Bakic for their valuable contribution to the editing and smooth publication of this book. We hope that it will become a valuable reference and a further inspiration for basic and practical research on the implementation of NGS technologies and bioinformatics and assist in elucidating all the wonders of the genetic code still waiting to be deciphered at the many different levels of biology, now and into the future.

Jerzy K Kulski

[1] Department of Molecular Life Science,
Division of Basic Medical Science and Molecular Medicine,
Tokai University School of Medicine, Isehara, Japan

[2] Centre for Forensic Science,
The University of Western Australia,
Nedlands, WA, Australia

Genomics, Transcriptomics and Methylomics: Tools and Applications

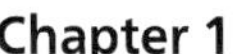

Next-Generation Sequencing — An Overview of the History, Tools, and "Omic" Applications

Jerzy K. Kulski

Additional information is available at the end of the chapter

http://dx.doi.org/10.5772/61964

Abstract

Next-generation sequencing (NGS) technologies using DNA, RNA, or methylation sequencing have impacted enormously on the life sciences. NGS is the choice for large-scale genomic and transcriptomic sequencing because of the high-throughput production and outputs of sequencing data in the gigabase range per instrument run and the lower cost compared to the traditional Sanger first-generation sequencing method. The vast amounts of data generated by NGS have broadened our understanding of structural and functional genomics through the concepts of "omics" ranging from basic genomics to integrated systeomics, providing new insight into the workings and meaning of genetic conservation and diversity of living things. NGS today is more than ever about how different organisms use genetic information and molecular biology to survive and reproduce with and without mutations, disease, and diversity within their population networks and changing environments. In this chapter, the advances, applications, and challenges of NGS are reviewed starting with a history of first-generation sequencing followed by the major NGS platforms, the bioinformatics issues confronting NGS data storage and analysis, and the impacts made in the fields of genetics, biology, agriculture, and medicine in the brave, new world of "omics."

Keywords: Next-generation sequencing, tools, platforms, applications, omics

1. Introduction

Next-generation sequencing (NGS) refers to the deep, high-throughput, in-parallel DNA sequencing technologies developed a few decades after the Sanger DNA sequencing method first emerged in 1977 and then dominated for three decades [1, 2]. The NGS technologies are different from the Sanger method in that they provide massively parallel analysis, extremely high-throughput from multiple samples at much reduced cost [3]. Millions to billions of DNA

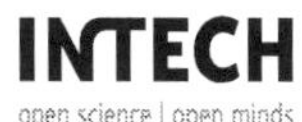

nucleotides can be sequenced in parallel, yielding substantially more throughput and minimizing the need for the fragment-cloning methods that were used with Sanger sequencing [4]. The second-generation sequencing methods are characterized by the need to prepare amplified sequencing libraries before undertaking sequencing of the amplified DNA clones, whereas third-generation single molecular sequencing can be done without the need for creating the time-consuming and costly amplification libraries [5]. The parallelization of a high number of sequencing reactions by NGS was achieved by the miniaturization of sequencing reactions and, in some cases, the development of microfluidics and improved detection systems [6]. The time needed to generate the gigabase (Gb)-sized sequences by NGS was reduced from many years to only a few days or hours, with an accompanying massive price reduction. For example, as part of the Human Genome Project, the J. C. Venter genome [7] took almost 15 years to sequence at a cost of more than 1 million dollars using the Sanger method, whereas the J. D. Watson (1962 Nobel Prize winner) genome was sequenced by NGS using the 454 Genome Sequencer FLX with about the same 7.5x coverage within 2 months and for approximately 100th of the price [8]. The cost of sequencing the bacterial genome is now possible at about $1000 (https://www.nanoporetech.com), and the large-scale whole-genome sequencing (WGS) of 2,636 Icelanders [9] has brought some of the aims of the 1000 Genomes Project [10] to abrupt fruition.

Rapid progress in NGS technology and the simultaneous development of bioinformatics tools has allowed both small and large research groups to generate *de novo* draft genome sequences for any organism of interest. Apart from using NGS for WGS [11], these technologies can be used for whole transcriptome shotgun sequencing (WTSS) — also called RNA sequencing (RNA-seq) [12], whole-exome sequencing (WES) [13], targeted (TS) or candidate gene sequencing (CGS) [14–16], and methylation sequencing (MeS) [17]. RNA-seq can be used to identify all transcriptional activities (coding and noncoding) or a select subset of targeted RNA transcripts within a given sample [12], and it provides a more precise and sensitive measurement of gene expression levels than microarrays in the analysis of many samples [18–21]. In contrast to WGS, WES provides coverage for more than 95% of human exons to investigate the protein-coding regions (CDS) of the genome and identify coding variants or SNPs when WGS and WTSS are not practical or necessary [13]. Since the exome represents less than 2% of the human genome, it is the cost-effective alternative to WGS and RNA-seq in the study of human genetics and disease [13]. However, WGS may be preferred over WES because it provides more data with better uniformity of read coverage on disease-associated variants and reveals polymorphisms outside coding regions and genomic rearrangements [19, 22]. The analysis of the methylome by MeS complements WGS, WES, and CGS to determine the active methylation sites and the epigenetic markers that regulate gene expression, epistructural base variations, imprinting, development, differentiation, disease, and the epigenetic state [23–30]. The impact of NGS technology is indeed egalitarian in that it allows both small and large research groups the possibility to provide answers and solutions to many different problems and questions in the fields of genetics and biology, including those in medicine, agriculture, forensic science, virology, microbiology, and marine and plant biology.

The aim of this chapter is to provide an overview of the advances, applications, and challenges of NGS, starting with a history of first-generation sequencing followed by the major NGS platforms, the bioinformatics issues confronting NGS data storage and analysis, and the applications and challenges for biology and medicine in the world of "omic" expansion.

2. First-generation sequencing: A brief history

Twelve years after the publication of the Watson and Crick double-helix DNA structure in 1953 [31], the first natural polynucleotide sequence was reported [32]. It was the 77-nt yeast alanine tRNA with a proposed cloverleaf structure, although the anticodon, the three nucleotides that bind to the mRNA sequence, was not yet identified in the sequence [32]. It took 7 years to prepare up to 1 g of the tRNA from commercial baker's yeast by countercurrent distribution before fragmenting the RNA into short oligonucleotides with various RNase enzymes to reconstruct and identify the nucleotide residues using two-dimensional chromatography and spectrophotometric procedures [33]. At that time, scientists could sequence only a few base pairs per year, not nearly enough to sequence an entire gene. Nevertheless, despite the time-consuming and laborious nature of these very first sequencing methods that were developed for tRNA and other oligonucleotides, there was a flurry of RNA and DNA sequencing for the next 10 years that improved the sequencing procedures of fragmented DNA and provided new information on the sequences of more than 100 different tRNA. These initial labor-intensive sequencing efforts resulted also in the first complete genome sequence — the 3,569-nucleotide-long bacteriophage MS2 RNA, the lysozyme gene sequence of bacteriophage T4 DNA, and the 24-bp lac operator sequence [33–36]. This eventually led to the Maxam and Gilbert chemical degradation DNA sequencing method that chemically cleaved specific bases of terminally labeled DNA fragments and separated them by electrophoresis [37]. New data on how to sequence bacteriophage DNA by specific primer extension methods resulted in Sanger et al. [1] using primer-extension and chain-termination methods for sequencing polynucleotides longer than oligonucleotide lengths. Subsequently, the new Sanger DNA chain-termination sequencing method [1], known simply as the Sanger sequencing method, prevailed over the Maxam and Gilbert chemical degradation method [37] because of its greater simplicity and reliability and the use of fewer toxic chemicals and lower amounts of radioactivity. The first-generation automated DNA sequencers developed by Applied Biosystem Instruments (ABI) used the Sanger method with fluorescent dye-terminator reagents for single-reaction sequencing rather than the usual four separate reactions [34–36]. These sequencers were later improved by including computers to collect, store, and analyze the sequencing data [38]. The invention of the PCR technology [39] and thermal cyclers and the use of a heat-resistant enzyme such as Taq polymerase from *Thermus aquaticus* between 1985 and 1990 enabled the generation of random or specific sequences for *de novo* sequencing, filling gaps, and resequencing particular regions of interest [35]. The discovery of reverse transcriptase in 1970 [40, 41] led to the development of RNA sequencing using cDNA reverse transcribed from RNA. In 1991, Adams et al. [42] initiated a systematic cDNA sequencing project using the Sanger method and the 373A DNA semiautomated sequencers to generate large batches of cDNA sequences with an average length of 397 bases, which they named "expressed sequence tags" (ESTs) and used as substrates and markers for RNA contig and transcriptome mapping. These improvements, together with the establishment of GenBank (http://www.ncbi.nlm.nih.gov/genbank) in 1982, resulted in the generation of hundreds of thousands of more DNA sequences throughout the 1980s, 1990s [34–36], and right up to the beginning of the new millennium, with the publication of the first draft sequence of the human genome [43, 44].

A sudden increase in the number of DNA and RNA sequences generated for GenBank between 1992 and 2004 (http://www.ncbi.nlm.nih.gov/genbank/statistics) resulted mostly from three main initiatives: the development of automated sequencers and the emergence of service providers, the industrialization and the establishment of sequencing centers and international consortiums, and the continued development of computing hardware and software to store and analyze nucleotide sequences. The automated-industrialized approach based on random or shotgun sequencing was initiated by The Institute for Genomic Research (TIGR) in Rockville, Maryland, and resulted in the publication of 337 new human genes and 48 homologous genes from other organisms [42]. By 1999, the TIGR venture generated 83 million nucleotides of cDNA sequence, 87,000 human cDNA sequences, and the complete genome sequences of two bacterial species, *Haemophilus influenzae* [45] and *Mycoplasma genitalium* [46]. This success was in part due to the development of the TIGR sequence assembler, an innovative computer program to assemble vast amounts of EST data [47]. By the end of 2001, the automated sequencers, such as the fully automated Prism 3700 with 96 capillaries that could produce 1.6×10^5 bases of sequence data per day, sequencing centers and international consortiums, such as the TIGR in the USA, the Sanger Centre in the United Kingdom, and RIKEN in Japan, produced the complete genomic sequences of the bacteria *E. coli* and *Bacillus subtilis*, the yeast *Saccharomyces cerevisiae*, the nematode *C. elegans*, the fruit fly *Drosophila melanogaster*, the plant *Arabidopsis thialiana*, and the human genome (see references cited by Stein [48]). Although sequencing was still hugely expensive and time consuming, Sanger sequencing was by then the dominant method. Pundits now placed DNA sequencing into a postgenomic era and predicted functional genomics, SNPs, and transcript arrays as the future of biological investigation [49, 50]. Indeed, after the establishment of the first Affymetrix and GeneChip microarrays in 1996, the decade saw a rapid growth in DNA array technology and applications for various gene expression studies in prokaryotes and eukaryotes [21, 51, 52]. Nevertheless, the outputs for genomic and/or RNA sequencing had neither finished nor slowed; new sequencing methods continued to emerge after 2005 to challenge the cost and supremacy of the Sanger dideoxy method [34–36]. These new methods became known as next-generation sequencing because they were designed to employ massively parallel strategies to produce large amounts of sequence from multiple samples at very high-throughput and at a high degree of sequence coverage to allow for the loss of accuracy of individual reads when compared to Sanger sequencing. These different approaches brought the cost of sequencing the genome down from $100 million in 2001 to less than $10,000 in 2014 [53].

3. Second-generation sequencing

A more detailed history of the development of the first- and next-generation sequencing platforms has been presented in a number of previous reviews [2–6, 11, 34–36, 54]. Table 1 outlines the basic features and performances of the common next-generation sequencing platforms. The basic characteristics of second-generation sequencing technology are the following. Shotgun sequencing of random fragmented genomic (fg) DNA or cDNA reverse transcribed from RNA is performed without the need for cloning via a foreign host cell: instead, linker and/or adapter sequences are ligated to the fgDNA or cDNA for construction of template libraries. Library amplification is performed on a solid surface or on beads while isolated within miniature emulsion droplets or arrays. Nucleotide incorporation is monitored directly by luminescence detection or by changes in electrical charge during the sequencing procedure. NGS generates many millions of nucleotide short reads in parallel in a much shorter time than by the Sanger sequencing method. The read types generated by NGS are digital and therefore enable direct quantitative comparisons. Either single or pair end reads can be obtained at fragment ends.

3.1. DNA and RNA library preparations for second-generation sequencing

The general workflow for second-generation sequencing is the preparation and amplification of libraries prepared from DNA or RNA samples, clonal formation, sequencing, and analysis [55–59]. Head et al. [55] have reviewed the methods and problems encountered for preparing NGS libraries for whole-genome sequencing, exome sequencing, target sequencing, RNA-seq, ChIP-seq, RIP-seq, and methylation sequencing (methyl-seq). Prior to library preparation, the genomic DNA is fragmented by acoustic shearing, sonication, or enzymatic digestion with DNase I or fragmentase and then labeled with adapters, tags, barcodes, and primers using established ligation and PCR methods. Alternatively, Illumina's fragmentation technology, called Nextera Tagmentation, can be implemented using a transposase enzyme to simultaneously fragment and insert adapter sequences into the ds DNA and thereby reduce sample handling and preparation time [57]. For targeted sequencing, the exomes or regions of interest within the fragmented DNA can be captured and enriched by probe-hybridization-capture kits or by PCR amplification with custom-designed primers. For RNA-seq of mRNA, polyA-RNA is isolated usually from total RNA or rRNA-depleted RNA and reverse transcribed to cDNA with reverse transcriptase and polyT or polyU primers before being treated much the same way as the fragmented genomic DNA. RNA sequencing libraries also can be created from immunoprecipitated RNA-binding proteins. To isolate noncoding RNAs (micro, small, and long) from total RNA, these sequences are selectively ligated to 3' and 5' adapters and reverse transcribed to cDNA. For methylation sequencing, the genomic DNA is reacted usually with bisulfite chemicals prior to library construction. On the other hand, ChIP-seq and RIP-seq use antibody capture to enrich the relevant sequences before preparation of the genomic DNA fragments for sequencing. In comparison to high-input gDNA libraries, the RNA and ChIP libraries may be limited by low cell numbers as starting material and consequently result in a low input of extracted DNA from the immunoprecipitated histones or DNA-binding proteins and in a limited sequence coverage.

Numerous DNA and RNA library kits and machines are available for the semiautomated or fully automated preparation of DNA libraries both for second- and/or third-generation sequencing. Some of these are GemCode from x10 (http://10xgenomics.com) and Raindrop's Thunderstorm (http://raindancetech.com) for all sequencing platforms, cBot for the Illumina platform [58], and Ion Chef and Ion OneTouch for the Ion Torrent platform [59]. All of these kits and auxiliary machines attempt to reduce workload and costs for the main platform sequencers. The DNA libraries are labeled with barcode sample tags, such as the multiplex identifier (MID) for Roche/454 sequencing, to enable the libraries to be pooled and therefore maximize the sequence output as a multiplex amplicon sequencing step for each sequencing run. After library construction, the DNA fragments are clonally amplified by emulsion PCR with microbeads [4, 6, 60] or by solid-phase PCR using primers attached to a solid surface [4, 61, 62] in order to generate sufficient single-stranded DNA molecules and detectable signal for producing sufficiently reliable sequencing data [54]. Roche 454, Life Technologies' SOLiD, and Ion Torrent platforms use emulsion PCR, whereas Illumina's HiSeq/MiSeq platforms use solid-phase PCR [4]. More recently, isothermal PCR amplification on a solid surface of a flow cell [62] was developed for the SOLiD 5500 W series of sequencing machines.

A problem with preparing sequencing libraries by PCR amplification is that PCR introduces GC bias, a major source of unwanted variation and errors in the sequencing coverage [63]. Using alternative methods to PCR amplification improves library complexity and the coverage of high GC regions and reduces the number of duplicate reads [64]. A number of different PCR-free library preparation kits are available commercially, such as NEXTflex PCR-Free from Bioo Scientific, Accel NGS 2S PCR-free library kit from Swift Biosciences, and the Illumina TruSeq DNA PCR-Free Sample Preparation Kit that uses ligation amplification for Illumina and other sequencing platform systems.

3.2. NGS platforms

The main features and performances of five commonly used second-generation sequencing technologies that have been reviewed in detail by others [2–4, 11, 36, 54] are shown in Table 1.

NGS platforms/company/max output per run	Read length per run (bp)	No. reads per run	Time (h or days)	Cost per 10^6 bases	Raw error rate (%)	Platform cost (USD approx.)	Chemistry
First generation							
Sanger/Life Technologies/84 kb	800	1	2 h	2400	0.3	95,000	Dideoxy terminator
Second generation							
454 GS FLX+/Roche/0.7 Gb	700	1×10^6	24/48 h	10	1	500,000	Pyrosequencing
GS Junior/Roche/70 Mb	500	1×10^5	18 h	9		100,000	Pyrosequencing
HiSeq/Illumina/1500 Gb	2x150	5×10^9	27/240 h	0.1	0.8	750,000	Reversible terminators
MiSeq/Illumina/15 Gb	2x300	3×10^8	27 h	0.13	0.8	125,000	Reversible terminators
SOLiD/Life Technologies/120 Gb	50	1×10^9	14 days	0.13	0.01	350,000	Ligation
Retrovolocity/BGI/3000 Gb	50	1×10^9	14 days	0.01	0.01	12×10^6	Nanoball/ligation

NGS platforms/company/max output per run	Read length per run (bp)	No. reads per run	Time (h or days)	Cost per 10^6 bases	Raw error rate (%)	Platform cost (USD approx.)	Chemistry
Ion Proton/Life Technologies/100 Gb	200	6×10^7	2–5 h	1	1.7	215,000	Proton detection
Ion PGM/Life Technologies/2 Gb	200	5×10^6	2–5 h	1	1.7	80,000	Proton detection
Third generation							
SMRT/Pac Bio/1 Gb	>10,000	1×10^6	1–2 h	2	12.9	750,000	Real-time SMS
Heliscope/Helicos/25 Gb	35	7×10^9	8 days	0.01	0.2	1.35×10^6	Real-time SMS
Nanopore/Oxford Nanopore Technologies/1 Gb	>5000	6×10^4	48/72 h	<1	34	1000	Real-time SMS
Electron microscopy/ZS	7200		14 h	<0.01		1×10^6	Real-time SMS
Genia nanopore (http://www.geniachip.com)							Real-time SMS

Table 1. Basic features and performances of NGS platforms. Sources are [4, 11, 20, 54, 115]. For comparison of the NGS outputs, the human genome has 3×10^9 bp or 3 Gb.

3.2.1. Roche 454 pyrosequencing

Roche 454 pyrosequencing by synthesis (SBS) was the first commercially successful second-generation sequencing system developed by 454 Life Sciences in 2005 and acquired by Roche in 2007 (http://www.my454.com). This technology uses sequencing chemistry, whereby visible light is detected and measured after it is produced by an ATP sulfurylase, luciferase, DNA polymerase enzymatic system in proportion to the amount of pyrophosphate that is released during repeated nucleotide incorporation into the newly synthesized DNA chain [2, 4, 6]. The system was miniaturized and massively parallelized using PicoTiterPlates to produce more than 200,000 reads at 100 to 150 bp per read with an output of 20 Mb per run in 2005 [6]. The upgraded 454 GS FLX Titanium system released by Roche in 2008 improved the average read length to 700 bp with an accuracy of 99.997% and an output of 0.7 Gb of data per run within 24 h. The GS Junior bench-top sequencer produced a read length of 700 bp with 70 Mb throughput and runtime of 10 to 18 h. The major drawbacks of this technology are the high cost of reagents and high error rates in homopolymer repeats. The estimated cost per million bases is $10 by Roche 454 compared to $0.07 by Illumina HiSeq 2000 [54]. A more serious challenge for those using this technology is the announcement by Roche that they will no longer supply or service the 454 sequencing machines or the pyrosequencing reagents and chemicals after 2016 [65].

3.2.2. Illumina (Solexa) HiSeq and MiSeq sequencing

Illumina (http://www.illumina.com) purchased the Solexa Genome Analyzer in 2006 and commercialized it in 2007 [66, 67]. Today, it is the most successful sequencing system with a claimed >70% dominance of the market, particularly with the HiSeq and MiSeq platforms. The Illumina sequencer is different from the Roche 454 sequencer in that it adopted the technology of sequencing by synthesis using removable fluorescently labeled chain-terminating nucleotides that are able to produce a larger output at lower reagent cost [4, 6, 66]. The clonally enriched template DNA for sequencing is generated by PCR bridge amplification (also known as cluster generation) into miniaturized colonies called polonies [66]. The output of sequencing data per run is higher (600 Gb), the read lengths are shorter (approximately 100 bp), the cost is cheaper, and the run times are much longer (3-10 days) than most other systems [54]. Illumina provides six industrial-level sequencing machines (NextSeq 500, HiSeq series 2500, 3000, and 4000, and HiSeq X series five and ten) with mid to high output (120–1500 Gb) as well as a compact laboratory sequencer called the MiSeq, which, although small in size, has an output of 0.3 to 15 Gb and fast turnover rates suitable for targeted sequencing for clinical and small laboratory applications [68]. The MiSeq uses the same sequencing and polony technology such as the high-end machines, but it can provide sequencing results in 1 to 2 days at much reduced cost [54]. Illumina's new method of synthetic long reads using TruSeq technology apparently improves *de novo* assembly and resolves complex, highly repetitive transposable elements [69].

3.2.3. Sequencing by Oligonucleotide Ligation and Detection (SOLiD)

Supported Oligonucleotide Ligation and Detection (SOLiD) is a next-generation sequencer instrument marketed by Life Technologies (http://www.lifetechnologies.com) and first released in 2008 by Applied Biosystems Instruments (ABI). It is based on 2-nucleotide sequencing by ligation (SBL) [4, 6, 66]. This procedure involves sequential annealing of probes to the template and their subsequent ligation. Sequencers on the market today, such as the 5500 W series, are suitable for small- and large-scale projects involving whole genomes, exomes, and transcriptomes. Previously, sample preparation and amplification was similar to that of Roche 454 sequencing [66]. However, the upgrades to Wildfire chemistry have enabled greater throughput and simpler workflows by replacing beads with direct *in situ* amplification on FlowChips and paired-end sequencing [62]. The SOLiD 5500 W series sequencing reactions still use fluorescently labeled octamer probes in repeated cycles of annealing and ligation that are interrogated and eventually deciphered in a complex subtractive process using Exact Call Chemistry that has been well described by others [2, 36, 66]. The advantage of this method is accuracy with each base interrogated twice. The major disadvantages are the short read lengths (50–75 bp), the very long run times of 7 to 14 days, and the need for state-of-the-art computational infrastructure and expert computing personnel for analysis of the raw data.

3.2.4. DNA nanoball sequencing by BGI Retrovolocity

Complete Genomics (http://www.completegenomics.com) developed DNA nanoball sequencing (DNBS) as a hybrid of sequencing by hybridization and ligation [70]. Small fragments (440–500 bp) of genomic DNA or cDNA are amplified into DNA nanoballs by rolling-circle replication that requires the construction of complete circular templates before the generation of nanoballs. The DNA nanoballs are deposited onto an arrayed flow cell, with one nanoball per well sequenced at high density. Up to 10 bases of the template are read in 5′ and 3′ direction from each adapter. Since only short sequences, adjacent to adapters, are read, this sequencing format resembles a multiplexed form of mate-pair sequencing similar to using Exact Call Chemistry in SOLiD sequencing [2, 36, 66]. Ligated sequencing probes are removed, and a new pool of probes is added, specific for different interrogated positions. The cycle of annealing, ligation, washing, and image recording is repeated for all 10 positions adjacent to one terminus of one adapter. This process is repeated for all seven remaining adapter termini. Although the developers have sequenced the whole human genome, the major disadvantage of DNBS is the short length of reads and the length of time for the sequencing projects. Claimed cost of the reagents for sequencing of the whole human genome is under $5000. The major advantage of this approach is the high density of arrays and therefore the high number of DNBs (~350 million) that can be sequenced. In 2015, the Chinese genomics service company BGI-Shenzhen acquired Complete Genomics and introduced the Retrovolocity system for large-scale, high-quality whole-genome and whole-exome sequencing with 50x coverage per genome and with the sample to assembled genome produced in less than 8 days [71]. Complete Genomics claims to have sequenced more than 20,000 whole human genomes over 5 years and published widely on the use of their NGS platform. They provide public access to a human repository of 69 genomes data and a cancer data set of two matched tumor and normal sample pairs at http://www.completegenomics.com/public-data/.

3.2.5. Ion torrent

Ion Torrent technology (http://www.iontorrent.com) was developed by the inventors of 454 sequencing [60], introducing two major changes. Firstly, the nucleotide sequences are detected electronically by changes in the pH of the surrounding solution proportional to the number of incorporated nucleotides rather than by the generation of light and detection using optical components. Secondly, the sequencing reaction is performed within a microchip that is amalgamated with flow cells and electronic sensors at the bottom of each cell. The incorporated nucleotide is converted to an electronic signal detected by the electronic sensors. The two sequencers in the market that use Ion Torrent technology are the high-throughput Proton sequencer with more than 165 million sensors and the Ion Personal Genome Machine (PGM), a bench-top sequencer with 11.1 million sensors. There are four sequencing chips to choose from [72]. The Ion PI Chip is used with the Proton sequencer, and the Ion 314, 316, or 318 Chips are used with the Ion PGM. The Ion 314 Chip provides the lowest reads at 0.5 million reads per chip, whereas the Ion 318 Chip provides the highest reads of up to 5.5 million reads per chip. The Proton sequencer provides a higher throughput (10–100 Gb vs. 20 Mb–1 Gb) and more reads per run (660 Mb vs. 11 Mb) than the PGM chips, but the read lengths (200–500 bp), run time (4–5 h), and accuracy (99%) are similar [54, 72]. Sample preparation for the generation of DNA libraries is similar to the one used for Roche 454 sequencing but can be simplified with the use of the Ion Chef system for automated template preparation and chip loading. The Ion Torrent chip is used with an ion-sensitive field-effect transistor sensor that has been engineered to detect individual protons produced during the sequencing reaction. The chip is placed within the flow cell and is sequentially flushed with individual unlabeled dNTPs in the presence of the DNA polymerase. Incorporation of nucleotide into the DNA chain releases H protons and changes the pH of the surrounding solution that is proportional to the number of incorporated nucleotides. The major disadvantages of the system are problems in reading homopolymer stretches and repeats. The major advantages seem to be the relatively longer read lengths, flexible workflow, reduced turnaround time, and a cheaper price than those provided by the other platforms [54, 73].

4. Third-generation sequencing: Emerging technologies for single-molecule sequencing

Third-generation single-molecule sequencing technologies have emerged to reduce the price of sequencing and to simplify the preparatory procedures and sequencing methods [4, 74, 75].

4.1. Single-molecule real-time (SMRT) sequencing by pacific biosciences

Pacific Biosciences (http://www.pacificbiosciences.com) markets the PacBio RS II sequencer and the SMRT real-time sequencing system [74, 75]. SMRT sequencing is performed in SMRT cells that contain 150,000 ultra-microwells at a zeptoliter scale where one molecule of DNA polymerase is immobilized at the bottom of each well using the biotin-streptavidin system in nanostructures known as zero-mode waveguides (ZMWs). Once the template single-strand DNA is coupled with immobilized DNA polymerase, fluorescently labeled dNTP analogs are added and detected when the nucleotide is incorporated into the growing strand. CCD cameras continuously monitor the 150,000 ZMWs as a series of observed pulses that are converted into single molecular traces representing the template sequences. Since all four nucleotides are added simultaneously and measured in real time, the speed of sequencing is much increased compared to technologies where individual nucleotides are flushed sequentially. Although the reported accuracy was 99.3% initially with read lengths of about 900 bp [4], circularizing the template and sequencing it several times using a technology called SMRTbell templates provided longer reads and improved the accuracy to >99.999% [76, 77]. Once sequencing is initiated, the system's computational Blade Center performs real-time signal processing, base calling, and quality assessment. Primary analysis data, including trace and pulse data, read-length, distribution, polymerase speed, and quality measurement, is streamed directly to the secondary analysis software called SMRT Analysis that is capable of processing sequencing data in real time. The secondary analysis tools also include a full suite of tools to analyze single-molecule sequencing data for a broad range of applications.

4.2. Helicos sequencing by the genetic analysis system

The Helicos sequencing system was the first commercial implementation of single-molecule fluorescent sequencing [66, 78], marketed by the now bankrupt Helicos Biosciences. Today, the sequencing provider Seqll (http://seqll.com) sequences genomic DNA and RNA using the Helicos sequencing system and HeliScope single-molecule sequencers. DNA is sheared, tailed with polyA, and hybridized to a flow cell surface containing oligo-dT for sequencing-by-synthesis of billions of molecules in parallel. The polyA-tailed fragments of DNA molecules are hybridized directly to the oligo-dT50 bound on the surface of disposable glass flow cells. The addition of fluorescent nucleotides with a terminating nucleotide pauses the cyclical process until an image of one nucleotide for each DNA sequence has been captured, and then the process is repeated until the fragments have been completely sequenced [75, 76]. This sequencing system is a combination of sequencing by hybridization and sequencing by synthesis using a DNA polymerase [79]. Sample preparation does not require ligation or PCR amplification and, therefore, largely avoids the GC content and size biases observed in other technologies [56]. The HeliScope sequencing read lengths range from 25 to over 60 bases, with 35 bases being the average. This method has successfully sequenced the human genome [80] to provide disease signatures in a clinical evaluation [81] and sequenced RNA to produce quantitative transcriptomes of tissues and cells [82].

4.3. Nanopore sequencing by Oxford Nanopore Technologies (MinION and PromethION)

Oxford Nanopore Technologies provides the latest single-molecule sequencing system [83, 84]. The MinION Mkl is a portable handheld device for DNA and RNA sequencing that attaches directly to a laptop/computer using a USB port, whereas the PromethION is a small bench-top system. Nanopore sequencing uses pores formed from proteins, such as haemolysin, a biological protein channel system in *Staphylococcus aureus* [85]. The idea behind DNA and RNA sequencing using nanopores is that the conductivity of ion currents in the pore changes when the strand of nucleic acid passes through it [83]. The flow of ion current depends on the shape of the molecule translocating through the pore. Since nucleotides have different shapes, each nucleotide is recognized by its effect on the change of the ionic current [86]. The key advantage of this approach is that sample preparation is minimal compared to second-generation sequencing methods, and long read lengths can be obtained in the kbp range. In addition, there are no amplification or ligation steps required before sequencing. The main problem with this technology is the requirement to optimize the speed of DNA translocation through the nanopore to ensure reliable measurement of the ionic current changes and reduce the high error rates of base calling [83–86]. At this time, Oxford Nanopore Technologies is in the beta testing phase, and users are required to join the MinION Access Programme and pay a fee of $1000 [83] to access a MinION starter pack (3 MinION MkI flow cells, a Nanopore sequencing kit, and a wash kit). Laver et al. [87] have assessed the performance of an earlier version of the MinION sequencing device and concluded that "the MinION is an exciting prospect; however, the current error rate limits its ability to compete with existing sequencing technologies, though we do show that MinION sequence reads can enhance contiguity of *de novo* assembly when used in conjunction with Illumina MiSeq data." They resequenced three bacterial genomes and estimated the error rate to be 38.2%, with mean and median reads of 2 and 1 kb, respectively, and with the longest single read of 98 kb. The low depth of coverage provided by the present nanopore technology is a possible barrier to accurate eukaryotic genome sequencing at the moment. Nevertheless, these are not intangibles and nanopore nucleic acid sequencing is envisaged to include methylation and direct RNA sequencing in the near future [83].

4.4. NGS by electron microscopy

The sequence of long, intact DNA molecules can be visualized and identified by using electron microscopy. The first report on the successful application of electron microscopy for NGS was for the partial sequencing of DNA base pairs within intact DNA molecules using synthesized genomes of 3.3 and 7.2 kb length that were sequenced by enzymatically incorporating modified bases that contained atoms of increased atomic number and allowed for the direct visualization and identification of individually labeled bases [88]. In this sequencing process, the double strands of the DNA sample are separated into single strands using common enzymes and reactions. Then, the single-stranded DNA is labeled by PCR using dNTPs attached to heavy-atom metal labels that can be separated into identifiable electron microscope-generated images showing large black dots, small black dots, and large gray dots along the DNA molecule linearized by ZSG threading. Standard image-based technologies perform the reads and analysis of the labeled DNA using image analysis software that provides sequence data in real time. The sequenced molecules are reads in the range of 5 to 50 kb in length that are useful for *de novo* genome assembly and for analysis of full haplotypes and copy number variants. The company ZS Genetics (http://www.zsgenetics.com) offers a service to provide accurate, long-read, single-molecule DNA sequences using the NGS electron microscopy platform.

5. NGS service providers

Researchers who cannot afford to purchase NGS machines at prices varying between $80,000 and over 1 million USD (depending on the platform) plus the many add-ons, computing requirements, and infrastructure changes, instead, might consider using one of the many available sequencing service providers. For example, Novogene, which was founded in Beijing in 2011 and now is located also in Great Britain and the USA, provides NGS for human, animal, plant, and microbe applications using Illumina MiSeq, HiSeq, and X platforms for whole-genome *de novo* sequencing and resequencing, exome sequencing, targeted sequencing, transcriptomics for mRNA and small RNA, and metagenomics. Similarly, the South Korean company Macrogen provides all the NGS services using Illumina platforms as well as epigenome sequencing for methylations by bisulfite conversion, methyl-CpG binding domain, or chromatin immunoprecipitation. Prices may vary between $500 and $2,000 USD per sample depending on the sequencing project and the project workflow from sample preparation to bioinformatics analysis (https://www.scienceexchange.com). Table 2 lists some of the service providers, and others can be accessed at http://omicsmaps.com.

Service provider	Platforms	DNA sequencing (TS WG WES)	RNA-seq	Methyl-seq	Web address
BGI	All	+ + +	+	+	bgiamericas.com
Novogene	Illumina	+ + +	+	+	novogene.com
Macrogen	Illumina	+ + +	+	+	macrogen.com
	Ion Torrent	+ + +	+	+	
CD Genomics	Illumina	+ + +	+	+	cd-genomics.com
	Ion Torrent	+ + +	+	+	

Service provider	Platforms	DNA sequencing (TS WG WES)	RNA-seq	Methyl-seq	Web address
	PacBioRS II	+ + +	+	+	
	CEA**			+	
SeqWright Genomic	Illumina	+ + +	+	+	seqwright.com/researchservices
	Ion Torrent	+ + +	+	+	
	Roche 454	+ + +	+		
EpigenDx	Ion Torrent			+	epigendx.com
Centrillion Genomic	Illumina	+ + +	+		centrillionbio.com
NXT-DX	Illumina		+	+	nxt-dx.com
AGRF***	Illumina	+ + +	+	+	agrf.org.au
	CEA**			+	
Broad Institute	Illumina	+ + +	+	+	genomics.broadinstitute.org
Illumina	Illumina	+ + +	+	+	illumina.com
Exiqon	Illumina		+		exiqon.com
SEQLL	Helicos	+ + +	+	+	seqll.com
Eurofins Genomics	Illumina	+ + +	+		eurofinsgenomics.eu
	Roche 454	+ + +			
	Ion Torrent	+ - +			
	PacBioRS II	+ - +			
Millennium Science	PacBioRS II	+ + +		+	mscience.com.au/view/
Oxford Nanopore Technologies	MINion	+ + +	+		nanoporetech.com
Complete Genomics	Nanoball arrays	+ +			completegenomics.com

Table 2. NGS service providers. In the DNA sequencing column, TS is targeted sequencing, WG is whole-genome sequencing, and WES is whole-exome sequencing. *RNA-seq includes whole transcriptome, mRNA, long, small, and microRNA sequencing. **Methyl-seq (methylation sequencing) or epigenetic analysis is usually performed by bisulfite sequencing and either NGS or capillary electrophoresis analysis (CEA). Other analyses such as MBD, MeDIP-seq, or ChIP-seq may be provided. Helicos and PacBio platforms also enable the detection of methylation sites. ***AGRF = Australian Genomic Research Facility. Most of the listed service providers also may perform sample and library preparation, Sanger sequencing, specialist genotyping, data analysis, and bioinformatics service. Other service providers can be accessed via the High-Throughput Sequencing Map site at http://omicsmaps.com.

6. Performance of NGS platforms and sequencing errors

All NGS systems produce unique sequencing errors and biases that need to be identified and corrected. The major sequencing errors are largely related to high-frequency indel polymorphisms, homopolymeric regions, GC- and AT-rich regions, replicate bias, and substitution errors [89–91]. While the PGM quality scores underestimate the base accuracy, the Roche 454 quality scores tend to overestimate the base accuracy. A key consideration for generating high-quality, unbiased, and interpretable data from next-generation sequencing studies is to achieve sufficient sequence depth and coverage for statistical certainty. Low sequencing depth can contribute to high error rates stemming from base calling and mapping errors, which in turn can affect the statistical significance for identifying true genotypes, nucleotide variants, and single nucleotide polymorphism. Increased depth of coverage can help sequence alignment mapping to differentiate between true variants and errors, although it might not resolve errors due to assembly gaps. Good sequence library preparation is paramount to producing good sequence depth and coverage. A number of different library methods are available to achieve this goal depending on the NGS applications [55]. Sims et al. [92] reviewed in critical detail the guidelines and precedents for optimal sequencing depth and coverage in regard to sequencing genomes, exomes, transcriptomes, methylomes, and epigenomes by chromatin immunoprecipitation and sequencing and/or chromosome conformation capture.

No single study has compared the performance of all the available NGS platforms simultaneously using the same control genomic sequences. However, a comparison of three bench-top sequencers, the Roche GS Junior, the Illumina MiSeq, and Ion PGM, revealed large differences in cost, sequence capacity, and performance outcomes of genome depth, stability of coverage and read lengths, and quality for sequencing bacterial genomes [54, 93]. Most sequencing errors arose with indel polymorphisms, GC-rich regions, and homopolymeric regions. Overall, the two laboratories concluded that all the machines had certain limitations that needed to be taken into account when designing sequencing experiments [54, 93]. In a comparison of bacterial genome sequencing between PacBio, Ion Torrent, and three Illumina machines (MiSeq, GAIIx, and HiSeq 2000), the sequencers all provided high accuracy for GC-rich, neutral, and moderately AT-rich genomes [94]. The main exception was the poor coverage in the extremely AT-rich region of *Plasmodium falciparum* with a single 316 chip for the Ion Torrent PGM that resulted in no coverage for 30% of the genome. In this study, PacBio generated the longest reads but produced the least accurate SNP detection and the highest error rate of 13% compared to 1.78% for Ion Torrent and less than 0.04% for the Illumina platforms. In a different comparison, the performance of whole-genome sequencing platforms Illumina's HiSeq2000, Life Technologies' SOLiD 4 and 5500xl SOLiD, and Complete Genomics' sequencing system were evaluated for their ability to call SNVs and to evenly cover the genome and specific genomic regions [95]. The authors concluded that all the platforms had their shortfalls with a pronounced GC bias in GC-rich regions and false-positive rates and that the best solution is to integrate the sequencing data from the four different platforms because it combined the strengths of different technologies. In an analysis of bacterial CREBBP exons, three different NGS platforms appear to have worked comparably well for targeted exomic sequencing with the percentage of total read numbers aligned to a reference sequence resulting in 99.8% for Roche 454, 98.1% for Illumina MiSeq, and 90.7% for Ion Torrent PGM sequence reads [96]. However, the Illumina MiSeq data showed the highest substitution error rate, whereas the PGM data revealed the highest indel error rate. On the other hand, there was little difference between the Junior Roche and the Ion PGM platforms for "in phase" sequence genotyping of HLA loci, and either platform could be used with excellent results [16]. In this case, the lower cost of reagents and a slightly quicker turnaround time favored the Ion PGM platform [97].

Five sequencing platforms, Illumina HiSeq, Ion PGM, Ion Proton, PacBio RS, and Roche 454, were tested in a comparative evaluation of RNA-seq reproducibility using reference RNA standards at 19 laboratory sites [20]. The results showed high intraplatform and interplatform concordance for expression measures across the deep-count regions but highly variable reproducibility for splice junction and variant detection between all platforms. Despite fewer bases sequenced, the Proton, PGM, and 454 platforms detected more known junctions compared to Illumina HiSeq.

7. Bioinformatics: DNA and RNA data analysis and storage

Bioinformatics is a major rate-limiting step for NGS technology with respect to overcoming the growing challenges of storage, analysis, and interpretation of NGS data [98–100]. There are at least four tiers of nucleotide sequence analysis to consider when using the NGS platforms [98–104]. The first is generation of sequence reads using the software integrated within the sequencing instruments that convert the raw signals into base calling with short reads of nucleotide sequences and associated quality scores. The second is the alignment and assembly of contigs and scaffolds and variant detection. The third is annotation, data integration, and visualization of the assembled sequence. The fourth is the amalgamation of all the data from the different NGS platforms into a single, coherent, bioinformatic output with accessible links and tools for general and particular biological or forensic interest. The Internet-web addresses to source the bioinformatics tools and databases for NGS data analysis from the original raw sequencing data to functional biology can be obtained from the following references [99–104] and Table 3.

The raw sequencing signals produced by the manufacturer's sequencing machine or system are converted into nucleotide bases of short read data (base calling) with base quality scoring using the system's FASTQ format or the native raw data file formats (Illumina, SFF, HDF5, CG, or SOLID). Storage of raw signal (image) and sequencing data as short read archives in the FASTQ format or native raw data file formats is a problem in regard to computing resources for many research sequencing laboratories and commercial service providers. Thus, the conversion of FASTQ files to the more compact Sequence Alignment Map (SAM) format and its compressed Binary Alignment Map (BAM) format is recommended because it is easier to read and process for later bioinformatics analysis [99, 102]. The safe storage of the original raw sequences is important for bioinformatics analysis and corrections because it is the source of the initial sequencing errors that are either filtered out or left within the final assembled sequence. Quality checks are necessary to remove reads with low phred levels, sequence errors, and sequences such as primers, vectors, adapters, tags, and tails that were introduced exper-imentally during the preparation of the sequencing libraries [101]. Errors or biases associated with raw reads from the Illumina, Roche, and SOLiD platforms are mainly fluorophore-dependent errors, whereas the non-fluorophore platforms such as Ion Torrent produce their own unique errors and biases [99, 101]. Therefore, many different signal and image detection programs and base calling algorithms still need to be developed and tested in an attempt to improve the accuracy of base calling [101]. The raw sequence data (a mixture of raw files and other metadata) from the NGS technologies can be submitted to the NCBI Sequence Read Archive database for DNA studies and to Gene Expression Omnibus and ArrayExpress for mRNA-seq or ChIP-Seq studies in order to receive a database accession number and to reference the raw sequence data in scientific publications [105]. The Sequence Read Archive (SRA) at NCBI also provides a fee-free, downloadable SRA computing toolkit to read the raw graphs and files from the different NGS platforms and to convert between different file formats (Table 3). Archive files in the SRA format (.sra) are converted into the FASTQ or SAM/BAM formats for input to downstream analysis using software programs (Table 3) to undertake the second tier analysis of sequence alignment (spliced and genomic), assembly, and variant detection.

The requirement for sequence alignment and variant detection at the second tier of bioinformatics depends on the complexity of the NGS project. Small sequence reads from small genomes (e.g., viruses) are less complex and easier to compute and align and assemble than the many more reads generated from large genomes of mammals or higher plants. The transfer of the preedited DNA data in the correct format to alignment and variant detection software is generally straightforward and there are many free and commercial software packages available to perform these tasks [99–104]. As often is the case, a single package does not suit all analytical requirements. There may need to be a degree of interchange and testing to find the best solutions as well as using appropriate and informative controls for standardization and normalization. Schlotterer et al. [104] have reviewed programs for genotype and SNP calling. ANGSD is a new multithreaded program suite that was developed recently to perform association mapping, population genetic analyses (population structure measures, allele frequency for cases and controls, admixture, and neutrality tests), SNP discovery, and genotype calling using the raw sequence data and genotype likelihoods in NGS data of human DNA samples for the 1000 Genomes Project [106].

The alignment of sequences to provide long assemblies (contigs and/or scaffolds) may take two different paths. One is comparative mapping of short reads aligned to reference sequences and the other is *de novo* assembly of overlapping reads [101]. The accuracy of *de novo* assembly can be confirmed or improved by integrating it with comparative alignment mapping to reference genomic sequences. Sequencing assemblers may employ different graph construction algorithms and preprocessing and postprocessing filter computations to flag, correct, or eliminate sequencing errors with no single computation solution. Some genome assemblers forgo the preprocess filtering step and they all differ in their ease of use, in the accuracy, efficiency, and quality of assembly, ability to fill gaps, and differentiate between error driven variants and true variants or SNPs and in the detection and elimination of repeats and sequencing errors [99]. According to El-Metwally et al. [99], an ideal assembler should have a set of layers with clearly defined inputs, communication output messages to facilitate the development of innovative, interactive, independent assemblers using the SAM/BAM file formats and the language of FASTG (http://fastg.sourceforge.net) for the next-generation environment. Another way to improve the quality of sequencing and assembly is to adopt a hybrid approach by using two or more different sequencing platforms and assembly software. A new software package *anytag* that fills gaps between paired-end reads to generate near-error-free contigs of up to 190 kb appears to be a fivefold improvement over existing *de novo* genome assemblers such as *soap* and *Newbler* [107].

In a recent evaluation of the most commonly used *de novo* genome assemblers to assemble the genomes of three vertebrate species (snake, bird, and fish) by Assemblathon, the authors recommended not to trust the results of any single assembly, nor place too much faith in a single metric of quality or accuracy, but instead to choose an assembler that excels in the area of interest and expectation to provide sufficient coverage, continuity, and error-free bases [108]. End users were reminded that the use of the assembly tools is not straightforward and that they should first gain considerable familiarity with the computing hardware and software and become aware of the "ease of installation, use, and management" of each assembly tool. Many problems with *de novo* genome assembly remain inherent with recognizing and evaluating highly heterozygous and repetitive regions, segmental duplications, and sequencing errors and gaps. This is complicated further by the different read lengths, read counts, and error profiles that are produced by different NGS technologies. In addition, most assembled genomic sequences in publicly accessible databases are at the level of or below a standard draft (minimum standards for submission to public databases) rather than a "high-quality draft" assembly that is completed to at least 90% of the expected genome size.

The third tier of bioinformatics is to annotate, transcribe, and translate the genomic sequences to a higher informatics level, such as defining gene exon coding (CDS) and noncoding (5′ noncoding, introns, and 3′ terminal end) untranslated regions (UTRs), alternate transcript isoforms, signal peptides, repeat elements, and other nontranscribed regions such as viral integration sites and chromosomal common fragile sites [103]. Genomic sequences of prokaryotes are a thousand times smaller and less complex than those of eukaryotes and consequently are easier to assemble and annotate. A typical methodology for prokaryote annotation suggested by the National Pathogen Data Resource to annotate 1000 genomes is to first submit the genomic sequence to the Rapid Annotation Server (RAST) at the Argonne National Laboratory and receive back the protein-encoded genes (CDS), the RNA-encoded genes (tRNAs and rRNAs), and identified subsystems such as metabolic pathways, complex structures, and phenotypes (Table 3). This initial annotation should then be reanalyzed in detail to find discrepancies between the sequence and the translation using any other public or commercial genomic tools to fix miscalled genes and variants, frameshifts, insertion sequences, and pseudogenes. The public web server CRISPRfinder detects and annotates the bacterial CRISPRs and tandem repeat sequences that may impact on genes and pseudogenes (Table 3). After the reanalysis and final fixes, the annotated and curated genome should be rerun through RAST to update the subsystems output. Other useful web-based microbial annotation servers can be accessed at MicroScope, BASys, and NCBI's Prokaryotic Genome Annotation Pipeline (PGAP), with additional software provided at Prokka (Table 3). A typical prokaryotic genome annotation process is outlined at NCBI (http://www.ncbi.nlm.nih.gov/genome/annotation_prok/process/).

Eukaryote genome annotation is more complex and challenging than prokaryote genome annotation. In an overview of the available tools and best practices for eukaryotic genome annotation, Yandell and Ence [103] pointed to five basic categories of annotation software: (1)

ab initio and evidence-drivable gene predictors; (2) EST, protein, and RNA-seq aligners and assemblers; (3) choosers and combiners; (4) genome annotation pipelines; and (5) genome browsers for curation. A typical eukaryotic genome annotation pipeline is outlined by NCBI at http://www.ncbi.nlm.nih.gov/genome/annotation_euk/process/. The essential first step for eukaryote genome annotation and gene determination is to identify and mask repeat elements (microsatellites, retrotransposons, and transposons) using RepeatMasker, Censor, or WindowMasker (Table 3). Without the initial masking step, the repeats would seed millions of spurious BLAST alignments and create incorrect gene annotations and corrupt the genome annotation with artifacts and false metadata. After masking, the annotation pipeline includes the following steps: transcript, RNA-seq read, protein/domain alignments; guided/*ab initio* gene model predictions; curated genomic sequence alignments; selection of the best evidence based models; gene naming and locus typing; assignment of GeneIDs; and annotation of small RNAs. In addition, there are the special considerations such as annotation of multiple assemblies and updated assemblies before the annotated products can obtain an Annotation Release number and a release date for availability in various NCBI resources, including the databases for nucleotides, proteins, BLAST, gene, Map Viewer, and FTP sites. Other websites and tools considered important for eukaryote annotation are BUSCO for assessing the "core" eukaryote genes, Babelomics for the functional analysis of transcriptomic and genomic data, the PASA and MAKER tools for updating annotations with RNA-seq data, and other data and information (Table 3). The annotated and mapped data can then be integrated, visualized, and presented at a fourth tier of bioinformatics with genome browsers such as those displayed at UCSC, Ensembl, JBrowse, Web Apollo (Table 3), and others such as Genome Maps [109]. The new Emsembl 2015 provides an up-to-date genomic interpretation system for annotations, query tools, and access methods for chordates and key model organisms [110].

Gene ontology is a bioinformatics initiative that provides (a) defined terms representing gene product properties and pathways covering biological domains such as cellular components, molecular function, and biological processes with their various subcategories and (b) functional annotation tools to find functions for large gene lists. It sits somewhere between the third tier (annotation) and the fourth tier of bioinformatic analyses and structures. The first major Gene Ontology (GO) project was founded in 1998 to address a need for standard filtered descriptions of gene products across different databases. GO is a collaborative effort that started between three model organism databases, FlyBase (*Drosophila*), the *Saccharomyces* Genome Database (SGD) and the Mouse Genome Database (MGD) but now incorporates many databases for plant, animal, and microbial genomes. The GO Contributors page lists all member organizations (http://geneontology.org/page/go-consortium-contributors-list). Some other ontology providers among many are the Open Biological and Biomedical Ontologies (OBBO), Reactome, DAVID, and the KEGG Pathway database (Table 3).

NGS manufacturers provide their own unique software for the first tier analysis to process the raw acquisition data and produce read files that contain high-quality consensus reads for the draft assemblies. However, only a few have attempted to include all three tiers of nucleotide sequence analysis into a fourth tier that is an easily accessible single integrated package. Illumina has provided the BaseSpace genomics cloud-computing program for integrated data storage and analysis (Table 3). This cloud storage and analysis program permits instrument integration with sequence analysis viewing and access to a wide range of software applications to align, assemble, and analyze reads and variants for RNA and DNA. These apply to various workflows, including basic analyses for prokaryotic and eukaryotic genomics and transcriptomics, metagenomics, and for more specialist interests such as detection and analysis of tumor variants, haplotype analysis, pathways and networks, forensic profiles, and many others, too numerous to list here. In comparison, Ion Torrent has storage devices and servers with a web browser driving the Torrent Suite Software (Table 3) on computers attached to their respective sequencing instruments. The manufacturer's software can be used to preprocess the DNA sequencing read data before transferring the preedited data onto other analytical software systems that are either provided by the manufacturer (vendor) or obtained from elsewhere. The National Center for Biotechnology Information (NCBI) is an example of a fourth tier bioinformatics provider (Table 3) that is a free, one-stop shop for DNA and RNA sequence data, analysis, and information. There are direct links at NCBI to 65 accessible databases, 35 download sites (for databases, tools, and utilities), 17 public submission portals, and 60 computing tools for sequence and data analysis, reports, and tutorials. In addition, NCBI is a resource for books and journals through its online library and the PubMed webpage.

Program	Website
1. Aligner, assembly, and postassembly tools	
MUMmer aligner	http://mummer.sourceforge.net
Bowtie aligner	http://bowtie-bio.sourceforge.net/index.shtml
TopHat RNA-seq aligner	https://ccb.jhu.edu/software/tophat/index.shtml
Anytag aligner	http://sourceforge.net/projects/anytag/files/anytag2.0/
Soap *de novo* assembler	http://soap.genomics.org.cn/soapdenovo.html
Allpaths-LG assembler	http://www.broadinstitute.org/software/allpaths-lg/blog/
Celera assembler	http://wgs-assembler.sourceforge.net/wiki/index.php?title=Main_Page
Velvet assembler	https://www.ebi.ac.uk/~zerbino/velvet/
SPAdes assembler	http://bioinf.spbau.ru/spades
Galaxy tools	https://usegalaxy.org
Genomic tools	http://molbiol-tools.ca/Genomics.htm
BaseSpace Illumina	https://basespace.illumina.com/home/sequence
Torrent Suite Software	http://www.lifetechnologies.com/torrentsuite
RATT: rapid annotation transfer tool	http://ratt.sourceforge.net
2. Prokaryote annotation web servers	
RAST	http://www.nmpdr.org/FIG/wiki/view.cgi/FIG/RapidAnnotationServer
	http://rast.nmpdr.org

Program	Website
CRISPRfinder	http://crispr.u-psud.fr/Server/CRISPRfinder.php
Mreps	http://bioinfo.lifl.fr/mreps/mreps.php
MicroScope	https://www.genoscope.cns.fr/agc/microscope/home/index.php
BaSys	https://www.basys.ca
PGAP	http://www.ncbi.nlm.nih.gov/genome/annotation_prok/
Prokka	http://www.vicbioinformatics.com/software.prokka.shtml
3. Eukaryote annotation web servers	
NCBI pipeline	http://www.ncbi.nlm.nih.gov/genome/annotation_euk/process/
RepeatMasker	http://www.repeatmasker.org/
Censor	http://www.girinst.org/censor/
WindowMasker	http://nebc.nerc.ac.uk/bioinformatics/docs/windowmasker.html
CEGMA tool	http://korflab.ucdavis.edu/datasets/cegma/
BUSCO	http://busco.ezlab.org
PASA	http://pasapipeline.github.io
MAKER	http://www.yandell-lab.org/software/maker.html
Babelomics	http://www.babelomics.org
4. Archives and databases	
DDBJ	http://www.ddbj.nig.ac.jp
EMBL	http://www.embl.org
GenBank	http://www.ncbi.nlm.nih.gov/genbank/
REPBASE	http://www.girinst.org
dbSNP	http://www.ncbi.nlm.nih.gov/projects/SNP/snp_summary.cgi
dbGAP	http://www.ncbi.nlm.nih.gov/gap
Complete Genomics data	http://www.completegenomics.com/public-data/
SRA	http://www.ncbi.nlm.nih.gov/sra
OMIM	http://www.ncbi.nlm.nih.gov/omim
COSMIC	http://cancer.sanger.ac.uk/cosmic
ENCODE	https://www.encodeproject.org
GTEx	http://www.gtexportal.org
FANTOM	http://fantom.gsc.riken.jp
Roadmap epigenomics	http://www.roadmapepigenomics.org
Blueprint epigenomics	http://www.blueprint-epigenome.eu
Regulome DB	http://regulomedb.org

Program	Website
ExPASy proteomics	http://www.expasy.org/proteomics/protein-protein_interaction
PRIDE proteomics	http://www.ebi.ac.uk/pride/archive/
FAME metabolomics	http://f-a-m-e.fame-vu.cloudlet.sara.nl
Metabolomexpress	https://www.metabolome-express.org
MetaboAnalyst	http://www.metaboanalyst.ca
AromaDeg	http://aromadeg.siona.helmholtz-hzi.de
EGA phenome	https://www.ebi.ac.uk/ega/home
GOLD	https://gold.jgi-psf.org
MG-RAST	https://metagenomics.anl.gov
ViralZone	http://viralzone.expasy.org
UCNEbase UC elements	http://ccg.vital-it.ch/UCNEbase/
UCbase 2.0 UC elements	http://ucbase.unimore.it/
DEG database	http://www.essentialgene.org
PhylomeDB	http://phylomedb.org/
Compara GeneTrees	http://asia.ensembl.org
TreeFam	http://treefam.genomics.org.cn
PANTHER	http://pantherdb.org
FATCAT	http://phylogenomics.berkeley.edu
HOGENOM database	http://doua.prabi.fr
5. *Gene ontology databases and tools*	
Gene Ontology Consortium	http://geneontology.org
OBBO	http://www.obofoundry.org, http://obofoundry.github.io
Reactome	http://www.reactome.org/
DAVID 6.7	https://david.ncifcrf.gov/
KEGG Pathway database	http://www.genome.jp/kegg/pathway.html
6. *Genome browsers, projects, and fourth tier providers*	
Kbase	http://kbase.us/glossary/systems-biology/
Earth Microbiome Project	http://www.earthmicrobiome.org
Terragenome Project	http://www.terragenome.org
Tara Oceans Project	http://ocean-microbiome.embl.de/companion.html
MetaHit project	http://www.metahit.eu
Vertebrate Genome 10K	http://genome10k.org
Human Microbiome	http://hmpdacc.org

Program	Website
Personal Genome Project	http://www.personalgenomes.org
1000 Genomes Project	http://www.1000genomes.org
HapMap	http://hapmap.ncbi.nlm.nih.gov/
UCSC browser	https://genome.ucsc.edu
Ensembl browser	http://www.ensembl.org
Jbrowse browser	http://jbrowse.org
Web Apollo browser	http://genomearchitect.org
NCBI mapview	http://www.ncbi.nlm.nih.gov/projects/mapview/
NCBI resources	http://www.ncbi.nlm.nih.gov/guide/all/ - tab-all_
KEGG	http://www.genome.jp/kegg/
7. Optical mappers	
BioNano mapper	http://www.bionanogenomics.com
Whole-Genome Mapping	http://opgen.com/genomic-services/what-is-whole-genome-mapping
8. NGS and bioinformatics software providers and biological databases	
Omicsmap for NGS	http://omicsmaps.com/
The NGS WikiBook	http://en.wikibooks.org/wiki/Next_Generation_Sequencing_(NGS)
The Sequencing Marketplace	http://allseq.com
Genomeweb	https://www.genomeweb.com
Bioinformatic software	http://seqanswers.com/wiki/Software/list
	https://en.wikipedia.org/wiki/List_of_open-source_bioinformatics_software
	http://bioinformaticssoftwareandtools.co.in
Bioinformatics Web	http://www.bioinformaticsweb.net
Biological databases	https://en.wikipedia.org/wiki/List_of_biological_databases
Applied Bioinformatics	http://www.appliedbioinformatics.com.au

Table 3. Useful websites for NGS tools, browsers, portals, providers, and online databases.

8. Impact and applications of NGS: Opening the doors into the world of "omics"

All hereditary information is contained within the structure, organization, and function of an organism's genome. The continual emergence of many new public bioinformatics databases (Table 3) on the World Wide Web demonstrates and reflects the impact of NGS on the life sciences and our need to constantly develop new methods to interrogate and decode hereditary information in and around DNA (or RNA for some viruses) and its nucleotide sequences (http://www.bioinformaticsweb.net).

Although genomics is a relatively young field, arguably starting sometime between 1976 with the publication of the bacteriophage MS2 RNA genome [111] and 1986 when the word "genomics" was first used [112], it already has made an enormous impact on the life sciences. The term "genomics" coined by Thomas Roderick in 1986 encompassed the structure and function of genes, and comparative genomics elucidated the hereditary relationships and evolution within and between different species [112]. Since the advent of NGS, the meaning of "genomics" has been narrowed more towards mapping the structure and organization of genomes and differentiating between *de novo* sequences, resequenced genomes, exonic or targeted sequences, and metagenomic sequences. The other implied meanings of "genomics" are attributed now to the suffix "-omics," added to integrated fields undertaken on a large or genome-wide scale such as transcriptomics, haplomics, methylomics, epigenomics, proteomics, metabolomics, nutrigenomics, physiomics, evolomics, epidemiomics, systeomics, personomics, multinomics, etc. [113]. Thus, NGS broadens our understanding of structural and functional genomics through the concepts of "omics" to provide new insight into the workings and meaning of genetic conservation and diversity of living things (http://www.nature.com/omics/index.html). It is more than ever about how different organisms use genetics and molecular biology to survive and reproduce with and without mutations, disease, and diversity within their own life cycles and within their population networks and changing environmental conditions.

8.1. Genomics

A detailed organizational analysis and an understanding of the full landscape of a genome are possible only after *de novo* whole-genome shotgun sequencing and annotation has been performed [11]. WGS has had an enormous impact on viral, bacterial, and archaeal genomics [114–117]. Some of these successes are provided in the metagenomics section (see section *8.5*). Others have reviewed the impact of WGS and genomics on fungi [118, 119], algae [120], animals [121, 122], and humans [10, 13, 123–127]. WGS has become increasingly easier, faster, and cheaper because of technological improvements and the availability of hundreds of sequenced genomes that can be used as references for annotation. Although it seems unlikely that the genomes of all the 11 million extant worldwide species will ever be or need to be sequenced, the genomic sequences for a large number of eukaryote species are already available for scientific scrutiny, including the genomes of some endangered vertebrate species that may need assistance in the management of their breeding and survival [122]. In 2009, an international consortium established the Genome 10K Project to sequence and analyze the complete genomes of 10,000 vertebrate species (http://genome10k.org).

NGS has blasted human genomics into an exciting new era of genetic investigation geared towards humanomics and disease (see section *8.9*) and the management of an individual's life cycle and health issues by way of personal genomes or personomics [123]. Targeted or whole-genome resequencing of individuals from within the same or different species is aimed to detect and catalogue SNPs, mutations, and sequence variants such as indels, copy number, and structural variations [14–16]. PCR-based candidate gene and whole-exome analysis are two widely used methods that can be performed with higher coverage and at much lower cost than whole-genome resequencing. Genotyping HLA genes of humans for clinical diagnosis or research by sequencing the entire gene [97, 128] or just the exons [129] is an example of targeted resequencing to identify polymorphisms that are important in tissue or cell matching for transplantation [130]. Exomics is targeted specifically towards coding genes and discovering exonic mutations responsible for rare Mendelian disorders such as hearing loss, intellectual disabilities, and movement disorders and for investigating common disorders such as heart disease, hypertension, diabetes, and cancer [13, 123, 125], and many others that are listed at the Online Mendelian Inheritance in Man (OMIM) database (Table 3, [49]). In contrast to WES, WGS can assess alterations in the coding genes and the regulatory and noncoding regions [123, 126], especially multiallelic copy number variations [127]. Cancer research has shown that it is important to target all types of somatic/germ-line genetic alterations, including nucleotide substitutions, small insertions and deletions (indels), CNVs, and chromosomal rearrangements in the noncoding regions [13, 15, 123]. WGS has been used to identify variants, indels, and multiple numbers of genes involved in rare and common diseases such as Charcot-Marie-Tooth neuropathy, dopa-responsive dystonia, acquired essential thrombocytosis, erythrocytosis, and many others [123, 126].

8.2. Transcriptomics and RNA sequencing

RNA-seq is the NGS method that sequences the transcriptome, that is, all the RNA transcript sets expressed by the genome in cells, tissues, and organs at different stages of an organism's life cycle [12, 18, 19, 20, 30]. High-throughput RNA sequencing using cDNA fragments was first employed in mammalian cells [131] and yeast [132], and now it is used for a wide range of organisms [133]. Without transcriptome data, the genome sequence alone is of limited use for understanding the intricacies of genome function in biology. RNA-seq provides technical reliability and sensitivity and unambiguous maps of the transcribed regions of the genome with high accuracy in quantitative expression levels, identification of tissue-specific transcript variants and isoforms (SNPs and mutations), transcription boundaries and splicing events, transcription factors, and small and large noncoding RNAs (ncRNA) involved in the regulation of gene expression [131–137].

At least 90% of the mammalian genome is actively transcribed to produce different classes of ncRNAs [135, 136], including ribosomal RNA (rRNA), transfer RNA (tRNA), microRNA (miRNA), small nuclear RNA (snRNA), small nucleolar RNA (snoRNA), small interfering RNA (siRNA), PIWI-interacting RNA (piRNA), and large intergenic noncoding RNA (lincRNA) [138–141] and retrotransposons [142–146]. The known classes of functional ncRNAs consists largely of those supporting protein translation (ribosomal, transfer, and small nucleolar RNAs), transcript splicing (snRNAs) [137, 138], and miRNA that target conserved binding sites of mRNAs to decrease their stability [139]. The new class of small piRNA was discovered to interact with PIWI regulatory proteins and RNA to silence transposons in the germ line and regulate gene expression in the soma [140]. The lincRNAs are expressed by a different class of actively transcribed RNA genes and they have diverse roles in processes such as cell cycle regulation, immune responses, brain processes, and gametogenesis [147–150]. A substantial fraction of lincRNAs binds to chromatin-modifying proteins and may modulate gene expression by bringing together protein complexes for specific functions [150].

Defective splicing of transcripts and expression levels are believed to contribute to at least 50% of inherited human diseases [151]. Altered expression levels of specific isoforms or alleles have been identified in ischemic stroke, type 2 diabetes, colorectal cancer, chronic lymphocytic leukemia, and many other diseases [30]. Dysregulation of gene expression, splicing, and other editing events in specific cell types have been associated also with the pathogenesis of cardiovascular diseases, neurological disorders, and different cancers [137, 151–153]. Similarly, different classes of small and large ncRNAs have been found to be associated with different diseases and cancers [147–149]. The expressed information of the transcriptome varies enormously between different cells of a multicellular organism and depends on the cell type and its functional and temporal state. At least two important databases, the Encyclopedia of DNA Elements (ENCODE) and Genotype-Tissue Expression (GTEx) (Table 3), have focused on mapping functional elements at high resolution and the regulation of gene expression and the transcriptome in different tissues of humans. The GTEx project is one of the most recent projects that have generated a large amount of RNA sequence data by RNA-seq technology to investigate the patterns of transcriptome variation across 43 tissues and 1641 samples from 175 postmortem individuals [153]. The analysis included 20,110 protein-coding genes and 11,790 lncRNAs with 88% and 71%, respectively, detected in at least one sample. A relatively small number of genes (a few hundred) were expressed for most tissues with a definite, differential modular profile showing tissue-preferential expression. In addition, 3,046 protein-coding genes were expressed together with an adjoining repeat element such as Alu, L1, ERV, Tigger, and Charlie [153]. These findings provide a better systematic understanding of the heterogeneity among a diverse set of human tissues and the enormous complexity and variation involved in the regulation of genome expression.

8.3. Methylomics and epigenomics

Epigenomics is the study of heritable gene regulation that does not involve the DNA nucleotide coding sequence itself but acts on a genome-wide scale via DNA nucleotide methylation and posttranslational modifications of histones, the interaction between transcription factors and their targets, and nucleosome positioning [23–30]. Methylomics is the genome-wide analysis of DNA methylations and their effects on gene expression and heredity [28]. Methyl-seq uses NGS to analyze and map DNA cytosine methylation at single-base resolution usually by employing bisulfite DNA sequencing [24, 25]. Treatment of genomic DNA with sodium bisulfite converts cytosines but not methylcytosines to uracils so that the uracils are PCR converted and sequence differentiated at the SNP locations as thymidines and the methylcytosines are sequenced as cytosines. Bisulfite DNA sequencing is used widely for DNA methylation profiling in various organisms as well as humans for assessing disease genes [23, 27, 29].

ChIP-seq is chromatin immunoprecipitation (ChIP) that is followed by NGS sequencing. It permits genome-wide profiling of DNA-binding proteins and histone and nucleosome modifications [30]. The ChIP-seq technology was partly adapted from microarray ChIP-chip technology and first implemented in 2007 and since then has been used widely to analyze transcription factor binding sites, histone modifications, and chromatin-modifying complexes and sequences in a wide variety of organisms [154]. ChIP-seq provides higher resolution, less noise, and greater coverage than the array-based ChIP-chip method that was previous used, and therefore, it has become the preferred tool for studying gene regulation and epigenetic mechanisms. Two other NGS tools commonly used for epigenetic studies are Hi-C and ChIA-PET that provide insights into the global 3D organization of eukaryote genomes [30]. Hi-C utilizes NGS on cross-linked DNA fragments to identify the DNA regions such as promoters, enhancers, and insulators that come together to mediate their regulatory activities. ChIA-PET uses immunoprecipitation of crosslinked-interacting protein-DNA and paired-end sequencing to reveal the interaction between enhancer and promoter regions located at intergenic distances away from each other but either on the same (*cis*) or different (*trans*) chromosomes [30]. de Wit and de Laat [155] provided an overview of the various derived chromosomal conformation capture (3C) methods, including 4C (chromosome conformation capture-on-chip) and 5C (chromosome conformation carbon copy) and their application in the study of chromatin interactions. Two epigenomic databases on the Internet, the NIH Roadmap Epigenomics Project and Blueprint (Table 3), catalogue the chemical modifications to the genome and how they activate gene expression in human tissues and cell types.

8.4. Proteomics, metabolomics, and systeomics

Proteomics is the large-scale study of the structure, function, identification, and characterization of peptides and proteins [113, 156, 157]. This includes information on protein abundance, variations and polymorphisms, modifications, and their interactions and networks in cellular processes. As a first step, the sequence translation of open reading frames of genomes, exons, and transcripts using a codon table and one or more bioinformatics tools is the simplest way of constructing proteomic profiles from NGS data. However, this is not the only analytical protocol used in the domain of proteomics, and protein specialists often employ a variety of other hardware and software tools to build up an organism's peptide and protein profiles. Among these are the detection and analysis of proteins and their functions by two-dimensional polyacrylamide gels, liquid chromatography coupled with tandem mass spectrometry, affinity-tagged proteins, and yeast two-hybrid assays [156, 157]. A number of public databases for proteomics and protein-protein interactions are available on the Internet such as ExPASy and PRIDE (Table 3).

Metabolomics is the study of an organism's total metabolic response to an environmental stimulus or a genetic modification [113]. The metabolomics of organisms are drawn indirectly from NGS data, mainly from the known functions of enzymes and proteins involved in metabolic and biochemical pathways. Metabolomics data also provide biochemical and physiological snapshots of processes that are obtained from cellular and tissue experimental studies using various technologies of separation (gas chromatography, high-performance liquid chromatography, and capillary electrophoresis) and detection (mass spectrophotometry, NMR spectrometry, ion mobility, and thin-layer chromatography) [158]. Metabolomics is an important part of functional genomics for determining the phenotypic effects of genetic manipulations such as gene deletions, insertions, and mutations. Nutrigenomics is an arm of metabolomics that links genomics, transcriptomics, proteomics, metabolomics, and microbiomics together in an examination of the effects of nutrition and energy metabolism on gene expression in relation to an organism's genotype [113, 159]. The use of constraint-based methods such as the Flux Balance Analysis to design models of metabolite flow in microbes has connected "omic" to phenotypes in the science of Fluxomics [160]. Some web-based metabolomic resources include FAME, AromaDeg, Metabolomexpress, and MetaboAnalyst (Table 3).

Systeomics is the integration of genomics, proteomics, metabolomics, and phenomics into a single network system. It is a branch of biology that uses computational techniques to analyze and model how the components of a biological system such as cells or organisms interact with each other to produce the characteristics and behavior of that system [160–162]. Systeomics is a biology-based interdisciplinary field applied to biomedical and biological scientific research that focuses on complex interactions within biological systems using a holistic approach. For example, the U.S. Department of Energy's Genomic Science program uses microbial and plant genomic data, high-throughput analytical technologies, and modeling and simulation to develop a predictive understanding of biological systems behavior relevant to solving energy and environmental challenges (http://doegenomestolife.org). The U.S. Department of Energy Systems Biology Knowledgebase (KBase) is a software and data platform for systems biology mechanisms (Table 3) to assist with the prediction and design of biological functions of microbes and plants. KBase integrates data, tools, and their associated interfaces into one unified, scalable environment to allow users to upload their own data for analysis, to build models, and to share and publish their workflows and conclusions. Another example is the Kyoto Encyclopedia of Genes and Genomes (KEGG), which is a database resource to integrate high-level functions and utilities of biological systems from molecular-level information (Table 3). Other "omics" that contribute to the "omic" lexicon and biology are epidemiomics [163], physionomics [113], variomics [164], and phenomics [165–167]. In the case of phenomics, the European Genome-phenome Archive (EGA) provides accession numbers that refer to the relationship between genomics and phenotype/traits, such as the physical and biochemical traits of humans (Table 3). It integrates physical traits or phenotypes with genomics, transcriptomics, methylomics, proteomics, and metabolomics [166].

8.5. Metagenomics and microbiomes

Metagenomics, or beyond genomics, is the study of the total genomic content of a microbial community that bridges the three domains of life, Archaea, Bacteria, and Eukaryotes [100, 114–118, 168–179]. The total DNA and/or RNA is isolated from a microbial population without prior cultivation, sequenced, and compared with previously known sequences to identify known species or to discover previously unknown species. Some of the environments from which microbial communities are isolated and studied include aquatic and terrestrial environments, host-associated ecosystems, and various human engineered systems such as those involved with food, water, and waste production, agriculture, animal husbandry, and various human and animal habitations [100, 115, 168, 169]. Hospitals are a worrying source of pathogenic microorganisms, especially those that develop resistance to commonly used medical antibiotics [115, 168]. Thus, NGS is an important growing application for epidemiological studies of various pathogens, such as mycobacteria, *S. aureus*, *E. coli*, cholera, influenza, HIV, Ebola virus, etc. [169–171]. The Earth Microbiome Project (http://www.earthmicrobiome.org) is an ambitious multidisciplinary attempt to analyze microbial communities across the globe using approximately 500,000 reconstructed microbial genomes.

The earliest metagenomic studies targeted 16S rRNA genes to genotype and identify the different species within the environment before the first NGS microbial studies using the Roche pyrosequencing and Illumina platforms targeted mining sites and the surface waters of the gulfs, seas, and oceans [114, 169]. Many big projects and consortia for sequencing metagenomes have been launched in the past 10 years, such as the TerraGenome project for soils (Table 3) and the *Tara* Oceans project on the microbiome, eukaryotic plankton, and viromes of the global oceans [172–174].

Microbes colonize the human body (microbiome) in numbers that are estimated to outnumber human genes and somatic cells by more than 100-fold [175]. These microbes (viruses, prokaryotes, and eukaryotic microbes) occupy various anatomical habitats including gut, skin, vagina, and oral mucosa and are believed to markedly influence human physiology, nutrition, and health [175–177]. Advances in NGS and computing methods have enabled human microbiome studies such as the MetaHit project and the Human Microbiome Project (HMP) (Table 3). In May 2015, SRA that was established by NCBI in 2008 to store raw sequence data from the NGS technologies had over 2,068 trillion open access nucleotides in its database to massively outgrow GenBank, EMBL, and DDBJ for bacterial sequence storage. The genomic sequences continue to accumulate in other databases as well [114], such as 47,083 prokaryotic genomes projected for Genomes Online Database (GOLD) [178] and 152,927 metagenomes for the MG-RAST server [179]. As of October 2014, the GOLD database contained 544 metagenomics studies associated with 6726 metagenome samples, whereas MG-RAST held 150,039 metagenomic samples, of which 20,415 were publicly available (Table 3). Recently, Zelezniak et al. [180] gathered and modeled NGS 16S rRNA sequence data to map interspecies metabolic exchanges and resource competition based on the genomic potential encoded by the microbial communities. They analyzed more than 1,297 communities and 261 species in soil, water, and human gut samples and concluded that the interplay between competitive and cooperative strategies for resources and the ability to exchange metabolites, such as amino acids and sugars, shapes the composition of microbial communities.

8.6. Comparative genomics, phylogenomics, and the phylomes of life

Comparative genomics and phylogenomics via NGS and the phylome (complete collection of all gene phylogenies in a genome) provide powerful applications for classifying and understanding the differences and similarities of all life forms and for unraveling their evolutionary histories [100, 116, 176, 181–186]. The three basic domains of life, Bacteria, Archaea, and Eukarya, were first identified and classified phylogenetically on the basis of ribosomal RNA sequences [181]. Although Bacteria and Archaea are both placed into the kingdom of the Prokaryotes or Monera (lacking a membrane-bound nucleus, mitochon-dria, and chloroplasts but containing a cell wall), their separate rRNA sequence clusters clearly divided them into distinct domains [181]. The Eukarya (eukaryotes) have been subdivided into four basic kingdoms, Protista, Fungi (Mycota), Plantae (Metaphyta), and Animalia (Metazoa) [182]. However, on the basis of metagenomic and phylogenomic studies and NGS data, the classifications and nomenclatures of eukaryotes continue to be revised and organized into other supergroups such as Amoebozoa, Opsthokonta, Ecavata, Archae-plastida (Plantae), SAR (Stra/Alveo/Rhizaria), and Incertae sedis [183, 184]. On the other hand, because viruses do not have rRNA genes, they have missed out on a life-domain classification [185, 186]. There is still a strong debate about whether or not viruses without rRNA genes should be classified as a separate life form (a fourth domain) or simply be viewed as exogenous parasites, infectious agents, and endogenous mobile elements that are dependent on and exist within the life forms of the three defined domains [185, 186]. Viruses impact greatly on all life forms, so they are a major interest for NGS applications and phylogenomics [34, 114, 174, 187–189], especially emerging viruses such as dengue, Ebola, Chikungunya, MERS, lyssavirus, and norovirus (http://viralzone.expasy.org), which are of a great concern to human health [114, 171, 189].

NGS, phylogenomics, and taxonomy profiling during the past decade has greatly expand-ed our knowledge of the diversity of bacterial genomes from the same and different species [116, 190], with the discovery of many DNA sequence repeats and transposons that contribute to at least 10% of the genome and play an important role in immunity [100, 191]. Archaea and thermophiles have a large proportion of their genomes consisting of defense genes often localized in genomic islands as a consequence of horizontal gene transfers [191, 192]. For example, the family of clustered regularly interspaced short palindromic repeats (CRISPRs) and the CRISPR-associated proteins in the CRISPR-Associated System (CAS) that have an important role in the host's adaptive immunity to pathogens and as responders to environmental stress [192–194] have been translocated between different prokaryote strains and species [191, 192]. CAS includes distinct gene families of 50 or more that show strong evidence of extensive plasticity and horizontal gene transfer to protect prokaryote cells against the replication of phage and plasmids that integrate into the CRISPR locus [193–195]. Moreover, the CRISPR/CAS systems have been developed as an "in vitro" genetic engineering tool to be transfected into the cells of various organisms to manipulate their genes [196], including the foreign defense system introduced into human cells against HIV-1 infection [197]. Other bacterial defense systems that have been studied or discovered by NGS include the toxin/anti-toxin, antigen, novel restriction-modification, and DNA phosphorathioation systems as well as those involved with infection-induced dormancy or programmed cell death [192]. Genomic sequencing also has revealed new bacterial microcompartments, protein structures, or organelles that are used in metabolic pathways [198], such as those involved in carbon fixation and metabolism of amino alcohols, ethanol, rhamnose, and fucose [199]. Bacterial genomes also provide sequences for phylogenetic and gene comparisons, taxonomic classification, transcriptomics, and methylomics and for the assessment of sequence diversity and variants for a better understanding of gene functions [100]. Although the classical operon structure predominates in bacteria and archaea, a variety of other transcription unit architectures have been elucidated [100]. More than 4,661 transcription units have been described with an average of 1.7 promoters per operon, and transcription factor binding sites have been determined for virtually all the transcription factors in *E. coli* [100]. DNA methylation was first discovered in bacterial restriction-modification systems with diverse functions in addition to cellular defense [200], and it is now seen as an evolutionarily conserved form of transcriptional repression and an ancestral form of defense against foreign DNA molecules and transposons and other mobile elements in all life forms [201].

Phylogenomics has been used to reevaluate the evolutionary affiliation between archaea and eukaryotes and to infer that the nuclear lineage in eukaryotes emerged from the archaeal radiation and most probably from the archaeal TACK superphylum [202]. Recently, Spang et al. [203] sequenced uncultivated metagenomes from a deep-sea vent and discovered novel archaeal genomes in the new phylum that they named "Lokiarchaeota." These novel archaea contain homologues of many eukaryotic proteins that function in the endomembrane system and in phagocytosis, including actin and related proteins, and Ras superfamily GTPases, suggesting that this newly discovered phylum is the missing link in eukaryogenesis. Although eukaryotes possess the membrane-enclosed mitochondrial organelle and prokaryotes do not, the eukaryotic mitochondria are believed to have evolved from a bacterial system, probably by endosymbiosis [204] involving an ancestor within the bacterial phylum Alphaproteobacteria [205]. Although mitochondrial phylogenomics suggests a monophyletic origin and assemblage, it is now evident that the mitochondria are genetic chimeras and functional mosaics with the bulk of the mitochondrial proteome originating during eukaryote evolution outside the Alphaproteobacteria and other bacterial phyla. It seems that the mitochondrial genome has expanded and contracted in various lineages during evolution with much of the original mitochondrial genetic information transferred to the nucleus [205]. Eukaryotic diploid cells appear to have evolved 2 billion years after haploid prokaryotes, and their evolution from proto-eukaryotic cells, such as the multinucleated *Giardia* organism [206], seems to have involved chromosomal crossing over from mitotic recombination to meiosis and to sexual reproduction where a set of chromosomes is inherited from each parent [207]. The genomes of diploid eukaryotes are usually larger than those in haploid prokaryotes probably because greater information complexity is needed by multicellular organisms to regulate and coordinate the multiple stages of their life cycles with the added requirement for more molecular regulatory systems to communicate and interact between multiple tissues and organs [206].

Eukaryotic genomes vary markedly in size and gene number and appear to be variable in their susceptibility to polyploidy (a doubling of the diploid sets of chromosomes), redundancy, duplication, and the persistent accumulation of interspersed repeats and mobile elements [208–210]. For example, the genomes of plants can range from the simplest like *Ostreococcus tauri* with a 12.6 Mb genome, containing less than 8,000 genes and minimal genome duplication [211], to the highly complex such as the canopy and pale-petal flowering plant *Paris japonica*, with a 150 Gb genome and eight sets of chromosomes derived by allopolyploidy and hybridization of four species [212]. The genomic size of *Paris japonica*, which has still to be fully sequenced, is 50 times larger than the human genome and extends the range of genome sizes to 2,400-fold across angiosperms and 66,000-fold across eukaryotes [212]. Genome duplication and polyploidy, both recent and ancient, have contributed to the considerable genomic complexity in eukaryotes, particularly in plants, amoeba, fungi, and vertebrates [208–223]. Following ancient polyploidization, most duplicated genes are deleted by intrachromosomal recombination, a process referred to as fractionation, and any remaining evidence for the polyploidy event is not easy to find by phylogenomic analysis [214]. Nevertheless, a phylogenomic comparison of gene duplications in a four-way comparison of paralogous regions in tunicate, fish, mouse, and human provided unmistakable evidence of two distinct genome duplication events (the 2R event) early in vertebrate evolution and before the divergence of fish and mammalian lineages [215], as was proposed by Ohno in 1970 [216]. Interestingly, polyploidy also can occur in humans during normal development and cancer [208, 209]. Fetal polyploidy in the form of triploidy (69,XXX chromosomes) and tetraploidy (92,XXXX chromosomes) is a rare and lethal event, resulting in spontaneous abortions or brief postpartum survival times [208], whereas polyploidy is common in stressed tissues and cells and in tumor development [208, 209]. On the other hand, comparative genomic studies have revealed that polyploidy is common in the evolutionary history of many different flowering plants [208, 214], for example, between different species of the allopolyploid tobacco plants, *Nicotiana* section Repandae [217]. In comparing the allotetraploid genomes of *Nicotiana repanda* and *Nicotiana nudicaulis*, it was assessed that the loss of low-copy sequences along with the loss of duplicate copies of genes and upstream regulators reflects genome diploidization, whereas genome size divergence between the allopolyploids is manifested through differential accumulation and/or deletion of high-copy-number sequences and transposable elements [217]. Diploidization and genome size change in *Nicotiana* allopolyploids is associated with differential dynamics of low- and high-copy sequences [218]. The induction of polyploidy is a common technique to overcome the sterility of a hybrid species during plant breeding; therefore, many agriculturally important plants such as the genus *Brassica* are polyploids [219-221]. Wheat, after millennia of hybridization and modification by humans, has strains that are diploid (2 sets of chromosomes), tetraploid (4 sets of chromosomes), and hexaploid (6 sets of chromosomes) [222, 223], whereas the invasive weed *Spartina anglica* has up to 12 sets of chromosomes [224].

A recent comparative genomic study has revealed how genomes change with speciation in an examination of genomes from five cichlid fish species, an ancestral lineage from the Nile, and four species from the East Africa lakes, Tanganyika, Malawi, and Victoria [225]. Compared to the ancestral Nile lineage, the East African cichlid genomes had many alterations in regulatory elements, accelerated evolution of protein-coding elements in genes for pigmentation, an excess of gene duplications, and other distinct features that affect gene expression associated with transposable element insertions and novel microRNA. Each species contains a reservoir of mutations different from the other species [225]. Much of the diversity between species evolves in a nonparallel manner often rapidly due to sexual selection and genetic conflicts between males and females and between different regions of the genome at a regulatory level rather than by the slower and weaker forces of classical natural selection [226].

Most genomes range between newly derived genes and the ultraconserved or the essential core coding and noncoding genes [100, 227, 228]. Comparative genomics has resulted in the discovery of ultraconserved noncoding elements (UCNE) across different phyla, starting with 481-long segments (>200 bp) that are 100% conserved between orthologous regions of the human, rat, and mouse genomes and 95% to 99% conserved in chicken and dog genomes [229]. A more recent comparison of 28 vertebrate genomes identified millions of additional con- served elements with distinct types of functional elements including regulatory motifs present in the promoters and untranslated regions of coregulated genes, insulators that constrain domains of gene expression, and conserved secondary structures in RNAs and in develop- mental regulators [230]. A webpage at http://ultraconserved.org provides study protocols, computer software, and references dedicated to ultraconserved elements [229]. Also, there are at least two databases for the conserved noncoding elements and the genomic regulatory blocks (Table 3), the UCNEbase for human and chicken [231], and the UCbase 2.0 for the 481 UCNE that were longer than 200 bp and that were discovered in the genomes of mammals [229]. The UCNEbase suggests that the evolution of species depends more on innovation and change in regulatory sequences than in proteins [231]. Indeed, there are essential genes that are indispensable for the survival of an organism and therefore are considered a foundation of life. The database of essential genes (DEG) (Table 3) catalogues known essential genomic elements, such as protein-coding genes and noncoding RNAs, within the bacteria, archaea, and eukaryotes that constitute a minimal genome and are useful for annotating newly sequenced genomes [232].

Phylomes provide the combined analysis of genome-wide collections of phylogenetic trees to aid in the inference of orthological and paralogical relationships and the detection of evolu- tionary events such as whole-genome duplication (polyploidization), gene family expansion and contraction, horizontal gene transfer, recombination, inversion, and incomplete lineage sorting [233, 234]. The online PhylomeDB v4 database was created as a phylogenomic reposi- tory and is useful for preliminary phylogenetic data analysis of genomes of interest from various phyla as well as for annotating newly derived genomic sequences [234]. As an example, Fig. 1 shows the PhylomeDB analysis of the duplications of the RLTPR gene, a gene that was first discovered in humans in 2004 [235]. The PhylomeDB analysis shows that the RLTPR gene has two paralogs, LRRC16B and LRRC16, which were generated by two separate duplication events at least prior to the divergence of mice and humans (Fig. 1). The functions of RLTPR are not well characterized, but its distinct functional domains suggest that it may multitask in protein-protein interactions, as recently demonstrated in the development of regulatory T cells in mice [236]. The analytical approach to find orthologous and paralogous relationships with maximum genomic coverage for the RLTPR gene is both gene-centric and genome-wide in PhylomeDB. Also of particular interest are the well-conserved genomic mechanisms of innate immunity, such as Apolipoprotein B Editing Catalytic subunit proteins 3 (APOBEC3s) in mammals that mutate and inactivate viral genomes [237]. Other phylogenetic databases that complement PhylomeDB in a comparative analysis are Ensembl Compara GeneTrees, TreeFam, PANTHER, PhyloFacts FATCAT, and the HOGENOM database (Table 3).

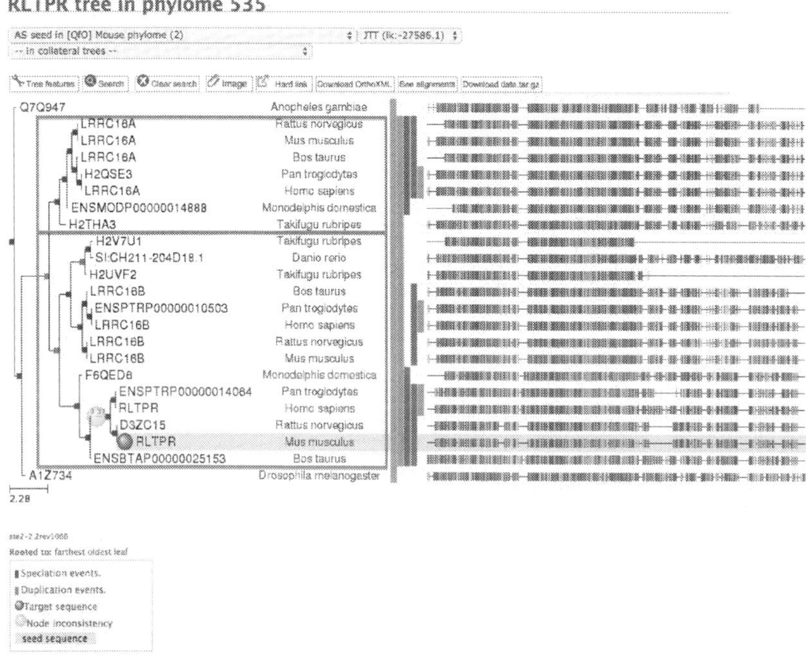

Figure 1. RLTPR gene tree shows the RLTPR gene orthologs and paralogs in 10 vertebrate species. The human gene RLTPR (NCBI Gene ID: 146206), first reported in 2004 [235], was used as the search query for the Phylome tree at http://phylomedb.org with the phylome data settings of AS seed in (Qf0) mouse phylome (2) and JTT (lk:-27586.1). The tree shows the speciation events (blue squares) and three duplication events (red squares) at the nodes with the first duplication event arising early in vertebrate evolution before the divergence of fish and mammalian lineages [215].

8.7. Mobilomics and Horizontal Gene Transfer (HGT)

The science of mobile genetic elements (mobilomics) developed long before the advent of genomics and NGS [238]. The 1983 Nobel Prize winner Barbara McClintock first reported the existence of mobile elements as jumping genes in maize in the late 1940s [239]. The discovery of new classes and families of DNA transposons and autonomous and nonautonomous retrotransposons continued slowly for the next five decades until the first online repeat element screening webserver CENSOR and database REPBASE (Table 3) was established by Jerzy Jurka and his colleagues between 1992 and 1996 [240, 241]. Since then, RepeatMasker (Table 3) and other tools such as Mobster [242], Red [243], and Visual TE [244] have followed on to help define the mobilome, the totality of mobile genetic elements in a particular genome. A list and description of some of the families, types, and classes of transposons and retro-transposons in prokaryotes and eukaryotes can be found in the following reviews [238, 245–251]. A recent survey of repeats and mobile elements that affect genomic stability has eluci-dated how some bacteria can control the mobilome through postsegregation killing systems

[192–195, 247]. Different classes of TEs are found in the genomes of different eukaryotes that contribute to at least 50% of the human genome [237] and up to 90% of the maize genome [252]. In humans, there are solitary Long Terminal Repeats (LTR) and LTR retrotransposons (endogenous retroviruses) that are characterized by the presence of LTR at both ends; Long Interspersed Nuclear Elements (LINEs) like L1 that represent families of non-LTR TEs about 6 kb in length and encode two proteins, a nucleic acid chaperone, and a reverse transcriptase/nuclease for retrotransposition; Nonautomomous Miniature Inverted-Repeat Transposable Elements (MITEs); Mammalian-wide Interspersed Repeats (MIRs), an ancient family of tRNA-derived SINEs exapted as enhancers and regulatory sequences; and Short Interspersed Nuclear Elements (SINEs) like Alu that are usually less than 300 bp and need a helper transposon element like L1 for transposition [245]. Most ERVs, SINEs, and LINEs in the human genome are now remnants of past insertions and are no longer capable of actively "jumping" like functional TEs [238, 245, 248]. Indeed, many of the TE ancient relics have undergone exaptation and developed new functions, such as transcript repeat elements, within regulatory gene networks to generate lineage-specific adaptation [145, 249].

The importance of widespread HGT in creating genomic diversity in microbes has been highlighted by the many comparative genomic studies using metagenome data [191]. Comparative genomic analysis of different strains of *E. coli* revealed that up to 30% of genes in pathogenic strains were acquired by HGT often creating duplication events and modifying metabolic networks by adding operons that encode two or more enzymes [253]. Comparative genomics of photosynthetic prokaryotes revealed that they have evolved as complex mosaics via multiple HGT events [254]. Similarly, photosynthetic gene clusters and gene clusters that encode various toxins, resistance genes, metabolic genes, and components of secretion systems appear to be the products of HGT [247, 253–255]. Indeed, many HGT events probably were mediated by genomic mobile elements, such as bacteriophages, plasmids, viruses, transposable elements, and toxin/antitoxin systems that are persistent in all life forms [191, 228, 246, 255, 256].

Before the new millennium, transposons and repeat elements were largely viewed as junk and as parasites that created unnecessary burden on the genome. Comparative genomics and online databases dedicated to transposons and repeat elements such as SINES, LINES, and ERVs, however, began to change this picture in the 1990s, and it soon became evident that these elements were the drivers of evolutionary innovation. Many integrated transposons mutate with time to interact with the host transcriptional machinery and therefore provide a useful substrate for evolution of novel regulatory elements [145, 228, 255–258]. Moreover, some of the ancient integrated retrotransposons appear to have been involved in advantageous segmental genomic duplications such as in the major histocompatibility complex region [259–261], and others have dispersed regulatory controls to provide coordinated regulation across the genome [257, 258].

8.8. Agrigenomics

Agrigenomics or agricultural genomics can be defined as the research and development activities that translate NGS and genomics technology into a better understanding of plant biology and advancing crop improvements. During the past decade, NGS had an enormous impact on developing fundamental genome resources to directly address many of today's concerns in agriculture and agronomics. Since the publication in 2000 of the first plant genome, *Arabidopsis thaliana*, 54 new plant genomes were published by 2013 [221] followed by at least another 6 plant genomes including the hexaploid bread wheat genome [223]. In reviewing the first 55 plant genomes, Michael and Jackson [221] concluded that, although these genomes have provided a glimpse at the gene number, types, and numbers of repeats and genomic growth, contraction, and rearrangement, we are only just at the beginning of defining the functional aspects of plant genomes "and various other 'omics' data layered on genomes."

8.9. Humanomics, personomics, and health

The accumulation of knowledge on the human genome and its genetic and molecular processes (humanomics) has amplified considerably since the first draft assembly was published in 2001 [262]. The first human hybrid genome took about 15 years to sequence and assemble, and when released to the public, it covered 90% of the euchromatic genome, contained about 250,000 gaps, and had many errors in the nucleotide sequence [43, 44]. Ten years after the publication of the first human draft sequence, six more human genome sequences were completed with a much greater coverage and accuracy, enabling more informative comparisons to be made between them [7, 8, 79]. Studies by the 1000 Genomes Project [10], the Personal Genome Project [263], the HapMap Consortium [264], and the Pan-Asian Single Nucleotide Polymorphism Project [265] revealed the enormous sequence diversity that exists between individuals. Since then, 225 Ethiopian and Egyptian genomes were compared to reconstruct their population history out of Africa [266], 911 genomes from 10 populations of African, East Asian, and European ancestries were sequenced to elucidate novel patterns and signatures of genetic differentiation [267], and whole-exome sequences from 951 genomes of a ClinSeq cohort were compared to discover new loss-of-function mutations [268]. Today, there are many 1000 human genome projects, and WGS of the human genome for personalized medicine (personomics) is already a reality for 2,638 Icelanders [9] and for some others [269, 270] of the 7.3 billion individuals currently populating the globe (http://www.worldometers.info/world-population).

Veeramah and Hammer [271] recently reviewed the usefulness of NGS to sequence ancient DNA samples for phylogenetic and evolutionary studies and for the reconstruction of human population history. Some of these NGS studies have helped to refine the demographic histories of human evolution. These studies include those of the ancient DNA of extinct hominins (Neanderthals, Denisovans) and ancient modern humans such as 7,000-year-old Mesolithic hunter-gathers in northwestern Spain, Neolithic and post-Neolithic (5,300- to 4,000-year-old) hunter-gathers and farmers in Scandinavia, a 4,000-year-old Paleo-Eskimo from southern Greenland, and a 24,000- and 17,000-year-old South-Central Siberian [271]. NGS of ancient nonhuman genomes such as those of pathogens, parasites, and domesticated animals and plants also can provide new information about human history in regard to life styles, health, and the spread of agriculture [272].

NGS has allowed a detailed analysis of single nucleotide variants (SNVs), structural variants (SV), and methylations in coding and noncoding regions and to assess their role in human disease [9, 14, 15, 19, 22, 25, 29, 30, 123, 125–127, 144, 148, 151, 152]. The establishment of the International HapMap Project in 2003 (Table 3) to develop a "hapmap" of human haplotype genomes from samples of large populations was an important initiative to find genes and genomic variations (SNP and CNV frequencies, genotypes, and phased haplotypes) that affect health and disease [264]. More than 97 million validated SNPs (dbSNP) have been discovered from human genome sequencing projects and many of the variants have been linked to a range of medical and phenotypic conditions and catalogued at dbGAP (Table 3), the database of genotype and phenotype [273]. In July 2015, dbGAP had links to 592 disease and phenotype studies and 3,711 data sets. In addition to SNV, small and large SVs that are duplicated, deleted, or rearranged relative to the reference sequences and individuals have been identified in NGS studies and associated with various diseases [9, 30, 127]. NGS has been used to diagnose rare Mendelian diseases and genetically heterogeneous complex disorders, such as X-linked intellectual disability, congenital disorders, cancer genome heterogeneity, and fetal aneuploidy [13, 15, 123, 125, 208, 209, 274, 275]. The impact of NGS on the diagnosis of rare genetic diseases is evidenced by the growth of the genes and OMIM database [49, 276] that has doubled in data since 2007 [274]. However, it should be noted that NGS does not always reveal causative mutations but instead may provide a list of possible candidates. Many detected SNPs, SNVs, and SV have not been associated to disease or phenotype and many diseases still await a genetic or genomic cause. NGS in human studies must be used with caution because of the significant levels of false-positive and false-negative rates in sequencing errors and amplification biases.

Soon et al. [30] listed and reviewed the various NGS methods employed in the ENCODE project to annotate and analyze the transcriptome and map elements and identify the methylation patterns of the whole human genome. The information in ENCODE and other databases such as GTEx, FANTOM, NIH ROADMAP, and BLUEPRINT (Table 3) has enabled researchers to map genetic variants to gene regulatory regions and assess indirect links to disease. The Regulome DB based on the accumulation of nongenic functional regulatory regions obtained from ENCODE is a useful resource for the evaluation of polymorphisms of regulatory regions [276]. Although disease-associated SNPs obtained from GWAS studies may point to gene coding regions, they actually might reside in regulatory sites of downstream genes that are in linkage disequilibrium with the reported SNPs [262]. RNA-seq and NGS has confirmed that 98% of the human genome is transcribed from noncoding genomic regions, that only about 2% of the human genome codes for peptides and proteins with about 20,000 distinct protein-coding genes, and that alternative splicing seems to occur for 90% of protein-coding genes to yield many more different types of proteins than genes [134, 135, 151, 152]. The vast majority of the human genome is not functionless "junk DNA" as previously thought [262], but rather, it can be viewed as DNA/RNA "dark matter" expressing hundreds to millions of transcribed short and long noncoding RNA molecules that have important regulatory roles in transcription, translation, transport, metabolism, and innate immunity [133]. Some of these are the interspersed retroelements such as Alu and L1 and endogenous retroviruses (ERVs) that have evolved before and during primate history to function as regulators of transcription and translation [24, 25, 142, 145, 257, 258].

NGS has especially revolutionized the field of cancer genomes revealing mutations, amplifications, deletions, translocations, and dysregulation of noncoding and coding RNAs to provide a better understanding of the complex genetics and loss of regulation in cancer [15, 25, 29, 208, 209, 275]. For example, paired end sequencing showed that about half of structural rearrangements in breast cancer genomes were fusion transcripts resulting from the rearrangements of segmental tandem duplications involving multiple genes [277]. Similarly, other cancer types were found to be dominated by duplications, translocations, structural variations, and complex rearrangements called "chromothripsis" that involve chromosomal rearrangements as single events confined to genomic regions in one or a few chromosomes [278]. NGS also has been applied to circulating tumor cells isolated from the body fluids (blood, urine, sputum, saliva, and stools) [30, 274]. A genomic landscape and a catalogue of somatic mutations in cancer are provided on the Internet at COSMIC (Table 3, [275]). Thus, NGS potentially provides cancer patients with opportunities for personalized diagnosis and optimized therapeutic treatment [279, 280].

The integration of NGS data obtained from whole genome, exome, transcriptome, and methylome to build up individual genomic profiles is a growing reality in human health care. Recently, Chen et al. [269] developed "integrated personal omic profiling" in an individual by sequencing their genome at high accuracy and profiling their transcriptome, metabolome, and proteome over a 14-month period. In the study, they tracked the emergence of type 2 diabetes and assessed the individual's genetic make-up and disease risks. Others have performed similar studies demonstrating that monitoring the longitudinal trends and changes within individuals is an important future protocol for the diagnosis, management, and treatment of disease [9, 81, 270]. The challenges for "person omics," however, remain formidable at many levels, not least the time, cost, and effort required to gather, process, and interpret the data [101]. The cost benefits of NGS for personomics have still to be assessed with many economic, securities, personal, familial, social, and ethical issues to be considered and resolved.

9. Futuromics

The first-generation sequencing technologies and the pioneering computing and bioinformatics tools produced the initial sequencing data and information within a framework of structural and functional genomics in readiness for the following NGS developments. NGS provides substantially cheaper, friendlier, and more flexible high-throughput sequencing options with a quantum leap towards the generation of much more data on genomics, transcriptomics, and methylomics that translate more productively into proteomics, metabolomics, and systeomics. This major progression towards a more comprehensive characterization of genomes, epigenomes, and transcriptomes of humans and other species provides even more data as a proxy to probe diverse molecular interactions in the era of "omics" in many fields of biology, industry, and health care. A few years ago, the McKinsey Global Institute produced a report predicting that NGS and genomics, including the sequencing of a million human genomes, would become an economically and socially disruptive technology as well as an annual trillion dollar industry by 2025 [281]. The authors assessed that next-generation genomics would affect many high impact areas of molecular biology and bioindustry such as improving genetic engineering tools to custom build organisms, genetically engineer biofuels, modify crops to improve farming practices and food stocks, and develop drugs to treat cancers and other diseases. Although these technologies promise huge benefits, they also come with social, ethical, and regulatory risks in regard to privacy and security of personal genetic information, the dangerous effects of modified organisms on the environment, the spectre of bioterrorism, eugenics, and concerns about the ownership and commercialization of genomic information. The application of prenatal genome sequencing for genetic screening already points to the potential of producing genetically modified babies with desired traits. Much will need to be done to educate and inform regulators and society about the risks and benefits when formulating the regulatory policies about the advances and applications of these next-generation technologies.

Today, NGS is the science of biological information systems and "Big Data,", but many challenges still remain in regard to NGS data acquisition, storage, analysis, integration, and interpretation [282, 283]. Future advancements will undoubtedly rely on new technologies and large-scale collaborative efforts from multidisciplinary and international teams to continue generating comprehensive, high-throughput data production and analysis. The availability of economically friendlier bench-top sequencers and third-generation sequencing tools will allow smaller laboratories and individual scientists to participate in the genomics revolution and contribute new knowledge to the different fields of structural and functional genomics in the life sciences. The authors of the following chapters in this book present additional examples, more detailed information, and a broader view of the methods and many advances, applications, and challenges of NGS that were either missed or not covered adequately in this opening chapter, particularly in regard to the RNA sequencing and transcriptome methods and data that provide us with a better understanding of functional genomics in microorganisms, plants, animals, and humans. *Te volo, bonam lectionem.*

Author details

Jerzy K. Kulski[1,2*]

Address all correspondence to: kulski@me.com

1 Department of Molecular Life Science, Division of Basic Medical Science and Molecular Medicine, Tokai University School of Medicine, Isehara, Japan

2 Centre for Forensic Science, The University of Western Australia, Nedlands, WA, Australia

References

[1] Sanger F, Nicklen S, Coulson AR: DNA sequencing with chain-terminating inhibitors. Proc Natl Acad Sci USA. 1977;74:5463–7. PMCID: PMC431765

[2] Mardis ER: Next-generation DNA sequencing methods. Annu Rev Genomics Hum Genet. 2008;9:387–402. DOI: 10.1146/annurev.genom.9.081307.164359

[3] Mardis ER: A decade's perspective on DNA sequencing technology. Nature. 2011;470:198–203. DOI: 10.1038/nature09796

[4] Metzker ML: Sequencing technologies — The next generation. Nat Rev Genet. 2010;11:31–46. DOI: 10.1038/nrg2626

[5] Thompson JF, Milos PM: The properties and applications of single-molecule DNA sequencing. Genome Biol. 2011;12:217. DOI: 10.1186/gb-2011-12-2-217

[6] Margulies M, Egholm M, Altman WE, et al: Genome sequencing in microfabricated high-density picolitre reactors. Nature. 2005;437:376–80. PMID: 16056220

[7] Levy S, Sutton G, Ng PC, et al: The diploid genome sequence of an individual human. PLoS Biol. 2007;5:e254. PMID: 17803354

[8] Wheeler DA, Srinivasan M, Egholm M, et al: The complete genome of an individual by massively parallel DNA sequencing. Nature. 2008;452:872–6. DOI: 10.1038/nature06884

[9] Gudbjartsson DF, Helgason H, Gudjonsson SA, et al: Large-scale whole-genome sequencing of the Icelandic population. Nat Genet. 2015;47:435–44. DOI: 10.1038/ng.3247

[10] The 1000 Genomes Project Consortium: An integrated map of genetic variation from 1,092 human genomes. Nature. 2012;491:56–65. DOI: 10.1038/nature11632

[11] Lam HY, Clark MJ, Chen R, et al: Performance comparison of whole-genome sequencing platforms. Nat Biotechnol. 2012;30:78–83. DOI: 10.1038/nbt.2065

[12] Wang Z, Gerstein M, Snyder M: RNA-Seq: a revolutionary tool for transcriptomics. Nat Rev Genet. 2009;10:57–63. DOI: 10.1038/nrg2484

[13] Rabbini B, Tekin M, Mahdieh N: The promise of whole-exome sequencing in medical genetics. J Hum Genet. 2014;59:5–15. DOI: 10.1038/jhg.2013.114

[14] Leo VC, Morgan NV, Bern D, et al: Use of next-generation sequencing and candidate gene analysis to identify underlying defects in patients with inherited platelet function disorders. J Thromb Haemost. 2015;13:643–50. DOI: 10.1111/jth.12836

[15] Mardis ER, Wilson RK: Cancer genome sequencing: A review. Hum Mol Genet. 2009;18(R2):R163–8. DOI: 10.1093/hmg/ddp396

[16] Kulski JK, Suzuki S, Ozaki Y, Mitsunaga S, Inoko H, Shiina T: Phase HLA genotyping by next generation sequencing — A comparison between two massively parallel sequencing bench-top systems, the Roche GS Junior and Ion Torrent PGM. In: Xi Y, editor. HLA and Associated Important Diseases. Croatia: Intech; 2014. p. 141–81.

[17] Pelizzola M, Ecker JR: The DNA methylome. FEBS Lett. 2011;585:1994–2000. DOI: 10.1016/j.febslet.2010.10.061

[18] Ozsolak F, Milos PM: RNA sequencing: Advances, challenges and opportunities. Nat Rev Genet. 2011;12:87–98. DOI: 10.1038/nrg2934

[19] Wang K, Kim C, Bradfield J, et al: Whole-genome DNA/RNA sequencing identifies truncating mutations in RBCK1 in a novel Mendelian disease with neuromuscular and cardiac involvement. Genome Med. 2013;5:67. DOI: 10.1186/gm471

[20] Li S, Tighe SW, Nicolet CM, et al: Multi-platform and cross-methodological reproducibility of transcriptome profiling by RNA-seq in the ABRF next generation sequencing study. Nat Biotechnol. 2014;32:915–25. DOI: 10.1038/nbt.2972

[21] Kulski JK, Kenworthy W, Bellgard M, et al: Gene expression profiling of Japanese psoriatic skin reveals an increased activity in molecular stress and immune response signals. J Mol Med (Berl). 2005;83:964–75. PMID: 16283139

[22] Meynert AM, Ansari M, FitzPatrick D, Taylor MS: Variant detection sensitivity and biases in whole genome and exome sequencing. BMC Bioinform. 2014;15:247. DOI: 10.1186/1471-2105-15-247

[23] Chang G, Gao S, Hou X, et al: High-throughput sequencing reveals the disruption of methylation of imprinted gene in induced pluripotent stem cells. Cell Res. 2014;24:293–306. DOI: 10.1038/cr.2013.173

[24] Ekram MB, Kim J: High-Throughput Targeted Repeat Element Bisulfite Sequencing (HT-TREBS): Genome-wide DNA methylation analysis of IAP LTR retrotransposon. PLoS One. 2014;9:e101683. DOI: 10.1371/journal.pone.0101683

[25] Bakshi A, Ekram MB, Kim J: Locus-specific DNA methylation analysis of retrotransposons in ES, somatic and cancer cells using high-throughput targeted repeat element bisulphite sequencing. Genomics Data. 2015;3:87–9. PMID: 25554740

[26] Corley MJ, Zhang W, Zheng X, Lum-Jones A, Maunakea AK: Semiconductor-based sequencing of genome-wide DNA methylation states. Epigenetics. 2015;10:2:153–66. DOI: 10.1080/15592294.2014.1003747

[27] Farlik M, Sheffield NC, Nuzzo A, et al: Single-cell DNA methylome sequencing and bioinformatics inference of epi-genomic cell-state dynamics. Cell Rep. 2015;10:1386–97. DOI: 10.1016/j.celrep.2015.02.001

[28] Hirst M: Epigenomics: Sequencing the methylome. Methods Mol Biol. 2013;973:39–54. DOI: 10.1007/978-1-62703-281-0_3

[29] Li Y, Zhang Y, Li S, et al: Genome-wide DNA methylome analysis reveals epigenetically dysregulated non-coding RNAs in human breast cancer. Sci Rep. 2015;5:8790. DOI: 10.1038/srep08790

[30] Soon WW, Hariharan M, Snyder MP: High-throughput sequencing for biology and medicine. Mol Syst Biol. 2013;9:640. DOI: 10.1038/msb.2012.61.

[31] Watson JD, Crick FH: Molecular structure of nucleic acids; a structure for deoxyribose nucleic acid. Nature. 1953;171:737–8. PMID: 13054692

[32] Holley RW, Apgar J, Everett GA, et al: Structure of a ribonucleic acid. Science. 1965;147:1462–5. PMID: 5898068

[33] RajBhandary UL, Kohrer C: Early days of tRNA research: Discovery, function, purification and sequence analysis. J BioSci. 2006;31:439–51. PMID: 17206064

[34] Barba M, Czosnek H, Hadidi A: Historic perspective, development and applications of next-generation sequencing in plant virology. Viruses. 2014;6:106–36. DOI: 10.3390/v6010106

[35] Franca LTC, Carrilho E, Kist TBL: A review of DNA sequencing techniques. Q Rev Biophys. 2002;35:169–200. DOI: 10.1017/S0033583502003797

[36] Guzvic M: The history of DNA sequencing. J Med Biochem. 2013;32:301–12. DOI: 10.2478/jomb-2014-0004

[37] Maxam AM, Gilbert W: A new method for sequencing DNA. Proc Natl Acad Sci USA. 1977;74(2):560–4. PMID: 265521

[38] Smith LM, Sanders JZ, Kaiser RJ, et al: Fluorescence detection in automated DNA sequence analysis. Nature. 1986;321:674–9. PMID: 3713851

[39] Saiki RK, Scharf S, Faloona F, et al: Enzymatic amplification of beta-globin genomic sequences and restriction site analysis for diagnosis of sickle cell anemia. Science. 1985;230:1350–4. PMID: 2999980

[40] Temin HM, Mizutani S: RNA-dependent DNA polymerase in virions of Rous sarcoma virus. Nature. 1970;226:1211–3. DOI: 10.1038/2261211a0

[41] Baltimore D: Viral RNA-dependent DNA polymerase: RNA-dependent DNA polymerase in virions of RNA tumour viruses. Nature. 1970;226:1209–11. PMID: 4316300

[42] Adams MD, Kelley JM, Gocayne JD, et al: Complementary DNA sequencing: Expressed sequence tags and human genome project. Science. 1991;252:1651–6. DOI: 10.1126/science.2047873

[43] International Human Genome Sequencing Consortium: Initial sequencing and analysis of the human genome. Nature. 2001;409:860–921. PMID: 11237011

[44] Venter JC, Adams MD, Myers EW, et al: The sequence of the human genome. Science. 2001;291:1304–51. PMID: 11181995

[45] Fleischmann RD, Adams MD, White O, et al: Whole-genome random sequencing and assembly of *Haemophilus influenzae Rd*. Science. 1995;269:496–512. PMID: 7542800

[46] Fraser CM, Gocayne JD, White O, et al: The minimal gene complement of *Mycoplasma genitalium*. Science. 1995;270:397–404. PMID: 7569993

[47] Sutton GG, White O, Adams MD, Kerlavage AR: TIGR assembler: A new tool for assembling large shotgun sequencing projects. Genome Sci Technol. 1995;1:9–19.

[48] Stein L: Genome annotation. From sequence to biology. Nat Rev Genet. 2001;2:493–503. PMID: 11433356

[49] Peltonen L, McKusick VA: Dissecting human disease in the postgenomic era. Science. 2001;291:1224–9. PMID: 11233446

[50] Kiechle FL, Zhang X: The postgenomic era. Implications for the clinical laboratory. Arch Pathol Lab Med. 2002;126:255–62. PMID: 11860296

[51] Zhu T: Global analysis of gene expression using GeneChip microarrays. Curr Opin Plant Biol. 2003;6:418–25. PMID: 12972041

[52] Lenoir T, Giannella E: Case study. The emergence and diffusion of DNA microarray technology. J Biomed Discov Collab. 2006;1:11. DOI: 10.1186/1747-5333-1-11

[53] Wetterstrand K: DNA Sequencing Costs: Data from the NHGRI Genome Sequencing Program (GSP) [Internet]. Available from: https://www.genome.gov/sequencingcosts [Accessed: 2015-07-13].

[54] Liu L, Li Y, Li S, et al: Comparison of next-generation sequencing systems. J Biomed Biotechnol. 2012;2012:251364. DOI: 10.1155/2012/251364

[55] Head SR, Komori HK, LaMere SA, et al: Library construction for next-generation sequencing: Overviews and challenges. BioTech. 2014;56:61–77. DOI: 10.2144/000114133

[56] Hart C, Lipson D, Ozsolak F, et al: Single-molecule sequencing: sequence methods to enable accurate quantitation. Methods Enzymol. 2010;472:407e430. DOI: 10.1016/S0076-6879(10)72002-4

[57] Nextera XT DNA sample preparation guide [Internet]. Available from: http://www.liai.org/files/nextera_xt_sample_preparation_guide_15031942_c.pdf [Accessed: 2015-07-01].

[58] Illumina cBot [Internet]. Available from: http://www.illumina.com/documents/products/datasheets/datasheet_cbot.pdf (Accessed: 2015-07-01].

[59] Ion ChefTM or the Ion OneTouchTm 2 [Internet]. Available from: http://www.life-technologies.com/au/en/home/brands/ion-torrent.html [Accessed: 2015-07-01].

[60] Rothberg JM, Hinz W, Rearick TM, et al: An integrated semiconductor device enabling non-optical genome sequencing. Nature. 2011;475:348–52. DOI: 10.1038/nature10242

[61] Bentley DR, Balasubramanian S, Swerdlow HP, et al: Accurate whole human genome sequencing using reversible terminator chemistry. Nature. 2008;456:53–9. DOI: 10.1038/nature07517

[62] Ma Z, Lee RW, Li B, et al: Isothermal amplification method for next-generation sequencing. Proc Natl Acad Sci USA. 2013;110:14320–3. DOI: 10.1073/pnas.1311334110

[63] Aird D, Ross MG, Chen WS, et al: Analyzing and minimizing PCR amplification bias in Illumina sequencing libraries. Genome Biol. 2011;12:R18. DOI: 10.1186/gb-2011-12-2-r18

[64] Kozarewa, I, Kozarewa I, Ning Z, et al: Amplification-free Illumina sequencing-library preparation facilitates improved mapping and assembly of (G+C)-biased genomes. Nat Methods. 2009;6:291–5. DOI: 10.1038/nmeth.1311

[65] Bio-IT World Staff. Six Years After Acquisition, Roche Quietly Shutters 454 [Internet]. Available from: http://www.bio-itworld.com/2013/10/16/six-years-after-acquisition-roche-quietly-shutters-454.html [Accessed: 2015-06-16].

[66] Shendure J, Ji H: Next-generation DNA sequencing. Nat Biotechnol. 2008;26:1135–45. DOI: 10.1038/nbt1486

[67] Balasubramanian S: Solexa sequencing: Decoding genomes on a population scale. Clin Chem. 2015;61:21–4. DOI: 10.1373/clinchem.2014.221747

[68] Illumina Sequencer Comparison Table [Internet]. Available from: http://www.illumina.com/systems/sequencing.html [Accessed: 2015-06-16].

[69] McCoy RC, Taylor RW, Blauwkamp TA, et al: Illumina TruSeq synthetic long-reads empower *de novo* assembly and resolve complex, highly-repetitive transposable elements. PLoS One. 2014;9(9):e106689. DOI: 10.1371/journal.pone.0106689

[70] Drmanac R, Sparks AB, Callow MJ, et al: Human genome sequencing using unchained base reads on self-assembling DNA nanoarrays. Science. 2010;327:78–81. DOI: 10.1126/science.1181498

[71] Retrovolocity [Internet]. Available from: http://www.completegenomics.com/revolocity/ [Accessed: 2015-06-26].

[72] Wang Y, Wen Z, Shen J, et al: Comparison of the performance of Ion Torrent chips in noninvasive prenatal trisomy detection. J Hum Genet. 2014;59:393–6. DOI: 10.1038/jhg.2014.40

[73] Diekstra A, Bosgoed E, Rikken A, et al: Translating Sanger-based routine DNA diagnostics into generic massive parallel ion semiconductor sequencing. Clin Chem. 2015;61:154–62. DOI: 10.1373/clinchem.2014.225250

[74] Schadt EE, Turner S, Kasarskis A: A window into third-generation sequencing. Hum Mol Gene. 2010;19:R227–40. DOI: 10.1093/hmg/ddq416

[75] Eid J, Fehr A, Gray J, et al: Real-time DNA sequencing from single polymerase molecules. Science. 2009;323:133–8. DOI: 10.1126/science.1162986

[76] Travers KJ, Chin C-S, Rank DR, Eid JS, Turner SW: A flexible and efficient template format for circular consensus sequencing and SNP detection. Nucleic Acids Res. 2010;38(15):e159. DOI: 10.1093/nar/gkq543

[77] Koren S, Harhay GP, Smith TP, et al: Reducing assembly complexity of microbial genomes with single-molecule sequencing. Genome Biol. 2013;14:R101.

[78] Thompson JF, Steinmann KE: Single molecule sequencing with a HeliScope Genetic Analysis System. Curr Protoc Mol Biol. 2010;Chapter 7:Unit7.10. DOI: 10.1002/0471142727.mb0710s92

[79] Fuller CW, Middendorf LR, Benner SA, et al: The challenges of sequencing by synthesis. Nat Biotechnol. 2009;27:1013–23. DOI: 10.1038/nbt.1585

[80] Pushkarev D, Neff NF, Quake SR: Single-molecule sequencing of an individual human genome. Nat Biotechnol. 2009;27:847–52. PubMed: 19668243

[81] Ashley EA, Butte AJ, Wheeler MT, et al: Clinical assessment incorporating a personal genome. Lancet. 2010;375:1525–35. DOI: 10.1016/S0140-6736(10)60452-7

[82] Hickman SE, Kingery ND, Ohsumi T, et al: The microglial sensome revealed by direct RNA sequencing. Nat Neurosci. 2013;16:1896–905. DOI: 10.1038/nn.3554

[83] Bayley H: Nanopore sequencing: From imagination to reality. Clin Chem. 2015;61:25–31. DOI: 10.1373/clinchem.2014.223016

[84] Wang Y, Yang Q, Wang Z: The evolution of nanopore sequencing. Front Genet. 2005;5:1–20. DOI: 10.3389/fgene.2014.00449

[85] Bayley H, Cremer PS: Stochastic sensors inspired by biology. Nature. 2001;413:226–30. PMID: 11557992

[86] Stoddart D, Heron A, Mikhailova E, Maglia G, Bayley H: Single nucleotide discrimination in immobilized DNA oligonucleotides with a biological nanopore. Proc Natl Acad Sci USA. 2009;106:7702–7. DOI: 10.1073/pnas.0901054106

[87] Laver T, Harrison J, O'Neill PA, et al: Assessing the performance of the Oxford Nanopore Technologies MinION. Biomol Detect Quant. 2015;3:1–8.

[88] Bell DC, Thomas WK, Murtagh KM, et al: DNA base identification by electron microscopy. Microsc Microanal. 2012;18:1049–53. DOI: 10.1017/S1431927612012615

[89] Bragg LM, Stone G, Butler MK, Hugenholtz P, Tyson GW: Shining a light on dark sequencing: Characterising errors in Ion Torrent PGM Data. PLoS Comput Biol. 2013;9:e1003031. DOI: 10.1371/journal.pcbi.1003031

[90] Gilles A, Meglecz E, Pech N, et al: Accuracy and quality assessment of 454 GS-FLX Titanium pyrosequencing. BMC Genomics. 2011;12:245. DOI: 10.1186/1471-2164-12-245

[91] Huse SM, Huber JA, Morrison HG, Sogin ML, Welch DM: Accuracy and quality of massively parallel DNA pyrosequencing. Genome Biol. 2007;8:R143. PMID: 17659080

[92] Sims D, Sudbery I, Ilott NE, Heger A, Ponting CP: Sequencing depth and coverage: key considerations in genomic analyses. Nat Rev Genet. 2014;15:121–32. DOI: 10.1038/nrg3642

[93] Loman NJ, Misra RV, Dallman TJ, et al: Performance comparison of benchtop high-throughput sequencing platforms. Nat Biotechnol. 2012;30:434–9. DOI: 10.1038/nbt. 2198. Erratum in Nat Biotechnol. 2012;30:562.

[94] Quail M, Smith M, Coupland P, et al: A tale of three next generation sequencing platforms: comparison of Ion Torrent, Pacific Biosciences and Illumina MiSeq sequencers. BMC Genomics. 2012;13:341. DOI: 10.1186/1471-2164-13-341

[95] Rieber N, Zapatka M, Lasitschka B, et al: Coverage bias and sensitivity of variant calling for four whole-genome sequencing technologies. PLoS One. 2013;8:e66621. DOI: 10.1371/journal.pone.0066621

[96] Fuellgrabe MW, Herrmann D, Knecht H, et al: High-throughput, amplicon-based sequencing of the CREBBP gene as a tool to develop a universal platform-independent assay. PLoS One. 2015;10:e0129195. DOI: 10.1371/journal.pone.0129195

[97] Ozaki Y, Suzuki S, Kashiwase K, et al: Cost-efficient multiplex PCR for routine genotyping of up to nine classical HLA loci in a single analytical run of multiple samples by next generation sequencing. BMC Genomics. 2015;16:318. DOI: 10.1186/ s12864-015-1514-4

[98] Horner DS, Pavesi G, Castrignano T, et al: Bioinformatics approaches for genomics and post genomics applications of next generation sequencing. Brief Bioinform. 2010;11:181–97. DOI: 10.1093/bib/bbp046

[99] El-Metwally S, Hamza T, Zakaria M, Helmy M: Next-generation sequence assembly: four stages of data processing and computational challenges. PLoS Comput Biol. 2013;9:e1003345. DOI: 10.1007/s10142-015-0433-4

[100] Land M, Hauser L, Jun SR, et al: Insights from 20 years of bacterial genome sequencing. Funct Integr Genomics. 2015;15:141–61. DOI: 10.1007/s10142-015-0433-4

[101] Hong HX, Zhang WQ, Shen J, et al: Critical role of bioinformatics in translating huge amounts of next-generation sequencing data into personalized medicine. Sci China Life Sci. 2013;56:110–8. DOI: 10.1007/s11427-013-4439-7

[102] Oliver GR, Hart SN, Klee EW: Bioinformatics for clinical next generation sequencing. Clin Chem. 2015;61:124–35. DOI: 10.1373/clinchem.2014.224360

[103] Yandell M, Ence D: A beginner's guide to eukaryotic genome annotation. Nat Rev Genet. 2012;13:329–42. DOI: 10.1038/nrg3174

[104] Schlotterer C, Tablerm R, Kofler R, Nolte V: Sequencing pools of individuals—Mining genome wide polymorphism data without big funding. Nat Rev Genet. 2014;15:749–63. DOI: 10.1038/nrg3803

[105] Shumway M, Cochrane G, Sugawara H: Archiving next generation sequencing data. Nucleic Acids Res. 2010;38:D870–1. DOI: 10.1093/nar/gkp1078

[106] Korneliussen TS, Albrechtsen A, Nielsen R: ANGSD: Analysis of next generation sequencing data. BMC Bioinform. 2014;15:356. DOI: 10.1186/s12859-014-0356-4

[107] Ruan J, Jiang L, Chong Z, et al: Pseudo-Sanger sequencing: massively parallel production of long and near error-free reads using NGS technology. BMC Genomics. 2013;14:711. DOI: 10.1186/1471-2164-14-711

[108] Bradnam Fass JN, Alexandrov A, et al: Assemblathon 2: Evaluating *de novo* methods of genome assembly in three vertebrate species. Gigascience. 2013;2:10. DOI: 10.1186/2047-217X-2-10

[109] Medina I, Salavert F, Sanchez R, et al: Genome Maps, a new generation genome browser. Nucleic Acids Res. 2013;41:W41–6. DOI: 10.1093/nar/gkt530

[110] Cunningham F, Amode MR, Barrell D, et al: Ensembl 2015. Nucleic Acids Res. 2015;43:D662–9. DOI: 10.1093/nar/gku1010

[111] Fiers W, Contreras R, Duerinck F, et al: Complete nucleotide sequence of bacteriophage MS2 RNA: primary and secondary structure of the replicase gene. Nature. 1976;260:500–7. PMID: 1264203

[112] Kuska B: Beer, Bethesda and biology: How "genomics" came into being. J Natl Cancer Inst. 1998;80:93. PMID: 9450566

[113] Hocquette JF, Cassar-Malek, Scalbert A, Guillou F: Contribution of genomics to the understanding of physiological functions. J Physiol Pharmacol. 2009;60(Suppl 3):5–16. PMID: 19996478

[114] Wylie KM, Weinstock GM, Storch GA: Virome genomics: A tool for defining the human virome. Curr Opin Microbiol. 2013;16(4):479–84. DOI: 10.1016/j.mib.2013.04.006

[115] Kwong JC, McCallum, Sintchenko V, Howden BP: Whole genome sequencing in clinical and public health microbiology. Pathol. 2015;47:199–210. DOI: 10.1097/PAT.0000000000000235

[116] Chun J, Rainey FA: Integrating genomics into taxonomy and systematics of the Bacteria and Archaea. Int J Syst Evol Microbiol. 2014;64:316–24. DOI 10.1099/ijs.0.054171-0

[117] Ladner JT, Beitzel, Chain PSG: Standards for sequencing viral genomes in the era of high-throughput sequencing. mBio. 2014;5:e01360–14. DOI: 10.1128/mBio.01360-14

[118] Galagan JE, Henn MR, Ma L-J, Cuomo CA, Birren B: Genomics of the fungal kingdom: Insights into eukaryotic biology. Genome Res. 2005;15:1620–31. PMID: 16339359

[119] Stajich JE, Harris T, Brunk BP, et al: FungiDB: an integrated functional genomics database for fungi. Nucleic Acids Res. 2012;40(Database issue):D675–81. DOI: 10.1093/nar/gkr918

[120] Kim KM, Park J-H, Bhattacharya D, Yoon HS: Applications of next-generation sequencing to unraveling the evolutionary history of algae. Int J Syst Evol Microbiol. 2014;64:333–45. DOI: 10.1099/ijs.0.054221-0

[121] Pareek CSP, Smoczynski R, Tretyn A: Sequencing technologies and genome sequencing. J Appl Genet. 2011;52:413–35. DOI: 10.1007/s13353-011-0057-x

[122] Ekblom R, Wolf JBW: A field guide to whole-genome sequencing, assembly and annotation. Evol Appl. 2014;7:1026–42. DOI: 10.1111/eva.12178

[123] Gonzaga-Jauregui C, Lupski JR, Gibbs RA: Human genome sequencing in health and disease. Annu Rev Med. 2012;63:35–61. DOI: 10.1146/annurev-med-051010-162644

[124] Tewhey R, Bansal V, Torkamani A, Topol EJ, Schork NJ: The importance of phase information for human genomics. Nat Rev Genet. 2011;12:215–23. DOI: 10.1038/nrg2950

[125] Green RC, Berg JS, Grody WW, et al: ACMG recommendations for reporting of incidental findings in clinical exome and genome sequencing. Genet Med. 2013;15:565–74. DOI: 10.1038/gim.2013

[126] Taylor JC, Martin HC, Lise S, et al: Factors influencing success of clinical genome sequencing across a broad spectrum of disorders. Nat Genet. 2015;47:717–26. DOI: 10.1038/ng.3304

[127] Handsaker RE, Van Doren V, Berman JR, et al: Large multiallelic copy number variations in humans. Nat Genet. 2015;47:296–303. DOI: 10.1038/ng.3200

[128] Ammar R, Paton TA, Torti D, Shlein A, Bader GD: Long read nanopore sequencing for detection of HLA and CYP2D6 variants and haplotypes. F1000Res. 2015;4:17. DOI: 10.12688/f1000research.6037.1

[129] Erlich HA: HLA typing using next generation sequencing: An overview. Hum Immunol. 2015;pii: S0198-8859(15)00093-2. DOI: 10.1016/j.humimm.2015.03.001

[130] Shiina T, Hosomichi K, Inoko H, Kulski JK: The HLA genomic loci map: Expression, interaction, diversity and disease. J Hum Genet. 2009;54:15–39. DOI: 10.1038/jhg.2008.5

[131] Mortazavi A, Williams BA, McCue K, Schaeffer L, Wold B: Mapping and quantifying mammalian transcriptomes by RNA-Seq. Nat Methods. 2008;5:621–8. DOI: 10.1038/nmeth.1226

[132] Nagalakshmi U, Wang Z, Waern K, et al: The transcriptional landscape of the yeast genome defined by RNA sequencing. Science. 2008;320:1344–9. DOI: 10.1126/science.1158441

[133] Kapranov P, St. Laurent G: Dark matter RNA: Existence, function, and controversy. Front Genet. 2012;3:article 60:1–9. DOI: 10.3389/fgene.2012.00060

[134] Birney E. Stamatoyannopoulos, JA, Dutta A, et al: Identification and analysis of functional elements in 1% of the human genome by the encode pilot project. Nature. 2007;447:799–816. PMID: 17571346

[135] Clamp, M. Fry B, Kamal M, et al: Distinguishing protein-coding and noncoding genes in the human genome. Proc Natl Acad Sci USA. 2007;104:19428–33. PMID: 18040051

[136] Marioni JC, Mason CE, Mane SM, Stephens M, Gilad Y: RNA-seq: An assessment of technical reproducibility and comparison with gene expression arrays. Genome Res. 2008;18:1509–17. DOI: 10.1101/gr.079558.108

[137] Costa V, Angelini C, de Feis I, Ciccodicola A: Uncovering the complexity of transcriptomes with RNA-seq. J. Biomed. Biotechnol. 2010;2010:853916. DOI: 10.1155/2010/853916

[138] The RNAcentral Consortium: RNAcentral: an international database of ncRNA sequences. Nucleic Acids Res. 2015;43:D123–9. DOI: 10.1093/nar/gku991

[139] Huntzinger E, Izaurrralde E: Gene silencing by microRNAs: contributions of translational repression and miRNA decay. Nat Rev Genet. 2011;12:99–110. DOI: 10.1038/nrg2936

[140] Ross RJ, Weiner MM, Lin H: PIWI proteins and PIWI-interacting RNAs in the soma. Nature. 2014;505:353–9. DOI: 10.1038/nature12987

[141] Lindblad-Toh K, Garber M, Zuk O: A high-resolution map of human evolutionary constraint using 29 mammals. Nature. 2011;478:476–82. DOI: 10.1038/nature10530

[142] Fujii YR: RNA genes: Retroelements and virally retroposable microRNAs in human embryonic stem cells. Open Virol J. 2010;4:63–75. DOI: 10.2174/1874357901004010063

[143] Kelley D, Rinn J: Transposable elements reveal a stem cell-specific class of long noncoding RNAs. Genome Biol. 2012;13:R107. DOI: 10.1186/gb-2012-13-11-r107

[144] Amaral PP, Dinger ME, Mattick JS: Non-coding RNAs in homeostasis, disease and stress responses: An evolutionary perspective. Brief Funct Genomics. 2013;12:254–78. DOI: 10.1093/bfgp/elt016

[145] Moolhuijzen P, Kulski JK, Dunn DS, et al: The transcript repeat element: The human Alu sequence as a component of gene networks influencing cancer. Funct Integr Genomics. 2010;10:307–19. DOI: 10.1007/s10142-010-0168-1

[146] Costa FF: Non-coding RNAs, epigenetics and complexity. Gene. 2008;410:9–17. DOI: 10.1016/j.gene.2007.12.008

[147] Derrien T, Johnson R, Bussotti G, et al: The GENCODEv7 catalog of human long noncoding RNAs: Analysis of their gene structure, evolution and expression. Genome Res. 2012;22:1775–89. DOI: 10.1101/gr.132159.111

[148] Yarmishyn AA, Kurochkin IV: Long noncoding RNAs: a potential novel class of cancer biomarkers. Front Genet. 2015;6:Article 145:1–10. DOI: 10.3389/fgene.2015.00145

[149] Iyer MK, Niknafs YS, Malik R: The landscape of long noncoding RNAs in the human transcriptome. Nat Genet. 2015;47:199–208. DOI: 10.1038/ng.3192

[150] Vance KW, Ponting CP: Transcriptional regulatory functions of nuclear long noncoding RNAs. Trends Genet. 2014;30:348–55. DOI: 10.1016/j.tig.2014.06.001

[151] Ward AJ, Cooper TA: The pathobiology of splicing. J Pathol. 2010;220:152–63. DOI: 10.1002/path.2649

[152] Poulos MG, Batra R, Charizanis K, Swanson MS: Developments in RNA splicing and disease. Cold Spring Harb Perspect Biol. 2011;3:a000778. DOI: 10.1101/cshperspect.a000778

[153] Melé M, Ferreira PG, Reverter F, et al: Human genomics. The human transcriptome across tissues and individuals. Science. 2015;348:660–5. DOI: 10.1126/science.aaa0355

[154] Landt SG, Marinov GK, Kundaje A, et al: ChIP-seq guidelines and practices of the ENCODE and modENCODE consortia. Genome Res. 2012; 22:1813–31. DOI: 10.1101/gr.136184.111

[155] de Witt E, de Laat W: A decade of 3C technologies: Insights into nuclear organization. Genes Dev. 2012;26:11–24. DOI: 10.1101/gad.179804.111

[156] Berggard T, Linse S, James P: Methods for the detection and analysis of protein-protein interactions. Proteomics. 2007;7:2833–42. DOI: 10.1002/pmic.200700131

[157] Malm EK, Srivastava V, Sundqvist G, Bulone V: APP: An Automated Proteomics Pipeline for the analysis of mass spectrometry data based on multiple open access tools. BMC Bioinform. 2014;15:441. DOI: 10.1186/s12859-014-0441-8

[158] Chagoyen M, Pazos F: Tools for functional interpretation of metabolomics experiments. Brief Bioinform. 2013;14:737–44. DOI: 10.1093/bib/bbs055

[159] Pavlidid C, Patrinos GP, Katsila T: Nutrigenomics: A controversy. Appl Transl Genomics. 2015;4:50–3. DOI: 10.1016/j.atg.2015.02.003

[160] Winter G, Krömer JO: Fluxomics — Connecting "omics" analysis and phenotypes. Environ Microbiol. 2013;15:1901–16. DOI: 10.1111/1462-2920.12064

[161] Stanberry L, Mias GI, Haynes W, Higdon R, Snyder M, Kolker E: Integrative analysis of longitudinal metabolomics data from a personal multi-omics profile. Metabolites. 2013;3:741–60. DOI: 10.3390/metabo3030741

[162] Hernández-Prieto MA, Semeniuk TA, Futschik ME: Toward a systems-level understanding of gene regulatory, protein interaction, and metabolic networks in cyanobacteria. Front Genet. 2014;5:191. DOI: 10.3389/fgene.2014.0019

[163] Wang Q, Lu Q, Zhao H: A review of study designs and statistical methods for genomic epidemiology studies using next generation sequencing. Front Genet. 2015:6:149. DOI: 10.3389/fgene.2015.00149

[164] Editorial: Marshaling the variome. Nat Genet. 2015;47:849. DOI: 10.1038/ng.3377

[165] Groza T, Kohler S, Moldenhauer D, et al: The human phenotype ontology: Semantic unification of common and rare disease. Am J Hum Genet. 2015;97:111–24. DOI: 10.1016/j.ajhg.2015.05.020

[166] Paltoo DN, Rodriguez LL, Feolo M, et al: Data use under the NIH GWAS data sharing policy and future directions. Nat Genet. 2014;46:934–8. DOI: 10.1038/ng.3062

[167] Lappalainen I, Almeida-King J, Kumanduri V, et al: The European Genome-phenome Archive of human data consented for biomedical research. Nat Genet. 2015;47:692–5. DOI: 10.1038/ng.3312

[168] Bashir Y, Singh SP, Konwar BK: Metagenomics: an application based perspective. Chin J Biol. 2014;ID146030:7 pages, http://dx.doi.org/10.1155/2014/146030

[169] Gilbert JA, Dupont CL: Microbial metagenomics: Beyond the genome. Annu Rev Mar Sci. 2011;3:347–71. PMID: 21329209

[170] Croucher NJ, Harris SR, Grad YH, Hanage WP: Bacterial genomes in epidemiology — Present and future. Phil Trans R Soc B. 2013;368:20120202. http://dx.doi.org/10.1098/rstb.2012.0202

[171] Grad YH, Lipsitch M: Epidemiologic data and pathogen genome sequences: a powerful synergy for public health. Genome Biol. 2014;15:538. http://genomebiology.com/2014/15/11/538

[172] Sunagawa S, Coelho LP, Chaffron S, et al: Ocean plankton. Structure and function of the global ocean microbiome. Science. 2015;348:1261359. DOI: 10.1126/science.1261359

[173] de Vargas C, Audic S, Henry N, et al: Ocean plankton. Eukaryotic plankton diversity in the sunlit ocean. Science. 2015;348:1261605. DOI: 10.1126/science.1261605

[174] Brum JR, Ignacio-Espinoza JC, Roux S, et al: Ocean plankton. Patterns and ecological drivers of ocean viral communities. Science. 2015;348:1261498. DOI: 10.1126/science. 1261498

[175] Weinstock GM: Genomic approaches to studying the human microbiota. Nature. 2012;489:250–6. DOI: 10.1038/nature11553

[176] Morgan XC, Segata N, Huttenhower C: Biodiversity and functional genomics in the human microbiome. Trends Genet. 2013;29:51–8. DOI: 10.1016/j.tig.2012.09.005

[177] Ursell LK, Metcalf JL, Parfrey LW, Knight R: Defining the human microbiome. Nutr Rev. 2012;70 Suppl 1:S38–44. DOI: 10.1111/j.1753-4887.2012.00493.x

[178] Reddy TBK, Thomas A, Stamatis D, et al: The Genomes OnLine Database (GOLD) v. 5: a metadata management system based on a four level (meta)genome project classification. Nucleic Acids Res. 2014;97:111–24. DOI: 10.1093/nar/gku950

[179] Myer F, Paarmann D, D'Souza M, et al: The metagenomics RAST server—A public resource for the automatic phylogenetic and functional analysis of metagenomes. BMC Bioinform. 2008;9:386. DOI: 10.1186/1471-2105-9-386

[180] Zelezniak A, Andrejev S, Ponomarova O, Mende DR, Bork P, Patil KR: Metabolic dependencies drive species co-occurrence in diverse microbial communities. Proc Natl Acad Sci USA. 2015;112:6449-54. http://dx.doi.org/10.1073/pnas.1421834112 (2015)

[181] Olsen GJ, Woese C: Archael genomics: An overview. Cell. 1997;89:991–4. PMID: 9215619

[182] Hagen JB: Five kingdoms, more or less: Robert Whittaker and the broad classification of organisms. BioScience. 2012;62:67–74. DOI: 10.1525/bio.2012.62.1.11

[183] Pawlowski J: The new micro-kingdoms of eukaryotes. BMC Biol. 2013;11:40. DOI: 10.1186/1741-7007-11-40

[184] Adl SM, Simpson AGB, Lane CE, et al: The revised classification of eukaryotes. J Eukaryot Microbiol. 2012;59:429–93. DOI: 10.1111/j.1550-7408.2012.00644.x

[185] Villarreal LP: How viruses shape the tree of life. Future Virol. 2006;1:587–95.

[186] Moreira D, Lopez-Garcia P: Ten reasons to exclude viruses from the tree of life. Nat Rev Microbiol. 2009;7:306–11. DOI: 10.1038/nrmicro2108

[187] Philippe N, Legendre M, Doutre G, et al: Pandoraviruses: Amoeba viruses with genomes up to 2.5 Mb reaching that of parasitic eukaryotes. Science. 2013;341:281–6. DOI: 10.1126/science.1239181

[188] Legendre M, Bartoli J, Shmakova L, et al: Thirty-thousand-year-old distant relative of giant icosahedral DNA viruses with a pandoravirus morphology. Proc Natl Acad Sci USA. 2014;111:4274–9. DOI: 10.1073/pnas.1320670111

[189] Beerenwinkel N, Gunthard HF, Roth V, Metzner KJ: Challenges and opportunities in estimating viral genetic diversity from next-generation sequencing data. Front Microbiol. 2012;3:329. DOI: 10.3389/fmicb.2012.00329

[190] Shah V, Zakrzewski M, Wibberg D, Eikmeyer F, Schlüter A, Madamwar D: Taxonomic profiling and metagenome analysis of a microbial community from a habitat contaminated with industrial discharges. Microb Ecol. 2013;66:533-50. DOI: 10.1007/s00248-013-0244-x

[191] Soucy SM, Huang J, Gogarten JP: Horizontal gene transfer: Building the web of life. Nat Rev Genet. 2015;16:472–82. DOI: 10.1038/nrg3962

[192] Makarova KS, Wolf YI, Koonin EV: Comparative genomics of defense systems in archaea and bacteria. Nucleic Acids Res. 2013;41:4360–77. DOI: 10.1093/nar/gkt157

[193] Haft DH, Selengut J, Mongodin EF, Nelson KN: A guild of 45 CRISPR-associated (Cas) protein families and multiple CRISPR/Cas subtypes exist in prokaryotic genomes. PLoS Comput Biol. 2005;1:e60. DOI: 10.1371/journal.pcbi.0010060

[194] Louwen R, Staals RHJ, Endtz HP, van Baarlen P, van der Oost J: The role of CRISPR-Cas systems in virulence of pathogenic bacteria. Microbiol Mol Biol Rev. 2014;78:74–88. DOI: 10.1128/Mmbr. 00039- 13

[195] Makarova KS, Haft DH, Barrangou R, et al: Evolution and classification of the CRISPR-Cas systems. Nat Rev Microbiol. 2011;9:467–77. DOI: 10.1038/nrmicro2577

[196] Shalem O, Sanjana NE, Zhang F: High-throughput functional genomics using CRISPR-Cas9. Nat Rev Genet. 2015;16:299–310. DOI: 10.1038/nrg3899

[197] Liao, HK, Gu Y, Diaz A, et al: Use of the CRISPR-Cas9 system as an intracellular defense against HIV-1 infection in human cells. Nat Commun. 2015;6:6413. DOI: 10.1038/ncomms7413

[198] Chowdhury C, Sinha S, Chun S, Yeates TO, Bobik TA: Diverse bacterial microcompartment organelles. Microbiol Mol Biol Rev. 2014;78:438–68. DOI: 10.1128/mmbr. 00009-14

[199] Jorda J, Lopez D, Wheatley NM, Yeates TO: Using comparative genomics to uncover new kinds of protein-based metabolic organelles in bacteria. Protein Sci. 2013;22:179–95. DOI: 10.1002/pro.2196

[200] Vasu K, Nagaraja V: Diverse functions of restriction-modification systems in addition to cellular defense. Microbiol Mol Biol Rev. 2013;77:53–72. DOI: 10.1128/MMBR. 00044-12

[201] Zilberman D: The evolving functions of DNA methylation. Curr Opin Plant Biol. 2008;11:554–9. DOI: 10.1016/j.pbi.2008.07.004

[202] Guy L, Ettema TJG: The archaeal 'TACK' superphylum and the origin of eukaryotes. Trends Microbiol. 2011;19:580–7. DOI: 10.1016/j.tim.2011.09.002

[203] Spang A, Saw JH, Jørgensen SL, et al: Complex archaea that bridge the gap between prokaryotes and eukaryotes. Nature. 2015;521:173–9. DOI: 10.1038/nature14447

[204] Margulis L: Origin of Eukaryotic Cells. New Haven, CT: Yale University Press; 1970.

[205] Gray MW: Mitochondrial evolution. Cold Spring Harb Perspect Biol. 2012;4:a01140. DOI: 10.1101/cshperspect.a011403

[206] Kabnick KS, Peattie DA: *Gardia*: A missing link between prokaryotes and eukaryotes. Am Sci. 1991;79:34–43.

[207] Wilkins AS, Holliday R: The evolution of meiosis from mitosis. Genetics. 2009;181:3–12. DOI: 10.1534/genetics.108.099762

[208] Otto SP: The evolutionary consequences of polyploidy. Cell. 2007;13:452–62. PMID: 17981114

[209] Davoli T, de Lange T: The causes and consequences of polyploidy in normal development and cancer. Annu Rev Cell Dev Biol. 2011;27:585–610. DOI: 10.1146/annurev-cellbio-092910-154234

[210] Madlung A: Polyploidy and its effect on evolutionary success: old questions visited with new tools. Heredity. 2013;110:99–104. DOI: 10.1038/hdy.2012.79

[211] Hindle MM, Martin SF, Noordally ZB, et al: The reduced kinome of *Ostreococcus tauri*: core eukaryotic signally components in a tractable model species. BMC Genomics. 2014;15:640. DOI: 10.1186/1471-2164-15-640

[212] Pellicer J, Fay MF, Leitch IJ: The largest eukaryotic genome of them all? Botanical J Linnean Soc. 2010;164:10–5. DOI: 10.1111/j.1095-8339.2010.01072.x

[213] Katju V, Bergthorsson U: Copy-number changes in evolution: rates, fitness effects and adaptive significance. Front Genet. 2013;4:273. DOI: 10.3389/fgene.2013.00273

[214] Garsmeur O, Schnable JC, Almeida A, Jourda C, D'Hont A, Freeling M: Two evolutionary distinct classes of paleopolyploidy. Mol Biol Evol. 2014;31:448–54. DOI: 10.1093/molbev/mst230

[215] Dehal P, Boore JL: Two rounds of whole genome duplication in the ancestral vertebrate. PLoS Biol. 2005;3:e314. DOI: 10.1371/journal.pbio.0030314

[216] Ohno S. Evolution by Gene Duplication. New York: Springer-Verlag; 1970.

[217] Parisod C, Mhiri C, Lim KY, et al: Differential dynamics of transposable elements during long-term diploidization of *Nicotiana* Section *Repandae* (Solanaceae) allopolyploid genomes. PLoS One. 2012;7:e50352. DOI: 10.1371/journal.pone.0050352

[218] Renny-Byfield S, Kovarik A, Kelly LJ, et al: Diploidization and genome size change in allopolyploids is associated with differential dynamics of low- and high-copy sequences. Plant J. 2013;74:829–39. DOI: 10.1111/tpj.12168

[219] Wang X, Freeling M: The Brassica genome. Front Plant Sci. 2013;4:148. DOI: 10.3389/fpls.2013.00148

[220] Shikari AB, Parray GA, Sofi NR, Hussain A, Dar ZA, Iqbal AM: Group balanced block design for comparisons among oilseed *Brassicae*. Sci Res Essays. 2015;10:302–5. DOI: 10.3389/fpls.2013.00148

[221] Michael TP, Jackson S: The first 50 plant genomes. Plant Genome. 2013;6:1–7.

[222] Feldman M, Levy AA: Genome evolution due to allopolyploidization in wheat. Genetics. 2012;192:763–74. DOI: 10.1534/genetics.112.146316

[223] Chapman, Mascher M, Buluc A, et al: A whole-genome shotgun approach for assembling and anchoring the hexaploid bread wheat genome. Genome Biol. 2015;16:26. DOI: 10.1186/s13059-015-0582-8

[224] Ainouche ML, Fortune PM, Salmon A, et al: Hybridization, polyploidy and invasion: Lessons from *Spartina* (Poaceae). Biol Inv. 2008;11:1159–73. DOI: 10.1007/s10530-008-9383-2

[225] Brawand D, Wagner CE, Li YI, et al: The genomic substrate for adaptive radiation in African cichlid fish. Nature. 2014;513:375–81. DOI: 10.1038/nature13726

[226] Seehausen O, Butlin RK, Keller I, et al: Genomics and the origin of species. Nat Rev Genet. 2014;15:176–92. DOI: 10.1038/nrg3644

[227] Alvarez-Ponce D, Lopez P, Bapteste E, McInerney JO: Gene similarity networks provide tools for understanding eukaryote origins and evolution. Proc Natl Acad Sci USA. 2013;110:E1594–603. DOI: 10.1073/pnas.1211371110

[228] Feschotte C: The contribution of transposable elements to the evolution of regulatory networks. Nat Rev Genet. 2008;9:397–405. DOI: 10.1038/nrg2337

[229] Bejerano G, Pheasant M, Makunin I, et al: Ultraconserved elements in the human genome. Science. 2004;304:1321–5. DOI: 10.1126/science.1098119

[230] Miller W, Rosenbloom K, Hardison RC, et al: 28-way vertebrate alignment and conservation track in the UCSC genome browser. Genome Res. 2007;17:1797–808. PMID: 17984227

[231] Dimitrieva S, Bucher P: UCNEbase—A database of ultraconserved non-coding elements and genomic regulatory blocks. Nucleic Acids Res. 2013;41(Database issue):D101-9. DOI: 10.1093/nar/gks1092

[232] Luo H, Lin Y, Gao F, Zhang C-T, Zhang R: DEG 10, an update of the Database of Essential Genes that includes both protein-coding genes and non-coding genomic elements. Nucleic Acids Res. 2014;42:D574–80. DOI: 10.1093/nar/gkt1131

[233] Huerta-Cepas J, Dopazo H, Dopazo J, Gabaldón T: The human phylome. Genome Biol. 2007;8:R109. PMID: 17567924

[234] Huerta-Cepas J, Capella-Gutiérrez S, Pryszcz LP, Marcet-Houben M, Gabaldón T: PhylomeDB v4: Zooming into the plurality of evolutionary histories of a genome. Nucleic Acids Res. 2014;42(Database issue):D897–902. DOI: 10.1093/nar/gkt1177

[235] Matsuzaka Y, Okamoto K, Mabuchi T, et al: Identification, expression analysis and polymorphism of a novel RLTPR gene encoding a RGD motif, tropomodulin domain and proline/leucine-rich regions. Gene. 2004;343:291–304. PMID: 15588584

[236] Liang Y, Cucchetti M, Roncagalli R, et al: The lymphoid lineage-specific actin-uncapping protein Rltpr is essential for costimulation via CD28 and the development of regulatory T cells. Nat Immunol. 2013;14:858–66. DOI: 10.1038/ni.2634

[237] Willems L, Gillet NA: APOBEC3 interference during replication of viral genomes. Viruses. 2015;7:2999–3018. DOI: 10.3390/v7062757

[238] Richard GF, Kerrest A, Dujon B: Comparative genomics and molecular dynamics of DNA repeats in eukaryotes. Microbiol Mol Biol Rev. 2008;72:686–727. DOI: 10.1128/MMBR.00011-08

[239] McClintock B: The significance of responses of the genome to challenge. Science. 1984;226:792–801. PMID: 15739260

[240] Jurka J, Klonowski P, Dagman V, Pelton P: CENSOR—A program for identification and elimination of repetitive elements from DNA sequences. Comput Chem. 1996;20:119–21. PMID: 8867843

[241] Kohany O, Gentles AJ, Hankus L, Jurka J: Annotation, submission and screening of repetitive elements in Repbase: Rep baseSubmitter and Censor. BMC Bioinform. 2006;7:474. DOI: 10.1186/1471-2105-7-474

[242] Thung DT, de Ligt J, Vissers LEM, et al: Mobster: Accurate detection of mobile element insertions in next generation sequencing data. Genome Biol. 2014:15:488. PMID: 25348035

[243] Girgis HZ: Red: An intelligent, rapid, accurate tool for detecting repeats *de-novo* on the genomic scale. BMC Bioinform. 2015;16:227. DOI 10.1186/s12859-015-0654-5

[244] Tempel S, Talla E. VisualTE: a graphical interface for transposable element analysis at the genomic scale. BMC Genomics. 2015;16:139. DOI 10.1186/s12864-015-1351-5

[245] Burns KH, Boeke JD: Human transposon tectonics. Cell. 2012;149:740–52. DOI: 10.1016/j.cell.2012.04.019

[246] Feschotte C, Pritham EJ: DNA transposons and the evolution of eukaryotic genomes. Annu Rev Genet. 2007;41:331–48. PMID: 18076328

[247] Frost LS, Leplae R, Summers AO, Toussaint A: Mobile genetic elements: The agents of open source evolution. Nat Rev Microbiol. 2005;3:722–32. PMID:16138100

[248] Giordano J, Ge Y, Gelfand Y, Abrusa'n G, Benson G, et al: Evolutionary history of mammalian transposons determined by genome-wide defragmentation. PLoS Comput Biol. 2007;3:e137. DOI: 10.1371/journal.pcbi.0030137

[249] Hoen DR, Bureau TE: Discovery of novel genes derived from transposable elements using integrative genomic analysis. Mol Biol Evol. 2015;32(6):1487–506. DOI: 10.1093/molbev/msv042

[250] Bao W, Kojima KK, Kohany O: Repbase Update, a database of repetitive elements in eukaryotic genomes. Mob DNA 2015;6:11. DOI: 10.1186/s13100-015-0041-9

[251] Menconi G, Battaglia G, Grossi R, Pisanti N, Marangoni R: Mobilomics in *Saccharomyces cerevisiae* strains. BMC Bioinform. 2013;14:102. DOI: 10.1186/1471-2105-14-102

[252] SanMiguel P, Tikhonov A, Jin YK, et al: Nested retrotransposons in the intergenic regions of the maize genome. Science. 1996;274:765–8. PMID: 12021852

[253] Koonin EV, Wolf YI: Genomics of bacteria and archaea: The emerging dynamic view of the prokaryotic world. Nucleic Acids Res. 2008;36:6688–719. DOI: 10.1093/nar/gkn668

[254] Raymond J, Zhaxybayeva O, Gogarten JP, Gerdes SY, Blankenship RE: Whole-genome analysis of photosynthetic prokaryotes. Science. 2002;298:1616–20. PMID: 12446909

[255] Rankin DJ, Rocha EPC, Brown SP: What traits are carried on mobile genetic elements, and why? Heredity. 2011;106:1–10. DOI: 10.1038/hdy.2010.24

[256] Boto L: Horizontal gene transfer in the acquisition of novel traits by metazoans. Proc R Soc B. 2014;281:20132450. http://dx.doi.org/10.1098/rspb.2013.2450

[257] Jjingo D, Conley AB, Wang J, et al: Mammalian-wide interspersed repeat (MIR)-derived enhancers and the regulation of human gene expression. Mobile DNA. 2014;5:14. DOI: 10.1186/1759-8753-5-14

[258] Wang J, Vicente-García C, Seruggia D, et al: MIR retrotransposon sequences provide insulators to the human genome. Proc Natl Acad Sci USA. 2015;112:E4428–37. DOI: 10.1073/pnas.1507253112

[259] Kulski JK, Gaudieri S, Inoko H, Dawkins RL: Comparison between two human endogenous retrovirus (HERV)-rich regions within the major histocompatibility complex. J Mol Evol. 1999;48:675–83. PMID: 10229571

[260] Kulski JK, Gaudieri S, Martin A, Dawkins RL: Coevolution of PERB11 (MIC) and HLA class I genes with HERV-16 and retroelements by extended genomic duplication. J Mol Evol. 1999;49:84–97. PMID: 15269276

[261] Kulski JK, Anzai T, Shiina T, Inoko H: Rhesus macaque class I duplicon structures, organization, and evolution within the alpha block of the major histocompatibility complex. Mol Biol Evol. 2004;21:2079–91. PMID:15269276

[262] Lander E: Initial impact of the sequencing of the human genome. Nature. 2011;470:187–97. DOI: 10.1038/nature09792

[263] Ball MP, Bobe JR, Chuo MF, et al: Harvard Personal Genome Project: Lessons from participatory public research. Genome Med. 2014;6:10. DOI: 10.1186/gm527

[264] The International HapMap Consortium: Integrating common and rare genetic variation in diverse human populations. Nature. 2010;467:52-58. DOI: 10.1038/nature09298

[265] HUGO Pan-Asian SNP Consortium, Abdulla MA, Ahmed I, et al: Mapping human genetic diversity in Asia. Science. 2009;326:1541-5. DOI: 10.1126/science.1177074

[266] Pagini L, Schiffels S, Gurdasani D, et al: Tracing the route of modern humans out of Africa by using 225 human genome sequences from Ethiopians and Egyptians. Am J Hum Genet. 2015;96:986–91. DOI: 10.1016/j.ajhg.2015.04.019

[267] Colonna V, Ayub Q, Chen Y, et al: Human genomic regions with exceptionally high levels of population differentiation identified from 911 whole-genome sequences. Genome Biol. 2014;14:R88. DOI: 10.1186/gb-2014-15-6-r88

[268] Johnson JJ, Lewis KL, Ng D, et al: Individualized iterative phenotyping for genome-wide analysis of loss-of-function mutations. Am J Hum Genet. 2015;96;913–25. DOI: 10.1016/j.ajhg.2015.04.013

[269] Chen R, Mias GI, Li-Pook-Than J, et al: Personal omics profiling reveals dynamic molecular and medical phenotypes. Cell. 2012;148:1293–307. DOI: 10.1016/j.cell.2012.02.009

[270] Frese KS, Katus HA, Meder B: Next generation sequencing. From understanding biology to personalized medicine. Biology. 2013;2:378–98. DOI: 10.3390/biology2010378

[271] Veeramah KR, Hammer MF: The impact of whole-genome sequencing on the reconstruction of human population history. Nat Rev Genet. 2014;15:162. DOI: 10.1038/nrg3625

[272] Hofreiter M, Paijmans LA, Goodchild H, et al: The future of ancient DNA: Technical advances and conceptual shifts. Bioessays. 2014;37:284–93. DOI: 10.1002/bies.201400160

[273] Tryka KA, Hao L, Sturcke A, et al: The Database of Genotypes and Phenotypes (dbGaP) and PheGenI. The NCBI Handbook [Internet]. 2nd ed., 2013. Available from: http://www.ncbi.nlm.nih.gov/books/NBK154410/ [Accessed: 2015-07-25].

[274] Koboldt DC, Steinberg KM, Larson DE, Wilson RK, Mardis ER: The next-generation sequencing revolution and its impact on genomics. Cell. 2013;155:27–38. DOI: 10.1016/j.cell.2013.09.006

[275] Forbes SA, Bindal N, Bamford S, et al: COSMIC: Mining complete cancer genomes in the Catalogue of Somatic Mutations in Cancer. Nucleic Acids Res. 2011;39:D945–50. DOI: 10.1093/nar/gkq929

[276] Boyle AP, Araya CL, Brdlik C, et al: Comparative analysis of regulatory information and circuits across distant species. Nature. 2014;512:453–6. DOI: 10.1038/nature13668

[277] Inaki K, Hillmer AM, Ukil L, et al: Transcriptional consequences of genomic structural aberrations in breast cancer. Genome Res. 2011;21:676–87. DOI: 10.1101/gr.113225.110

[278] Zhang C-Z, Spektor A, Comils, et al: Chromothripsis from DNA damage in micronuclei. Nature. 2015;522:179–84. DOI: 10.1038/nature14493

[279] Mardis ER: Genome sequencing and cancer. Curr Opin Genet Dev. 2012;22:1–6. http://dx.doi.org/10.1016/j.gde.2012.03.005

[280] Jones S, Anagnostou V, Lytle K, et al: Personalized genomic analyses for cancer mutation discovery and interpretation. Sci Transl Med. 2015;7:283ra53. DOI: 10.1126/scitranslmed.aaa7161

[281] Manyika J, Chui M, Bughin J, Dobbs R, Bisson P, Marrs A: Disruptive technologies: Advances that will transform life, business, and the global economy. McKinsey Global Institute, May 2013. Available from: http://www.mckinsey.com/insights/business_technology/disruptive_technologies [Accessed: 2015-08-10].

[282] Tang H, Zhao Z: Bioinformatics drives the applications of next-generation sequencing in translational biomedical research. Methods. 2015;79–80:1–2. DOI: 10.1016/j.ymeth.2015.04.035

[283] Stephens ZD, Lee SY, Faghri F, et al: Big Data: Astronomical or genomical? PLoS Biol. 2015;13:e1002195. DOI: 10.1371/journal.pbio.1002195

Chapter 2

Next Generation Sequencing in Aquatic Models

Yuan Lu, Yingjia Shen, Wesley Warren and Ronald Walter

Additional information is available at the end of the chapter

http://dx.doi.org/10.5772/61657

Abstract

The most valuable application of next generation sequencing (NGS) technology is genome sequencing. Genomes of several aquatic models had been sequenced in the past few years due to their importance in genomics, development biology, toxicology, pathology, and cancer research. NGS technology is greatly advanced in sequencing length and accuracy, which facilitate the sequencing process, but sequence assembly, especially for the species with complicated genomes, is still the biggest challenge for bench-top scientists.

This chapter will focus on the application of NGS in aquatic genome and transcriptome assemblies. However, the associated techniques, problems, concerns, and solutions can also be applied to genome sequencing of other eukaryotic systems. Using our *Xiphophorus* genome and transcriptome sequencing as examples, this chapter will cover the technical details of NGS, data processing, genome assembly, and different methods of transcriptome assembly, as well as genome/transcriptome annotation. Additionally, the problems that were confronted in genome sequencing of several fish models and alternative approaches to assemble these genomes will be discussed. Lastly, the problems that remain to be the bottleneck of genome sequencing will be discussed, and a plan of what needs to be fulfilled is proposed.

Keywords: NGS, genome, aquatic models

1. Introduction

Next generation sequencing (NGS) technology has been broadly used in biomedical research. The most valuable application of this technology is genome and transcriptome sequencing, which form a bridge to link fundamental discoveries in research using disease model systems

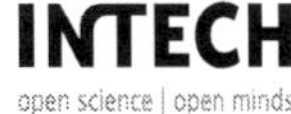

to clinical application. Aquatic animal models are widely used in genomics, development biology, toxicology, pathology, and cancer research (for a recent review, see [1]). The genomes of several aquatic models had been sequenced using NGS technology over the past few years [2, 3]. NGS technology has been trending toward reduced cost with greater sequencing length and accuracy. While this has facilitated the sequencing process, sequence assembly remains a significant challenge for bench-top scientists, and especially for species with complicated genomes.

In this chapter, we will focus on the application of NGS in aquatic genome and transcriptome assemblies. Although our focus will be on the genome sequencing of aquatic models, the associated techniques, problems, concerns, and solutions can also be applied to genome sequencing of other model systems. Using *Xiphophorus maculatus* (*X. maculatus*), *X. couchianus*, and *X. hellerii* genome sequencing as examples, we will discuss the technical details of NGS, data processing, and genome assembly using guided approaches. We will also discuss the problems encountered in genome sequencing of several feral fish models (ice fish, blind cave fish, etc.) and alternative approaches to sequence and assemble these genomes. Some problems remain and these are causing a bottleneck to broadening the representation of aquatic models with genome assemblies. These problems are summarized and methods to address them in the next five years are proposed.

2. Aquatic animal models in biomedical research

In recent years, aquatic animal models have been widely used in human disease research. These model systems have demonstrated the usefulness for improving our understanding of disease pathology at the molecular and cellular biology levels and have facilitated the development of new diagnostic and therapeutic methods. A few examples of diseases modeled by aquatic models are summarized in Table 1.

An example of the use of an aquatic model for human disease research is the *Xiphophorus* model. In the 1920s, it was found that F_1 interspecies hybrids between *X. maculatus* (*X. maculatus*) and *X. hellerii*, when backcrossed to *X. hellerii*, result in melanoma development among 25% of the backcross progeny (Gordon-Kosswig cross [4–6]). The melanoma develops from naturally occurring macromelanophores that are found in *Xiphophorus*. In this cross, melanoma development is the result of interaction of a melanoma locus *Tu* and a tumor suppressor locus (*R/Diff*) that is capable of inhibiting *Tu*'s oncogenic effect in the parental *X. maculatus* fish. Since *Tu* and *Diff* are on different chromosomes, the segregation of *Tu* and *Diff* into backcross hybrids results in 25% of the animals with inherited *Tu* but do not inherit melanoma suppression by the *R/Diff* and thus exhibit melanomagenesis. The gene corresponding to *Tu* was discovered to be a mutant copy of the human epidermal growth factor receptor (EGFR) termed *Xmrk*, while a candidate gene for *R/Diff* is a *Xiphophorus* homologue of human *cdkn2a/b* (i.e., p15/16) [7–9]. It has been found that the mutational inactivation of human *cdkn2a* (p16) is associated with human melanoma (for a review, see [10]), and EGFR-driven downstream signaling by Ras-Raf-MAPK activation is a marker of human melanoma

Model Organism	Scientific names	Modeled Disease	Genomic Sequence Availability
Amazon molly	*Poecilia formosa*	Melanoma, thyroid cancer, infectious deseases	Genome is available (http://www.ncbi.nlm.nih.gov/genome/?term=Poecilia+formosa)
Antarctic icefish	*Notothenioidei* Species	Anemia; Osteopenis	Not yet
Blind cavefish	*Astyanax mexicanus*	Retinal Degeneration; pigmentation disorders; sleep disorders	Genome is available (http://www.ncbi.nlm.nih.gov/genome/?term=Astyanax+mexicanus)
California sea hare	*Aplysia californica*	Neurobiology	Genome is available (http://www.ncbi.nlm.nih.gov/genome/?term=Aplysia+californica)
Cichlid fish	*Cichlidae* species	craniofacial malformations	Genome is available (Not public available)
Damselfish	*Stegastes partitus*	Viral cancerl neruofibromatosis	Genome is available (http://www.ncbi.nlm.nih.gov/genome/?term=Stegastes+partitus)
Eel	*Anguilla anguilla, Anguilla japonica*	Bone demineralization	Not yet
Medaka	*Oryzias latipes*	Toxicology	Genome is available (http://www.ncbi.nlm.nih.gov/genome/?term=Oryzias+latipes)
Mummichog	*Fundulus heteroclitus*	Environmental toxicology and intoxication; cystic fibrosis	Genome is available (http://www.ncbi.nlm.nih.gov/genome/?term=Fundulus+heteroclitus)
Platy fish and sword tails	*Xiphophorus maculatus* *Xiphophorus hellerii* *Xiphophorus couchianus*	Melanoma; sexual maturation disorders	*X. maculatus, X. couchianus* and *X. hellerii* genomes are available (http://www.ncbi.nlm.nih.gov/genome/?term=xiphophorus)
Rainbow trout	*Oncorhynchus mykiss*	Carcinogen-induced cancer	Not yet
Sheepshead minnow	*Crprinodon variegatus*	Environmental toxicology	Genome is available (Not public available)
Toadfish	*Porichhthys notatus* *Opsanus beta*	Hepatic encephalipathy; Skickle cell anemia	Not yet
Turquoise killifish	*Nothobranchius furzeri*	Aging and aging related disease	Genome is available (http://www.ncbi.nlm.nih.gov/genome/?term=Nothobranchius+furzeri)
Western clawed frog	*Xenopus tropicalis*	Congenital malformations	Genome is available available(http://www.ncbi.nlm.nih.gov/genome/?term=Xenopus+tropicalis)

Table 1. Aquatic models for human diseases

(for a review, see [11, 12]). This makes *Xiphophorus* a good model for geﾠnetic study of melanoma, a cancer that shows increasing worldwide incidence but has forwarded very few experimentally tractable animal models [13–15]. In addition to this spontaneous melanoma model, different *Xiphophorus* interspecies hybrids have been shown to be melanoma inducible after exposure to DNA damaging agents such as UVB light. Some of these inducible melanoma models involve hybridization of *X. maculatus* and *X. couchianus* with a following backcross of the F_1 hybrid to the *X. couchianus* parent. Both the heavy pigmented backcross progeny and F_1 hybrids can develop melanoma after UVB or MNU exposure in their early life stage [16–20].

Genomes of aquatic disease models serve as bridges to link phenotypic changes to genetic responses and allow physiological and pathophysiological discoveries from animal models to be applied to human disease research. The sequencing of model system genomes offers researchers great resources for biomedical research. Genome sequences allow researchers to (a) find sequence variation among genomes and transcriptomes between different species and populations; (b) compare genetic response between different phenotypes, development stages, disease conditions, drug treatment, etc.; and (c) discover gene/gene and gene/environment interactions and use these findings to direct medical applications.

For *Xiphophorus*, genome sequencing, assembly, and annotation for 3 *Xiphophorus* species (*X. maculatus*, *X. couchianus*, and *X. hellerii*) were accomplished in 2014 ([3, 21] and unpublished data). In the post-*Xiphophorus* genome era, these genomes resources have strengthened the *Xiphophorus* melanoma models by establishing high similarity in gene expression patterns for *Xiphophorus* and human melanoma tumors. The genome assemblies for both parents of an interspecific disease model are now allowing regulatory dissection of melanoma relevant gene expression in hybrids and after tumor-inducing treatments [22]. The gene expression features that characterize metastatic melanoma progression in humans closely mimic those found in *Xiphophorus* melanoma tumors (unpublished data). For the purpose of screening potential anti-melanoma compounds, a mutant *Xmrk* gene has been used to make a transgenic medaka (*Oryzias latipes*) fish model that develops melanoma very early after hatching [23, 24]. Whole transgenic melanoma medaka at 3–4 weeks post hatch are being utilized to characterize melanoma disease markers and for use in screening of small compounds for inhibitors of melanoma progression. In this way, several aquatic models systems represent a direct connection from "fish tank" discovery to "bedside" therapeutic application (for additional information on this topic, see https://dpcpsi.nih.gov/sites/default/files/orip/document/zebrafish_workshop_final_report_orip_website.pdf).

3. *Xiphophorus* genome assembly

3.1. Next generation sequencing

The NGS technique produces millions of short sequences (typical read length of 125 bp), which represent many unconnected small pieces of a genome or transcriptome, in each flow cell of the sequencing platform per sequence run. With these short sequences, one may *de novo* construct transcripts or genomes, characterize sequence variation (i.e., single nucleotide variation (SNV), insertion, and deletion), quantify sequence architecture (i.e., sequence repeats, copy numbers, and gene expression), and most importantly provide a sequence reference to expand discoveries from one species to another. Over the past decade, the sequence length of NGS (specifically Illumina technology) has significantly increased from 35 bp to current commonly produced 125 bp (Illumina HiSeq), and new long single sequence technology platforms are delivering sequence lengths of up to 40 kb in size (e.g., Pacific Bioscience RSII at 20 kb) that are changing the paradigm for whole genome *de novo* assembly.

It is beyond the scope of this chapter to examine all of the current and upcoming sequencing technologies, and thus we focus on the most common NGS platform that is currently being employed to establish genomic and transcriptomic resources in aquatic models systems.

The Illumina genome analyzer platform is currently the most widely used NGS system accounting for over 70% of the NGS market [25]. In Figure 1, we illustrate the basic steps of Illumina sequencing technology. The sequencing process starts with preparation of a library. The DNA (for genomic sequencing) or cDNA (for RNA sequencing) sample is sheared, usually by physical, enzymatic, or chemical method, into short fragments predetermined to be a specific size, and then sequencing adaptors are ligated to both ends of each short fragment by annealing. The fragments are then loaded onto a flow cell. The flow cell has oligonucleotides bound to the surface of the flow cell, and their sequences are complementary to the adaptors such that the free end of the fragment is attached to the flow cell via base pairing. A PCR step converts the initial fragment to its complementary sequence, and now both the forward strand and the reverse strand of fragments are bound to the surface of the flow cell (Figure 1). To amplify the signal, PCR is repeated for several rounds resulting in a cluster of copies around the initial copy of a fragment. Cyclic sequencing of these fragment clusters is very similar to Sanger sequencing and utilizes a sequence-by-synthesis process. One of two unique primers is attached to the free end of the bound fragments, and then nucleotides that each carries a different fluorescent reporter tag and a reversible terminator are flowed onto the flow cell. Since each nucleotide contains an elongation terminator, only a single nucleotide can be incorporated into newly synthesized sequences per sequencing cycle. After the nucleotide incorporation, laser sources excite the fluorescent reporter, and an optical sensor scans the entire flow cell to capture colors that represent newly added bases in every cluster. This optical information is converted to a base call for each growing sequence. At the end of each cycle, the terminator is removed and the next cycle continues until the desired sequence length is attained. In paired-end sequencing, after the forward strand sequence is attained, another sequence primer initiates the sequencing of the reverse strand of each fragment.

This massively parallel sequencing platform allows high throughput sequencing. Each flow cell contains 8 lanes with each lane producing 250 million reads (i.e., up to 500 GB/flow cell) with length of each sequence read ranging from 35 bp to 250 (Illumina HiSeq-2500) or 300 bp (Illumina MiSeq). Each sequencing adaptor has incorporated into it a unique barcode in the format of oligonucleotides. Thus, multiple samples from different sources can be pooled together in one lane, and this greatly facilitates the sequencing throughput.

Before subsequent sequence assembly or reference sequence alignment, a quality control step is usually necessary to attain sequences that best represent the biology being studied. A short sequencing result file contains two types of "contaminants" that can hinder the sequence assembly and result in misrepresentation of actual nucleotide sequence: adaptor sequence and low quality base calls. For paired-end sequencing, the length of DNA fragment between the

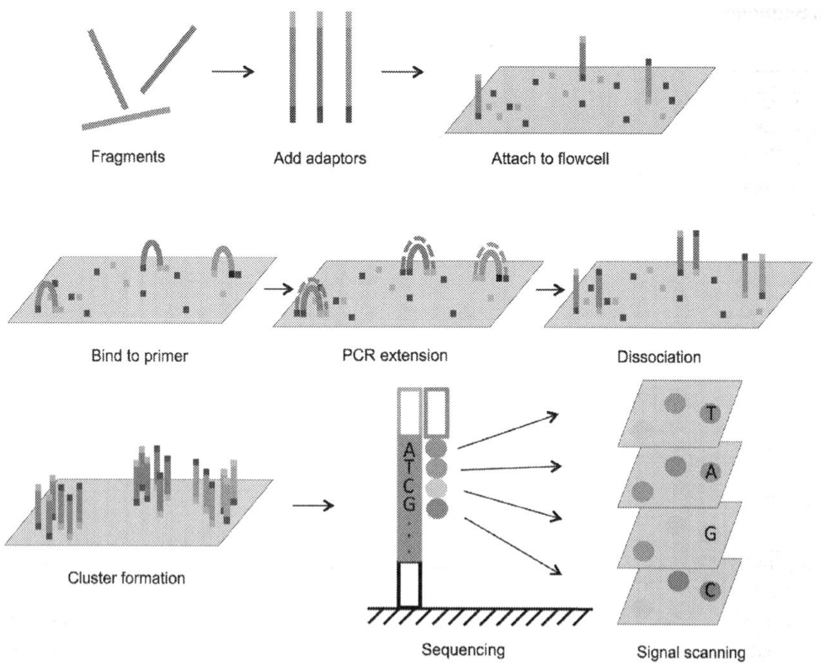

Figure 1. Outline of Illumina genome analyzer sequencing process. (1) Adaptors are annealed to the ends of sequence fragments. (2) Fragments bind to primer-loaded flow cell and bridge PCR reactions amplify each bound fragment to produce clusters of fragments. (3) During each sequencing cycle, one fluorophore attached nucleotide is added to the growing strands. Laser excites the fluorophores in all the fragments that are being sequenced and an optic scanner collects the signals from each fragment cluster. Then the sequencing terminator is removed and the next sequencing cycle starts.

two adaptor sequences is defined as "insertion size." When the desired sequencing length is longer than insertion size, the short sequencing can contain adaptor sequence in it. This artificial sequence must be trimmed off, so as not to produce significant sequence error in sequence assemblies. Another contaminant, the low quality base call, has many sources, from equipment to sequencing glitches. The quality of a base call is defined as Phred quality score (Q_{Phred} score). If we assign P as base calling error probabilities [26], then

$$Q_{Phred} = -10 \; log_{10} P$$

To retain the most usable as high-quality sequencing reads, the adaptor sequences are first clipped off, subsequently trim off low-quality base calls at the end of sequencing reads, and finally filter out sequence reads that contain a certain percentage of base calls that are below a defined Q_{Phred} score. Several tool software packages are available that can be utilized to perform the read filtering steps (e.g., fastx_toolkit: http://hannonlab.cshl.edu/fastx_toolkit/).

3.2. Sequence assembler algorithms

There are two major types of sequence assembly methods, Overlap-Layout-Consensus assembly and De Bruijn graph assembly. Current efficient and successful sequence assembly programs, including the ones employed for *Xiphophorus* genome assemblies (i.e., ALLPATHS), utilize the De Bruijn graph as a central data processing structure (De Bruijn-based assemblers are summarized in Table 2).

Software Name	Location
EULER-SR	euler-assembler.ucsd.edu/protal/
Velvet	www.ebi.ac.ik/~zerbino/velvet
ALLPATHS-LG	ftp.broadinstitute.org/pub/crd/ALLPATHS/Release-LG/
Abyss	www.bcgsc.ca/platform/bioinfo/software/abyss
SOAPdenovo	soap.genomics.org.cn/soapdenovo.html

Table 2. De Bruijn-based sequence assembler

De Bruijn graph-based assembler begins the assembling process by breaking the sequencing reads into k-mers, which in a genome is defined as a sequence of k consecutive bases. To build a De Bruijn graph, each k-mer is split into two parts, the left $(k-1)$ base x and right $(k-1)$ base y. Then all the x and the possible y are joined together by directed edges $(x \rightarrow y)$. A De Bruijn graph is obtained by taking the x and the y as nodes and the adjacencies as edges. The edges represent $(k-1)$ overlap between the connected nodes. In DNA sequencing, each node can have 8 possible connections, 4 are from the upstream sequence and 4 are to the downstream sequence, respectively. Actual connections are recorded in the memory as they are observed in the sequencing data. As sequencing data runs through the graph-building algorithm, discrete seed graphs are joined as the reads connecting to them are identified. In Figure 2, we present a simplified assembly and a sequence feature that can lead to problems in the sequence assembling process.

In Figure 2, 4 short DNA fragments that were attained from a randomly sheared 21 nt genome are sequenced. The k-mer length of 5 was chosen for this assembly. In the De Bruijn graph, there are 11 balanced nodes, where the number of indegree equals that of outdegree, and two semibalanced nodes, where indegree differs from outdegree. This graph is directed, connected, and considered as Eulerian since it has and only has at most 2 semibalanced nodes. The node in this directed graph that has more outdegree than indegree is considered to be the staring site of the assembly, while the other semibalanced node is the end of the assembly. At the end of the graph, where a cyclic edge forms, a problem for short sequence assemblers when repetitive sequence regions are encountered is presented. De Bruijn algorithms cannot resolve this problem and will simply ignore it, resulting in gaps in the contigs assembled. Long repeats present in the genome constantly cause assembly issues in practice. A detailed solution to this will be discussed in the following part of this chapter.

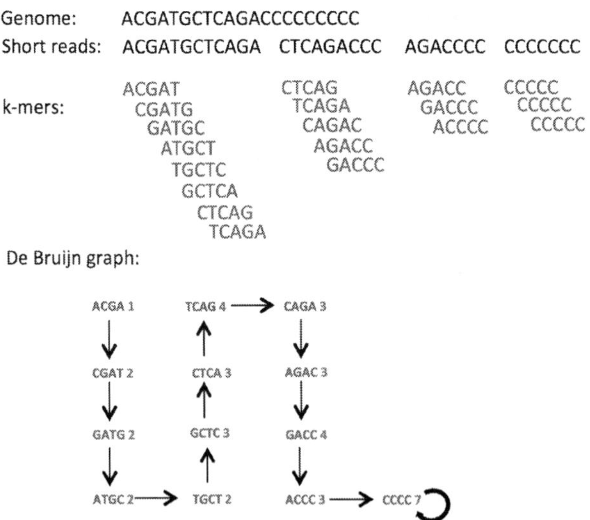

Figure 2. Outline of De Bruijn graph build during the sequence assembling process. A short model genome is sequenced. Four short reads were generated from template. The *k*-mer length of 5 was chose to be used in sequence assembly. For each *k*-mer, the left *k*– 1 and right *k*– 1 were represented as nodes in the De Bruijn graph, and all left parts are connected to possible right parts by directed edges. The red digit shows the number of occurrence of each node. The cyclic edge at the rightmost end of the graph causes the gap of contig assembly. Thus, the final assembly does not fully represent the "repeat" in the genome sequence.

Taking ALLPATHS for instance, the memory use is estimated to be roughly 1.7 bytes per read base, which equals to a 102-GB RAM of a 60× coverage 1-GB genome. This level of RAM requirement can be fully fulfilled nowadays. Alternatively, this RAM requirement can be solved by sharing memory from different computer nodes, or by distributing the workload to different nodes within a computer cluster, which is normally accessible in most universities and research institutions. In addition, the development of cloud computing allows one to gain access to high-speed computer clusters in a pay-as-you-go manner, and there are several recently developed cloud-based sequence assemblers (summarized in Table 3).

Software Name	Location
MERmaid	http://aws.amazon.con/ec2/
Contrail	http://contrail-bio.svn.sourceforge.net/
Crossbow	http://bowtie-bio.sourceforge.net/crossbow/

Table 3. Cloud computing-based sequence assemblers

3.3. *Xiphophorus* genome sequencing and assembly

Sequencing of *X. maculatus* genome is of great value to the aquatic model community [3, 21]. A problem encountered by those using the *Xiphophorus* model was that a genome sequence of one single *Xiphophorus* parent used in an interspecies cross did not allow the regulation of allele-specific gene expression to be determined in interspecies hybrid. The interspecies crosses are important in disease model research for both spontaneous and induced melanoma and other life history traits that involve complex genetic interactions. Therefore, 2 additional *Xiphophorus* species genomes (*X. couchianus* and *X. hellerii)* have been sequenced and assembled. In this section, sequencing and assembling multiple *Xiphophorus* species genomes is used as real-world example of the process of genome sequencing.

3.3.1. Biological sample

X. couchianus were maintained by sibling inbreeding, and the fish that were sequenced were in their 77th generation of inbreeding. *X. hellerii* was maintained by reciprocal cross breeding between 2 distinct *X. hellerii* strains, differing by sword color. All the fish that were used for genome sequencing were female since the high degree of repetitive DNA generally found to make up Y-chromosomes can confound the downstream assembly.

3.3.2. Genome sequencing and assembly

The Illumina HiSeq-2000 platform was chosen for *Xiphophorus* genome sequencing. Sequencing libraries with different insert sizes (300 bp, 500 bp, 3 kb, and 8 kb) were prepared. The purpose of using different insert size libraries is to using the paired-end reads that span different lengths of genome to estimate the gap size in a higher level of assembly. Over 700 (*X. couchianus*) and 360 (*X. hellerii*) million 100 bp paired-end short sequence reads were obtained from sequencer.

Genomes of *X. couchianus* and *X. hellerii* were constructed at three stages: contig, scaffold, and chromosome. The contigs were assembled in a *de novo* manner to maximally capture any sequences that are not present in *X. maculatus*, while scaffolds and chromosomes were assembled using the *X. maculatus* genome as a reference to guide assembly.

The first stage contig assembly was carried out by ALLPATHS using only the Illumina sequencing reads. This step generated contig-level assembly with N50 of 60 kb and 30 kb for *X. couchianus* and *X. hellerii*, respectively.

These contigs were further grouped into scaffolds using the *X. maculatus* scaffolds assembly as reference. *X. couchianus* and *X. hellerii de novo* assembled contigs, as well as the sequencing reads, were aligned to *X. maculatus* genome scaffold assembly using a multi-phase aligner SRprism (ftp://ftp.ncbi.nlm.nih.gov/pub/agarwala/srprism/). The sequence gaps between consecutive contigs were filled with long-insertion paired-end Illumina reads that bridge the upstream ends and downstream ends of contigs that are right next to the gaps. Scaffolding of contigs and gap fillings increased the length of both assemblies to N50s of 1.8 Mb and 1.6 Mb, respectively.

The construction of chromosomal level genome was accomplished by aligning *de novo* assembled contigs to the *X. maculatus* chromosome assembly using Mummer 3 package Nucmer3.0 (http://mummer.sourceforge.net). For each species, sequences of contigs and the location of *X. maculatus* chromosome alignments were recorded. By using a customized Perl script, these sequences and alignment information were organized into chromosomes.

3.3.3. Genome annotation

To annotate the newly assembled *X. couchianus* and *X. hellerii* genome, two methods, rapid annotation of transfer tool (RATT) and *de novo* assembled transcriptome, were used and the result from each were compared to each other.

Transcript sequences and associated functional annotations can be transferred between closely related species. A modified gene annotation method, RATT, was applied using the *X. maculatus* genome and gene model as a reference to quickly transfer genome annotation [27]. Since the *X. maculatus* genome was already available, using RATT to transfer annotation can minimize computational and human resources that are required for genome annotation. Both *X. couchianus* and *X. hellerii* genomic scaffold sequences were used as query species to be aligned to the well annotated *X. maculatus* genome using Nucmer3.0 with parameters implemented by RATT for annotation transfer. To avoid frame shift between two species, the synteny between both species and reference was established and insertions/deletions were also identified, respectively. *X. maculatus* gene models were then transferred and corrected to both query species. Of the 20,482 gene models annotated in *Xiphophorus* genome, 20,300 and 20,325 of them were transferred to *X. couchianus* and *X. hellerii*, respectively (Table 4).

To compare to this RATT annotation transfer method, *X. couchianus* and *X. hellerii* genome annotations were also annotated with a different method using *de novo* assembled transcriptomes. This method is reference genome independent. Briefly, RNA samples from one month old whole fish of *X. hellerii* and *X. couchianus* and a collection of tissues of mature individuals of each species were sequenced using Illumina GAIIx platform as 60 bp paired-end reads as well as HiSeq-2000 platform as 100 bp paired-end reads. *De novo* transcript assemblies and reports of putative transcripts were performed using velvet v1.1.05 and Oases v0.1.22 [28, 29]. The transcriptome assembly resulted in 110,604 and 242,675 transcripts for *X. couchianus* and *X. hellerii*, respectively.

	Species	# of transcripts	N50(nt)	Average size(nt)	Size(Mb)	RAM requirement	Cost(USD)
De novo	*X. couchianus*	110,604	3,922	2,197	243	> 100 Gb	10,000
	X. hellerii	242,675	3,280	1,991	483		10,000
RATT	*X. couchianus*	20,300	3,609	2,575	51	~ 10Gb	4,000
	X. hellerii	20,325	3,635	2,581	52		4,000

Table 4. Comparisons between reference-based annotation and *de novo*-based annotation

Comparing these two methods of annotation to each other in perspective of transcriptome quality, *de novo* method produced very larger transcriptomes in number of transcripts and final assembly size (Table 4). Many transcripts produced this way are unverified isoforms of same genes and redundant splicing isoforms of the same gene. In contrast, the RATT gene model transfer produced transcriptomes are similar to the reference [27]. In addition, both methods produced comparable N50s; however, reference-based method had longer average length, suggesting this method is superior.

In conclusion, the *de novo* assembly of a species transcriptome and its use in biological inference studies is appropriate, when a reference genome is not available and assuming tissue diversity is adequately captured. Nonetheless, reference-based gene model transfer is a reliable, economical, and efficient means to annotate closely related species.

3.3.4. Transposable elements analysis

As found previously, *X. maculatus* transposable elements (TEs) make up ~5% of the transcriptome [3]. Although the percentage of TEs is only slightly higher than the compact genomes of puffer fishes and is close to that of chicken genome, there is a high diversity of TE families in *X. maculatus* genome [3, 30, 31].

To annotate the TEs in *X. couchianus* and *X. hellerii* genomes, a previously established library was further completed employing RepeatScount (http://bix.ucsd.edu/repeatscout/) and RepeatModeler (http://www.repeatmasker.org/RepeatModeler.html) software. Redundant sequences were discarded, leaving 1019 sequences in the new library. RepeatMasker (http://www.repeatmasker.org/) was subsequently utilized to mask genome assemblies. Custom Perl script was then used to establish repeat coverage and copy numbers. After removing TE sequences that are smaller than 80 nt and share less than 80% identity with reference library, TEs were found to make up ~12% of each *Xiphophorus* genome (*X. maculatus*, 12.11%; *X. couchianus*, 12.61%; *X. hellerii*, 12.14%; unpublished data). A detailed classification of TEs in each *Xiphophorus* genome is shown in Table 5.

Species	Coverage(%)		
	X. couchianus	*X. maculatus*	*X. hellerii*
DNA transposons	6.212	6.023	6.022
LINE retrotransposons	1.678	1.672	1.536
LTR retrotransposons	0.316	0.253	0.333
SINE retrotransposons	0.395	0.315	0.347
Unknown	4.012	3.947	3.903
Total	12.613	12.11	12.141

Table 5. Transposable elements in *Xiphophorus* genomes

4. Problems and potential resolutions in genome assembly

4.1. Repetitive sequences in genome result in gaps of assembly

Several aquatic model genomes have been sequenced, assembled, and annotated for public use due to the activities of the aquatic model community. During the genome sequencing and assembling process for many of these model systems, several problems have been encountered. Specific sequence architecture (e.g., repetitive sequences) may confuse assembly algorithms and results in gaps in sequence contiguity that ultimately lead to a poorly-assembled genome or no assembly at all. For example, *k*-mer frequency estimation showed the toadfish genome consisted of ~48% repetitive sequences, which account for the rather high assembly fragmentation. Regions that have assembling difficulties typically include repeats (repetitive sequences of varied lengths, usually found in intergenic regions), telomere sequences (short sequence repeated thousands of times), centromere sequences (large array of repetitive DNA), segmental duplication of loci (segments of DNA with near-identical sequence), and closely organized gene families (portion of genome with genes of very similar sequences). The problems in assembling these regions are also present in genome sequencing projects of other model organisms. During the sequence assembly of aquatic models listed in Table 6, a conservative estimation of missing bases in each draft genome shows a range of 66 to 239 Mb within scaffolds, and 14 Mb to 26 Mb between scaffolds, respectively.

Species	Assembled size	Scaffold gap size	Remaining base loss*	N50 contigs length
Xiphophorus maculatus	730Mb	66Mb	14Mb	22kb
Aystanax mexicanus	1225Mb	222Mb	24Mb	15kb
Fundulus heteroclitus	932Mb	239Mb	18Mb	18kb
Aplysia californica	927Mb	189Mb	18Mb	9.5kb
Oryzias latipes	700Mb	169Mb	14Mb	9.6kb
Xenopus tropicalis	1358Mb	153Mb	26Mb	17kb

*Estimates of bases missing between scaffolds at 2% of assembled genome size.

Table 6. Reference assembly gap sequence estimates from NCBI or Ensembl

Although the length of sequencing reads continues to expand, repetitive sequences are still the main barrier encountered, toward a goal of uninterrupted consensus base counts. It is well known no graphical-based assembly method completely resolve repeat structure. Both graphical approaches, De Bruijn and Overlap-Layout-Consensus, will exclude repetitive sequence by truncating the assembly when certain repeat types are encountered or alternatively collapse unique repeats into a single representation (Figure 2). This leaves gaps in sequence assembly and collapses long repeat sequences. Some of the gaps can be closed by using proper oriented paired-end reads with long insertion sizes, such as bacteria artificial chromosome or P1-derived artificial chromosome clones. However, in most cases, such long insert resources are not available. During scaffold assembly of X. *couchianus* and X. *hellerii* genomes, consensus contigs were built by locating consecutive contigs bridged by mate pairs having 30-mers on each side of the gap, followed by *de novo* assembly in gaps using the bridged contigs and 30-mers from reads that were used in the first-level contig assembly. However, repetitive regions that expand hundreds of Mb can still not be resolved by this method.

4.2. Long sequencing reads are possible solution to assembly issues

Since repetitive sequences are the major causes of gaps in sequence assemblies, one way to maximize assembly contiguity is to employ long reads that are capable of covering the entire repetitive regions. The Pacific Bioscience (PacBio, www.pacificbiosciences.com) P6-C4 sequencing platform now offers the longest sequencing reads in the field, with longest sequence read length of 40 kbp and an average length of ~10 kbp (Figure 3).

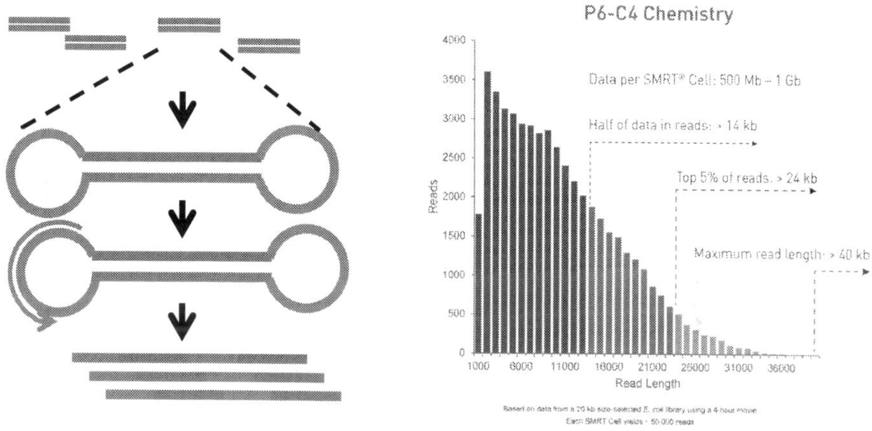

Figure 3. Outline of PacBio Single Molecule Real Time sequencing (SMRT) technology. Unlike Illumina sequencing platform, the sequencing adaptor form loops at the ends of double-stranded DNA fragments and ultimately form a circular sequencing template. After removing the adaptor sequences from raw reads, the genomic sequence information can be retained for *de novo* assembly. P6-C4 chemistry offers currently longest sequence reads. (The figure on the right is from Pacific Biosciences, http://www.pacificbiosciences.com/products/smrt-technology.)

Since PacBio long sequencing reads are capable of traveling through the repeat regions, therefore gaps are less likely to be present when assembling the genome. In several recent aquatic genome-sequencing projects, the incorporation of PacBio sequencing technology in concert with very deep Illumina 100 bp paired-end reads (60× coverage) significantly improved the quality of genome assembly. For example, using 8×–30× PacBio sequence coverage, 62% of gaps could be closed with a 2-fold increase in N50 contig length for the blind cavefish genome build (unpublished data). Similarly, gap filling using long sequencing reads almost tripled the N50 contig length (from 5 kb to 14 kb) for the ice fish genome, but this genome assembly remains plagued with difficult regions that have yet to be resolved (unpublished data).

The usage of long sequencing reads to improve the current genome builds is not limited to aquatic genome research as this application has also been utilized in the improvement of genome quality of other model organisms as well (e.g., avian models [32]). For example, the current chicken reference genome has 8106 gaps within scaffolds. After PacBio's long sequence reads (10× coverage) were incorporated, 6888 of these gaps were closed, along with 6.3 Mb of new sequence added (unpublished data).

For small genomes (<200 Mb haploid size), long sequencing read technology has advanced to a stage where near complete genomes can be represented. For example, the *Drosophila* genome has 139.5 million base pairs located on 4 pairs of chromosomes that can be covered once by 10,000 averaged-length PacBio sequencing reads [33]. One concern of PacBio long sequencing technology is its high error rate (median error rare of ~11%) in base calls. However, this "error-prone" problem can be addressed. First, PacBio sequencing technology utilizes a circular template. It allows the polymerase to travel through the template multiple times, thus generating several copies of reads that represent the same genome fragment. Second, although the error rate of "single-pass" PacBio sequencing reads is high, the errors are distributed randomly and can be filtered out upon building consensus for all sequence copies of a given fragment. Quiver (www.pacbiodevnet.com/Quiver) was developed to deliver high-quality consensus sequences by averaging the sequence information for each base call vertically to each other. Based on the error rate, 9 out of 10 reads will contain a correctly sequenced base, making it straightforward to distinguish the correct base call. This error correction is capable of generating >99.9% accurate consensus sequence [34, 35].

In addition to improving current genome assembly quality, long sequencing reads are capable of sequencing full-length transcripts, thus facilitating gene expression analyses and transcriptome assembly. Current RNA-Seq tasks apply short reads (50 bp single-end to 125 bp paired-end depends on experiment design) to fragmented cDNA libraries. These short reads are then aligned to either reference genome or an array of reference transcripts for statistical analysis of gene expression. Uniquely aligned short reads provide solid evidence of the expression levels of the aligned genes. However, inappropriate treatment of ambiguously aligned reads can lead to biased or even mistaken expression profiles in complicated vertebrate genomes (e.g., zebrafish genome and human genome). This problem severely affects transcript variance discovery such as alternative splicing and relative expression of alternative splicing isoforms, which play significant roles in pathological processes (e.g., Bcl11b1). Alternative splicing isoform expression quantification heavily relies on distribution of short reads on each exon; thus, low-coverage splicing isoforms cannot be distinguished [36]. The utilization of PacBio long-read sequencing platform can eliminate this problem by providing long reads that are capable of covering all connected exons in one single read, thus avoiding mistakes in assigning reads to a certain exons [37].

5. Perspectives in aquatic genome research

The availability of aquatic genome models in the past few years significantly expends the resources for biological and biomedical discovery. However, as detailed, problems persist in the current aquatic model draft assemblies (i.e., gaps in and between scaffold and repetitive sequence). Over the next few years, there should be a concerted effort to (a) *de novo* assemble genomes by combining standard Illumina library builds with new PacBio long-read sequencing and (b) developing new assembly routines to resolve assembly errors and create chromosome builds for each species.

5.1. *De novo* genome assembly using long sequencing reads

In Table 6, we show estimated sequence gaps missing from within scaffolds. It is estimated that 2–5% of each genome is not sequenced or assembled outside of scaffold gaps (unpublished result). Previous tasks to close gaps in the assemblies of other species genomes have shown that structurally variant alleles, simple tandem repeats, and high GC content regions account for the majority of these gaps. The new PacBio sequencing technology, if used to produce high coverage (at least 60×) fragments, may be expected to overcome many of these assembly problems and should result in better-represented genome models. Assembling genomes using PacBio sequencing reads requires special treatment to the raw reads, as well as the sequence assembling processes. For example, the multiple-pass raw reads from circular sequencing template need to be clipped into subreads that represent the DNA fragment. The PacBio sequencing reads also need to be error-corrected using Quiver. The sequence assembling process with these very long reads requires different tools than what were discussed above. MinHash Alignment Process (MHAP) that is included in Celera Assembler PBcR pipeline is a reference implementation of a probabilistic sequence overlapping algorithm that is designed for detecting overlaps between long-read sequence data [33]. It is therefore a proper tool for sequence assembly that employs long sequencing reads.

During the process of *de novo* genome assembly using long sequencing read technology, higher-quality genome models are expected. This will provide animal disease model communities much better genome references (longer N50, less gaps and less missing bases) in newly developed draft *de novo* assemblies. In addition, re-sequencing to enhance the contiguity of current genome assemblies by incorporating PacBio reads promises to produce much improve reference genomes in the next few years.

5.2. Chromosome level aquatic genome assembly

Accurate chromosome assemblies require correctly ordered contigs in scaffolds for gene functional interpretation. During chromosome construction, the placement and order of scaffolds on chromosomes relies on a genetic map, which is based on meiotic recombination. Among the aquatic genome models created in the past few years, the *Xiphophorus* genome assembly has been aligned to chromosomes using a Rad-Tag approach to generate a meiotic gene map having over 16,000 markers ([21] and unpublished data). The RAD-tag markers and microsatellite makers from older studies were used to guide the placement of scaffolds into the *Xiphophorus* chromosomes (for RAD-tag method, see [38]). However, the RAD-tag map method is resource and labor intensive, for examples, 267 backcross *Xiphophorus* hybrids were used for genetic mapping and sequence alignment [21].

Recently, new optical mapping technology has been provided by BioNano (http://www.bionanogenomics.com). The optical mapping improves the process of constructing whole genome physical map. In this process, high molecular weight genomic DNA is immobilized onto the positively charged glass surface of a chip-like device having engraved nano-channels that are only wide enough to stretch a single DNA molecule. Buffer fluid that flows though the channel stretches a single DNA molecule to maintain its orientation and integrity. The DNA molecules are subsequently sheared by a restriction enzyme into fragments that are stained with florescent dye. An imaging system then measures the florescent light intensity that represents the length of each DNA fragment. Accompanied with the restriction enzyme site sequence, the length of each fragment is linked to form a single-molecule optical restriction map.

During chromosome assembly, the scaffold sequences can be converted to *in silico* restriction map. The location of the restriction enzyme digestion sequence and the distance between these sequences can then be used to assign scaffolds into chromosomes [39]. Using this approach, incorrect joining errors of contigs may be corrected to improve the current reference genome continuity concurrent with scaffolds alignment into chromosomes.

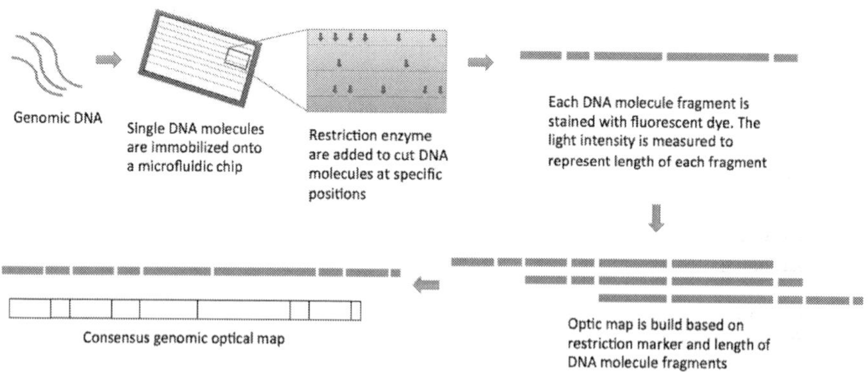

Figure 4. Illustration of optic mapping technology. Genomic DNA is obtained from lysed cells and is loaded onto a chip-like channel-forming device. DNA molecules are stretched onto a positively changed glass surface by buffer fluid that flows through the channels. This step maintains the integrity and orientation of the DNA molecule for subsequent steps. The stretched and immobilized DNA molecules are digested with a restriction enzyme and subsequently stained with florescent dye. The florescent light intensity of each DNA fragment was imaged, and the images are analyzed to measure the size of DNA fragments. Using the restriction enzyme digestion site sequence and the distance between digestion sites, a single-molecule restriction map can be generated to guide scaffold assignment.

6. Conclusion

Aquatic models are proven to be as important and useful as other animal models to study the etiology and progression of human disease. Aquatic models have gained the attention of funding agencies, and the overall research community using aquatic models has grown rapidly. This growth has resulted in the availability of genome and reference transcriptome resources. The aquatic genome models that were constructed in the past few years are available through NCBI or Ensembl with new updates constantly being made. Although problems persist in genome assembly of complicated structures, newer sequencing platforms, mapping technologies, and sequence assembly algorithms are expected to rapidly address these problems and soon offer the community much improved resources.

Author details

Yuan Lu[1*], Yingjia Shen[2], Wesley Warren[3] and Ronald Walter[1]

*Address all correspondence to: y_l54@txstate.edu

1*Xiphophorus* Genetic Stock Center, Texas State University, San Marcos, TX, USA

2 Xiamen University, Shenzhen, China

3 The Genome Institute at Washington University, St. Louis, MO, USA

References

[1] Schartl, M., *Beyond the zebrafish: diverse fish species for modeling human disease.* Dis Model Mech, 2014. 7(2): p. 181–92.

[2] McGaugh, S.E., et al., *The cavefish genome reveals candidate genes for eye loss.* Nat Commun, 2014. 5: p. 5307.

[3] Schartl, M., et al., *The genome of the platyfish, Xiphophorus maculatus, provides insights into evolutionary adaptation and several complex traits.* Nat Genet, 2013. 45(5): p. 567–72.

[4] Gordon, M., *The genetics of a viviparous top-minnow platypoecilus; the inheritance of two kinds of melanophores.* Genetics, 1927. 12(3): p. 253–83.

[5] Häussler, G., *Über Melanombildungen bei Bastarden von Xiphophorus Helleri und Platypoecilus Maculatus var. Rubra.* J Mol Med, 1928. 7: p. 1561–1562.

[6] K., K., *Über Bastarde der Teleostier Platypoecilus und Xiphophorus. Z Indukt.* Abstamm Vererbungsl, 1928. 44: p. 150–158.

[7] Adam, D., W. Maueler, and M. Schartl, *Transcriptional activation of the melanoma inducing Xmrk oncogene in Xiphophorus.* Oncogene, 1991. 6(1): p. 73–80.

[8] Kazianis, S., et al., *Localization of a CDKN2 gene in linkage group V of Xiphophorus fishes defines it as a candidate for the DIFF tumor suppressor.* Genes Chromosomes Cancer, 1998. 22(3): p. 210–20.

[9] Kazianis, S., et al., *Comparative structure and characterization of a CDKN2 gene in a Xiphophorus fish melanoma model.* Oncogene, 1999. 18(36): p. 5088–99.

[10] Mehnert, J.M. and H.M. Kluger, *Driver mutations in melanoma: lessons learned from bench-to-bedside studies.* Curr Oncol Rep, 2012. 14(5): p. 449–57.

[11] Daud, A. and B.C. Bastian, *Beyond BRAF in melanoma.* Curr Top Microbiol Immunol, 2012. 355: p. 99–117.

[12] Kraehn, G.M., M. Schartl, and R.U. Peter, *Human malignant melanoma. A genetic disease?* Cancer, 1995. 75(6): p. 1228–37.

[13] Reed, D., et al., *Controversies in the evaluation and management of atypical melanocytic proliferations in children, adolescents, and young adults.* J Natl Compr Canc Netw, 2013. 11(6): p. 679–86.

[14] Herlyn, M. and M. Fukunaga-Kalabis, *What is a good model for melanoma?* J Invest Dermatol, 2010. 130(4): p. 911–2.

[15] Ha, L., et al., *Animal models of melanoma.* J Investig Dermatol Symp Proc, 2005. 10(2): p. 86–8.

[16] Kazianis, S., et al., *Genetic analysis of neoplasia induced by N-nitroso-N-methylurea in Xiphophorus hybrid fish.* Mar Biotechnol (NY), 2001. 3(Supplement 1): p. S37–43.

[17] Nairn, R.S., et al., *A CDKN2-like polymorphism in Xiphophorus LG V is associated with UV-B-induced melanoma formation in platyfish-swordtail hybrids.* Proc Natl Acad Sci U S A, 1996. 93(23): p. 13042–7.

[18] Rahn, J.J., et al., *Etiology of MNU-induced melanomas in Xiphophorus hybrids.* Comp Biochem Physiol C Toxicol Pharmacol, 2009. 149(2): p. 129–33.

[19] Setlow, R.B., et al., *Wavelengths effective in induction of malignant melanoma.* Proc Natl Acad Sci U S A, 1993. 90(14): p. 6666–70.

[20] Setlow, R.B., A.D. Woodhead, and E. Grist, *Animal model for ultraviolet radiation-induced melanoma: platyfish-swordtail hybrid.* Proc Natl Acad Sci U S A, 1989. 86(22): p. 8922–6.

[21] Amores, A., et al., *A RAD-tag genetic map for the platyfish (Xiphophorus maculatus) reveals mechanisms of karyotype evolution among teleost fish.* Genetics, 2014. 197(2): p. 625–41.

[22] Lu, Y., et al., *Molecular genetic response of Xiphophorus maculatus–X. couchianus interspecies hybrid skin to UVB exposure.* Comp Biochem Physiol C Toxicol Pharmacol, 2015.

[23] Schartl, M., et al., *Conserved expression signatures between medaka and human pigment cell tumors.* PLoS One, 2012. 7(5): p. e37880.

[24] Schartl, M., et al., *A mutated EGFR is sufficient to induce malignant melanoma with genetic background-dependent histopathologies.* J Invest Dermatol, 2010. 130(1): p. 249–58.

[25] Thayer, A.M., *Next-Gen sequencing is a numbers game.* Chem Eng News, 2014. 92(33): p. 11–15.

[26] Ewing, B. and P. Green, *Base-calling of automated sequencer traces using phred. II. Error probabilities.* Genome Res, 1998. 8(3): p. 186–94.

[27] Otto, T.D., et al., *RATT: Rapid Annotation Transfer Tool.* Nucleic Acids Res, 2011. 39(9): p. e57.

[28] Schulz, M.H., et al., *Oases: robust de novo RNA-seq assembly across the dynamic range of expression levels*. Bioinformatics, 2012. 28(8): p. 1086–92.

[29] Zerbino, D.R. and E. Birney, *Velvet: algorithms for de novo short read assembly using de Bruijn graphs*. Genome Res, 2008. 18(5): p. 821–9.

[30] Wicker, T., et al., *The repetitive landscape of the chicken genome*. Genome Res, 2005. 15(1): p. 126–36.

[31] Aparicio, S., et al., *Whole-genome shotgun assembly and analysis of the genome of Fugu rubripes*. Science, 2002. 297(5585): p. 1301–10.

[32] Ganapathy, G., et al., *High-coverage sequencing and annotated assemblies of the budgerigar genome*. Gigascience, 2014. 3: p. 11.

[33] Berlin, K., et al., *Assembling large genomes with single-molecule sequencing and locality-sensitive hashing*. Nat Biotechnol, 2015. 33(6): p. 623–30.

[34] Carneiro, M.O., et al., *Pacific biosciences sequencing technology for genotyping and variation discovery in human data*. BMC Genomics, 2012. 13: p. 375.

[35] Koren, S., et al., *Hybrid error correction and de novo assembly of single-molecule sequencing reads*. Nat Biotechnol, 2012. 30(7): p. 693–700.

[36] Hiller, D. and W.H. Wong, *Simultaneous isoform discovery and quantification from RNA-seq*. Stat Biosci, 2013. 5(1): p. 100–18.

[37] Au, K.F., et al., *Characterization of the human ESC transcriptome by hybrid sequencing*. Proc Natl Acad Sci U S A, 2013. 110(50): p. E4821–30.

[38] Lewis, Z.A., et al., *High-density detection of restriction-site-associated DNA markers for rapid mapping of mutated loci in Neurospora*. Genetics, 2007. 177(2): p. 1163–71.

[39] Dong, Y., et al., *Sequencing and automated whole-genome optical mapping of the genome of a domestic goat (Capra hircus)*. Nat Biotechnol, 2013. 31(2): p. 135–41.

Chapter 3

MHC Genotyping in Human and Nonhuman Species by PCR-based Next-Generation Sequencing

Takashi Shiina, Shingo Suzuki and Jerzy K. Kulski

Additional information is available at the end of the chapter

http://dx.doi.org/10.5772/61842

Abstract

The major histocompatibility complex (MHC) is a highly polymorphic genomic region that encodes the transplantation and immune regulatory molecules. It receives special attention for genetic investigation because of its important role in the regulation of innate and adaptive immune responses and its strong association with numerous infectious and/or autoimmune diseases. Recently, genotyping of the polymorphisms of MHC genes using targeted next-generation sequencing (NGS) technologies was developed for humans and some nonhuman species. Most species have numerous highly homologous MHC loci so the NGS technologies are likely to replace traditional genotyping methods in the near future for the investigation of human and animal MHC genes in evolutionary biology, ecology, population genetics, and disease and transplantation studies. In this chapter, we provide a short review of the use of targeted NGS for MHC genotyping in humans and nonhuman species, particularly for the class I and class II regions of the Crab-eating Macaque MHC (Mafa).

Keywords: HLA, MHC, polymorphism, genotyping, NGS

1. Introduction

The major histocompatibility complex (MHC) genomic region consists of a large group of evolutionary-related genes involved functionally with the innate and adaptive immune systems in jawed vertebrates [1]. In humans, the MHC is located on the short arm of chromosome 6, band p21.3, and the MHC class I and class II genomic regions encode the highly polymorphic gene complex classified as the human leukocyte antigen (HLA) complex [2, 3]. The HLA class I and class II molecules expressed by the MHC play important roles in restricted

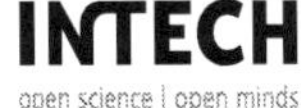

cellular interactions and tissue histocompatibility due to cellular discrimination of "self" and "nonself" that require an essential knowledge of the effects of HLA allele matched and mismatched donors in transplantation medicine [4] and transfusion therapy [5]. While the HLA class I molecules are expressed by all nucleated cells to present processed peptides of intracellular origin to CD8+ cytotoxic T cells and serve as ligands for natural killer cells, the class II molecules are expressed by antigen-presenting cells such as B cells, dendritic cells, or macrophages to present exogenous peptides to CD4+ helper T cells of the immune system [6]. In addition, the classical HLA class I genes, HLA-A, HLA-B, and HLA-C, and the classical HLA class II genes, HLA-DR, HLA-DQ, and HLA-DP are distinguished by their extraordinary polymorphisms, whereas the nonclassical HLA class I genes, HLA-E, HLA-F, and HLA-G, are distinguished by their tissue-specific expression and limited polymorphism [2, 3, 7].

The highly polymorphic HLA genomic region is critically involved in the rejection and graft-versus-host disease (GVHD) of hematopoietic stem cell transplants [8, 9], the pathogenesis of numerous autoimmune diseases [10–13], and infectious diseases [14]. Apart from regulating immunity, the MHC genes may have a role in reproduction and social behavior, such as pregnancy maintenance, mate selection, and kin recognition [15]. The MHC genomic region also appears to influence drug adverse reactions [16, 17], CNS development and plasticity [18–22], neurological cell interactions [23, 24], synaptic function and behavior [25, 26], cerebral hemispheric specialization [27], and neurological and psychiatric disorders [28–32]. Hence, the MHC is one of the most biomedically important genomic regions that warrant special attention for genetic investigation.

In general, the study of the diversity and polymorphic variation of the MHC genomic region has been focused more on humans than any other species and animal population [1] largely because of the high cost and limited throughput of the first generation Sanger sequencing method [33, 34]. However, this is now changing because the next-generation sequencing (NGS) technologies are becoming the method of choice for lower-cost, high-throughput genotyping of MHC genes that are composed of highly homologous multiple loci such as those found in the macaque primate species [35]. Thus, the NGS technologies are expected to perform precise MHC genotyping in human and model animals that already have a collection of MHC allele references, and to facilitate MHC genotyping of wild animals that as yet have no MHC allele references. In addition, the NGS technologies are likely to replace traditional genotyping methods such as subcloning, Sanger sequencing, and previously developed PCR-based MHC typing methods (PCR-RFLP, PCR-SSP, and so on) in the near future. Recently, many articles concerning the development of NGS technologies for precise MHC genotyping and genotyping data of MHC genes using the new NGS technologies have been published on the investigations of human and nonhuman MHC polymorphisms in various fields of study such as medical science, evolutionary biology, ecology, and population genetics.

In this chapter, we provide a short review of the current HLA polymorphism information and the use of PCR-based NGS for MHC genotyping in human and nonhuman species, particularly for the Filipino crab-eating macaque MHC (*Mafa*) class I (Mafa-A, -B, -E, -F, and -I) and class II loci (Mafa-DPA1, -DPB1, -DQA1, -DQB1, and -DRB1).

2. HLA allele number

A total of 13,840 HLA allele sequences, 10,297 in the class I and 3543 in the class II gene regions, were released by the IMGT/HLA database [7] release 3.22 in October 2015 (Table 1).

Category	Locus	Allele no.	Protein no.
Class I	HLA-A	3285	2313
	HLA-B	4077	3011
	HLA-C	2801	1985
	HLA-E	18	7
	HLA-F	22	4
	HLA-G	51	17
	Pseudogene	43	0
	Total	10,297	7337
Class II	HLA-DRA	7	2
	HLA-DRB1	1825	1335
	HLA-DRB3	60	48
	HLA-DRB4	17	10
	HLA-DRB5	22	19
	HLA-DQA1	54	32
	HLA-DQB1	876	595
	HLA-DPA1	42	21
	HLA-DPB1	587	480
	HLA-DMA	7	4
	HLA-DMB	13	7
	HLA-DOA	12	3
	HLA-DOB	13	5
	Pseudogene	8	0
	Total	3543	2561

Table 1. Number and genomic distribution (loci) of HLA alleles

The IMGT/HLA database is a specialist database for HLA sequences. Ten years ago, the allelenumbers were only 2182, but since then, the numbers have increased by 1000 allele sequenceseach year. Of 10,297 HLA class I alleles, 3285, 4077, 2801, 18, 22, and 51 alleles were countedin HLA-A, HLA-B, HLA-C, HLA-E, HLA-F, and HLA-G genes, respectively (Table 1);

10,163 and91 alleles were counted in the classical and nonclassical HLA class I genes, respectively.Of the 3543 HLA class II alleles, 7, 1825, 99, 54, 876, 42, 587, 7, 13, 12, and 13 alleles were countedin HLA-DRA, HLA-DRB1, HLA-DRB3/4/5, HLA-DQA1, HLA-DQB1, HLA-DPA1, HLA-DPB1, HLA-DMA, HLA-DMB, HLA-DOA, and HLA-DOB genes, respectively (Table 1), with3490 and 45 alleles in the classical and nonclassical HLA class II genes, respectively.

3. History of HLA genotyping methods

Many variations of the conventional HLA genotyping methods such as incorporating restriction fragment polymorphisms (RFLP) [36], single strand conformation polymorphism (SSCP) [37], sequence-specific oligonucleotides (SSOs) [38], sequence-specific primers (SSPs) [39], and sequence-based typing (SBT), like the Sanger method [33], have been used for the efficient and rapid HLA matching in transplantation therapy [40–43], research into HLA-related diseases [2, 3], population diversity studies [44–46], and in forensic and paternity testing [47]. The HLA genotyping methods mainly applied today are PCR-SSOP, such as the Luminex commercial methodology [48, 49], and SBT by the Sanger method employing capillary sequencing based on chain–termination reactions [33, 34]. However, both methods often detect more than one pair of unresolved HLA alleles because of chromosomal phase (*cis*/*trans*) ambiguity [50, 51]. To solve the phase ambiguity problem, new HLA genotyping technologies have been reported and commercialized that combine the PCR amplification of targeted HLA genomic regions with NGS platforms such as the ion PGM system (Life Technologies), GS Junior system (Roche), and the MiSeq system (Illumina) [52]. The PCR/NGS methods are expected to produce genotyping results that detect new and null alleles efficiently without phase ambiguity.

4. Summary of NGS-based human MHC genotyping methods

Table 2 shows list of publications on NGS-based human MHC genotyping that includes information for PCR range, targeted HLA locus, NGS platform, and allele assignment method. The MHC genotyping methods in human are basically composed of three steps, PCR, NGS, and allele assignment. We summarize the important points in each of the three steps below. The more detailed information is described in our previous publication [52].

4.1. PCR step

4.1.1. Long- and short-range PCR

PCR methods produce amplicons of different sequence lengths depending on the primer design and the type of DNA polymerase used for the PCR. The amplicon sizes are usually classified into two size ranges: the short-range system where the amplicon size is <1 kb and the long-range system where the amplicon size is >1 kb as shown in Figure 1.

No.	PCR range	Sorting from PCR range	Targeted HLA locus	NGS platform	Allele assignment method	Ref.
1	410–790 bp	Short-range system	A, B, C, DRB1/3/4/5, DQA1, DQB1, DPB1	454 GS FLX	Conexio Assign ATF	[66]
2	400–900 bp	Short-range system	A, B	454 GS FLX	GS-FLX amplicon variant analyzer	[67]
3	Unknown	Long-range system	A, B, C, DRB1, DQB1	454 GS FLX	Conexio Assign-NG	[51]
4	410–790 bp	Short-range system	A, B, C, DRB1/3/4/5, DQA1, DQB1, DPB1	454 GS FLX	Conexio Genomics ATF	[68]
5	381–537 bp	Short-range system	A, B, C	454 GS FLX	SSAHA2	[69]
6	**4.6–11.2 kb**	**Long-range system**	**A, B, C, DRB1, DQA1, DQB1, DPA1, DPB1**	**454 GS Junior, Ion PGM**	**SeaBass**	[70]
7	2.7–4.1 kb	Long-range system	A, B, C, DRB1	HiSeq2000, Miseq	Alignment with IMGT/HLA data	[71]
8	410–790 bp	Short-range system	A, B, C, DRB1/3/4/5, DQA1, DQB1, DPB1	454 GS FLX, (or GS Junior)	Conexio Assign ATF 454	[72]
9	3.4–13.6 kb	Long-range system	A, B, C, DRB1, DPB1, DQB1	MiSeq	BWA, Samtools, GATK, PerlScript	[73]
10	**5.1–5.6 kb**	**Long-range system**	**DRB3, DRB4, DRB5**	**454 GS Junior**	**SeaBass**	[74]
11	250–270 bp	Short-range system	A, B, C, DRB1, DPB1, DQB1	MiSeq	neXtype	[75]
12	250–270 bp	Short-range system	DRB1/3/4/5, DQA1, DQB1, DPA1, DPB1	MiSeq	Genetics Management System	[76]
13	Unknown	Long-range system	A, B, DRB1	PacBio	Bayes' theorem, NGSengine	[77]
14	**4.0–7.2 kb**	**Long-range system**	**A, B, C, DRB1/3/4/5, DQB1, DPB1**	**Ion PGM**	**SeaBass**	[54]

Table 2. Publication list of NGS-based MHC genotyping in human. Bold letter shows publications from the author's group

The short-range PCR system is a method based on PCR amplification of each exon that includes polymorphic exons 2 and 3 in HLA-A, HLA-B, and HLA-C and exon 2 in HLA-DR, HLA-DQ, and HLA-DP. One of the advantages of the short-range system is that it is the most suitable for application of physically fragmented DNA samples as templates such as those extracted from swabs because the PCR length is relatively short, ranging from 250 bp to 900 bp, per

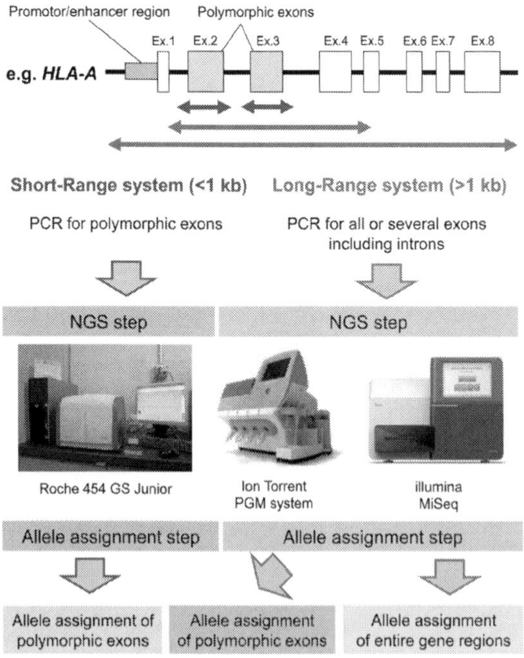

Figure 1. Outline of NGS-based human MHC typing.

amplicon. On the other hand, the short-range system is less effective for genotyping recombinant alleles that have been generated by recombination events of the HLA genes because it is difficult to avoid the phase ambiguities generated by recombinations. For example, in Figure 2, B*15:20 has an identical nucleotide sequence with B*15:01 in exon 2 and B*35:01 in exon 3, but B*35:43 has an identical nucleotide sequence with B*35:01 in exon 2 and B*15:01 in exon 3. When we genotype a DNA sample that has B*15:01 or B*15:20 and B*35:01 or B*35:43, ambiguous genotyping can result in assignments such as B*15:01/20 and B*35:01/43 that are difficult to assign correctly and definitively.

The long-range PCR system is a method based on PCR amplification of the entire HLA gene region including the promotor-enhancer region, 5′ untranslated region (UTR), all exons, all introns, and the 3′ UTR or partial gene regions that include polymorphic exons and adjacent introns (Figure 1). Primer sets for long-range systems have already been developed and published for HLA-A, HLA-B, HLA-C, HLA-DRB1/3/4/5, HLA-DQA1, HLA-DQB1, HLA-DPA1, and HLA-DPB1 (Table 2). The advantage of long-range PCR is that this system can easily solve phase ambiguity even if recombinant alleles such as those shown in Figure 2 are present in DNA samples. Also, the long-range PCR method is expected to detect new polymorphisms and variations throughout the entire HLA gene region. Therefore, the long-range

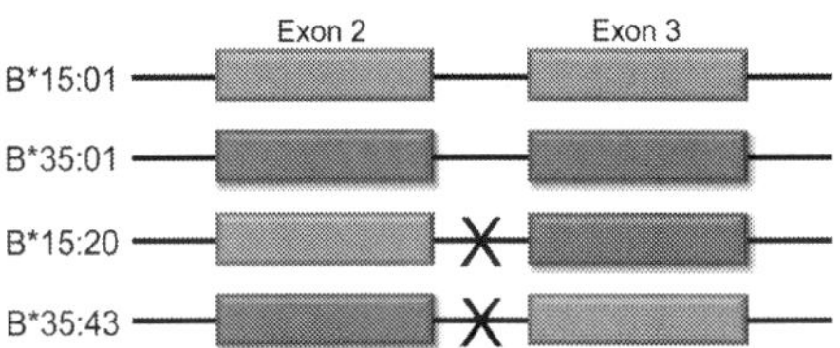

Figure 2. Example of recombinant HLA alleles. B*15:01 and B*15:20 and B*15:01 and B*35:43 have identical nucleotide sequences in exon 2 and in exon 3, respectively (red boxes), and B*35:01 and B*35:43 and B*35:01 and B*15:20 have identical nucleotide sequences in exon 2 and in exon 3, respectively (blue boxes). "X" indicates the recombination site.

system is an important and useful alternative to the short-range system for donor-recipient matching in bone marrow transplantation and HLA-related disease studies. In fact, one of the main themes of the upcoming 17th International HLA and Immunogenetics Workshop (IHIWS) in 2017 [53] is "NGS of full length HLA genes," with the following objectives: (1) to complete the sequence of all HLA alleles of the reference cell lines from the 13th IHIWS and (2) to perform HLA genotyping of 10,000 quartet families of varied ancestry, utilizing at least one NGS method.

4.1.2. Development of multiplex PCR methods

Recently, we developed four kinds of multiplex PCR methods based on the long-range system for genotyping nine HLA loci (HLA-A, -B, -C, -DRB1/3/4/5, -DQB1, and -DPB1) [54] (Figure 3).

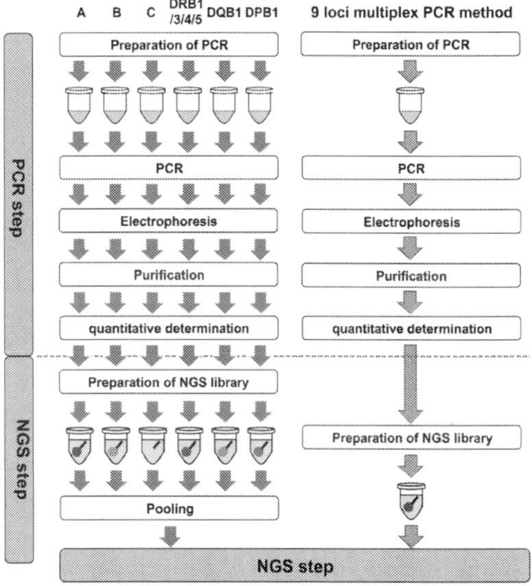

Figure 3. Two different nine loci HLA genotyping procedures at the PCR step.

The multiplex PCR methods contributed greatly to simplifying, accelerating, and reducing costs and the number of reagents for the PCR step that is used to prepare samples and libraries for NGS in the NGS-based HLA genotyping method. The multiplex methods also conserved on the amounts of DNA samples needed to genotype a multiple number of HLA loci. Overall, the multiplex PCR method is a powerful tool for providing precise genotyping data without phase ambiguity, with a strong potential to replace the current routine genotyping methods to find polymorphisms. Commercialized PCR amplification reagents such as NEType (One-Lambda) that are based on multiplex PCR methods will be made available in the near future, whereas those based on the one-locus, one-tube PCR methods (left side of Figure 3) such as the TruSight HLA panel (Illumina) and NGSgo (GenDX) are already available in the market place.

4.2. NGS step

Although the 454 GS FLX was used often in the early stages of development of NGS-based HLA genotyping, the benchtop next-generation sequencers such as the GS Junior system, Ion Torrent PGM system, and the MiSeq system have been used more recently for the development and application of the HLA genotyping methods (Table 2). At the moment, complicated operations such as the preparation of NGS libraries are necessary for each of the different second generation sequencing platforms. However, the NGS companies are attempting to overcome these procedural bottlenecks by simplifying, automating, and speeding-up of the preparatory steps for NGS. For example, a new protocol using Ion Isothermal Amplification Chemistry that enables sequence reads of up to and beyond 500 bp, and Ion Hi-Q™ Sequencing Chemistry that reduces consensus insertion and deletion (indel) errors, including homopolymer errors, might lead to further simplification and cost reduction with higher data quality.

4.3. Allele assignment step

A variety of different allele assignment methods have been developed with some allele assignment software packages such as Assign (CONEXIO), OMIXON Target (OMIXON), and NGSengine (GenDX) commercially available, and others such as TypeStream (Life Technologies) still to be made commercially available in the near future. From our knowledge, Assign and NGSengine only support NGS data obtained from the one-locus, one-tube PCR method, whereas OMIXON Target and TypeStream also support NGS data obtained by the multiplex PCR methods. However, accuracy rates of the assignment methods are not 100% with genotyping errors caused by (1) missing HLA allele sequences, (2) generation of excessive allelic imbalance (ratio of sequence read numbers of allele 1 and allele 2), and (3) interference of HLA-DRB1 genotyping by participation of sequence reads originating from highly homologous HLA-DRB3/4/5 and other HLA-DRB pseudogenes. To avoid the errors raised in point 1, it is necessary to have a full and proper collection of all the HLA allele sequences to achieve precise HLA genotyping. In this regard, a much greater collection of high-quality full-length HLA allele sequences are expected to be obtained by way of international collaborations at the 17th IHIWS meeting in 2017 [53].

4.3.1. In-house Sequence Alignment-Based Assigning Software (SeaBass)

Recently, we developed a new next sequence allele assignment program (Sequence Alignment-Based Assigning Software; SeaBass) to solve the problems previously outlined in points 2 and 3 above. The program includes (1) output of sequence reads, (2) homology search using the Blat program [55] with the "match" variable set to 100% to detect identical exons within the known HLA alleles released from the IMGT-HLA database [7], (3) selection of allele candidates, (4) mapping of the sequence reads to the selected allele candidates as references with the "match" set at 100% using Reference Mapper (Roche), (5) calculation of coverages, and (6) confirmation of the mapping data and allele assignment (Figure 4).

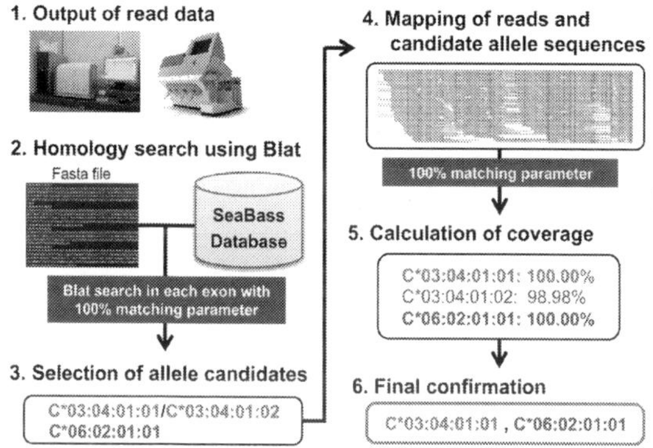

Figure 4. Allele assignment method using the newly developed Sequence Alignment-Based Assigning Software, SeaBass.

The operations from Eqs. (2) to (5) are automatically processed. If a new polymorphism is included in the exon, we can detect its presence at the Blat search stage as shown in Figure 5, and if a new polymorphism is included in the intron, we can detect its presence during the calculation of the coverage and the final confirmation stages (Figure 6).

After the detection of the new polymorphisms, we further confirm them by traditional methods such as Sanger sequencing and subcloning. In addition, we validated the use of the SeaBass assignment methods for three next-generation sequencers, the GS Junior system, the Ion Torrent PGM system, and the MiSeq system. To evaluate the SeaBass program, we used a total of 2414 HLA sequences from all the classical HLA loci that have frequent HLA alleles in Caucasians, African-Europeans, and Japanese, and we obtained an overall accuracy rate of >99.8% and 100% for the Japanese subjects (Table 3).

The accuracy rate was not 100% for HLA-DRB1/3/4/5 and HLA-DPB1 of the non-Japanese subjects because the complete coding sequences have not been determined as yet for some of their HLA-DRB and HLA-DPB1 alleles. Nevertheless, the allele assignment method that we developed for SeaBass appears to be the most accurate and efficient way to detect new and null alleles by NGS.

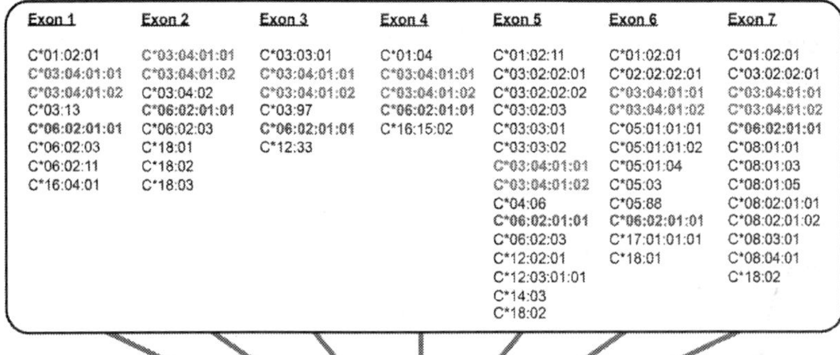

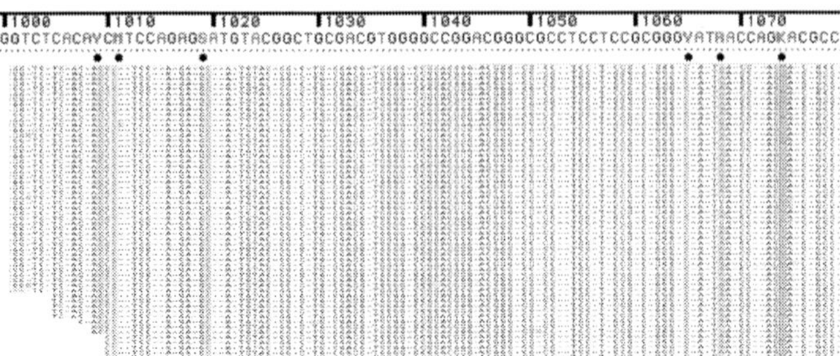

Figure 5. Detailed information concerning selection of allele candidates using the SeaBass computer program. (A) "Extraction of allele candidates" by Blat search. We select allele candidates that are extracted in all of the exons. (B-1) New allele detection. In this example, one allele was called B*15:18:01, but the other allele was called B*44:03:01 excluding the exon 3. (B-2) Confirmation of the new allele by NGS. Mapping of the sequence reads with B*44:03:01 as a reference suggested six nucleotide differences with B*44:03:01 were detected in exon 3. We confirmed the polymorphisms by Sanger sequencing and deposited the sequence to DDBJ and IMGT-HLA database. Now the formal allele name is B*44:184 [94].

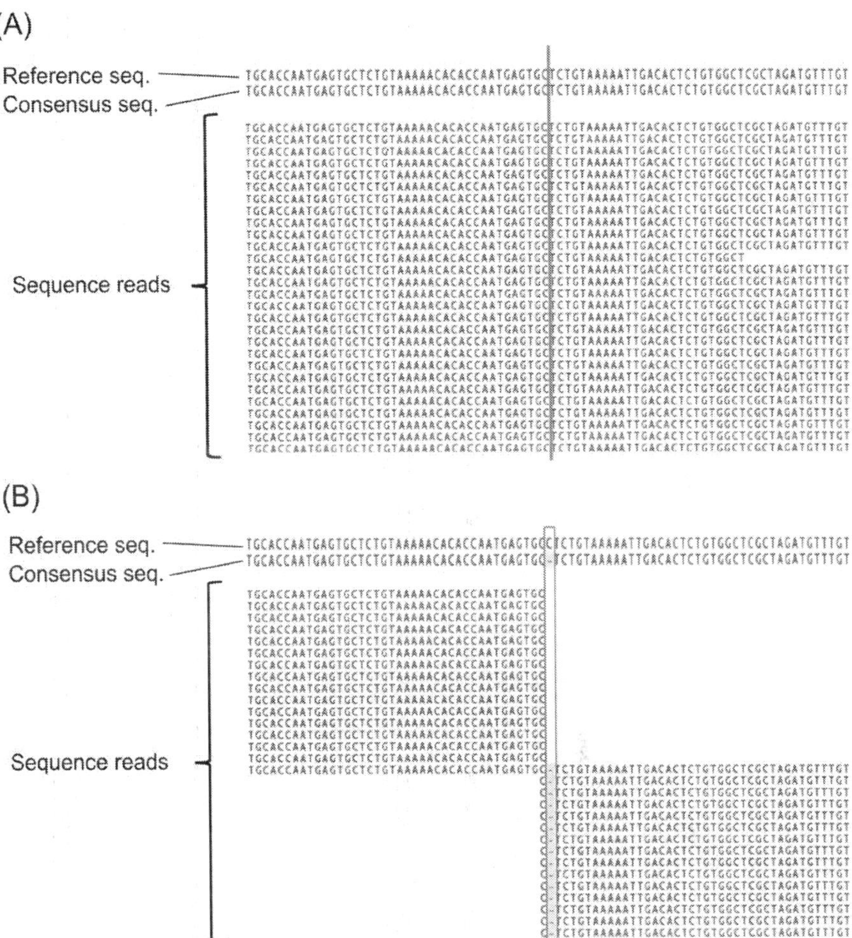

Figure 6. Detection of a new allele during the calculation of the coverage and final confirmation stages in SeaBass. Mapping results of the sequence reads using GS Reference Mapper are shown. (A) In this case, there is no mismatch between the reference and consensus sequence. (B) In this case, there is a mismatch between the reference and consensus sequence (reference: C; consensus: -) indicated by yellow background.

5. NGS-based MHC genotyping methods in nonhuman species

NGS technology provides the opportunity to genotype MHC sequences either by PCR targeted DNA sequencing or by PCR targeted RNA sequencing, that is, by DNA sequencing after converting the RNA samples to cDNA by reverse transcriptase. Usually, one or other of the

Worldwide subject (1916 loci)

	Total	A	C	B	DRB345	DRB1	DQA1	DQB1	DPA1	DPB1
Locus number	1916	250	250	242	186	239	140	234	140	235
Allele number	3832	500	500	484	372	478	280	468	280	470
Accuracy rate (%)	99.8	100	100	100	99.2	99.6	100	100	100	99.6

Japanese subject (498 loci)

	Total	A	C	B	DRB345	DRB1	DQA1	DQB1	DPA1	DPB1
Locus number	498	86	80	77	50	68	4	65	4	64
Allele number	996	172	160	154	100	136	8	130	8	128
Accuracy rate (%)	100	100	100	100	100	100	100	100	100	100

Table 3. Evaluation of the SeaBass program

sequencing methods is chosen rather than using both methods on the same samples. In the following sections, we compare the use and limitations of targeted NGS sequencing using DNA or RNA samples for MHC genotyping of MHC class I and class II genes in nonhuman species such as the Filipino cynomolgus macaques.

5.1. Advantage and disadvantage of using DNA and RNA samples for NGS

Table 4 shows a summary of the advantages and disadvantages of using DNA and RNA samples for NGS-based MHC genotyping.

	DNA	RNA
Difficulty of sampling	Easy	Difficult
Extraction cost of nucleic acid	Cheap	Expensive
Preparation before PCR	No	RT reaction
Primer location	Both of exons and introns	Exons only
Required sequence read number	Few	Many
Exclusion of pseudogene	Difficult	Easy
Estimation of expression level	Impossible	Possible

Table 4. Advantages and disadvantages of DNA and RNA samples for NGS-based MHC genotyping

The advantages of using DNA samples instead of RNA samples are that (1) the sampling and extraction of the DNA nucleic acids are easier and cheaper than RNA samples, (2) PCR amplification can be perform directly without an additional reaction such as the reverse transcriptase (RT) reaction, (3) design of primers in the exon and intron regions, and (4) fewer read sequences are required for DNA than RNA samples if all alleles are amplified without allelic imbalance. Although many more read sequences are necessary for RNA samples than DNA samples to genotype all the MHC alleles that have different transcription levels, the advantages of using RNA samples for genotyping are that (1) they provide an opportunity to examine MHC gene expression, (2) transcription levels are possible to be estimated for each of MHC alleles from the read sequence depth [56], and (3) only transcribed MHC genes are detected without contamination of PCR products originating from pseudogenes if the primer locations cross over to at least two homologous exons. Thus, the use of RNA samples is thought to be more effective for precise MHC genotyping on duplicated MHC genes that have high similarities among the genes. However, DNA and RNA samples have their own unique advantages and disadvantages for informative NGS-based MHC genotyping and widen the choices for experimentation and data collection.

5.2. Methodology

Table 5 shows a publication list of the MHC genotyping by PCR-based NGS methods in different animal species, and it includes the MHC species name, target gene, PCR method, degree of allele data accumulation, and the allele assignment method.

	Species	MHC name	Animal model or nonmodel type	Template	Target gene	NGS platform	Degree of allele data accumulation	Allele assignment method	Ref.
Mammal	Rhesus macaque	*Mamu*	Model	RNA	Class I and II	454, Illumina	Relatively rich	Mapping *de novo* assembly	[78, 79]
	Cynomolgus macaque	*Mafa*	Model	RNA	Class I and II	454, Illumina, PacBio	Relatively rich	Mapping *de novo* assembly	[35, 78, 80, 81]
	Pig-tailed macaque	*Mane*	Model	RNA	Class I and II	454, Illumina	Relatively rich	Mapping *de novo* assembly	[78, 82]
	Swine	*SLA*	Model	RNA	Class I	454	Relatively rich	Mapping *de novo* assembly	[56]
	Grey mouse lemur	*Mimu*	Nonmodel	DNA	DRB and DQB	454	Poor	*De novo* assembly	[83]

	Species	MHC name	Animal model or nonmodel type	Template	Target gene	NGS platform	Degree of allele data accumulation	Allele assignment method	Ref.
	Alpine marmots	*Mama*	Nonmodel	DNA	Class I and DRB	454	Poor	*De novo* assembly	[84]
	New Zealand sea lion	*Phho*	Nonmodel	DNA	DRB and DQB	454	Poor	*De novo* assembly	[85]
Avian	Collared flycatcher	*Fial*	Nonmodel	DNA	Class II	454	Poor	*De novo* assembly	[86]
	Great tit	*Pama*	Nonmodel	DNA	Class I	454	Poor	*De novo* assembly	[87]
	House Sparrows	*Pado*	Nonmodel	DNA	Class I	454	Poor	*De novo* assembly	[88]
	Berthelot's pipittawny pipit	*AnbeAnca*	Nonmodel	DNA	Class II	454	Poor	*De novo* assembly	[89]
	New Zealand passerine	*Peph*	Nonmodel	DNA	Class II	PGM	Poor	*De novo* assembly	[90]
	Eurasian Coot	*Fuat*	Nonmodel	DNA	Class II	454	Poor	*De novo* assembly	[91]
Reptile	Ornate dragon lizard	*Ctor*	Nonmodel	DNA	Class I	454	Poor	*De novo* assembly	[92]
Fish	Stickleback fish	*Gaac*	Nonmodel	DNA	Class II	454	Poor	*De novo* assembly	[93]

Table 5. Publication list of MHC genotyping by PCR-based NGS methods in nonhuman species

As discussed previously, for humans, the HLA alleles obtained by next-generation sequencers are mainly assigned by mapping to known allele sequences that are used as the read references because a large number of HLA allele sequences already have been collected in the IMGT-HLA database [7] (Table 2). On the other hand, *de novo* assembly of read sequences and subcloning of PCR products identifies novel allele sequences. Of the nonhuman species, RNA samples tend to be used for MHC genotyping in experimental animals (model animals) such as macaque species and swine, whereas DNA samples are mainly used for MHC genotyping wild (nonmodel) animals because collecting RNA samples from them in their natural environment is more difficult than sampling captured or domesticated experimental animals (Table 5).

5.2.1. MHC genotyping RNA samples collected from Filipino cynomolgus macaques

MHC alleles in humans and experimental animals such as the macaque species and swine are mainly assigned by mapping methods because of the large amount of MHC allele information already available for them than for most other species. This allele information is collected and released by the IPD-MHC database [57]. When novel alleles are detected, *de novo* assembly of the read sequences and subcloning of PCR products identifies the sequences.

We identified homozygous and heterozygous cynomolgus macaques (Mafa) that have specific Mafa MHC haplotypes by genotyping the MHC of more than 5000 Filipino animals, and we found that they have a smaller number of different Mafa-class I and Mafa-class II alleles than the Indonesian and Vietnamese populations. In this section, we outline the MHC genotyping method using RNA samples and provide some results as an example of the method. Figure 7 shows a comparative genomic map of MHC regions between human and Filipino cynomolgus macaque.

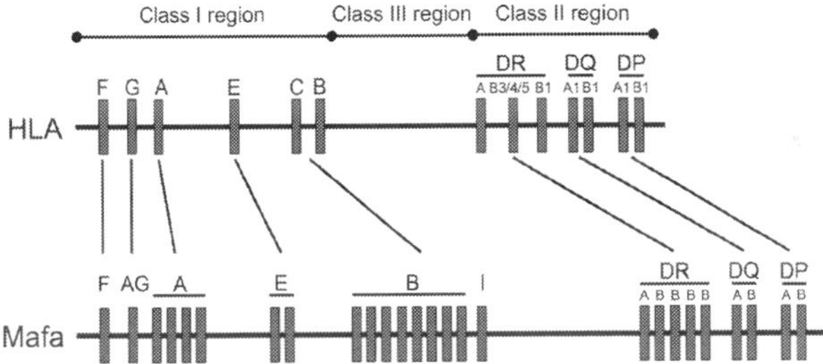

Figure 7. Comparative genomic map of the human (HLA) and the Filipino cynomolgus macaque (Mafa) Class I and Class II transcribed genes.

The MHC class I genomic region has many more Mafa-class I genes than HLA-class I genes generated by gene duplication events, whereas the organization of Mafa-class II genes are well conserved between the two species. Also, there are many Mafa-class I pseudogenes located in the Mafa-class I region. Therefore, we performed MHC genotyping by amplicon sequencing with the Roche GS Junior system using RNA samples from the Filipino cynomolgus macaques to prevent contamination of PCR products originating from the pseudogenes (Figure 8).

The workflow that we used is composed mainly of five steps: (1) RNA extraction and cDNA synthesis, (2) multiplex PCR amplification, (3) pooling of the PCR products, (4) amplicon NGS sequencing, and (5) allele assignment. In step 1, we usually extracted total RNA from the peripheral white blood cell samples using the TRIzol reagent (Invitrogen/Life Technologies/ Thermo Fisher Scientific, Carlsbad, CA) and synthesized cDNA by oligo d(T) primer using the ReverTraAce for the reverse transcriptase reaction (TOYOBO, Osaka, Japan) after treatment of the isolated RNA with DNase I (Invitrogen/Life Technologies/Thermo Fisher Scientific, Carlsbad, CA). In step 2, we designed a single Mafa-class I-specific primer set in exon 2 and exon 4 (PCR product size: 514 bp or 517 bp) that could amplify all known Mafa-class I alleles, whereas the Mafa-class II locus-specific primer sets included the polymorphic exon 2 in Mafa-DRB (420 bp), Mafa-DQA1 (435 bp), Mafa-DQB1 (396 bp), Mafa-DPA1 (407 bp), and Mafa-DPB1 (333, 336 or 339 bp) for massively parallel pyrosequencing (Figure 9).

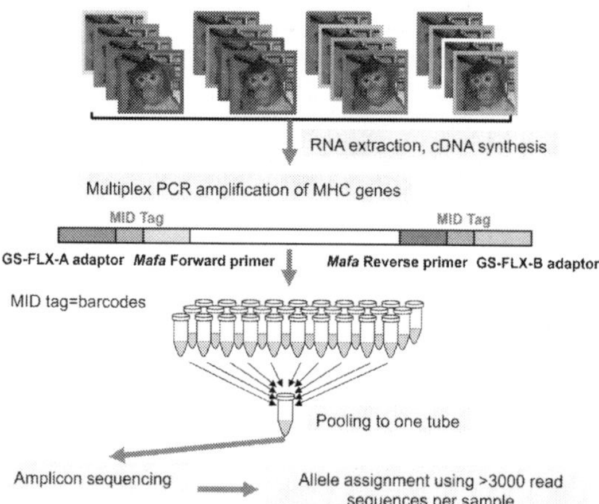

Figure 8. A schematic workflow of the successive steps of the MHC genotyping method by NGS amplicon sequencing for the Filipino cynomolgus macaques.

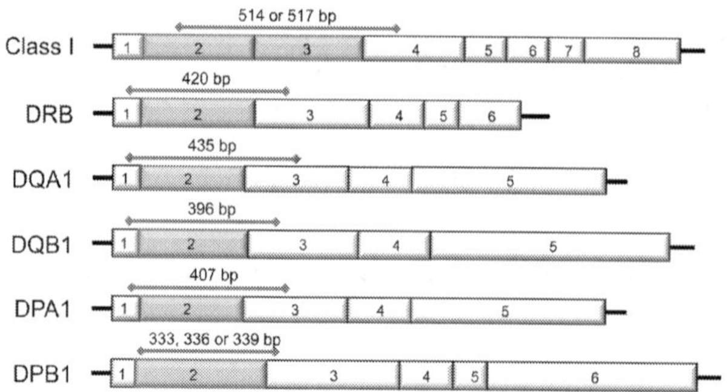

Figure 9. Location of primer sites to amplify Filipino cynomolgus macaque MHC genes. Yellow boxes and blue arrows indicate polymorphic exons and PCR regions, respectively. Numbers indicate exon numbers.

In addition to these primer sets, we also designed 50 different types of fusion primers that contained the 454 titanium adaptor (A in forward and B in reverse primer), 10 bp MID (multiple identifier), and MHC-specific primers (Figure 8). Moreover, we constructed a multiplex PCR method using the primer sets by carefully optimizing primer composition and PCR conditions and by comparing the sequence read data obtained by NGS (Figure 10).

As a result of these primer designs, 51.5%, 13.6%, and 8.6–8.9% of all read sequence numbers were detected in Mafa-class I, Mafa-DRB, and the other Mafa-class II genes, respectively, and we confirmed that the genotypes obtained by the multiplex PCR method were consistent with

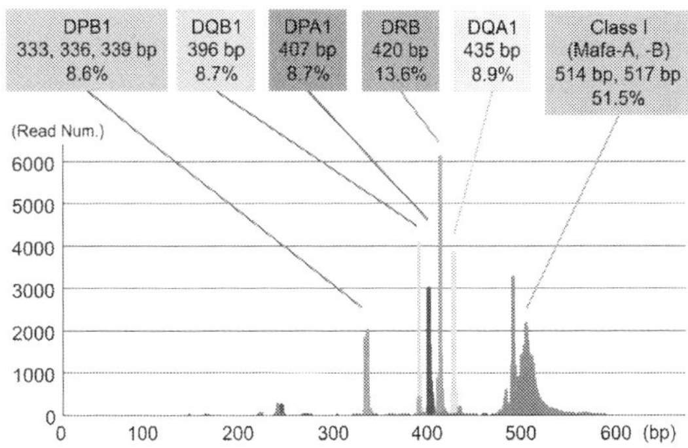

Figure 10. Ratio of read sequence numbers obtained by amplicon sequencing of multiplex PCR products.

our previous uniplex PCR methods. Therefore, the multiplex PCR method greatly simplified the procedures required in preparing the DNA samples for NGS by reducing the time of preparation and the amount and cost of reagents. In the pooling step of the PCR products, we quantified the purified PCR products by the Picogreen assay (Invitrogen) with a Fluoroskan Ascent micro-plate fluorometer (Thermo Fisher Scientific, Waltham, MA), mixed each of the PCR products at equimolar concentrations and then diluted them according to the manufacture's recommendation. In the NGS amplicon sequencing step, we perform emulsion PCR (emPCR) and emulsion-breaking according to the manufacturer's protocol (Roche, Basel, Switzerland). After the emulsion-breaking step, we enriched and counted the beads carrying the single-stranded DNA templates, and deposited them into a PicoTiterPlate to obtain the sequence reads.

A schematic workflow of the allele assignment process as a follow on from Figure 8 is shown in Figure 11.

After the sequencing run, image processing, signal correction, and base calling are performed by the GS Run Processor Ver. 3.0 (Roche) with full processing for shotgun or paired-end filter analysis. Quality-filter sequence reads that are passed by the assembler software (single sff file) are binned according to the MID labels into each separate sequence sff file using the sff file software (Roche). These files are further quality trimmed to remove poor sequence at the end of the reads with quality values (QVs) of less than 20. After separation of the trimmed and MID-labeled sequence reads in each of forward and reverse side read sequences, we independently detect the Mafa-class I and Mafa-class II allele candidates from both sides of the forward and reverse reads by using the BLAT program to match the trimmed and MID labeled sequence reads at 99% and 100% identity while setting the minimum overlap length at 200 and the alignment identity score parameter at 10 against all the known Mafa-class I and Mafa-class II allele sequences released in the IMGT/MHC-NHP database [58]. After the extraction of common allele candidates from both sequencing sides, we finally assign the "real alleles" by confirming nucleotide sequences of the allele candidates using the GS Reference Mapper Ver.

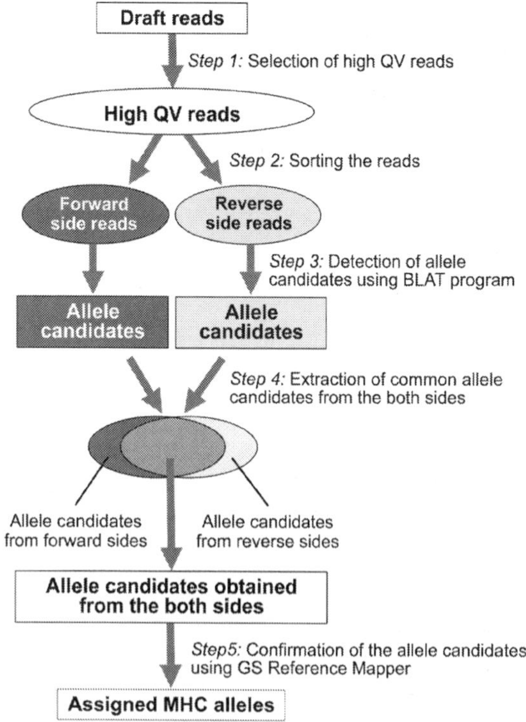

Figure 11. A schematic workflow of the allele assignment process using the SeaBass software.

3.0. To discover novel Mafa-class I sequences, we perform the de novo assembly set to detect >85% matches using the trimmed and MID-binned sequences after converting the outputs to ace files for the Sequencher Ver. 5.01 DNA sequence assembly software (Gene Code Co., Ann Arbor, MI). We then use the defined consensus sequence obtained from the de novo assembly as a reference sequence to identify and map the correct allele sequences. Using this process, we genotyped a set of 400 unrelated animals by the Sanger sequencing method and high resolution pyrosequencing and identified 190 different alleles, 28 at Mafa-A, 54 at Mafa-B, 12 at Mafa-I, 11 at Mafa-E, 7 at Mafa-F, 34 at Mafa-DRB, 13 at Mafa-DQA1, 13 at Mafa-DQB1, 9 at Mafa-DPA1, and 9 at Mafa-DPB1 alleles [35, 59].

On the basis of our large-scale project to genotype the MHC of 5000 Filipino cynomolgus macaques by NGS, we so far have detected 15 different types of Mafa haplotypes (HT1~HT15) in 45 homozygous animals. These Mafa homozygous animals provided the basis to efficiently estimate other Mafa haplotypes. For example, we estimated a variety of Mafa-A, Mafa-B/I, Mafa-E, and Mafa-class II (Mafa-DRB, Mafa-DQA1, Mafa-DQB1, Mafa-DPA1, and Mafa-DPB1) haplotypes by comparing the homozygous animals with heterozygous animals that carry the identical Mafa-class I and Mafa-class II alleles in the homozygous animals. In addition, we estimated the Mafa haplotypes and haplotype frequencies by the PHASE 2.1.1 program [60] using the allele data obtained by amplicon sequencing. From these procedures, we estimated a total of 84 Mafa-class I and 18 Mafa-class II haplotypes. Of the 15 different Mafa HT haplotypes, the haplotype frequencies of HT1, HT2, HT4, and HT8 were the highest. Of them, HT1 and HT8 have entirely different Mafa alleles, whereas HT2 and HT4 are thought to be recombinants of HT1 and HT8 (Figure 12).

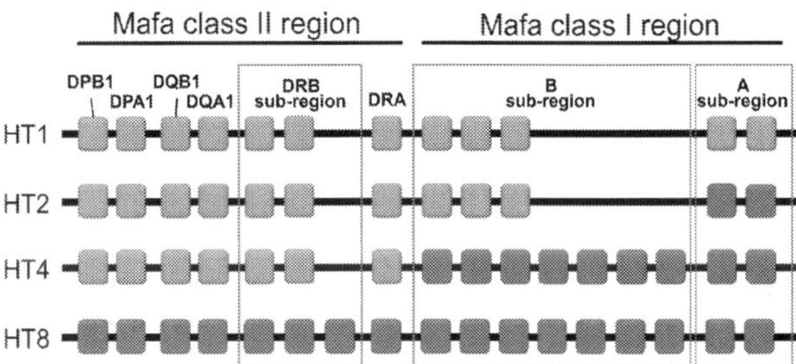

Figure 12. Gene composition of representative Mafa MHC haplotypes HT1 and HT8 and their recombinants HT2 and HT4.

Namely, the Mafa-A allele in HT2 is identical to that in HT8, whereas HT2 also has alleles at other loci that are identical with those in HT1. Similarly, HT4 has alleles in Mafa-class I loci that are identical with those in HT8, and alleles in the Mafa-class II loci that are identical with those in HT1. Therefore, Mafa homozygous animals with known haplotypes such as H1 and H2 are important for biomedical research, such as the transplantation outcomes of induced pluripotent stem (iPS) cells (Figure 13) because such studies are undertaken on animals with a defined genetic background and relatively well-characterized MHC haplotypes that might regulate the adaptive immune system in different ways and efficiencies.

5.2.2. MHC genotyping using DNA samples of wild animals

At this time in the development of MHC genotyping by NGS, it is difficult to apply the RNA-sequencing mapping method to accurately genotype the MHC of wild animals using known allele sequences as references. This is because the present allele information is relatively poor for most of them (Table 5). Therefore, MHC genotyping of wild animals or poorly studied species by NGS is based on *de novo* assembly of DNA sequences. In this case, the definition of "real alleles" and "artifact alleles" is important because NGS errors such as monostretch sequences are frequently observed in the assembled consensus sequences. Some of the allele assignment approaches based on *de novo* assembly that have been published include the allele validation threshold (AVT) method [61], clustering method [62–64], and the relative sequencing depth modeling methods [65]. These methods suppose that the contigs that have a sequence depth greater than the threshold level are the "real alleles," and they are determined by

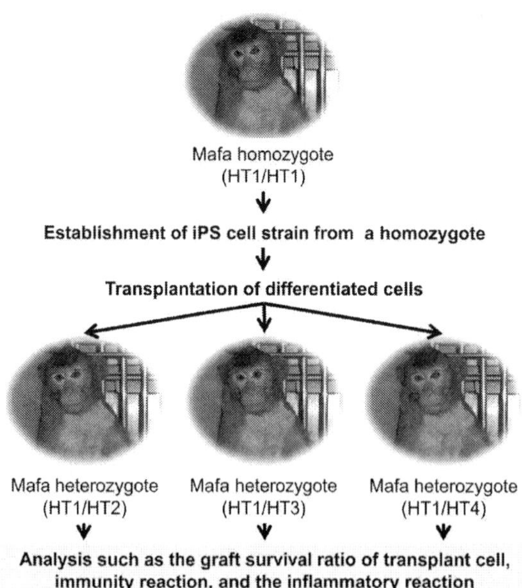

Figure 13. Application of Mafa homozygous and heterozygous animals for nonclinical trials of induced pluripotent stem (iPS) cells.

statistical calculation of the threshold using the sequence depth values of all contigs obtained in *de novo* assembly. Therefore, the detection of exact or "real" alleles depends largely on the setting of the threshold level and the quality of the sequence reads [65]. To enable the correct setting of the threshold level, it is important to use primers that can amplify all alleles of the target locus or loci without allelic imbalance. Furthermore, additional considerations such as repeating independent NGS experiments at least three times and detecting identical allele sequences in at least two animals are necessary to distinguish between real and artifactual alleles.

6. Conclusion

Genotyping the polymorphisms of MHC genes using targeted NGS technologies has been developed for humans and some nonhuman species to replace the use of other more cumbersome and less accurate procedures. We found that targeted NGS of DNA or RNA samples is feasible, productive, and generates high-quality MHC allele information from a large number of samples not easily achievable by other genotyping methods. We used second-generation sequencing protocols to target the DNA region and RNA subsets of interest in our NGS studies. It is likely that the longer sequence reads produced by third-generation platforms such as the

Pacific Biosciences single-molecule real-time sequencing or the Oxford nanopore sequencing platform will enable and improve the task of MHC sequence phasing and haplotyping, although this has yet to be demonstrated and proved to be advantageous and more economical. Continued allele data collection for different species, improvements to the reagents, protocols, and data analysis tools also are likely to simplify procedures and lower the costs of generating sequencing data in future. Most species have numerous highly polymorphic MHC loci; hence, the many benefits of using NGS technologies are likely, in the near future, to replace many of the traditional genotyping methods for the investigation of human and animal MHC genes and their role in evolutionary biology, ecology, population genetics, disease, and transplantation.

Author details

Takashi Shiina[1*], Shingo Suzuki[1] and Jerzy K. Kulski[1,2]

*Address all correspondence to: tshiina@is.icc.u-tokai.ac.jp

1 Division of Basic Medical Science and Molecular Medicine, Department of Molecular Life Science, Tokai University School of Medicine, Isehara, Kanagawa, Japan

2 Centre for Forensic Science, The University of Western Australia, Nedlands, WA, Australia

References

[1] Kulski JK, Shiina T, Anzai T, Kohara S, Inoko H. Comparative genomic analysis of the MHC: the evolution of class I duplication blocks, diversity and complexity from shark to man. Immunological Reviews. 2002;190:95–122. DOI: 10.1034/j.1600-065X. 2002.19008.x.

[2] Shiina T, Inoko H, Kulski JK. An update of the HLA genomic region, locus information and disease associations: 2004. Tissue Antigens. 2004;64(6):631–49. DOI: 10.1111/j.1399-0039.2004.00327.x.

[3] Shiina T, Hosomichi K, Inoko H, Kulski JK. The HLA genomic loci map: expression, interaction, diversity and disease. Journal of Human Genetics. 2009;54(1):15–39. DOI: 10.1038/jhg.2008.5.

[4] Claas FH, Duquesnoy RJ. The polymorphic alloimmune response in clinical transplantation. Current Opinion in Immunology. 2008;20(5):566–7. DOI: 10.1016/j.coi. 2008.08.001.

[5] Choo SY. The HLA system: genetics, immunology, clinical testing, and clinical implications. Yonsei Medical Journal. 2007;48(1):11–23. DOI: 10.3349/ymj.2007.48.1.11.

[6] Kulski JK, Inoko H. Major histocompatibility complex (MHC) genes. In: Cooper DN, editor. Nature Encyclopedia of the Human Genome. London: Nature Publishing Group; 2003. pp. 778–85.

[7] IMGT/HLA Database. Available from: http://www.ebi.ac.uk/imgt/hla/.

[8] Zinkernagel RM, Doherty PC. The discovery of MHC restriction. Immunology Today. 1997;18(1):14–7. DOI: http://dx.doi.org/10.1016/S0167-5699(97)80008-4.

[9] Sasazuki T, Juji T, Morishima Y, Kinukawa N, Kashiwabara H, Inoko H, et al. Effect of matching of class I HLA alleles on clinical outcome after transplantation of hematopoietic stem cells from an unrelated donor. Japan Marrow Donor Program. New England Journal of Medicine. 1998;339(17):1177–85. DOI: 10.1056/NEJM199810223391701.

[10] International MHC, Autoimmunity Genetics N, Rioux JD, Goyette P, Vyse TJ, Hammarstrom L, et al. Mapping of multiple susceptibility variants within the MHC region for 7 immune-mediated diseases. Proceedings of the National Academy of Sciences of the United States of America. 2009;106(44):18680–5. DOI: 10.1073/pnas.0909307106.

[11] Cotsapas C, Voight BF, Rossin E, Lage K, Neale BM, Wallace C, et al. Pervasive sharing of genetic effects in autoimmune disease. PLoS Genetics. 2011;7(8):e1002254. DOI: 10.1371/journal.pgen.1002254.

[12] International Multiple Sclerosis Genetics C, Wellcome Trust Case Control C, Sawcer S, Hellenthal G, Pirinen M, Spencer CC, et al. Genetic risk and a primary role for cell-mediated immune mechanisms in multiple sclerosis. Nature. 2011;476(7359):214–9. DOI: 10.1038/nature10251.

[13] Raychaudhuri S, Sandor C, Stahl EA, Freudenberg J, Lee HS, Jia X, et al. Five amino acids in three HLA proteins explain most of the association between MHC and seropositive rheumatoid arthritis. Nature Genetics. 2012;44(3):291–6.DOI: 10.1038/ng.1076.

[14] International HIVCS, Pereyra F, Jia X, McLaren PJ, Telenti A, de Bakker PI, et al. The major genetic determinants of HIV-1 control affect HLA class I peptide presentation. Science. 2010;330(6010):1551–7. DOI: 10.1126/science.1195271.

[15] Ziegler A, Kentenich H, Uchanska-Ziegler B. Female choice and the MHC. Trends in Immunology. 2005;26(9):496–502. DOI: 10.1016/j.it.2005.07.003.

[16] McCormack M, Alfirevic A, Bourgeois S, Farrell JJ, Kasperaviciute D, Carrington M, et al. HLA-A*3101 and carbamazepine-induced hypersensitivity reactions in Europeans. New England Journal of Medicine. 2011;364(12):1134–43. DOI: 10.1056/NEJMoa1013297.

[17] Illing PT, Vivian JP, Dudek NL, Kostenko L, Chen Z, Bharadwaj M, et al. Immune self-reactivity triggered by drug-modified HLA-peptide repertoire. Nature. 2012;486(7404):554–8. DOI: 10.1038/nature11147.

[18] Xiao BG, Link H. Immune regulation within the central nervous system. Journal of the Neurological Sciences. 1998;157(1):1–12. DOI: http://dx.doi.org/10.1016/S0022-510X(98)00049-5.

[19] Huh GS, Boulanger LM, Du H, Riquelme PA, Brotz TM, Shatz CJ. Functional requirement for class I MHC in CNS development and plasticity. Science. 2000;290(5499):2155–9. DOI:10.1126/science.290.5499.2155.

[20] Boulanger LM, Shatz CJ. Immune signalling in neural development, synaptic plasticity and disease. Nature Reviews Neuroscience. 2004;5(7):521–31. DOI: 10.1038/nrn1428.

[21] Cullheim S, Thams S. The microglial networks of the brain and their role in neuronal network plasticity after lesion. Brain Research Reviews. 2007;55(1):89–96. DOI: 10.1016/j.brainresrev.2007.03.012.

[22] Ohtsuka M, Inoko H, Kulski JK, Yoshimura S. Major histocompatibility complex (Mhc) class Ib gene duplications, organization and expression patterns in mouse strain C57BL/6. BMC Genomics. 2008;9:178. DOI: 10.1186/1471-2164-9-178.

[23] Matsuo R, Asada A, Fujitani K, Inokuchi K. LIRF, a gene induced during hippocampal long-term potentiation as an immediate-early gene, encodes a novel RING finger protein. Biochemical and Biophysical Research Communications. 2001;289(2):479–84. DOI: 10.1006/bbrc.2001.5975.

[24] Patino-Lopez G, Hevezi P, Lee J, Willhite D, Verge GM, Lechner SM, et al. Human class-I restricted T cell associated molecule is highly expressed in the cerebellum and is a marker for activated NKT and CD8+ T lymphocytes. Journal of Neuroimmunology. 2006;171(1–2):145–55. DOI: 10.1016/j.jneuroim.2005.09.017.

[25] Goddard CA, Butts DA, Shatz CJ. Regulation of CNS synapses by neuronal MHC class I. Proceedings of the National Academy of Sciences of the United States of America. 2007;104(16):6828–33. DOI: 10.1073/pnas.0702023104.

[26] Tonelli LH, Postolache TT, Sternberg EM. Inflammatory genes and neural activity: involvement of immune genes in synaptic function and behavior. Frontiers in Bioscience. 2005;10:675–80. DOI: http://dx.doi.org/10.2741/1562.

[27] Lengen C, Regard M, Joller H, Landis T, Lalive P. Anomalous brain dominance and the immune system: do left-handers have specific immunological patterns? Brain and Cognition. 2009;69(1):188–93. DOI: 10.1016/j.bandc.2008.07.008.

[28] O'Keefe GM, Nguyen VT, Benveniste EN. Regulation and function of class II major histocompatibility complex, CD40, and B7 expression in macrophages and microglia:

implications in neurological diseases. Journal of Neurovirology. 2002;8(6):496–512.DOI: 10.1080/13550280290100941.

[29] Raha-Chowdhury R, Andrews SR, Gruen JR. CAT 53: a protein phosphatase 1 nuclear targeting subunit encoded in the MHC Class I region strongly expressed in regions of the brain involved in memory, learning, and Alzheimer's disease. Brain Research. Molecular Brain Research. 2005;138(1):70–83. DOI: 10.1016/j.molbrainres. 2005.04.001.

[30] Cohly HH, Panja A. Immunological findings in autism. International Review of Neurobiology. 2005;71:317–41. DOI: 10.1016/S0074-7742(05)71013-8.

[31] Bailey SL, Carpentier PA, McMahon EJ, Begolka WS, Miller SD. Innate and adaptive immune responses of the central nervous system. Critical Reviews in Immunology. 2006;26(2):149–88. DOI: 10.1615/CritRevImmunol.v26.i2.40.

[32] McElroy JP, Oksenberg JR. Multiple sclerosis genetics. Current Topics in Microbiology and Immunology. 2008;318:45–72.

[33] Santamaria P, Lindstrom AL, Boyce-Jacino MT, Myster SH, Barbosa JJ, Faras AJ, et al. HLA class I sequence-based typing. Human Immunology. 1993;37(1):39–50. DOI: 10.1016/0198-8859(93)90141-M.

[34] Hutchison CA, 3rd. DNA sequencing: bench to bedside and beyond. Nucleic acids Research. 2007;35(18):6227–37. DOI: 10.1093/nar/gkm688.

[35] Shiina T, Yamada Y, Aarnink A, Suzuki S, Masuya A, Ito S, et al. Discovery of novel MHC-class I alleles and haplotypes in Filipino cynomolgus macaques (*Macaca fascicularis*) by pyrosequencing and Sanger sequencing : Mafa-class I polymorphism. Immunogenetics. 2015;67(10):563–78. DOI: 10.1007/s00251-015-0867-9.

[36] Ota M, Fukushima H, Kulski JK, Inoko H. Single nucleotide polymorphism detection by polymerase chain reaction-restriction fragment length polymorphism. Nature Protocols. 2007;2(11):2857–64. DOI: 10.1038/nprot.2007.407.

[37] Arguello JR, Madrigal JA. HLA typing by Reference Strand Mediated Conformation Analysis (RSCA). Reviews in Immunogenetics. 1999;1(2):209–19.

[38] Saiki RK, Walsh PS, Levenson CH, Erlich HA. Genetic analysis of amplified DNA with immobilized sequence-specific oligonucleotide probes. Proceedings of the National Academy of Sciences of the United States of America. 1989;86(16):6230–4.

[39] Olerup O, Zetterquist H. HLA-DR typing by PCR amplification with sequence-specific primers (PCR-SSP) in 2 hours: an alternative to serological DR typing in clinical practice including donor-recipient matching in cadaveric transplantation. Tissue Antigens. 1992;39(5):225–35. DOI: 10.1111/j.1399-0039.1992.tb01940.x.

[40] Sheldon S, Poulton K. HLA typing and its influence on organ transplantation. Methods in Molecular Biology. 2006;333:157–74. DOI: 10.1385/1-59745-049-9:157.

[41] Mahdi BM. A glow of HLA typing in organ transplantation. Clinical and Translational Medicine. 2013;2(1):6. DOI: 10.1385/1-59745-049-9:157.

[42] Petersdorf EW. Optimal HLA matching in hematopoietic cell transplantation. Current Opinion in Immunology. 2008;20(5):588–93. DOI: 10.1016/j.coi.2008.06.014.

[43] Erlich HA, Opelz G, Hansen J. HLA DNA typing and transplantation. Immunity. 2001;14(4):347–56. DOI: http://dx.doi.org/10.1016/S1074-7613(01)00115-7.

[44] Fernandez Vina MA, Hollenbach JA, Lyke KE, Sztein MB, Maiers M, Klitz W, et al. Tracking human migrations by the analysis of the distribution of HLA alleles, lineages and haplotypes in closed and open populations. Philosophical Transactions of the Royal Society of London Series: B. Biological Sciences. 2012;367(1590):820–9. DOI: 10.1098/rstb.2011.0320.

[45] Gourraud PA, Khankhanian P, Cereb N, Yang SY, Feolo M, Maiers M, et al. HLA diversity in the 1000 genomes dataset. PLoS One. 2014;9(7):e97282. DOI: 10.1371/journal.pone.0097282.

[46] Nakaoka H, Mitsunaga S, Hosomichi K, Shyh-Yuh L, Sawamoto T, Fujiwara T, et al. Detection of ancestry informative HLA alleles confirms the admixed origins of Japanese population. PLoS One. 2013;8(4):e60793. DOI: 10.1371/journal.pone.0060793.

[47] Grubic Z, Stingl K, Martinez N, Palfi B, Brkljacic-Kerhin V, Kastelan A. STR and HLA analysis in paternity testing. International Congress Series. 2004;1261:535–7. DOI: 10.1016/S0531-5131(03)01654-6.

[48] Itoh Y, Mizuki N, Shimada T, Azuma F, Itakura M, Kashiwase K, et al. High-throughput DNA typing of HLA-A, -B, -C, and -DRB1 loci by a PCR-SSOP-Luminex method in the Japanese population. Immunogenetics. 2005;57(10):717–29. DOI: 10.1007/s00251-005-0048-3.

[49] Itoh Y, Inoko H, Kulski JK, Sasaki S, Meguro A, Takiyama N, et al. Four-digit allele genotyping of the HLA-A and HLA-B genes in Japanese patients with Behcet's disease by a PCR-SSOP-Luminex method. Tissue Antigens. 2006;67(5):390–4. DOI: 10.1111/j.1399-0039.2006.00586.x.

[50] Adams SD, Barracchini KC, Chen D, Robbins F, Wang L, Larsen P, et al. Ambiguous allele combinations in HLA Class I and Class II sequence-based typing: when precise nucleotide sequencing leads to imprecise allele identification. Journal of Translational Medicine. 2004;2(1):30. DOI: 10.1186/1479-5876-2-30.

[51] Lind C, Ferriola D, Mackiewicz K, Heron S, Rogers M, Slavich L, et al. Next-generation sequencing: the solution for high-resolution, unambiguous human leukocyte antigen typing. Human Immunology. 2010;71(10):1033–42. DOI: 10.1016/j.humimm.2010.06.016.

[52] Kulski JK, Suzuki S, Ozaki Y, Mitsunaga S, Inoko H, Shiina T. In phase HLA genotyping by next generation sequencing—a comparison between two massively paral-

lel sequencing bench-top Systems, the Roche GS Junior and Ion Torrent PGM. In: Xi Y, editor. HLA and Associated Important Diseases. Croatia: Intech; 2014. p. 141–81.

[53] 17th International HLA and Immunogenetics Workshop (IHIWS) in 2017. Available from: http://ihiws.org/ngs-of-full-length-hla-genes/.

[54] Ozaki Y, Suzuki S, Kashiwase K, Shigenari A, Okudaira Y, Ito S, et al. Cost-efficient multiplex PCR for routine genotyping of up to nine classical HLA loci in a single analytical run of multiple samples by next generation sequencing. BMC Genomics. 2015;16:318. DOI: 10.1186/s12864-015-1514-4.

[55] Blat program. Available from: http://genome.ucsc.edu/

[56] Kita YF, Ando A, Tanaka K, Suzuki S, Ozaki Y, Uenishi H, et al. Application of high-resolution, massively parallel pyrosequencing for estimation of haplotypes and gene expression levels of swine leukocyte antigen (SLA) class I genes. Immunogenetics. 2012;64(3):187–99. DOI: 10.1007/s00251-011-0572-2.

[57] IPD-MHC database. Available from: http://www.ebi.ac.uk/ipd/mhc/.

[58] Robinson J, Halliwell JA, McWilliam H, Lopez R, Marsh SG. IPD—the Immuno Polymorphism Database. Nucleic Acids Research. 2013;41(Database issue):D1234–40. DOI: 10.1093/nar/gks1140.

[59] Blancher A, Aarnink A, Yamada Y, Tanaka K, Yamanaka H, Shiina T. Study of MHC class II region polymorphism in the Filipino cynomolgus macaque population. Immunogenetics. 2014;66(4):219–30. DOI: 10.1007/s00251-014-0764-7.

[60] Stephens M, Smith NJ, Donnelly P. A new statistical method for haplotype reconstruction from population data. American Journal of Human Genetics. 2001;68(4): 978–89. DOI: 10.1086/319501.

[61] Zagalska-Neubauer M, Babik W, Stuglik M, Gustafsson L, Cichon M, Radwan J. 454 sequencing reveals extreme complexity of the class II Major Histocompatibility Complex in the collared flycatcher. BMC Evolutionary Biology. 2010;10:395.DOI: 10.1186/1471-2148-10-395.

[62] Sommer S, Courtiol A, Mazzoni CJ. MHC genotyping of non-model organisms using next-generation sequencing: a new methodology to deal with artefacts and allelic dropout. BMC Genomics. 2013;14:542. DOI: 10.1186/1471-2164-14-542.

[63] Pavey SA, Sevellec M, Adam W, Normandeau E, Lamaze FC, Gagnaire PA, et al. Nonparallelism in MHCIIbeta diversity accompanies nonparallelism in pathogen infection of lake whitefish (*Coregonus clupeaformis*) species pairs as revealed by next-generation sequencing. Molecular Ecology. 2013;22(14):3833–49. DOI: 10.1111/mec. 12358.

[64] Lamaze FC, Pavey SA, Normandeau E, Roy G, Garant D, Bernatchez L. Neutral and selective processes shape MHC gene diversity and expression in stocked brook charr

populations (*Salvelinus fontinalis*). Molecular Ecology. 2014;23(7):1730–48. DOI: 10.1111/mec.12684.

[65] Lighten J, van Oosterhout C, Bentzen P. Critical review of NGS analyses for de novo genotyping multigene families. Molecular Ecology. 2014;23(16):3957–72. DOI: 10.1111/mec.12843.

[66] Bentley G, Higuchi R, Hoglund B, Goodridge D, Sayer D, Trachtenberg EA, et al. High-resolution, high-throughput HLA genotyping by next-generation sequencing. Tissue Antigens. 2009;74(5):393–403. DOI: 10.1111/j.1399-0039.2009.01345.x.

[67] Gabriel C, Danzer M, Hackl C, Kopal G, Hufnagl P, Hofer K, et al. Rapid high-throughput human leukocyte antigen typing by massively parallel pyrosequencing for high-resolution allele identification. Human Immunology. 2009;70(11):960–4. DOI: 10.1016/j.humimm.2009.08.009.

[68] Holcomb CL, Hoglund B, Anderson MW, Blake LA, Bohme I, Egholm M, et al. A multi-site study using high-resolution HLA genotyping by next generation sequencing. Tissue Antigens. 2011;77(3):206–17. DOI: 10.1111/j.1399-0039.2010.01606.x.

[69] Erlich RL, Jia X, Anderson S, Banks E, Gao X, Carrington M, et al. Next-generation sequencing for HLA typing of class I loci. BMC Genomics. 2011;12:42. DOI: 10.1111/j.1399-0039.2010.01606.x.

[70] Shiina T, Suzuki S, Ozaki Y, Taira H, Kikkawa E, Shigenari A, et al. Super high resolution for single molecule-sequence-based typing of classical HLA loci at the 8-digit level using next generation sequencers. Tissue Antigens. 2012;80(4):305–16. DOI: 10.1111/j.1399-0039.2012.01941.x.

[71] Wang C, Krishnakumar S, Wilhelmy J, Babrzadeh F, Stepanyan L, Su LF, et al. High-throughput, high-fidelity HLA genotyping with deep sequencing. Proceedings of the National Academy of Sciences of the United States of America. 2012;109(22):8676–81. DOI: 10.1073/pnas.1206614109.

[72] Moonsamy PV, Williams T, Bonella P, Holcomb CL, Hoglund BN, Hillman G, et al. High throughput HLA genotyping using 454 sequencing and the Fluidigm Access Array System for simplified amplicon library preparation. Tissue Antigens. 2013;81(3):141–9. DOI: 10.1111/tan.12071.

[73] Hosomichi K, Jinam TA, Mitsunaga S, Nakaoka H, Inoue I. Phase-defined complete sequencing of the HLA genes by next-generation sequencing. BMC Genomics. 2013;14:355. DOI: 10.1186/1471-2164-14-355.

[74] Ozaki Y, Suzuki S, Shigenari A, Okudaira Y, Kikkawa E, Oka A, et al. HLA-DRB1, -DRB3, -DRB4 and -DRB5 genotyping at a super-high resolution level by long range PCR and high-throughput sequencing. Tissue Antigens. 2014;83(1):10–6. DOI: 10.1111/tan.12258.

[75] Lange V, Bohme I, Hofmann J, Lang K, Sauter J, Schone B, et al. Cost-efficient high-throughput HLA typing by MiSeq amplicon sequencing. BMC Genomics. 2014;15:63.DOI: 10.1186/1471-2164-15-63.

[76] Smith AG, Pyo CW, Nelson W, Gow E, Wang R, Shen S, et al. Next generation sequencing to determine HLA class II genotypes in a cohort of hematopoietic cell transplant patients and donors. Human Immunology. 2014;75(10):1040–6. DOI: 10.1016/j.humimm.2014.08.206.

[77] Chang CJ, Chen PL, Yang WS, Chao KM. A fault-tolerant method for HLA typing with PacBio data. BMC Bioinformatics. 2014;15:296. DOI: 10.1186/1471-2105-15-296.

[78] Wiseman RW, Karl JA, Bimber BN, O'Leary CE, Lank SM, Tuscher JJ, et al. Major histocompatibility complex genotyping with massively parallel pyrosequencing. Nature Medicine. 2009;15(11):1322–6. DOI: 10.1038/nm.2038.

[79] Dudley DM, Karl JA, Creager HM, Bohn PS, Wiseman RW, O'Connor DH. Full-length novel MHC class I allele discovery by next-generation sequencing: two platforms are better than one. Immunogenetics. 2014;66(1):15–24. DOI: 10.1007/s00251-013-0744-3.

[80] Budde ML, Wiseman RW, Karl JA, Hanczaruk B, Simen BB, O'Connor DH. Characterization of Mauritian cynomolgus macaque major histocompatibility complex class I haplotypes by high-resolution pyrosequencing. Immunogenetics. 2010;62(11–12): 773–80. DOI: 10.1007/s00251-010-0481-9.

[81] Westbrook CJ, Karl JA, Wiseman RW, Mate S, Koroleva G, Garcia K, et al. No assembly required: full-length MHC class I allele discovery by PacBio circular consensus sequencing. Human Immunology. 2015. DOI: 10.1016/j.humimm.2015.03.022.

[82] O'Leary CE, Wiseman RW, Karl JA, Bimber BN, Lank SM, Tuscher JJ, et al. Identification of novel MHC class I sequences in pig-tailed macaques by amplicon pyrosequencing and full-length cDNA cloning and sequencing. Immunogenetics. 2009;61(10):689–701. DOI: 10.1007/s00251-009-0397-4.

[83] Huchard E, Albrecht C, Schliehe-Diecks S, Baniel A, Roos C, Kappeler PM, et al. Large-scale MHC class II genotyping of a wild lemur population by next generation sequencing. Immunogenetics. 2012;64(12):895–913. DOI: 10.1007/s00251-012-0649-6.

[84] Ferrandiz-Rovira M, Bigot T, Allaine D, Callait-Cardinal MP, Cohas A. Large-scale genotyping of highly polymorphic loci by next-generation sequencing: how to overcome the challenges to reliably genotype individuals? Heredity. 2015;114(5):485–93. DOI: 10.1038/hdy.2015.13.

[85] Osborne AJ, Zavodna M, Chilvers BL, Robertson BC, Negro SS, Kennedy MA, et al. Extensive variation at MHC DRB in the New Zealand sea lion (Phocarctos hookeri) provides evidence for balancing selection. Heredity. 2013;111(1):44–56. DOI: 10.1038/hdy.2013.18.

[86] Zagalska-Neubauer M, Babik W, Stuglik M, Gustafsson L, Cichon M, Radwan J. 454 sequencing reveals extreme complexity of the class II Major Histocompatibility Complex in the collared flycatcher. BMC Evolutionary Biology. 2010;10:395. DOI: 10.1186/1471-2148-10-395.

[87] Sepil I, Moghadam HK, Huchard E, Sheldon BC. Characterization and 454 pyrosequencing of major histocompatibility complex class I genes in the great tit reveal complexity in a passerine system. BMC Evolutionary Biology. 2012;12:68. DOI: 10.1186/1471-2148-12-68.

[88] Karlsson M, Westerdahl H. Characteristics of MHC class I genes in house sparrows *Passer domesticus* as revealed by long cDNA transcripts and amplicon sequencing. Journal of Molecular Evolution. 2013;77(1–2):8–21. DOI: 10.1007/s00239-013-9575-y.

[89] Gonzalez-Quevedo C, Phillips KP, Spurgin LG, Richardson DS. 454 screening of individual MHC variation in an endemic island passerine. Immunogenetics. 2015;67(3): 149–62. DOI: 10.1007/s00251-014-0822-1.

[90] Sutton JT, Robertson BC, Jamieson IG. MHC variation reflects the bottleneck histories of New Zealand passerines. Molecular Ecology. 2015;24(2):362–73. DOI: 10.1111/mec. 13039.

[91] Alcaide M, Munoz J, Martinez-de la Puente J, Soriguer R, Figuerola J. Extraordinary MHC class II B diversity in a non-passerine, wild bird: the Eurasian coot *Fulica atra* (Aves: Rallidae). Ecology and Evolution. 2014;4(6):688–98. DOI: 10.1002/ece3.974.

[92] Radwan J, Kuduk K, Levy E, LeBas N, Babik W. Parasite load and MHC diversity in undisturbed and agriculturally modified habitats of the ornate dragon lizard. Molecular Ecology. 2014;23(24):5966–78. DOI: 10.1111/mec.12984.

[93] Stutz WE, Bolnick DI. Stepwise threshold clustering: a new method for genotyping MHC loci using next-generation sequencing technology. PLoS One. 2014;9(7):e100587. DOI: 10.1371/journal.pone.0100587.

[94] Wada A, Shiina T, Michino J, Yasumura S, Sugiyama T. A novel HLA-B allele, HLA-B*44:184, identified by super high-resolution single-molecule sequence-based typing in a Japanese individual. Tissue Antigens. 2014;83(3):198–9. DOI: 10.1111/tan.12284.

Chapter 4

Transcriptomic Profiling Using Next Generation Sequencing - Advances, Advantages, and Challenges

Krishanpal Anamika, Srikant Verma, Abhay Jere and Aarti Desai

Additional information is available at the end of the chapter

http://dx.doi.org/10.5772/61789

Abstract

Transcriptome, the functional element of the genome, is comprised of different kinds of RNA molecules such as mRNA, miRNA, ncRNA, rRNA, and tRNA to name a few. Each of these RNA molecules plays a vital role in the physiological response, and understanding the regulation of these molecules is extremely critical for the better understanding of the functional genome. RNA Sequencing (RNASeq) is one of the latest techniques applied to study genome-wide transcriptome characterization and profiling using high-throughput sequenced data. As compared to array-based methods, RNASeq provides in-depth and more precise information on transcriptome characterization and quantification. Based upon availability of reference genome, transcriptome assembly can be reference-guided or *de novo*. Once transcripts are assembled, downstream analysis such as expression profiling, gene ontology, and pathway enrichment analyses can give more insight into gene regulation. This chapter describes the significance of RNASeq study over array-based traditional methods, approach to analyze RNASeq data, available methods and tools, challenges associated with the data analysis, application areas, some of the recent advancement made in the area of transcriptome study and its application.

Keywords: RNASeq, *de novo* and reference-based transcriptome assembly, Differential gene expression, Next Generation Sequencing

1. Introduction

Completion of the Human Genome Project in 2001 brought with it the realization that while understanding the genome is of great value, our understanding of biology is woefully incomplete without the knowledge of the functional elements of the genome. The functional element of the genome is the transcriptome, which is the set of RNA molecules such as mRNA, rRNA, tRNA, and various small RNAs. A large number of research projects are now focused

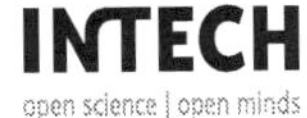

on the transcriptome rather than on genome and proteome as only 1-2% of genes are coding and 80-90% of the transcribed genes are not translated to proteins. However, these are known to be involved in epigenetic regulation and gene expression regulation [1-4]. Gene expression is a complex process regulated at multiple levels such as gene transcription, post-transcriptional modifications, and translation. Briefly, complexity at the transcription regulation arises from the presence of multiple Transcription Start Sites (TSSs), which can result in production of multiple transcripts from a single gene [5] and alternate splicing as well as alternate polyadenylation of the primary RNA to produce several different forms of transcripts originating from the same gene [6, 7]. Because of different TSSs, eventually each mature transcript will code for different protein [8]. Additionally, noncoding RNAs, which are not translated to proteins, play catalytic and structurally important roles. For example, tRNAs and rRNAs play a critical role in translation, small nuclear RNAs (snRNAs) participate in mRNA splicing, small nucleolar RNAs (snoRNAs) regulate rRNA splicing, guide RNAs (gRNAs) regulate RNA editing, and miRNA are involved in translational repression [9]. Study of the transcriptome provides an understanding of the regulation of gene expression pattern [10], alternative splicing and transcript structure [11], dynamic regulation of transcripts in different tissues [12], and detailed information about the gene regulation in normal and diseased conditions [13].

Transcriptome profiling is typically performed using hybridization or sequencing-based methodologies. Hybridization-based methods involve binding of fluorescently labeled fragments to complementary probe sequences either in solution or on a solid surface, e.g., microarray [14, 15]. These approaches, however, suffer from limitations such as low resolution, low specificity, and low sensitivity [16]. Later, Sanger sequencing-based approaches such as SAGE (Serial Analysis of Gene Expression) [17], CAGE (Cap Analysis of Gene Expression) [18], and MPSS (Massively Parallel Signature Sequencing) [19] were developed, but these approaches have serious limitations such as consideration of partial transcripts structure for gene expression and inability to distinguish between isoforms [20]. With the advent of Next Generation Sequencing (NGS), a technology that enables sequencing of millions of nucleotide fragments in parallel, RNA Sequencing (RNASeq) has emerged as a powerful method for studying the transcriptome. Though microarrays are high-throughput and economical, RNASeq offers numerous advantages over microarrays [15]. Some of the key benefits of using RNASeq over microarrays are:

a.   Genome-wide coverage of transcripts is offered by RNASeq.

b.   No prior knowledge of genome sequence is required in the case of RNASeq as opposed to microarray and hence RNASeq experiment can be performed in the absence of the reference genome.

c.   Improved sensitivity and specificity: RNASeq offers enhanced detection of transcripts and differentially expressed genes and isoforms. Moreover, RNASeq is known to be more accurate in terms of fold change detection for both high- and low-abundance genes.

d.   Detection of novel transcripts: Unlike microarray, RNASeq enables genome-wide unbiased study and is not dependent on transcript or region-specific probes and hence it investigates both known and novel transcripts.

e. Detection of low-abundance transcripts if sequencing is done at high depth.

f. No or minimal background signal: While mapping the reads to the genome, one can consider reads mapping unambiguously, which results in noise reduction. On the other hand, cross-hybridization increases noise-to-signal ratio in microarrays.

g. SNP detection: RNASeq data can be used for SNP detection especially for highly and medium expressed genes.

Because of its wider detection range, more sensitivity, genome-wide capture of expression profile, and rapidly decreasing cost, RNASeq technology is being preferred over array-based methods for transcriptome profiling. RNASeq has been widely used in the detection of differentially expressed genes between cancerous and normal tissue samples [21], identification of novel gene fusion events in melanoma [22], discovery of several novel miRNAs in cancerous cells [23], identification of differential gene expression and splicing events in Alzheimer's disease [24], identification of differential promoter usage, and higher expression of noncoding RNA in diabetes [25, 26]. RNASeq is now being used extensively for transcriptome assembly, thus enabling better characterization of economically important plants such as Garlic [27], Pea [28], Chickpea [29], Rice [30], Olive [31], Wheat [32], and many other plants [33]. Further, combination of molecular biology and biochemical techniques with sequencing has led to the study of different aspects of the transcriptome, such as mRNASeq, miRNASeq, GROSeq, CLIPSeq, NETSeq, PARESeq, and ChIRPSeq (additional information in Table 1). Projects such as ENCODE (ENCyclopedia of the DNA Elements) and TCGA (The Cancer Genome Atlas) have characterized transcriptome of several different human cell lines and tumor samples, respectively, using NGS-based transcriptome profiling. Goal of ENCODE (https://www.**encode**project.org/) is to identify genome-wide transcriptome profile to understand the downstream effects of gene regulation in the human genome. TCGA (www.cancergenome.nih.gov/), which contains information on cancer patient data, aims to understand the mechanism of tumor transformation and progression.

RNASeq methods	Description	Reference
mRNASeq	To identify messenger RNAs (mRNAs)	[12]
miRNASeq	To identify micro RNAs (miRNAs)	[167]
GROSeq (Global Run On Sequencing), PROSeq	To identify nascent RNAs that are actively transcribed by RNA Pol II	[168]
ChIRPSeq (Chromatin Isolation by RNA Purification)	To discover regions of the genome bound by a specific RNA	[169]
RiboSeq (Ribosome profile Sequencing)	To identify RNAs that are being processed by the ribosome and hence this method helps to monitor the translation process	[170]
CLIPSeq (Cross-Linking and Immunoprecipitation Sequencing)	To identify the binding sites of cellular RNA-binding proteins (RBPs) using UV light to cross-link RNA to RBPs without the incorporation of photoactivatable groups into RNA	[171]

RNASeq methods	Description	Reference
PAR-CLIP Seq(Photoactivatable-Ribonucleoside-Enhanced Cross-Linking and Immunoprecipitation Sequencing)	To identify and sequence the binding sites of cellular RNA-binding proteins (RBPs) and microRNA-containing ribonucleoprotein complexes (miRNPs)	[172]
NETSeq (Native Elongation Transcript Sequencing)	It sequences and captures nascent RNA transcripts after immunoprecipitation of RNA Pol II elongation complex	[173]
TRAPSeq (Targeted Purification of Polysomal mRNA Sequencing)	To detect and identify translating mRNAs	[174]
PARESeq (Parallel Analysis of RNA Ends Sequencing) and GMUCT (Genome-wide Mapping of Uncapped Transcripts)	To detect and identify miRNA cleavage sites and uncapped transcripts that undergo degradation	[175]
TIFSeq (Transcript Isoform Sequencing) or Paired-End Analysis of Transcription start site (PEAT)	RNA isoforms are identified after 5' and 3' paired-end sequencing	[176]
CELSeq (Cell Expression by Linear amplification and Sequencing), SMARTSeq (Switching Mechanism At the 5' end of the RNA Template Sequencing), STRT (Single-cell Tagged Reverse Transcription)	Single-cell transcriptomics methods	[177]

Table 1. Various RNASeq-based methods to study transcriptome

One of the first steps while designing the RNASeq experiment is choosing an appropriate sequencing platform. Several sequencing platforms such as Illumina, Roche, PacBio, and Ion Torrent, which are based on different sequencing chemistry and technology, are available [reviewed in 34, 35]. Current leading platform for RNASeq (and other NGS-based analyses) is the HiSeq series of sequencers from Illumina (https://www.illumina.com/systems.html) because it provides high throughput, deep sequencing, low sequence error, and long enough read data to be useful in multiple applications. Recently, the PacBio RS II (http://www.pacif-icbiosciences.com/) is gaining popularity for better transcriptome construction, because of its ability to generate long reads. Once the millions of reads are generated from an RNASeq experiment, the bioinformatics data analysis begins. In the following section, we briefly present the bioinformatics data analysis steps, tools, and methods.

2. Bioinformatics analysis of RNASeq data

Analysis of the RNASeq data is a multistep process that typically includes quality check, data preprocessing, transcriptome assembly (reference-guided and *de novo* transcriptome assembly), quantification, statistical analysis, and functional annotation (Figure 1). These steps are described in details in the following.

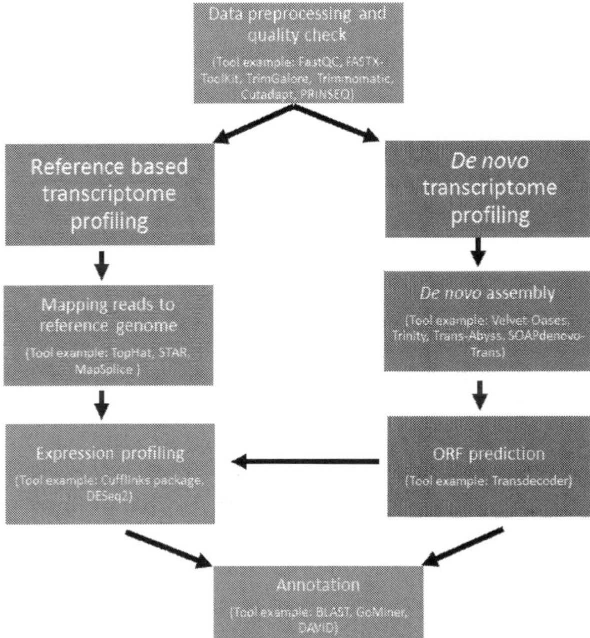

Figure 1. Basic RNASeq data analysis workflow. Firstly, raw sequenced data are checked for the quality and, if required, low-quality reads and artifacts are removed. In the case of reference-based assembly, the reads are mapped to the reference genome in order to know their location. All the mapped reads are then analyzed for expression profiling. Further, differentially expressed genes and isoforms can be annotated using Gene Ontology (GO) and Pathway enrichment analyses. In *de novo* assembly approach, after preprocessing of the raw reads, transcriptome can be assembled using different *de novo* transcriptome assemblers. Once transcripts are constructed and abundance estimate is obtained, the complete Open Reading Frames (ORFs) transcripts are predicted. The predicted ORFs can be annotated or analyzed for expression profiling and then annotated using remote homology search method, GO, and pathway enrichment analyses.

2.1. Quality check and data preprocessing

Next generation sequencers assign a Phred quality score, which is the probability of the base call being inaccurate, to the called bases. Low Phred scores (Q< 30) indicate read data of poor quality. Poor-quality read data can arise from problems in the library preparation or from sequencing itself. Additionally, PCR artifacts, sequence-specific biasness, untrimmed adapter sequences, and other possible contaminants can lead to poor data quality. These factors can affect the downstream analysis and data interpretation, and can give inaccurate results. In order to assess quality of raw sequenced data several tools such as FastQC (http://www.bioin-formatics.babraham.ac.uk/projects/fastqc/) and PRINSEQ [36] are available. Once the data are checked for quality, they should be processed to remove reads with low-quality bases, adapter sequences, and other contaminating sequences. Tools such as Cutadapt [37], Trimmomatic [38], TrimGalore (http://www.bioinformatics.babraham.ac.uk/projects/trim_galore/), FASTX-Toolkit (http://hannonlab.cshl.edu/fastx_toolkit/), which trim adapter or other contaminants based upon user-provided parameters, can be used for performing these operations. A brief description of some of these quality and data preprocessing tools is provided below:

FastQC: FastQC is a simple, easy-to-use tool that evaluates the quality of read data generated from the next generation sequencers. The input file/s for FastQC can be in Fastq, SAM, or BAM format either in the compressed or uncompressed form. FastQC reports basic statistics for the read data such as overrepresented sequences, k-mer content, base quality and content, adapter content, read duplication level, etc. FastQC is available as a stand-alone Java-based program with a graphical user interface and can be run from both Linux (using command line) and Windows systems.

PRINSEQ: PRINSEQ reports base quality, GC content, duplicates, adapters, presence of ambiguous sequences represented as "N," poly A tails, etc. Unlike FastQC, PRINSEQ also has the option of trimming and filtering reads. PRINSEQ is available as stand-alone as well as web application (http://prinseq.sourceforge.net/). It accepts uncompressed files in Fasta, Qual, and Fastq formats.

Trimmomatic: Trimmomatic is a Java-based program for the preprocessing of NGS read data (http://www.usadellab.org/cms/?page=trimmomatic). It can trim contaminant sequences, adapters, and filter reads based upon the quality. It supports compressed files in Fastq format and generates output in Fastq format. Because of its multithreading option, its data processing speed is higher than other tools available to perform the same function. Unlike some of the other tools, Trimmomatic can analyze both single-end as well as paired-end read data.

Cutadapt: Cutadapt is a python-based tool for read preprocessing and can be run as a command line application (https://cutadapt.readthedocs.org/en/stable). It accepts compressed files in Fasta, Qual, and Fastq formats, and supports both paired-end and single-end files. It trims low-quality bases, multiple adapter sequences from either 3', 5', or from both ends. In addition, Cutadapt can remove fixed number of bases from either ends of the sequences and supports demultiplexing, i.e., reads can be written to different output files depending upon the adapter sequence found in the reads. The demultiplexing feature is particularly useful since pooling multiple samples in a single run is an increasingly common practice as a result of increased sequencer throughput.

TrimGalore: TrimGalore is a wrapper tool written around FastQC and Cutadapt for quality check and adapter trimming for regular as well as MspI-digested RRBS-type (Reduced Representation Bisufite-Seq) libraries. It accepts compressed Fastq files and supports paired-end and single-end data.

FASTX-Toolkit: FASTX-Toolkit is a collection of tools that accepts read data in Fasta and Fastq file formats and trim the data based on base quality and adapter sequence contamination. Additionally, the toolkit has tools that can perform file format conversion, split sequences based upon barcodes, and generate reverse complement of sequences.

Once the read data are filtered and trimmed to remove low-quality bases, adapter sequence, and contaminants, they are ready for transcriptome assembly and profiling analysis. There are two different approaches for constructing full-length transcripts: reference-based assembly (when a reference genome is available) and *de novo* assembly (when the reference genome is not available), a computationally intensive and complex process (Table 2). Reference-based or genome-guided assembly refers to mapping sequenced reads to the reference genome followed by assembling the transcripts. In contrast, in *de novo* transcriptome assembly, transcripts are constructed directly from the overlapping sequenced reads. For the transcriptome assembly of organisms without reference genome, only *de novo* transcriptome assembly approach is available for transcriptome construction. However, for organisms with known reference genome, both reference-based and *de novo* transcriptome assembly can be employed for transcriptome construction. In fact, in this case, *de novo* transcriptome assembly will be more effective in filling in the gaps (observed due to variation in reference genome sequence and poor-quality annotation) and hence would complement the reference-based transcriptome assembly. More details on these two transcriptome assembly approaches are discussed in the following sections.

Reference-based assembly	*de novo* assembly
Reference genome is required to assemble the transcriptome	Transcriptome is assembled *de novo*
Relatively less computation- intensive	Computation- intensive
Contaminants and sequencing artifacts are not of major concern	Contaminants and sequencing artifacts can lead to poor quality of assembled transcriptome
Mapping quality of transcripts is dependent on splice aligners	Mapping is not required
Can assemble transcripts of low abundance	Difficult to assemble the transcripts of low abundance unless sequencing depth is high
Can work well with low sequencing depth data (~10X)	Work well with high sequencing depth data (~30X)
Less efficient in identifying novel isoforms and SNPs	Efficient in identifying novel isoforms and SNPs
Completeness and contiguity of transcriptome is relatively higher	Completeness and contiguity of transcriptome is relatively lower especially for low sequencing depth data

Table 2. Difference between reference-based and *de novo* assembly approaches

2.2. Transcriptome assembly

2.2.1. Reference-based transcriptome assembly and profiling

Typically, in a reference-based transcriptome profiling study, the computational workflow starts with aligning the quality-checked reads to the reference genome or transcriptome using a suitable read aligner. The aligned reads are then used to quantitate the genomic features (genes/isoforms). The quantity of the features needs to be normalized before comparison between different experimental conditions. The normalized feature counts are then used for drawing statistical inference on their difference in expression between samples under study. Finally, the differentially expressed set of genes is processed to derive biological insights relevant to the experimental setup. The success of this analysis depends very much on decisions that the user takes while choosing reference genome, annotation, tools, and associated parameter values at every step of the analysis. Steps involved in reference-based transcriptome assembly and analysis are described below.

2.2.1.1. Choice of reference build and annotation file

Reference genome and annotation files of a large number of species are available from a number of publicly available resources. Three of the most widely used resources are Ensembl (http://www.ensembl.org), the National Center of Biotechnology Information (NCBI; ftp:// ftp.ncbi.nih.gov/genomes), and UCSC genome browser (http://genome.ucsc.edu). Ensembl is jointly headed by the European Molecular Biology Laboratory – European Bioinformatics Institute (EMBL-EBI) and the Wellcome Trust Sanger Institute (WTSI). Ensembl generates genome annotation for vertebrates and other eukaryotic species, and the information is made freely available to the research community [39]. According to the latest Ensembl release 81, a total 23,636 genomes from 4,991 species are available. The NCBI also hosts genome sequence annotation data of over 1000 organisms including bacteria, archaea, eukaryote, viruses, phages, viroids, plasmids, and organelles. The UCSC genome browser is maintained by the UCSC Genome Bioinformatics group and provides data for over 90 organisms that belong to vertebrates, deuterostomes, insects, nematodes, yeast, viruses, and others [40]. In addition to the aforementioned data resources, Genome Reference Consortium (GRC), comprising of WTSI, the Genome Institute of Washington University (TGI), EBI, and NCBI ensures that the human, mouse, and zebrafish, and the genome assemblies of other model organisms are continuously updated and properly maintained.

Irrespective of the source, it is always recommended to use the latest genome sequence and its annotation. Zhao et al. [41] demonstrated that the choice of a gene model (annotation information/annotation catalog) has a dramatic effect on both gene quantification and differential analysis. We would recommend using Ensembl as it provides more detailed annotation of the genomic features.

2.2.1.2. Choice of read aligner

One of the most challenging parts of RNASeq analysis is mapping the sequencing reads to the genome correctly, especially for eukaryotes where presence of splicing events adds to the complexity. Multiple aligners, which can be divided into two categories, are available for aligning short-reads to the genome:

1. Non-spliced aligners: These aligners do not handle splicing events and are therefore suitable for prokaryotic RNASeq analysis only.

2. Spliced aligners: These aligners can place spliced reads across introns and determine exon–intron boundaries. Therefore, these are preferred for eukaryotic RNASeq analysis.

The non-spliced aligners can be further classified, on the basis of the algorithm used, into two categories:

• Hash table-based aligners: This set of aligners uses a seed sequence to identify alignment candidates, which are then either extended or discarded using more precise dynamic programming alignment algorithms. These aligners can be further divided, based upon the approach of finding a seed, into two groups:

   a. Reference indexing: Aligners create index using reference genome. Examples include BFAST [42], Novoalign (http://www.novocraft.com), GNUMAP [43], SHRiMP2 [44], Mosaik [45].

   b. Read indexing: Aligners use read-based index. Examples include MAQ [46], RMAP [47], and RazerS [48].

• FM-index-based aligners: This set of aligners creates FM-index of the genome using Burrows Wheeler Transform data compression algorithm. FM-index's compressed, yet searchable suffix array-like structure makes these aligners both memory-efficient and ultrafast. Examples include Bowtie1 [49], Bowtie2 [50], BWA [51], and SOAP2 [52].

Example of spliced aligners include GSNAP [53], MapSplice [54], SpliceMap [55], STAR [56], and TopHat2 [57]. GSNAP can identify a splice site in two ways: first, by evaluating the surrounding genomic sequence using probabilistic models of donor and acceptor splice site; second, by utilizing user-provided database of known exon–intron boundaries, which improves the sensitivity and specificity of the tool. Both MapSplice and TopHat2 use a two-step algorithm where in the first step potential splice sites are detected, which are then used in the second step to find correct map of reads. MapSplice is a *de novo* spliced aligner, whereas TopHat2 can perform both *de novo* and gene-annotation-based splice alignment. TopHat2 incorporates Bowtie1 or Bowtie2, in the back-end, for initial alignments. SpliceMap is also a *de novo* splice aligner, which is highly sensitive and specific in finding novel splice junctions without using any existing gene model information in arbitrary RNASeq read lengths. Another splice-aware aligner, STAR, utilizes sequential maximum mappable seed search in uncompressed suffix arrays followed by seed clustering and stitching procedure. It has been evaluated to be the fastest aligner among the above-listed spliced aligners with lowest false-positive rate at high sensitivity [56]. However, its RAM requirement is higher as compared to its counterparts.

The latest addition to the list of spliced aligners is HISAT (Hierarchical Indexing for Spliced Alignments of Transcripts) [58], which is claimed to be the fastest aligner currently available.

The reason for this highly efficient system is believed to be the indexing scheme it utilizes. As compared to its counterparts, HISAT uses two different types of indexes instead of a single index: (i) a whole-genome FM index to anchor each alignment, and (ii) numerous local FM indexes for very rapid extension of these alignments. HISAT is 50 times faster than TopHat2, 12 times faster than GSNAP, and slightly faster than STAR [56]. In addition, HISAT requires comparable amount of RAM as TopHat2 but maximum 20% of RAM as GSNAP or STAR needs. Similar to TopHat2, HISAT also uses Bowtie2 in the back-end. Furthermore, it is the only aligner that can work directly on an SRA file, which eliminates the sra to fastq file conversion requirement.

Considering the options available, selecting the right aligner is a nontrivial task and there are several publications comparing the read aligners. Fonseca et al. [59] published a feature-level comparison of 60 mappers and highlighted the difficulties in determining the best aligner (in terms of accuracy and speed). Other comparative studies include one by Lindner and Friedel [60] on non-spliced aligners and another by Engstrom et al. [61] on spliced aligners.

Answers to the following questions may help to choose a suitable aligner:

1.   Does the genome sequence belong to a prokaryote (where a gene lacks intron) or eukaryote (where a gene has introns)?

If the genome is bacterial (example of a prokaryote), then computationally intensive splice aligners such as TopHat2 or STAR are not required. In this case, non-splice aligners such as Bowtie1, Bowtie2, or BWA are more appropriate because of the contiguous read mapping to the reference genome. On the contrary, for eukaryotic genomes such as human/mouse, where the reads will span an exon boundary and therefore a part of it will not map contiguously on the reference genome; it is better to use a splice aligner that can identify splice sites.

2.   Are the sequence data available in base space or color space format?

If the data are generated from a SOLiD sequencing platform, they will be in color space format and almost all recently developed tools do not support color space data. In this case, the only available options are aligners such as BWA (older than 0.6.x), Bowtie1, and TopHat2.

3.   Does the aim of RNASeq experiment include calling variants in transcripts?

In experiments where the aim is to find variants in transcripts, mapping quality plays a crucial role, and hence it is advisable to use only aligners that provide accurate mapping quality. BWA and STAR aligners are suitable for this purpose; however, Bowtie 1 is not because it does not assign appropriate quality score to the mapped reads.

Additionally, one should also consider the comparative precision and recall statistics, CPU, and RAM requirements of the aligners. In addition to the aligners used, the data type itself plays a critical role in the quality of mapped data. For example, paired-end information improves mapping accuracy and, therefore, paired-end data are favored over single-end data for RNASeq experiment.

The aligned read data generated from aligners mentioned in the previous section are stored in Sequence Alignment/Map (SAM) file format, which is a gold standard to store alignment data. The SAM format has been created by the SAM/BAM format specification working group (https://samtools.github.io/hts-specs/SAMv1.pdf) for standardizing the format in which aligned data are stored. A SAM file contains information about the reference sequence name, query sequence name, alignment position and direction of the read on the genome, mapping quality, etc. However, SAM files are typically very large; hence, these files are converted into binary counterpart known as BAM (Binary of SAM) files. This is done typically using SAMtools [62], which provides a set of programs to manipulate the alignment files. Alignment files can be further manipulated with utilities such as SAMtools and Picard (http://broadinstitute.github.io/picard/) to efficiently retrieve reads and regions of interest.

2.2.1.3. Choice of annotation source

Depending upon the biological question of interest, one may wish to perform expression study either on known transcripts only, as per a given annotation catalog, or on reconstructed transcriptome built using a known reference annotation. This enables the quantification of novel genes/isoforms in addition to the known ones. In the first case, the mapped reads and the annotation catalog can be used to assign read counts to each feature (genes/transcripts) using a tool like htseq-count [63], and then perform statistical analysis to identify the differentially expressed genes/isoforms. In the second case, transcriptome reconstruction is required prior to differential expression analysis. It requires assembly of reads into transcription units using either the reference-based or de novo assembly approach. Given a reference genome and an annotation catalog, there are tools such as Cufflinks [64, 65] that first map all the reads to the genome and then use spliced reads directly to reconstruct the transcriptome. It generates a GTF file that contains the assembled isoforms along with isoform-level relative abundance in Fragments Per Kilobase of exon model per Million mapped fragments (FPKM) units [65].

2.2.2. De novo transcriptome assembly

Building a transcriptome using *de novo* methods is a powerful way to create the transcriptome of a divergent or novel species. Mainly three features affect the quality of assembled transcripts: a) type of transcript: presence of repeats, polymorphisms, splicing event, complexity of organism, e.g., ploidy level, GC content; b) sequencing technology: library preparation, sequencing accuracy; c) bioinformatics workflow: assembly algorithms and annotation. Currently available *de novo* assemblers have different sensitivity, and specificity in terms of transcript identification are error-prone, and lead to fused transcripts, splicing errors, and gaps [66]. In order to enhance the sensitivity and specificity one can take the combined approach, which employs *de novo* assembly method with reference-guided approach.

2.2.2.1. De novo assembly approaches

There are several algorithms available for *de novo* transcriptome assembly (Table 3). In *de novo* transcriptome assembly, contigs or transfragments are created from overlapping reads. Process of assembly involves either de Bruijn graphs construction using k-mers or overlap-layout-consensus (OLC) approach for short and long reads, respectively [67].

Tool name	Algorithm	Read type	Reference
Trinity	de Bruijn graph	Single and Paired end	[78]
Velvet-Oases	de Bruijn graph	Single and Paired end	[74, 77]
SOAPdenovo-Trans	de Bruijn graph	Single and Paired end	[80]
IDBA-tran	de Bruijn graph	Paired end	[178]
Trans-ABySS	de Bruijn graph	Single and Paired end	[79]
EBARDe novo	Extension, Bridging, and Repeat-sensing *de novo*	Paired end	[179]
Bayesembler	Bayesian model	Paired end	[180]
Mira	Overlap graph	Single and Paired end	[68]

Table 3. A list containing different *de novo* transcriptome assemblers

Overlap-Layout-Consensus (OLC) approach:

OLC approach was initially developed for reconstruction of the genome from Sanger sequence and EST (Expressed sequenced tag) data. As the name suggests, in the OLC approach, the read data are searched for overlapping sequences and merged to create longer reads. Depending on the volume of data and complexity of genome (e.g., repeats), the OLC approach is computation- intensive. Some of the OLC-based assemblers are MIRA [68], Newbler (from Roche/454 Life Sciences), and CAP3 [69]. The assemblers using the OLC approach are more suitable for small volume of data, not sensitive to repeat region detection and resolution, and cannot handle the high-depth short read data generated from sequencers such as Illumina. The Eulerian path assemblers, which are based on *de Bruijn* graph algorithms [70], are more suitable for the high-depth short read data and are discussed in detail below.

De Bruijn-graph-based approach:

De Bruijn graph is a mathematical graph that uses a substring of letters (here nucleotides) of length k to represent nodes. Nodes are connected if shifting a substring by one nucleotide creates an exact k-1 overlap between the nodes [70]. *De Bruijn* graph can be created for both small as well as large sequences. Based upon the defined k-mer (a nucleotide substring of length k) length, reads are broken in k-length to generate substrings. Using these substrings, *de Bruijn* graph is generated in which each unique substring represents a node (or vertex) connected with overlaps between the last k-1 nucleotides of the previous sequence with the first k-1 nucleotides of the subsequent sequence [71]. Identical overlaps of k-mers are merged and counted while creating the graph. If the assembler finds differences in the nodes, the graph is branched. Upon subsequent identity and overlap in the nodes, the graph will join the ends. Presence of single nucleotide difference between the sequence data gives rise to bubbles in the graph. In the case of RNASeq data, occurrence of large bubbles and open-ended branches in the graph suggests presence of alternative splicing and alternative transcription start and end. Occurrence of small bubbles can be due to single nucleotide variation or sequencing errors [72]. In most of the *de Bruijn*-graph-based assemblers, the preferred value of k-mer is usually an odd number in order to avoid reverse complement of k-mers. The chosen size of k-mer has great impact on the assembly process as using a large k-mer can result in a unique *de Bruijn* graph, but this approach is computationally intensive. On the other hand, using small k-mers can result in a fragmented assembly. According to some of the previous studies it has been observed that smaller k-mers can be useful in more accurate transcriptome assembly of lowly expressed genes whereas larger k-mers perform better for abundant transcripts [73-75]. It is therefore essential to identify the optimal k-mer for the sequence being assembled and it depends to a large extent on the read length, sequencing depth, sequencing error rate, and the complexity of the genome. Additionally, using directionality of the read from paired-end data, assemblers can generate more accurate assembly as compared to single-end data [76]. Some of the most commonly used *de Bruijn*-graph-based assemblers are: Velvet/Oases [74, 77], Trinity [78], Trans-Abyss [79], SOAPdenovo-Trans [80].

Oases: Oases has a set of algorithms that post-processes the assembly generated by Velvet at different k-mers such as dynamic filtering of the noise, resolution of alternative splicing transcripts, and merging of the multiple assemblies generated using different k-mers (www.ebi.ac.uk/~zerbino/oases/). Data generated from different k-mers are merged to generate a complete assembly. Oases works well for the correction of errors and resolution of repeats in the case of paired-end data.

Trinity: Trinity uses three steps to produce transcriptome assembly: inchworm, chrysalis, and butterfly. Inchworm builds initial sets of contigs using k-mer graphs. Chrysalis groups these contigs and builds *de Bruijn* graphs from them. Butterfly simplifies and resolves the graphs to generate the final set of transcripts containing spliced variants and isoforms.

Trans-Abyss: Trans-Abyss considers multiple assemblies generated from Abyss to optimize the assembly and can tackle varying coverage of the transcripts very well.

SOAPdenovo-Trans: SOAPdenovo-Trans is derived from the genome assembler, SOAPdenovo2 [81] and is known to construct transcriptome faster than the above-mentioned assemblers.

2.2.2.2. Choosing the transcriptome assembler

Choosing an assembly algorithm is difficult as it depends on a number of factors such as read type, length, and complexity of the genome. Some instrument vendors such as Roche provide assembly algorithms, e.g., Newbler, which can handle the long read data and the homopolymer issue frequently observed in the data generated from 454. A recent study using peanut plant RNASeq data suggests that performance of Trinity is better than TransAByss and SOAPdenovo-Trans when raw reads are mapped to the reconstructed assembly of the polyploidy transcriptome [82]. Another study suggested use of multiple k-mers and clustering of k-mer assemblies and at the same time identifying unique contigs from each assembly for effective extraction of biological information from transcriptome assembly [83].

2.2.2.3. Assessing quality and accuracy of de novo assembled transcriptome

Because of sequencing errors and presence of repeats in the genome, it is hard to achieve a perfect assembly. Moreover, different assemblers use different heuristic approaches to assemble the transcriptome, which results in different number of identified transcripts.

Quality and accuracy of assembled transcriptome are assessed in several different ways [84, 85]:

1. Assembly statistics: Most algorithms generate an assembly statistic that includes the number of contigs/transfragments generated, total contigs/transfragments length and singletons, size of the assembly (in number of nucleotides), percentage of reads assembled to transfragments, percent GC content, etc. Assembly statistics provide overview of the organisms' transcriptome.

2. Transfragments/contigs statistics: This statistics includes lengths of the largest and shortest transfragments, average and median length of transfragments, and N50 of assembled transcriptome. N50 of the assembly is calculated by sorting the contigs in descending order and the size of the contig that makes the total greater than or equal to 50% of the genome size is regarded as the N50 value. A large N50 is indicative of a more contiguous assembly.

3. Mis-assembly and variations: Some of the major reasons for mis-assembly of the transcriptome are presence of ambiguous bases, repeat regions, insertions, deletions, SNPs, and chromosomal rearrangements in the transcriptome. Percentage of mis-assembled contigs can be calculated by mapping the contigs back to the reference genome. QUAST, a tool, generates consolidated report on mis-assembly statistics [84].

4. Number of transfragments matching with the closest reference genome: Once transcripts are assembled, it can be compared against a closely related species/genome. Assembly is considered to be of high quality if the number of reference transcripts matching with the transfragments is high. However, the genes that are not expressed, or lowly expressed, might not be captured.

5. Hybrid or fused transcripts: Hybrid transcripts result from joining of two or more different transcripts and hence matching to different locations of the genome. Reasons for hybrid transcript generation are sequencing error, improper trimming of the adapter/contaminant from the raw read, similarity of the transcripts, assembly algorithm's parameters, etc. Low number of hybrid transcripts reflects better assembly.

2.3. Quantification

Choice of expression unit: CPM, RPKM, FPKM, TPM, or read count

Once the read data is aligned to the reference genome, the gene expression can be quantitated by read counting at exon, transcript, or gene-level. Here are few possible expression units:

a. Read Count: read counts are number of reads overlapping a genomic feature such as a gene or transcript.

b. CPM (Counts Per Million mapped reads): CPMs are read counts scaled by the number of fragments sequenced times one million. This unit is used in a differential expression analysis R package edgeR [86].

c. RPKM (Reads Per Kilobase of transcript per Million): RPKM for a feature is computed by dividing the number of read counts by it length and total number of reads sequenced, followed by multiplication with one billion [12]. Applicable only for single-end data.

d. FPKM (Fragments Per Kilobase of transcript per Million): similar as RPKM. But takes into account a fragment (not reads) [65]. For pair-end data, there will be two reads for a single fragment of genome while for single-end data, there will be one read for a single fragment. Both the situations will add only one count.

e. TPM (Transcripts Per Million): TPM for a transcript is calculated by dividing the ratio of its read counts over its length by the summation of ratios for all the transcripts, and multiplying with one million [87]. Especially for transcript abundance.

2.4. Normalization

Why should one normalize the expression data?

RNASeq experiments have multiple sources of systematic variations introduced through inter-sample differences such as difference in library size (sequencing depth) or unwanted variations due to batch effects such as sampling time or different sequencing technology [12] or through intra-sample differences such as difference in read length [88] or GC content between genes [89, 90]. These variations, if ignored, can dramatically reduce the accuracy of statistical inference and hence should be removed or controlled during statistical analysis. Therefore, read count and FPKM of a feature, as calculated for example by htseq-count and Cufflinks, respectively, may not be appropriate to compare across features and samples without normalization.

Normalization is a process that aims to ensure that expression estimates are comparable. There are a number of normalization methods, such as:

a. Total Count: each read count of a feature expression is divided by total number of mapped reads in that sample and multiplied by the average total count across all the samples.

b. Upper Quartile: each feature expression is divided by the upper quartile of expression values, other than 0, in that sample and multiplied by the average upper quartile across all the samples [91]. Upper quartile for FPKMs or fragment counts has been implemented in Cuffdiff2 tool from Cufflinks suite [92].

c. Median: each feature expression is divided by the median of these expression values (other than 0) in that sample and multiplied by the average median expression across all the samples.

d. Quantile: the distribution of expression values for each sample is made identical [93]. Quantile method is available in R package limma [94].

e. Trimmed Mean of M-values (TMM): TMM normalization factor for each sample is computed as the weighted mean of log ratios between a test sample and a reference sample after excluding the features with highest expressions and features with largest log ratios. These factors are rescaled by the mean of normalized library sizes. Finally, each feature expression value is divided by these rescaled normalization factors to get the normalized expression [86, 95]. TMM method has been implemented in R package edgeR [86].

f.   Median of ratio: the normalization factor for each sample is computed as the median of ratios of expressions of features over their geometric means across all samples. Finally, each feature expression is divided by this factor to get the normalized expression [96]. Median of ratio has been implemented in R packages DESeq [96], DESeq2 [97], and in Cuffdiff2 [92].

Several publications [98, 99] comparing normalization methods suggest that median of ratio is the best method for normalization in differential expression study for mRNASeq experiment.

In addition to normalization methods, several packages have been developed to control batch effects, for example, svaseq [100]. svaseq can work on both, count-based data (e.g., htseq-count generated data) as well as FPKMs (Cufflinks generated data).

2.5. Differential expression analysis

Differential expression analysis helps identify genes that are important in the experimental conditions being tested and hence is the most routine analysis performed using the RNASeq data. In RNASeq data, a linear relationship has been observed between the number of reads that map to a transcript and the abundance of the transcript [12]. The goal of differential expression analysis is to compare these read counts for a feature between distinct sample groups and perform a statistical test to determine whether the difference is significant. For this purpose, a distribution is required to be fitted to the count data using generalized linear model (GLM). Based upon the assumption that reads are independently sampled from a population with a given, fixed fractions of genes, it can be said that the read counts will follow a multinomial distribution. This multinomial distribution can be approximated by the Poisson distribution and therefore Poisson distribution has been used to test differential expression in several studies [101-103]. But it has been found that this distribution predicts smaller variations than what is seen in the data. To overcome this issue, negative binomial (NB) distribution and beta negative binomial distribution were proposed. NB has been used in several differential expression tools such as edgeR [86], DESeq [96], DESeq2 (an enhanced version of DESeq) [97], and BaySeq [104]. Though these tools use a common distribution, the method of variance (dispersion) estimation differs, which affects the final outcome of the analysis. Cuffdiff2 uses beta negative binomial distribution to fit fragment counts [92].

Recent advances in this area of research suggest that a combination of Poisson distribution and NB distribution may yield better results. Chen et al. [105] derived a novel algorithm XBSeq from DESeq, where they used Poisson distribution to fit read counts that map to nonexonic regions (considered as sequencing noise) and used NB distribution to fit read counts that map to exonic regions (considered as true signals).

Recently, limma [94], a well-known R package for performing differential expression analysis of microarray data, has been empowered with RNASeq data analysis ability. It does not use the above-mentioned distribution, rather converts count data (or normalized count data) to log-counts per million using voom transformation, then fits a linear model to this data and performs differential expression analysis using an empirical Bayes method.

There is no clear evidence as such about the best tool for differential expression analysis; however, multiple studies comparing available methods have been performed. Soneson and Delorenzi [106] evaluated and compared eleven methods for differential expression analysis on simulated and real RNASeq data, whereas Seyednasrollah et al. [107] compared eight widely used tools on real data sets. Both the studies concluded that no single method is optimal under all circumstances. Soneson and Delorenzi [106] observed that limma performed well under many different conditions and Seyednasrollah et al. [107] found limma and DESeq as the preferred choice. Additionally, these studies have suggested that the method of choice should depend on the experimental conditions that include the number of samples per condition.

2.6. Annotation and pathway analysis

2.6.1. Annotation of de novo assembled transcriptome

In addition to transcriptome abundance calculation after mapping the assembled contigs/ transfragments to the assembled transcriptome or reference genome and differential expression data analysis, coding regions within *de novo* assembled transcripts can be searched using ORF predictor tools such as Transdecoder (http://transdecoder.github.io/). Further, homologous gene/protein identification of assembled transcripts can be done using tools such as BLAT and BLAST [108].

2.6.2. Making sense of the differentially expressed gene list

List of differentially expressed genes is just the first tangible outcome of an RNASeq experiment. In order to derive biological insight from this list of genes, it is important to identify functional categories of the genes that are differentially expressed and the biological pathways that are enriched as a result of these differentially expressed genes. In order to do so, enrichment analysis is typically performed using publicly available resources such as GO (Biological Processes and Molecular Functions) databases [109], KEGG pathways [110], BioCarta (www.biocarta.com), and Reactome [111].

In a review article, Khatri et al. [112] elaborated the current approaches of pathway analysis and their challenges and divided the existing approaches into three generations:

a.   First Generation: Overrepresentation Analysis (ORA) approach

This approach statistically evaluates the fraction of genes, among the set of differentially expressed genes, in a particular pathway. There are many tools that follow this approach, for example, Onto-Express [113], GenMAPP [114], GoMiner [115], and DAVID [116, 117]. However, this approach has certain limitations. For example, it does not consider the fold change values associated with the genes, thereby ignoring the extent of regulation. Moreover, it does not consider the gene product interactions that are found in a pathway. This approach also ignores the dependency between the pathways.

b.   Second Generation: Functional Class Scoring (FCS) approach

This approach addresses few limitations of ORA. It considers all the genes and their expression for pathway enrichment, so as to take into consideration the coordinated changes (irrespective of the magnitude) unlike ORA where only differentially expressed genes were considered and that too without considering their expression levels. Example of such tools include global test [118], GSEA [119].

But this approach too has some limitations. Similar to ORA, this approach ignores the dependency between the pathways and the interaction between gene products in a given pathway.

c.   Third Generation: Pathway Topology (PT)-based approach

To overcome the limitations of ORA and FCS, the Pathway-Topology-based approach has been devised. It uses pathway knowledgebase to include pathway topology information for enrichment analysis [112]. This information includes genes that are interacting, their mode of interaction (e.g, activation, inhibition), and their location of interaction (e.g, cytoplasm, nucleus). SPIA [120], an R package, is an example of this category of pathway analysis approach, which combines evidence of pathway overrepresentation and unusual signaling perturbations. NetGSA [121] is another method in this category that takes into consideration the change in correlation as well as the change in network structure as experimental condition changes. However, in the absence of high-resolution knowledge databases that can provide knowledge for all conditions, tissue- and cell-specific functions of a gene product; the true pathway topology is rarely inferred. And hence this restricts a researcher to investigate the dynamic states of a system [112].

2.7. Visualization

Analyzed RNASeq data can be visualized in many different ways. Several tools such as Cummerbund (an R package), RNAseqViewer for single and multiple sample visualization [122], HeatmapGenerator for heatmap visualization, GOexpress for GO term enrichment visualization   (http://www.bioconductor.org/packages/devel/bioc/html/GOexpress.html), RNASeq-specific genome viewers such as RNASeqExpressionBrowse [123], and RNASeq-Browser [124] are available for RNASeq data visualization.

We have recently developed SanGeniX (www.sangenix.com), an easy-to-use client-server-based NGS data analysis application with a highly intuitive user interface (manuscript under preparation). SanGeniX supports primary, secondary, and tertiary analysis of sequence data from Illumina, Ion Torrent, SOliD, and PacBio RS. SanGeniX integrates multiple robust and validated algorithms in the form of predefined workflows and offers flexibility to construct custom workflows for RNASeq (reference-based as well as *de novo*), genome assembly, ChIPSeq and DNASeq (for SNP and CNV calling). For example, in the case of RNASeq workflow, the analysis starts with quality check (using tool FastQC), contaminant/adapter trimming and removal (using Cutadapt and in-house scripts), read mapping using splice aware aligners (using STAR, TopHat2), transcript quantification, differential expression analysis (using Cufflinks packages and DESeq2), and gene ontology, as well as pathway enrichment analysis (using GoMiner) (Figure 2). Further, graphically enriched visuals such as heatmap based on clustering, scatter plot, and volcano plot for differentially expressed genes, pie chart on gene-ontology-based annotation, visualization of read data in the genome viewer, etc., are generated for easy interpretation of the data (Figure 3). These figures and underlying data can be downloaded in svg, png, and tsv formats. Moreover, the raw output files such as output of mapping in SAM and BAM formats can also be downloaded. The executed workflows can be shared with peers, rerun after changing parameters or tools. SanGeniX is available as cloud-hosted as well as on premise solution and supported on multiple Linux platforms such as Ubuntu, CentOS, and RedHat.

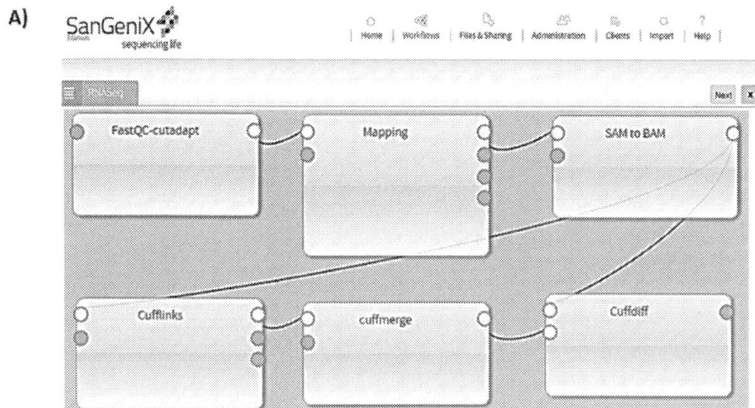

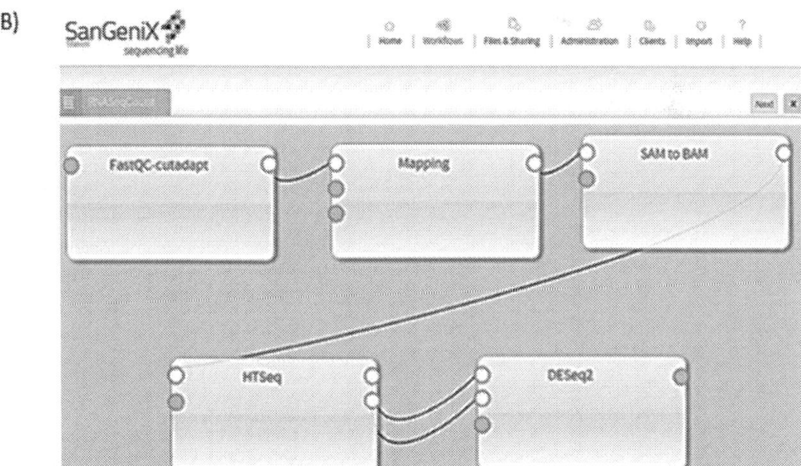

Figure 2. Snapshots of RNASeq data analysis workflow canvas in SanGeniX using (A) Cufflinks package and (B) HTSeq and DESeq2 are shown.

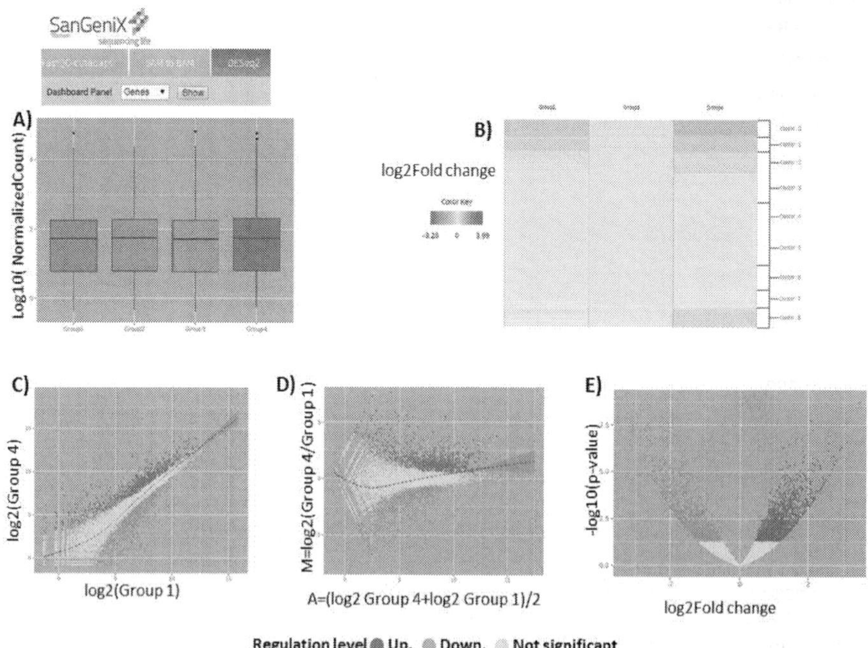

Figure 3. Snapshots from RNASeq results dashboard from SanGeniX for an experiment consisting of four groups (or samples). (A) Boxplot: It displays distribution of normalized expression values among different groups. Similar distribution of normalized expression values among the different groups of interest indicates that any technical biases due to difference in sequencing depth have been taken care of. (B) Heatmap is a convenient way to visualize cluster of genes based upon their expression. Here, log2 fold change of genes in three groups with respect to a reference group, Group1 has been plotted. The color-code helps to infer gene expression level. Scatter plot (C), MA plot (D), and Volcano plot (E) present visual investigation of differentially expressed genes between two conditions, for example, here Group 4 and Group 1. Scatter plot helps to quickly compare the expression of a gene between the two conditions, while MA plot depicts trends of difference in expression over the average expression, and Volcano plot helps to spot genes by considering both fold change and test statistic.

3. Challenges in RNASeq data generation and analysis

As described above, NGS-based transcriptomic data generation and analysis is a complex and multistep process. Every step has some key challenges that hinder the data analysis.

3.1. Library preparation

The process of library preparation is generating cDNA from the large RNA fragments, adding the adapters, and amplifying the cDNA for sequencing. Due to a series of experimental reactions, several biases can be introduced in the library preparation step. In majority of the cases, fragmentation of RNA or DNA, which plays an important role in the preparation of high-quality sequencing library, is done using physical or enzymatic methods or chemical shearing. The fragmentation of RNA has even coverage in the gene body and hence it is biased toward the gene body as compared to the 5′ and 3′ ends where the coverage is relatively depleted [20]. The library preparation step is further complicated by the presence of several identical short reads and hence duplicate sequences in the library could arise from abundance of RNA molecules. Another source of duplicate sequences in a library could be due to PCR artifacts. These two different scenarios can be assessed by considering biological replicates in the study. In the case of total RNAseq, abundance of ribosomal RNA (rRNA) dominates sequenced reads and hence creates bias if not removed.

3.2. Sequencing platform

Sequencing platforms are available from multiple vendors such as Illumina (http://www.illumina.com/), Life Technologies (https://www.lifetechnologies.com/), and Pacific Biosciences (www.pacificbiosciences.com/), and each of the platforms has its set of advantages and disadvantages [35]. In choosing a sequencing platform, some of the factors to be considered are sequencing length, sequencing type (single end or paired end), throughput, error rate, and type of errors in the generated sequence data. The gigabytes of short reads generated from the current platforms are not error-free, which affects the downstream analysis and interpretation. For transcriptome assembly, the larger read length (such as produced from 454, PacBio) is preferred over short read length (as produced by Illumina) as it will result in assembly of the high-quality and reliable transcripts. However, both 454 and PacBio platforms have limited throughput and hence the approach most commonly used is to generate data from multiple platforms and combine the data during analysis.

3.3. Mapping

Accurate mapping of RNASeq reads is a challenging issue because of large data volume, slow mapping speed, false-positive splicing events and incorrect estimation of exon–intron boundaries, large genome size, repeat sequences in the genome, and annotation quality of the genome. Usually, aligners search for introns smaller than a fixed length to reduce the computational power, which often leads to missing the splice reads spanning longer introns [66]. Multiple mapping of reads is another major problem that can be due to presence of repeat regions, similar sequences, and number of mismatches allowed in the mapping step. If such reads mapping to multiple regions are discarded, it will lead to gap in the regions that cannot be mapped uniquely, and if it is included, it can lead to false-positive transcription status. Reference-based assembly cannot efficiently detect trans-spliced genes that are formed from splicing and joining of two different precursor mRNAs and found in some disease conditions such as cancer [125, 126]. Additionally, aligners have to cope with sequencing errors, SNP, InDels, other genomics variations and parameters-based, suboptimal mapping outcome. In summary, mapping-based RNASeq analysis can be more effective and complete when reads are long, genome is well-annotated, and it can be combined with *de novo* genome assembly to identify novel transcripts.

3.4. Read quantification for the estimation of gene expression

Once the sequenced reads are aligned, gene expression is measured. The most common way of read quantification is counting the number of reads overlapping the exons of a gene and if the exon boundaries are not well-annotated, it may lead to false-positive hits. Another major challenge in read quantification is reads mapping to multiple locations.

3.5. Count normalization

There are several methods such as quantile-based normalization, GC-content-based normalization, Poisson model with variable rates for different positions, available to normalize and correct the biasness in the count data for the improved detection of differentially expressed genes [91, 127, 128]. The increasing number of normalization methods requires a state-of-the-art technique for comparing these methods. In the absence of such technique, there is no consensus on the best method for normalization. For example, Zyprych-Walczak et al. [99] found that TMM method worked poorly for them while Dillies et al. [98] found TMM and median of ratio methods to be the best as compared to other methods. The transcript length is another source of bias and leads to detection of more differential expression in longer transcripts compared to shorter transcripts [88].

3.6. Differential expression analysis

There are several tools and methods developed for the differential expression analysis comparing differences in gene expression in different conditions (see section 2). Nonparametric methods are not capable of better differential expression detection in the absence of sample replicates and hence parametric methods are preferred for differential expression analysis [129]. A study comparing various differential expression methods suggests that there is no optimized method that can serve well for all the different conditions. As compared to other tools, Cuffdiff performed poorly with large number of false-positives [130]. The accuracy of differentially expressed genes is statistically significant and makes more sense if multiple replicates are used in the analysis.

Similar to the situation as in normalization, picking up the best tool for differential analysis is a tricky job. This is because there is no consensus about the tool best-suited for all experimental setups. Soneson and Dolerenzi [106] found limma performing well under many conditions but it required at least three replicates. Furthermore, they found limma performing worse when dispersion differed between two conditions. They also observed that with large sample sizes DESeq was overly conservative, while edgeR was producing large number of false-positives.

3.7. *De novo* assembly

The performance and accuracy of the *de novo* transcriptome assembly is largely dependent on the complexity of the genome (e.g., genome size, number of paralogs, ploidy level), differential read coverage of the sequenced data, and sequencing error. Transcriptome assembly is complex and different from genome assembly in which read coverage is uniform. In contrast, in RNASeq, the abundance of reads vary based upon gene expression, in which case isoforms originating from same gene can have different expression levels and hence poses significant challenge in estimating the abundance especially for the lowly expressed genes if the sequencing depth is too low. In general, *de novo* transcriptome requires much higher sequencing depth than the reference-based transcriptome assembly.

The *de novo* transcriptome assembly generally consumes more time and is more computation-intensive than reference-based assembly [131]. The number of transfragments produced using the *de novo* approach is quite high, which can be due to multiple similar transcripts/isoforms at the locus from allelic variation, or could be due to artifacts. Additionally, the contiguity and completeness of the *de novo* assembled transcriptome is less than the reference-based assembly especially for the data with less sequencing depth [132].

3.8. Deep sequencing versus cost

Another challenge associated with the RNASeq technology is read coverage and cost associated with it. In order to detect lowly expressed genes or rare variants in the coding region, high read coverage is required. According to Nagalakshmi et al. [10], for simple organism such as yeast, which does not undergo alternative splicing, 30 million reads are sufficient to observe genome-wide transcriptome profile [10]. But for larger and complex genomes such as the human genome, higher-depth RNASeq data are required in order to capture the complete transcriptomes. Moreover, in a given organism the number of transcripts expressed in different conditions is different and hence same coverage may not be sufficient to capture all the transcripts expressed under different conditions. Hence, before designing an experiment, one should be aware of both sequencing depth required and the number of samples to be sequenced. If the aim of experiment is to detect rare variants or lowly expressed genes, one should go for high coverage of the transcriptome, whereas, if the aim of the experiment is focused on gene expression differences between different samples (or conditions), one should consider generating replicate data for statistical power [133].

There are other bioinformatics challenges such as data retrieval, storing, unavailability of optimized statistical methods, and high-end compute infrastructure requirement that add to the complexity of transcriptome analysis.

4. Applications of RNASeq

RNASeq provides an unprecedented view into the complexity of the transcriptome and hence is a powerful tool to characterize and profile transcriptome on a genome-wide scale. Some of these applications with detailed examples are discussed below.

4.1. Transcriptome profiling of economically important plants

Understanding the transcriptome and the functional elements of the economically important plants can provide tremendous insights into biological entities, critical for traits such as disease resistance, productivity, and characteristics such as flavor. Recently, Hu et al. [134] performed transcriptome assembly and annotation for the spice black pepper. Black pepper is one of the most widely used fruit for adding flavor to food as well for its medicinal properties. The authors were able to identify genes that might participate in piperidine, quinolizidine, indolizidine, and lycopodium alkaloid biosynthesis, of which piperidine alkaloids account for pungent taste and medicinal properties of black pepper. Similarly, Shudeesh et al. [135] performed assembly and annotation of field pea, a legume that is cultivated worldwide for human as well as livestock consumption. Studies have also been undertaken to identify transcriptomes of the pathogens that infect economically important plants and the defense mechanisms deployed by the plants. For example, the transcriptome of coffee leaf rust pathogen Hemileia vastatrix was sequenced by Talhinhas et al. [136] to identify genes/ pathways that play a key role in the early stage of the infection, and Yang et al. [137] sequenced the sand pear germplasm with differential resistance to infection by *Alternaria alternata* to identify genes that contribute toward the resistance.

4.2. Transcriptome profiling of economically important animals

Similar to the value provided by transcriptome profiling of plants, transcriptome profiling of economically important animals contributes toward better understanding of disease resistance, productivity, breeding, quality of meat, etc., in animals. Ropka-Molik et al. [138] have used the NGS transcriptome profiling approach to identify genes that are differentially expressed between two pig breeds with differences in muscularity that could contribute toward the quality of meat. Gene expression profiles have been generated from different breeds of cows to identify genes that contribute toward milk protein and fat percentage in cow milk [139, 140] and milk yield [141]. Transcriptome profiling has also been used very recently to identify the genes that are differentially expressed in silkworms (*B. mori*) undergoing thermal parthenogenesis [142]. Thermal parthenogenesis is a process that is used in silkworm breeding and selection.

4.3. Cancer

Cancer is a complex and heterogeneous genetic disorder that results from either inherited or somatic genetic variations such as single nucleotide variations (SNV), insertions, deletions, copy number variations, dysregulation of gene expression, and epigenetic modifications. As changes in the gene expression pattern play a key role in tumorigenicity [143], metastasis [144], prognosis [145], and relapse [146, 147], gene expression profiling has been used extensively in cancer research and diagnosis. OncotypeDx (http://www.oncotypedx.com/) is a gene-expression-based commercially available test that is used for breast cancer, colon cancer, and prostate cancer diagnosis and prognosis.

Contrary to microarrays and RT-PCR-based approaches used earlier, RNASeq, which can detect coding and noncoding RNA, strand orientation, and genetic variants all in one go, is a very powerful tool in deciphering the complex transcriptome changes usually found in cancer. One of the most comprehensive studies published recently is the transcriptome profiling of 4043 Cancers and 548 Normal Tissue Controls across 12 TCGA Cancer Types [148]. In this study, in addition to identifying tissue specific gene signature, the authors were able to identify a 14-gene signature that accurately distinguished the cancer samples from the normal. Using a whole transcriptome sequencing approach, Koh et al. [149] recently reported 14 candidate genes that are important in rhabdoid glioblastoma (R-GBM) tumor, a rare form of GBM. Similarly, RNASeq approach was used to identify gene signature in flow-sorted viable EpCAM + tumor epithelial cells and CD45+ tumor-infiltrating immune cells that were obtained from cervical cancer samples [150]. The authors identified TCL1A as a novel biomarker, found specifically in the immune cells, for predicting survival in cervical cancer patients.

The aforementioned studies highlight the varied approaches that can be used for identifying biomarkers or gene signatures associated with distinct cancer characteristics.

4.4. Reproductive health

With the advancing parental age and a desire to limit the number of pregnancies, many couples opt for assisted reproduction for childbearing. The advanced parental age is a key factor that contributes toward the complications in assisted reproduction, and genomics-based approaches are widely used to ensure a high success rate. Gene expression changes in ovarian granulosa cells in women >35 years of age include downregulation of polo-like kinase pathway, which plays an important role in cell cycle arrest of granulosa cells, and the G2/GM checkpoint pathway [151]. Another very recent study also used the RNASeq approach to identify differential gene expression profiles in women with successful pregnancy and a failed pregnancy through assisted reproduction [152]. The authors found that the genes that were differentially expressed played a role in immune response and inflammation, oocyte meiosis, and rhythmic process.

The application of RNASeq in reproductive health is relatively new and as more knowledge is gleaned through this, it might be possible to develop a signature that can be used for predicting the success of assisted reproductive approach.

4.5. Developmental disorders

Developmental disorders are ones in which the child develops slower than peers in areas such as motor function, social skills, and cognitive ability. Developmental disorders include Austism, Asperger's Syndrome, Attention Deficit Hyperactivity Disorder (ADHD), Rett Syndrome, and stereotypic movement disorder, to name a few. Gene expression profiling has been used extensively in Austism and genes involved in neuronal action potential, myelination, axon ensheathment, cellular development, and cellular proliferation have been found to be differentially expressed in autistic children [153]. Another study, using an *in vitro* model of Autism found expression differences in genes involved in cell proliferation, neuronal differentiation, and synaptic assembly [154]. Similarly, a gene expression study in Rett Syndrome [155], which is a rare variant of Austism, has identified genes involved in mitochondrial functions, cellular protein metabolic processes, and RNA processing and DNA organization to be differentially regulated.

In addition to the applications listed here, gene expression profiling can be used in number of other human disorders such as diabetes, hypertension, psychiatric disorders, and infectious diseases.

5. Future perspective

RNASeq technology is proving to be a valuable tool to study known and novel transcripts of an organism by providing more insights into the role of gene expression in development, differential expression between different conditions, changes in gene expression in disease progression, alternative splicing events, RNA editing, fusion transcripts, allele-specific expression, etc. This technology is revolutionizing the field of plant and animal transcriptome, where many of the species lack reference genome because of genome size and complexity. Metatranscriptomic-NGS technology employed to study microbial transcriptome is another emerging area of research in which construction of transcriptome assembly has led to simultaneous identification of thousands of transcripts from the microbial community of the human gastrointestinal tract [156], and the marine [157, 158] and soil [159]. Because of the fact that gene expression levels vary significantly from one cell to another, researchers are now moving toward single-cell transcriptomics, in which cell-to-cell variability on a genome-wide scale can be profiled. Hence, transcriptome of single cell can be probed more efficiently as compared to cell population where average transcript abundance of population is seen [160, 161]. A recent study by Sasagawa et al. developed the method Quartz-Seq for individual cell isolation followed by RNA sequencing and distinguished mouse embryonic stem cells from primitive endoderm based upon transcriptome profile as well as cell-to-cell stochastic variation [162]. Another recently developed method, RaceID, is very useful in identifying rare cell types in healthy and diseased tissues using mRNA sequencing [163]. Tissue-specific RNASeq is another emerging area of research that can reveal tissue-specific requirement of RNA expression. A recent study done on 13 different cell types discovered many tissue-specific and novel miRNAs, which suggests that the repertoire of human miRNA is more extensive than our current knowledge [164]. RNASeq is used as a powerful tool for clinical application as well. A recent study developed exome capture RNASeq protocol for degraded clinical formalin-fixed samples, which has shown to work successfully on prostate cancer samples suggesting that capture transcriptome study can be used beyond cell lines and in the clinical setting [165].

Moreover, there are several publicly available RNASeq data repositories such as ENCODE (https://www.**encode**project.org/), TCGA (www.cancergenome.nih.gov), and The Geuvadis Project (http://www.geuvadis.org/), which provide enormous amount of data to researchers to conduct genome-wide analyses beyond traditional gene expression and profiling analysis. Mining data from public repositories will provide new insights into the transcriptome and hence enable researchers to gain more information on gene regulation, which has been previously neglected.

Sequencing method and experimental protocols are also continuously improving to reduce the challenges associated with the technology. Platforms such as PacBio can produce a full-length transcript in a single read, which can eventually eliminate the transcript assembly step of the data analysis.

Additionally, to cater to the high volume of data and the demand for high-end computational resources for the transcriptome assembly, many assemblers have started supporting parallel data processing, which has significantly reduced the time required for the assembly (reviewed in [66]). Cloud computing is another lucrative approach for parallel computing, which is scalable and can be used as per the user requirement [166].

Author details

Krishanpal Anamika*, Srikant Verma, Abhay Jere and Aarti Desai

*Address all correspondence to: anamika_krishanpal@persistent.co.in

LABS, Persistent Systems Limited, Pingala - Aryabhata, Erandwane, Pune, India

References

[1] Elgar G, Vavouri T. Tuning in to the signals: noncoding sequence conservation in vertebrate genomes. *Trends Genet.* 2008;24(7):344–352. DOI: 10.1016/j.tig.2008.04.005

[2] Blignaut M. Review of non-coding RNAs and the epigenetic regulation of gene expression. *Epigenetics.* 2012;7(6):664–666. DOI: 10.4161/epi.20170

[3] Mattick JS, Dinger ME. The extent of functionality in the human genome. *HUGO J.* 2013;7:2. DOI: 10.1186/1877-6566-7-2

[4] Shabalina SA, Spiridonov NA. The mammalian transcriptome and the function of non-coding DNA sequences. *Genome Biol.* 2004;5(4):105. DOI: 10.1186/gb-2004-5-4-105

[5] Davuluri RV, Suzuki Y, Sugano S, Plass C, Huang TH. The functional consequences of alternative promoter use in mammalian genomes. *Trends Genet.* 2008;24(4):167-177. DOI: 10.1016/j.tig.2008.01.008

[6] Chen M, Manley JL. Mechanisms of alternative splicing regulation: insights from molecular and genomics approaches. *Nat Rev Mol Cell Biol.* 2009;10(11):741–754. DOI: 10.1038/nrm2777

[7] Tian B, Manley JL. Alternative cleavage and polyadenylation: the long and short of it. *Trends Biochem Sci.* 2013;38(6):312–320. DOI: http://dx.doi.org/10.1016/j.tibs.2013.03.005

[8] Kochetov AV. Alternative translation start sites and hidden coding potential of eukaryotic mRNAs. *Bioessays.* 2008;30(7):683–691. DOI: 10.1002/bies.20771

[9] Eddy S R. Non-coding RNA genes and the modern RNA world. *Nat Rev Genet.* 2001;2(12):919–929. DOI: 10.1038/35103511

[10] Nagalakshmi U, Wang Z, Waern K et al. The transcriptional landscape of the yeast genome defined by RNA sequencing. *Science.* 2008;320(5881):1344–1349. DOI: 10.1126/science.1158441

[11] Sultan M, Schulz MH, Richard H et al. A global view of gene activity and alternative splicing by deep sequencing of the human transcriptome. *Science.* 2008;321(5891):956–960. DOI: 10.1126/science.1160342

[12] Mortazavi A, Williams BA, McCue K, Schaeffer L, Wold B. Mapping and quantifying mammalian transcriptomes by RNASeq. *Nat Methods*. 2008;5(7):621–628. DOI: 10.1038/nmeth.1226

[13] Alizadeh AA, Eisen MB, Davis RE, Ma C, Lossos IS, et al. Distinct types of diffuse large B-cell lymphoma identified by gene expression profiling. *Nature*. 2000;403(6769):503–511. DOI: 10.1038/35000501

[14] Schena M, Shalon D, Davis R W, et al. Quantitative monitoring of gene expression patterns with a complementary DNA microarray. *Science*. 1995;270(5235):467–470. DOI: 10.1126/science.270.5235.467

[15] Okoniewski MJ, Miller CJ. Hybridization interactions between probesets in short oligo microarrays. *BMC Bioinformatics*. 2006;7:276. DOI: 10.1186/1471-2105-7-276

[16] Mantione KJ, Kream RM, Kuzelova H, Ptacek R, Raboch J, Samuel JM, Stefano GB. Comparing bioinformatic gene expression profiling methods: microarray and RNA-Seq. *Med Sci Monit Basic Res*. 2014;20:138–142. DOI: 10.12659/MSMBR.892101

[17] Velculescu VE, Zhang L, Vogelstein B, Kinzler KW. Serial analysis of gene expression. *Science*. 1995;270(5235):484–487. DOI: 10.1126/science.270.5235.484

[18] Kodzius R, Kojima M, Nishiyori H, Nakamura M, Fukuda S, Tagami M, Sasaki D, Imamura K, Kai C, Harbers M, Hayashizaki Y, Carninci P. CAGE: cap analysis of gene expression. *Nat Methods*. 2006;3:211–222. DOI: 10.1038/nmeth0306-211

[19] Brenner S, Johnson M, Bridgham J, Golda G, Lloyd DH, Johnson D, Luo S, McCurdy S, Foy M, Ewan M, Roth R, George D, Eletr S, Albrecht G, Vermaas E, Williams SR, Moon K, Burcham T, Pallas M, DuBridge RB, Kirchner J, Fearon K, Mao J, Corcoran K. Gene expression analysis by massively parallel signature sequencing (MPSS) on microbead arrays. *Nat Biotechnol*. 2000;18(6):630–634. DOI: 10.1038/76469

[20] Wang Z, Gerstein M, Snyder M. RNA-Seq: a revolutionary tool for transcriptomics. *Nat Rev Genet*. 2009;10:57–63. DOI: 10.1038/nrg2484

[21] Tuch BB, Laborde RR, Xu X et al. Tumor transcriptome sequencing reveals allelic expression imbalances associated with copy number alterations. *PLoS ONE*. 2010;5(2):e9317. DOI: 10.1371/journal.pone.0009317

[22] Berger MF, Levin JZ, Vijayendran K et al. Integrative analysis of the melanoma transcriptome. *Genome Res*. 2010;20(4):413–427. DOI: 10.1101/gr.103697.109

[23] Jima DD, Zhang J, Jacobs C, Richards KL, Dunphy CH et al. Deep sequencing of the small RNA transcriptome of normal and malignant human B cells identifies hundreds of novel microRNAs. *Blood*. 2010;116(23):e118–e127. DOI: 10.1182/blood-2010-05-285403

[24] Twine NA, Janitz K, Wilkins MR, Janitz M. Whole transcriptome sequencing reveals gene expression and splicing differences in brain regions affected by Alzheimer's disease. *PLoS ONE*. 2011;6:e16266. DOI: 10.1371/journal.pone.0016266

[25] Ku GM, Kim H, Vaughn IW et al. Research resource: RNASeq reveals unique features of the pancreatic β-cell transcriptome. *Mol Endocrinol*. 2012;26(10):1783–1792. DOI: 10.1210/me.2012-1176

[26] Morán I, Akerman I, van de Bunt M, Xie R, Benazra M, Nammo T, Arnes L, Nakić N, García-Hurtado J, Rodríguez-Seguí S, Pasquali L, Sauty-Colace C, Beucher A, Scharfmann R, van Arensbergen J, Johnson PR, Berry A, Lee C, Harkins T, Gmyr V, Pattou F, Kerr-Conte J, Piemonti L, Berney T, Hanley N, Gloyn AL, Sussel L, Langman L, Brayman KL, Sander M, McCarthy MI, Ravassard P, Ferrer J. Human β cell transcriptome analysis uncovers lncRNAs that are tissue-specific, dynamically regulated, and abnormally expressed in type 2 diabetes. *Cell Metab*. 2012;16(4):435–448. DOI: 10.1016/j.cmet.2012.08.010

[27] Sun X, Zhou S, Meng F, Liu S. De novo assembly and characterization of the garlic (Allium sativum) bud transcriptome by Illumina sequencing. *Plant Cell Rep*. 2012;31(10):1823–1828. DOI: 10.1007/s00299-012-1295-z

[28] Franssen SU, Shrestha RP, Bräutigam A, Bornberg-Bauer E, Weber AP. Comprehensive transcriptome analysis of the highly complex Pisum sativum genome using next generation sequencing. *BMC Genomics*. 2011;11:12:227. DOI: 10.1186/1471-2164-12-227

[29] Garg R, Patel RK, Tyagi AK, Jain M. De novo assembly of chickpea transcriptome using short reads for gene discovery and marker identification. *DNA Res*. 2011;18(1):53–63. DOI: 10.1093/dnares/dsq028

[30] Takehisa H, Sato Y, Igarashi M, Abiko T, Antonio BA, Kamatsuki K, Minami H, Namiki N, Inukai Y, Nakazono M, Nagamura Y. Genome-wide transcriptome dissection of the rice root system: implications for developmental and physiological functions. *Plant J*. 2012;69(1):126–140. DOI: 10.1111/j.1365-313X.2011.04777.x

[31] Alagna F, D'Agostino N, Torchia L, Servili M, Rao R, Pietrella M, Giuliano G, Chiusano ML, Baldoni L, Perrotta G. Comparative 454 pyrosequencing of transcripts from two olive genotypes during fruit development. *BMC Genomics*. 2009;10:399. DOI: 10.1186/1471-2164-10-399

[32] Pingault L, Choulet F, Alberti A, Glover N, Wincker P, Feuillet C, Paux E. Deep transcriptome sequencing provides new insights into the structural and functional organization of the wheat genome. *Genome Biol*. 2015;16:29. DOI: 10.1186/s13059-015-0601-9

[33] Chapman MA. Transcriptome sequencing and marker development for four underutilized legumes. *Appl Plant Sci*. 2015;3(2):1400111. DOI: 10.3732/apps.1400111.

[34] Metzker ML. Sequencing technologies – the next generation. *Nat Rev Genet*. 2010;11(1):31–46. DOI: 10.1038/nrg2626

[35] Liu L, Li Y, Li S, Hu N, He Y, Pong R, Lin D, Lu L, Law M. Comparison of next-generation sequencing systems. *J Biomed Biotechnol*. 2012;2012:251364. DOI: 10.1155/2012/251364

[36] Schmieder R, Edwards R. Quality control and preprocessing of metagenomic datasets. *Bioinformatics*. 2011;27(6):863–864. DOI: 10.1093/bioinformatics/btr026

[37] Martin M. Cutadapt removes adapter sequences from high-throughput sequencing reads. *EMBnet.journal*. 2011;17(1):10–12. DOI: 10.14806/ej.17.1.200

[38] Bolger AM, Lohse M, Usadel B. Trimmomatic: A flexible trimmer for Illumina Sequence Data. *Bioinformatics*. 2014;30(15):2114–2120. DOI: 10.1093/bioinformatics/btu170

[39] Cunningham F, Amode MR, Barrell D, Beal K, Billis K, Brent S, Carvalho-Silva D, Clapham P, Coates G, Fitzgerald S et al. Ensembl 2015. *Nucl Acids Res*. 2015;43:D662–D669. DOI: 10.1093/nar/gku1010

[40] Rosenbloom KR, Armstrong J, Barber GP, Casper J, Clawson H, Diekhans M, Dreszer TR, Fujita PA, Guruvadoo L, Haeussler M. et al. 2015. The UCSC Genome Browser database: 2015 update. *Nucl Acids Res*. 2015;43:D670–D681. DOI: 10.1093/nar/gku1177

[41] Zhao S, Zhang B. A comprehensive evaluation of ensembl, RefSeq, and UCSC annotations in context of RNASeq read mapping and gene quantification. *BMC Genomics*. 2015;16:97. DOI: 10.1186/s12864-015-1308-8

[42] Homer N, Merriman B, Nelson SF. BFAST: An alignment tool for large scale genome resequencing. *PLoS ONE*. 2009;4(11):e7767. DOI: 10.1371/journal.pone.0007767

[43] Clement NL, Snell Q, Clement MJ, Hollenhorst PC, Purwar J, Graves BJ, Cairns BR, Johnson WE. The GNUMAP algorithm: unbiased probabilistic mapping of oligonucleotides from next-generation sequencing. *Bioinformatics*. 2010;26(1):38–45. DOI: 10.1093/bioinformatics/btp614

[44] David M, Dzamba M, Lister D, Ilie L, Brudno M. SHRiMP2: Sensitive yet Practical Short Read Mapping, *Bioinformatics*. 2011;27(7):1011–1012. DOI: 10.1093/bioinformatics/btr046

[45] Lee W, Stromberg MP, Ward A, Stewart C, Garrison EP, Marth GT. MOSAIK: A Hash-based algorithm for accurate Next-Generation Sequencing short-read mapping. *PLoS ONE*. 2014;9(3):e90581. DOI: 10.1371/journal.pone.0090581

[46] Li H, Ruan J, Durbin R. Mapping short DNA sequencing reads and calling variants using mapping quality scores. *Genome Res*. 2008;18(11):1851–1858. DOI: 10.1101/gr.078212.108

[47] Smith AD, Chung W, Hodges E, Kendall J, Hannon G, Hicks J, Xuan Z, Zhang MQ. Updates to the RMAP short-read mapping software. *Bioinformatics*. 2009;25(21):2841–2842. DOI: 10.1093/bioinformatics/btp533

[48] Weese D, Emde A, Rausch T, Doring A, Reinert K. RazerS-fast read mapping with sensitivity control. *Genome Res*. 2009;19(9):1646–1654. DOI: 10.1101/gr.088823.108

[49] Langmead B, Trapnell C, Pop M, Salzberg SL. Ultrafast and memory-efficient align‐
ment of short DNA sequences to the human genome. *Genome Biol.* 2009;10:R25. DOI:
10.1186/gb-2009-10-3-r25

[50] Langmead B, Salzberg SL. Fast gapped-read alignment with Bowtie 2. *Natur Meth.*
2012;9:357–359. DOI: 10.1038/nmeth.1923

[51] Li H, Durbin R. Fast and accurate short read alignment with Burrows-Wheeler trans‐
form. *Bioinformatics.* 2009:25(14):1754–1760. DOI: 10.1093/bioinformatics/btp324

[52] Li R, Yu C, Li Y, Lam T, Yiu S, Kristiansen K, Wang J. SOAP2: an improved ultrafast
tool for short read alignment. *Bioinformatics.* 2009;25(15):1966–1967. DOI: 10.1093/
bioinformatics/btp336

[53] Wu TD, Nacu S. Fast and SNP-tolerant detection of complex variants and splicing in
short reads. *Bioinformatics.* 2010;26(7):873–881. DOI: 10.1093/bioinformatics/btq057

[54] Wang K, Singh D, Zeng Z, Coleman SJ, Huang Y, Savich GL, He X, Mieczkowski P,
Grimm SA, Perou CM, MacLeod JN, Chiang DY, Prins JF, Liu J. MapSplice: accurate
mapping of RNA-seq reads for splice junction discovery. *Nucl Acids Res.*
2010;38(18):e178. DOI: 10.1093/nar/gkq622

[55] Au KF, Jiang H, Lin L, Xing Y, Wong WH. Detection of splice junctions from paired-
end RNASeq data by SpliceMap. *Nucl Acids Res.* 2010:38(14): 4570–4578. DOI:
10.1093/nar/gkq211

[56] Dobin A, Davis CA, Schlesinger F, Drenkow J, Zaleski C, Jha S, Batut P, Chaisson M,
Gingeras TR. STAR: ultrafast universal RNASeq aligner. *Bioinformatics.* 2013;29(1):15–
21. DOI: 10.1093/bioinformatics/bts635

[57] Kim D, Pertea G, Trapnell C, Pimentel H, Kelley R, Salzberg SL. TopHat2: accurate
alignment of transcriptomes in the presence of insertions, deletions and gene fusions.
Genome Biol. 2013;14:R36. DOI: 10.1186/gb-2013-14-4-r36

[58] Kim D, Langmead B, Salzberg SL. HISAT: a fast spliced aligner with low memory re‐
quirements. *Nat Methods.* 2015;12(4):357–360. DOI: 10.1038/nmeth.3317

[59] Fonseca NA, Rung J, Brazma A, Marioni JC. Tools for mapping high-throughput se‐
quencing data. *Bioinformatics.* 2012;28(24):3169–3177. DOI: 10.1093/bioinformatics/
bts605

[60] Lindner R, Friedel CC. A comprehensive evaluation of alignment algorithms in the
context of RNASeq. *PLoS ONE.* 2012;7(12):e52403. DOI: 10.1371/journal.pone.0052403

[61] Engstrom PG, Steijger T, Sipos B, Grant GR, Kahles A, Ratsch G, Goldman N, Hub‐
bard TJ, Harrow J, Guigo R, Bertone P, The RGASP Consortium. Systematic evalua‐
tion of spliced alignment programs for RNA-seq data. *Natur Meth.* 2013;10(12):1185–
1191. DOI: 10.1038/nmeth.2722

[62] Li H, Handshakes B, Wysoker A, Fennell T, Ruan J, Homer N, Marth G, Abecasis G,
Durbin R, 1000 Genome Project Data Processing Subgroup. The Sequence Align‐

ment/Map format and SAMtools. *Bioinformatics*. 2009;25(16):2078–2079. DOI: 10.1093/ bioinformatics/btp352

[63] Anders S, Pyl PT, Huber W. Htseq-a Python framework to work high-throughput sequencing data. *Bioinformatics*. 2015;31(2):166–169. DOI: 10.1093/bioinformatics/btu638

[64] Roberts A, Pimentel H, Trapnell C, Pachter L. Identification of novel transcripts in annotated genomes using RNASeq. *Bioinformatics*. 2011;27(17):2325–2329. DOI: 10.1093/bioinformatics/btr355

[65] Trapnell C, Williams BA, Pertea G, Mortazavi A, Kwan G, van Baren MJ, Salzberg SL, Wold BJ. Pachter L. Transcript assembly and quantification by RNASeq reveals unannotated transcripts and isoform switching during cell differentiation. *Natur Biotechnol*. 2010;28:511–515. DOI: 10.1038/nbt.1621

[66] Martin JA, Wang Z. Next-generation transcriptome assembly. *Nat Rev Genet*. 2011;12(10):671–682. DOI: 10.1038/nrg3068

[67] Flicek P, Birney E. Sense from sequence reads: methods for alignment and assembly. *Nat Meth*. 2009;6:S6–S12. DOI: 10.1038/nmeth.1376

[68] Chevreux B, Pfisterer T, Drescher B, Driesel AJ, Müller WE, Wetter T, Suhai. Using the miraEST assembler for reliable and automated mRNA transcript assembly and SNP detection in sequenced ESTs. *Genome Res*. 2004;14:1147–1159. DOI: 10.1101/gr. 1917404

[69] Huang X, Madan A. CAP3: A DNA sequence assembly program. *Genome Res*. 1999;9:868–877. DOI: 10.1101/gr.9.9.868

[70] Pevzner PA, Tang H, Waterman MS. An Eulerian path approach to DNA fragment assembly. *Proc Natl Acad Sci U S A*. 2001;98(17):9748–9753. DOI: 10.1073/pnas. 171285098

[71] Compeau PEC, Pevzner PA, Tesler G. How to apply de Bruijn graphs to genome assembly. *Nat Biotechnol*. 2011;29:987–991. DOI: 10.1038/nbt.2023

[72] Schliesky S, Gowik U, Weber AP, Brautigam A. RNA-Seq assembly – Are we there yet? *Front Plant Sci*. 2012;3:220. DOI: 10.3389/fpls.2012.00220

[73] Surget-Groba Y, Montoya-Burgos JI. Optimization of de novo transcriptome assembly from next-generation sequencing data. *Genome Res*. 2010;20(10):1432–1440. DOI: 10.1101/gr.103846.109

[74] Schulz MH, Zerbino DR, Vingron M, Birney E. Oases: robust de novo RNASeq assembly across the dynamic range of expression levels. *Bioinformatics*. 2012;28(8):1086–1092. DOI: 10.1093/bioinformatics/bts094

[75] Gruenheit N, Deusch O, Esser C, Becker M, Voelckel C, Lockhart P. Cutoffs and k-mers: implications from a transcriptome study in allopolyploid plants. *BMC Genomics*. 2012;13:92. DOI: 10.1186/1471-2164-13-92

[76] Gongora-Castillo E, Buell CR. Bioinformatics challenges in de novo transcriptome assembly using short read sequences in the absence of a reference genome sequence. *Nat Prod Rep*. 2013;30(4):490–500. DOI: 10.1039/c3np20099j

[77] Zerbino DR, Birney E. Velvet: algorithms for de novo short read assembly using de Bruijn graphs. *Genome Res*. 2008;18(5):821–829. DOI: 10.1101/gr.074492.107

[78] Grabherr MG, Haas BJ, Yassour M, Levin JZ, Thompson DA, Amit I, Adiconis X, Fan L, Raychowdhury R, Zeng Q, Chen Z, Mauceli E, Hacohen N, Gnirke A, Rhind N, di Palma F, Birren BW, Nusbaum C, Lindblad-Toh K, Friedman N, Regev A. Full-length transcriptome assembly from RNASeq data without a reference genome. *Nat Biotechnol*. 2011;29:644–652. DOI: 10.1038/nbt.1883

[79] Robertson G, Schein J, Chiu R, Corbett R, Field M, Jackman SD, Mungall K, Lee S, Okada HM, Qian JQ, Griffith M, Raymond A, Thiessen N, Cezard T, Butterfield YS, Newsome R, Chan SK, She R, Varhol R, Kamoh B, Prabhu AL, Tam A, Zhao Y, Moore RA, Hirst M, Marra MA, Jones SJ, Hoodless PA, Birol I. De novo assembly and analysis of RNASeq data. *Nat Methods*. 2010;7(11):909–912. DOI: 10.1038/nmeth. 1517

[80] Xie Y, Wu G, Tang J, Luo R, Patterson J, Liu S, Huang W, He G, Gu S, Li S, Zhou X, Lam TW, Li Y, Xu X, Wong GK, Wang J. SOAPdenovo-Trans: de novo transcriptome assembly with short RNASeq reads. *Bioinformatics*. 2014;30(12):1660–1666. DOI: 10.1093/bioinformatics/btu077

[81] Luo R, Liu B, Xie Y, Li Z, Huang W et al. SOAPdenovo2: an empirically improved memory-efficient short-read de novo assembler. *Gigascience*. 2012;1:18. DOI: 10.1186/2047-217X-1-18

[82] Chopra R, Burow G, Farmer A, Mudge J, Simpson CE, Burow MD. Comparisons of de novo transcriptome assemblers in diploid and polyploid species using peanut (Arachis spp.) RNA-Seq data. *PLoS ONE*. 2014;9(12):e115055. DOI: 10.1371/journal.pone.0115055

[83] Haznedaroglu BZ, Reeves D, Rismani-Yazdi H, Peccia J. Optimization of de novo transcriptome assembly from high-throughput short read sequencing data improves functional annotation for non-model organisms. *BMC Bioinformatics*. 2012;13:170. DOI: 10.1186/1471-2105-13-170

[84] Gurevich A, Saveliev V, Vyahhi N, Tesler G. QUAST: quality assessment tool for genome assemblies. *Bioinformatics*. 2013;29(8):1072–1075. DOI: 10.1093/bioinformatics/btt086

[85] O'Neil ST, Emrich SJ. Assessing de novo transcriptome assembly metrics for consistency and utility. *BMC Genomics*. 2013;14:465. DOI: 10.1186/1471-2164-14-465

[86] Robinson MD, McCarthy DJ, Smyth GK. edgeR: a Bioconductor package for differential expression analysis of digital gene expression data. *Bioinformatics*. 2009;26(1):139–140. DOI: 10.1093/bioinformatics/btp616

[87] Li B, Ruotti V, Stewart RM, Thomson JA, Dewey CN. RNASeq gene expression estimation with read mapping uncertainty. *Bioinformatics*. 2009;26(4):493–500. DOI: 10.1093/bioinformatics/btp692

[88] Oshlack A, Wakefield MJ. Transcript length bias in RNASeq data confounds systems biology. *Biol Direct*. 2009;4:14. DOI:10.1186/1745-6150-4-14

[89] Pickrell JK, Marioni JC, Pai AA, Degner JF, Engelhardt BE, Nkadori E, Veyrieras J, Stephens M, Gilad Y, Pritchard JK. Understanding mechanisms underlying human gene expression variation with RNA sequencing. *Nature*. 2010;464(7289):768–772. DOI: 10.1038/nature08872

[90] Leek JT, Scharpf RB, Bravo HC, Simcha D, Langmead B, Johnson WE, Geman D, Baggerly K, Irizarry RA. Tackling the widespread and critical impact of batch effects in high-throughput data. *Natur Rev Genet*. 2010;11(10):733–739. DOI: 10.1038/nrg2825

[91] Bullard JH, Purdom E, Hansen KD, Dudoit S. Evaluation of statistical methods for normalization and differential expression in mRNASeq experiments. *BMC Bioinformatics*. 2010;11: 94. DOI: 10.1186/1471-2105-11-94

[92] Trapnell C, Hendrickson DG, Sauvageau M, Goff L, Rinn JL, Pachter L. Differential analysis of gene regulation at transcript resolution with RNASeq. *Natur Biotechnol*. 2013;31(1):46–53. DOI: 10.1038/nbt.2450

[93] Bolstad BM, Irizarry RA, Astrand M, Speed TP. A comparison of normalization methods for high density oligonucleotide array data based on variance and bias. *Bioinformatics*. 2003;19(2):185–193. DOI: 10.1093/bioinformatics/19.2.185

[94] Ritchie ME, Phipson B, Wu D, Hu Y, Law CW, Shi W, Symth GK. limma powers differential expression analyses for RNASequencing and microarray studies. *Nucl Acids Res*. 2015;43(7):e47. DOI: 10.1093/nar/gkv007

[95] Robinson MD, Oshlack A. A scaling normalization method for differential expression analysis of RNASeq data. *Genome Biol*. 2010;11(3):R25. DOI: 10.1186/gb-2010-11-3-r25

[96] Anders S, Huber W. Differential expression analysis for sequence count data. *Genome Biol*. 2010;11:R106. DOI: 10.1186/gb-2010-11-10-r106

[97] Love MI, Huber W, Anders S. Moderated estimation fold change and dispersion for RNASeq data with DESeq2. *Genome Biol*. 2014;15:550. DOI: 10.1186/s13059-014-0550-8

[98] Dillies MA, Rau A, Aubert J, Hennequet-Antier C, Jeanmougin M, Servant N, Keime C, Marot G, Castel D, Estelle J, Guernec G, Jagla B, Jouneau L, Laloe D, Gall CL, Schaeffer B, Crom SL, Guedj M, Jaffrezic F. A comprehensive evaluation of normali-

zation methods for Illumina high-throughput RNA sequencing data analysis. *Brief Bioinformatics*. 2013;14(6):671–683. DOI: 10.1093/bib/bbs046

[99] Zyprych-Walczak J, Szabelska Handschuh L, Gorczak K, Klamecka K, Figlerowicz M, Siat-kowski I. The impact of normalization methods on RNASeq data analysis. *Biomed Res Int*. 2015;2015:621690. DOI: 10.1155/2015/621690

[100] Leek JT. svaseq: removing batch effects and other unwanted noise from sequencing data. *Nucl Acids Res*. 2014:42(21):e161. DOI: 10.1093/nar/gku864

[101] Marioni JC, Mason CE, Mane SM, Stephens M, Gilad Y. RNASeq: An assessment of technical reproducibility and comparison with gene expression arrays. *Genome Res*. 2008;18(9):1509–1517. DOI: 10.1101/gr.079558.108

[102] Wang L, Feng Z, Wang X, Wang X, Zhang X. DEGseq: an R package for identifying differentially expressed genes from RNASeq data. *Bioinformatics*. 2010;26(1):136–138. DOI: 10.1093/bioinformatics/btp612

[103] Auer PL, Doerge RW. A two-stage Poisson model for testing RNASeq data. *Stat Appl Genet Mol Biol*. 2011;10(1):1–26. DOI: 10.2202/1544-6115.1627

[104] Hardcastle TJ, Kelly KA. baySeq: Empirical Bayesian methods for identifying differential expression in sequence count data. *BMC Bioinformatics*. 2010;11:422. DOI: 10.1186/1471-2105-11-422

[105] Chen HH, Liu Y, Zou Y, Zhao L, Sarkar D, Huang Y, Chen Y. Differential expression analysis of RNA sequencing data by incorporating non-exonic mapped reads. *BMC Genomics*. 2015;16(Suppl No. 7):S14. DOI: 10.1186/1471-2164-16-S7-S14

[106] Soneson C, Delorenzi M. A comparison of methods for differential expression analysis of RNA-se data. *BMC Bioinformatics*. 2013;14:91. DOI: 10.1186/1471-2105-14-91

[107] Seyednasrollah F, Laiho A, Elo LL. Comparison of software packages for detecting differential expression in RNASeq studies. *Brief Bioinform*. 2015;16(1):59–70. DOI: 10.1093/bib/bbt086

[108] Altschul SF, Gish W, Miller W, Myers EW, Lipman DJ. Basic local alignment search tool. *JMB*. 1990;215(3):403–410. DOI: 10.1016/S0022-2836(05)80360-2

[109] Ashburner M, Ball CA, Blake JA, Bostein D, Butler H, Cherry JM, Davis AP, Dolinski K, Dwight SS, Eppig JT, Harris MA, Hill DP, Issel-Tarver L, Kasarskis A, Lewis S, Matese JC, Richardson JE, Ringwald M, Rubin GM, Sherlock G. Gene ontology: tool for the unification of biology. The Gene Ontology Consortium. *Natur Genet*. 2000;25(1): 25–29. DOI: 10.1038/75556

[110] Kanehisa M, Goto S, Kawashima S, Okuno Y, Hattori M. The KEGG resource for deciphering the genome. *Nucl Acids Res*. 2004;32(Suppl 1):D277–D280. DOI: 10.1093/nar/gkh063

[111] Joshi-Tope G, Gillespie M, Vastrik I, D'Eustachio P, Schimdt E, Bono B, Jassal B, Gopinath GR, Wu GR, Matthews L, Lewis S, Birney E, Stein L. Reactome: a knowledge

base of biological pathways. *Nucl Acids Res.* 2005;33(Suppl. 1):D428–D432. DOI: 10.1093/nar/gki072

[112] Khatri P, Sirota M, Butte AJ. Ten years of pathway analysis: current approaches and outstanding challenges. *PLoS Comput Biol.* 2012;8(2):e1002375. DOI: 10.1371/journal.pcbi.1002375

[113] Khatri P, Draghici S, Ostemeier GC, Krawetz SA. Profiling gene expression using onto-express. *Genomics.* 2002;79(2):266–270. DOI: 10.1006/geno.2002.6698

[114] Dahlquist KD, Salomonis N, Vranizan K, Lawlor SC, Conkin BR. GenMAPP, a new tool for viewing and analyzing microarray data on biological pathways. *Natur Genet.* 2002;31:19–20. DOI: 10.1038/ng0502-19

[115] Zeeberg BR, Feng W, Wang G, Wang MD, Fojo AT, Sunshine M, Narasimhan S, Kane DW, Reinhold WC, Lababidi S, et al. GoMiner: a resource for biological interpretation of genomic and proteomic data. *Genome Biol.* 2003;4(4):R28. DOI: 10.1186/gb-2003-4-4-r28

[116] Dennis G, Sherman BT, Hosack DA, Yang J, Gao W, Lane HC, Lempicki RA. DAVID: Database for Annotation, Visualization, and Integrated Discovery. *Genome Biol.* 2003;4(9):R60. DOI: 10.1186/gb-2003-4-9-r60

[117] Huang DW, Sherman BT, Lempicki RA. Systematic and integrative analysis of large gene lists using DAVID bioinformatics resources. *Natur Protocols.* 2008;4(1):44–57. DOI: 10.1038/nprot.2008.211

[118] Goeman JJ, van de Geer SA, de Kort F, van Houwelingen HC. A global test for groups of genes: testing association with a clinical outcome. *Bioinformatics.* 2004;20(1):93–99. DOI: 10.1093/bioinformatics/btg382

[119] Subramanian A, Tamayo P, Mootha VK, Mukherjee S, Ebert BL, Gillette MA, Paulovich A, Pomeroy SL, Golub TR, Lander ES, Mesirov JP. Gene se enrichment analysis: a knowledge-based approach for interpreting genome-wide expression profiles. *Proc Natl Acad Sci U S A.* 2005;102(43):15545–15550. DOI: 10.1073/pnas.0506580102

[120] Tarca AL, Draghici S, Kathri P, Hasan SS, Mittal P, Kim J, Kim CJ, Kusanovic JP, Romero R. A novel signaling pathway impact analysis. *Bioinformatics.* 2009;25(1):75–82. DOI: 10.1093/bioinformatics/btn577

[121] Shojaie A, Michailidis G. Analysis of gene sets based on the underlying regulatory network. *J Comput Biol.* 2009;16(3):407–426. DOI: 10.1089/cmb.2008.0081

[122] Roge X, Zhang X. RNAseqViewer: visualization tool for RNA-Seq data. *Bioinformatics.* 2014 ;30(6):891–892. DOI: 10.1093/bioinformatics/btt649

[123] Nussbaumer T, Kugler KG, Bader KC, Sharma S, Seidel M, Mayer KF. RNASeqExpressionBrowser–a web interface to browse and visualize high-throughput expression data. *Bioinformatics.* 2014;30(17):2519–2520. DOI: 10.1093/bioinformatics/btu334

[124] An J, Lai J, Wood DL, Sajjanhar A, Wang C, Tevz G, Lehman ML, Nelson CC. RNA-SeqBrowser: a genome browser for simultaneous visualization of raw strand specific RNAseq reads and UCSC genome browser custom tracks. *BMC Genomics.* 2015;16:145. DOI: 10.1186/s12864-015-1346-2

[125] Kinsella M, Harismendy O, Nakano M, Frazer KA, Bafna V. Sensitive gene fusion detection using ambiguously mapping RNASeq read pairs. *Bioinformatics.* 2011;27(8): 1068–1075. DOI: 10.1093/bioinformatics/btr085

[126] McPherson A, Hormozdiari F, Zayed A, Giuliany R, Ha G et al. deFuse: an algorithm for gene fusion discovery in tumor RNASeq data. *PLoS Comput Biol.* 2011;7(5):e1001138. DOI: 10.1371/journal.pcbi.1001138

[127] Risso D, Schwartz K, Sherlock G, Dudoit S. GC-content normalization for RNASeq data. *BMC Bioinformatics.* 2011;12:480. DOI: 10.1186/1471-2105-12-480

[128] Benjamini Y, Speed TP. Summarizing and correcting the GC content bias in high-throughput sequencing. *Nucl Acids Res.* 2012;40: e72. DOI: 10.1093/nar/gks001

[129] Robles JA, Qureshi SE, Stephen SJ, Wilson SR, Burden CJ, Taylor JM. Efficient experimental design and analysis strategies for the detection of differential expression using RNA sequencing. *BMC Genomics.* 2012;13:484. DOI: 10.1186/1471-2164-13-484

[130] Rapaport F, Khanin R, Liang Y, Pirun M, Krek A, Zumbo P, Mason CE, Socci ND, Betel D. Comprehensive evaluation of differential gene expression analysis methods for RNASeq data. *Genome Biol.* 2013;14(9):R95. DOI: 10.1186/gb-2013-14-9-r95

[131] Garber M, Grabherr MG, Guttman M, Trapnell C. Computational methods for transcriptome annotation and quantification using RNASeq. *Nat Methods.* 2011;8:469–477. DOI: 10.1038/nmeth.1613

[132] Lu B, Zeng Z, Shi T. Comparative study of de novo assembly and genome-guided assembly strategies for transcriptome reconstruction based on RNASeq. *Sci China Life Sci.* 2013;56(2):143–155. DOI: 10.1007/s11427-013-4442-z

[133] Haas BJ, Chin M, Nusbaum C, Birren BW, Livny J. How deep is deep enough for RNA-Seq profiling of bacterial transcriptomes? *BMC Genomics.* 2012;13:734. DOI: 10.1186/1471-2164-13-734

[134] Hu L, Hao C, Fan R, Wu B, Tan L, Wu H. De novo assembly and characterization of fruit transcriptome in black pepper (*Piper nigrum*). *PLoS ONE.* 2015;10(6):e0129822. DOI: 10.1371/journal.pone.0129822

[135] Sudheesh S, Sawbridge TI, Cogan NO, Kennedy P, Forster JW, Kaur S. De novo assembly and characterisation of the field pea transcriptome using RNA-Seq. *BMC Genomics.* 2015;16(1):611. DOI: 10.1186/s12864-015-1815-7

[136] Talhinhas P, Azinheira HG, Vieira B, Loureiro A, Tavares S, Batista D, Morin E, Petitot AS, Paulo OS, Poulain J, Da Silva C, Duplessis S, Silva Mdo C, Fernandez D. Overview of the functional virulent genome of the coffee leaf rust pathogen *Hemileia*

vastatrix with an emphasis on early stages of infection. *Front Plant Sci.* 2014;5:88. DOI: 10.3389/fpls.2014.00088

[137] Yang X, Hu H, Yu D, Sun Z, He X, Zhang J, Chen Q, Tian R, Fan J. Candidate resistant genes of sand pear (*Pyrus pyrifolia* Nakai) to *Alternaria alternata* revealed by transcriptome sequencing. *PLoS ONE.* 2015;10(8):e0135046. DOI: 10.1371/journal.pone. 0135046

[138] Ropka-Molik K, Zukowski K, Eckert R, Gurgul A, Piorkowska K, Oczkowicz M. Comprehensive analysis of the whole transcriptomes from two different pig breeds using RNA-Seq method. *Anim Genet.* 2014;45(5):674–684. DOI: 10.1111/age.12184

[139] Cui X, Hou Y, Yang S, Xie Y, Zhang S, Zhang Y, Zhang Q, Lu X, Liu GE, Sun D. Transcriptional profiling of mammary gland in Holstein cows with extremely different milk protein and fat percentage using RNA sequencing. *BMC Genomics.* 2014;15:226. DOI: 10.1186/1471-2164-15-226

[140] Sandri M, Stefanon B, Loor JJ. Transcriptome profiles of whole blood in Italian Holstein and Italian Simmental lactating cows diverging for genetic merit for milk protein. *J Dairy Sci.* 2015;98(9):6119–6127.DOI: 10.3168/jds.2014-9049

[141] Wall EH, Bond JP, McFadden TB. Milk yield responses to changes in milking frequency during early lactation are associated with coordinated and persistent changes in mammary gene expression. *BMC Genomics.* 2003;14:296. DOI: 10.1186/1471-2164-14-296

[142] Liu P, Wang Y, Du X, Yao L, Li F, Meng Z. Transcriptome analysis of thermal parthenogenesis of the domesticated silkworm. *PLoS ONE.* 2015;10(8):e0135215. DOI: 10.1371/journal.pone.0135215

[143] Liu R, Wang X, Chen GY, Dalerba P, Gurney A, Hoey T, Sherlock G, Lewicki J, Shedden K, Clarke MF. The prognostic role of a gene signature from tumorigenic breast-cancer cells. *N Engl J Med.* 2007;356(3):217–226. DOI: 10.1056/NEJMoa063994

[144] van't Veer LJ, Dai H, van de Vijver MJ, He YD, Hart AA et al. Gene expression profiling predicts clinical outcome of breast cancer. *Nature.* 2002;415(6871):530–536. DOI: 10.1038/415530a

[145] van de Vijver MJ, He YD, van't Veer LJ, Dai H, Hart AA, Voskuil DW et al. A gene-expression signature as a predictor of survival in breast cancer. *N Engl J Med.* 2002;347(25):1999–2009. DOI: 10.1056/NEJMoa021967

[146] Huang L, Zheng M, Zhou QM, Zhang MY, Yu YH, Yun JP, Wang HY. Identification of a 7-gene signature that predicts relapse and survival for early stage patients with cervical carcinoma. *Med Oncol.* 2012;29(4):2911–2918. DOI: 10.1007/s12032-012-0166-3

[147] Hernández-Prieto S, Romera A, Ferrer M, Subiza JL, López-Asenjo JA, Jarabo JR, Gómez AM, Molina EM, Puente J, González-Larriba JL, Hernando F, Pérez-Villamil B, Díaz-Rubio E, Sanz-Ortega J. A 50-gene signature is a novel scoring system for tu-

mor-infiltrating immune cells with strong correlation with clinical outcome of stage I/II non-small cell lung cancer. *Clin Transl Oncol.* 2015;17(4):330–338. DOI: 10.1007/s12094-014-1235-1

[148] Peng L, Bian XW, Li DK, Xu C, Wang GM, Xia QY, Xiong Q. Large-scale RNA-seq transcriptome analysis of 4043 cancers and 548 normal tissue controls across 12 TCGA cancer types. *Sci Rep.* 2015;5:13413. DOI: 10.1038/srep13413

[149] Koh Y, Park I, Sun CH, Lee S, Yun H, Park CK, Park SH, Park JK, Lee SH. Detection of a distinctive genomic signature in rhabdoid glioblastoma, a rare disease entity identified by whole exome sequencing and whole transcriptome sequencing. *Transl Oncol.* 2015;8(4):279–287. DOI: 10.1016/j.tranon.2015.05.003.

[150] Punt S, Corver WE, van der Zeeuw SA, Kielbasa SM, Osse EM, Buermans HP, de Kroon CD, Jordanova ES, Gorter A. Whole-transcriptome analysis of flow-sorted cervical cancer samples reveals that B cell expressed TCL1A is correlated with improved survival. *Oncotarget.* 2015. DOI: 10.18632/oncotarget.4526

[151] Yu B, Russanova V, Gravina S, Hartley S, Mullikin JC, Ignezweski A, Graham J, Segars JH, DeCherney AH, Howard BH. DNA methylome and transcriptome sequencing in human ovarian granulosa cells links age-related changes in gene expression to gene body methylation and 3′-end GC density. *Oncotarget.* 2015;6(6):3627–3643. DOI: 10.18632/oncotarget.2875

[152] Zhang R, Yu C, Wu R, Zhang L, Zhu L, Xu A, Wang C. RNA-seq-based transcriptome analysis of changes in gene expression linked to human pregnancy outcome after in vitro fertilization-embryo transfer. *Reprod Sci.* 2015;pii: 1933719115597766. DOI: 10.1177/1933719115597766

[153] Jalbrzikowski M, Lazaro MT, Gao F, Huang A, Chow C, Geschwind DH, Coppola G, Bearden CE. Transcriptome profiling of peripheral blood in 22q11.2 deletion syndrome reveals functional pathways related to psychosis and autism spectrum disorder. *PLoS ONE.* 2015;10(7):e0132542. DOI: 10.1371/journal.pone.0132542

[154] Mariani J, Coppola G, Zhang P, Abyzov A, Provini L, Tomasini L, Amenduni M, Szekely A, Palejev D, Wilson M, Gerstein M, Grigorenko EL, Chawarska K, Pelphrey KA, Howe JR, Vaccarino FM. FOXG1-dependent dysregulation of GABA/glutamate neuron differentiation in autism spectrum disorders. *Cell.* 2015;162(2):375–390. DOI: 10.1016/j.cell.2015.06.034

[155] Pecorelli A, Leoni G, Cervellati F, Canali R, Signorini C, Leoncini S, Cortelazzo A, De Felice C, Ciccoli L, Hayek J, Valacchi G. Genes related to mitochondrial functions, protein degradation, and chromatin folding are differentially expressed in lympho-monocytes of Rett syndrome patients. *Mediators Inflamm.* 2013;2013:137629. DOI: 10.1155/2013/137629

[156] Gosalbes MJ, Durban A, Pignatelli M, Abellan JJ, Jimenez-Hernandez N, Perez-Cobas AE, Latorre A, Moya A. Metatranscriptomic approach to analyze the functional human gut microbiota. *PLoS ONE*. 2011;6(3):e17447. DOI: 10.1371/journal.pone.0017447

[157] Gilbert JA, Field D, Huang Y, Edwards R, Li W, Gilna P, Joint I. Detection of large numbers of novel sequences in the metatranscriptomes of complex marine microbial communities. *PLoS ONE*. 2008;3(8):e3042. DOI: 10.1371/journal.pone.0003042

[158] Frias-Lopez J, Shi Y, Tyson GW, Coleman ML, Schuster SC, Chisholm SW, Delong EF. Microbial community gene expression in ocean surface waters. *Proc Natl Acad Sci U S A*. 2008;105(10):3805–3810. DOI: 10.1073/pnas.0708897105

[159] Urich T, Lanzen A, Qi J, Huson DH, Schleper C, Schuster SC. Simultaneous assessment of soil microbial community structure and function through analysis of the meta-transcriptome. *PLoS ONE*. 2008;3(6):e2527. DOI: 10.1371/journal.pone.0002527

[160] Shapiro E, Biezuner T, Linnarsson S. Single-cell sequencing-based technologies will revolutionize whole-organism science. *Nat Rev Genet*. 2013;14:618–630. DOI: 10.1038/nrg3542

[161] Saliba AE, Westermann AJ, Gorski SA, Vogel J. Single-cell RNA-seq: advances and future challenges. *Nucl Acids Res*. 2014;42(14):8845–8860. DOI: 10.1093/nar/gku555

[162] Sasagawa Y, Nikaido I, Hayashi T, Danno H, Uno KD, Imai T, Ueda HR. Quartz-Seq: a highly reproducible and sensitive single-cell RNA-Seq reveals non-genetic gene expression heterogeneity. *Genome Biol*. 2013;14(4):R31. DOI: 10.1186/gb-2013-14-4-r31

[163] Grun D, Lyubimova A, Kester L, Wiebrands K, Basak O, Sasaki N, Clevers H, van Oudenaarden A. Single-cell messenger RNA sequencing reveals rare intestinal cell types. *Nature*. 2015;525:151–255. DOI: 10.1038/nature14966

[164] Londin E, Loher P, Telonis AG, Quann K, Clark P, Jing Y et al. Analysis of 13 cell types reveals evidence for the expression of numerous novel primate- and tissue-specific microRNAs. *Proc Natl Acad Sci U S A*. 2015;112(10):E1106–11015. DOI: 10.1073/pnas.1420955112

[165] Cieslik M, Chugh R, Wu YM, Wu M, Brennan C, Lonigro R, Su F, Wang R, Siddiqui J, Mehra R, Cao X, Lucas D, Chinnaiyan AM, Robinson D. The use of exome capture RNA-seq for highly degraded RNA with application to clinical cancer sequencing. *Genome Res*. 2015;25(9):1372–1381. DOI: 10.1101/gr.189621.115

[166] Taylor RC. An overview of the Hadoop/MapReduce/HBase framework and its current applications in bioinformatics. *BMC Bioinformatics*. 2010;11(Suppl 12):S1. DOI: 10.1186/1471-2105-11-S12-S1

[167] Ruby JG, Jan C, Player C, Axtell MJ, Lee W, Nusbaum C, Ge H, Bartel DP. Large-scale sequencing reveals 21U–RNAs and additional microRNAs and endogenous siRNAs in C. elegans. *Cell*. 2006;127(6):1193–1207. DOI: 10.1016/j.cell.2006.10.040

[168] Core LJ, Waterfall JJ, Lis JT. Nascent RNA sequencing reveals widespread pausing and divergent initiation at human promoters. *Science*. 2008;322(5909):1845–1848. 10.1126/science.1162228

[169] Chu C, Qu K, Zhong FL, Artandi SE, Chang HY. Genomic maps of long noncoding RNA occupancy reveal principles of RNA-chromatin interactions. *Mol Cell*. 2011;44(4):667–678. DOI: 10.1016/j.molcel.2011.08.027

[170] Ingolia NT, Ghaemmaghami S, Newman JR, Weissman JS. Genome-wide analysis in vivo of translation with nucleotide resolution using ribosome profiling. *Science*. 2009;324(5924):218–223. DOI: 10.1126/science.1168978

[171] Chi SW, Zang JB, Mele A, Darnell RB. Argonaute HITS-CLIP decodes microRNA-mRNA interaction maps. *Nature*. 2009;460:479–486. DOI: 10.1038/nature08170

[172] Hafner M, Landgraf P, Ludwig J, Rice A, Ojo T et al. Identification of microRNAs and other small regulatory RNAs using cDNA library sequencing. *Methods*. 2008;44(1):3–12. DOI: 10.1016/j.ymeth.2007.09.009

[173] Churchman LS, Weissman JS. Nascent transcript sequencing visualizes transcription at nucleotide resolution. *Nature*. 2011;469:368–373. DOI: 10.1038/nature09652

[174] Jiao Y, Meyerowitz EM. Cell-type specific analysis of translating RNAs in developing flowers reveals new levels of control. *Mol Syst Biol*. 2010;6:419. DOI: 10.1038/msb. 2010.76

[175] German MA, Pillay M, Jeong DH, Hetawal A, Luo S et al. Global identification of microRNA-target RNA pairs by parallel analysis of RNA ends. *Nat Biotechnol*. 2008;26(8):941–946. DOI: 10.1038/nbt1417

[176] Pelechano V, Wei W, Steinmetz LM. Extensive transcriptional heterogeneity revealed by isoform profiling. *Nature*. 2013;497(7447):127–131. DOI: 10.1038/nature12121

[177] Hashimshony T, Wagner F, Sher N, Yanai I. CEL-Seq: single-cell RNA-Seq by multiplexed linear amplification. *Cell Rep*. 2012;2(3):666–673. DOI: 10.1016/j.celrep. 2012.08.003

[178] Peng Y, Leung HC, Yiu SM, Lv MJ, Zhu XG, Chin FY. IDBA-tran: a more robust de novo de Bruijn graph assembler for transcriptomes with uneven expression levels. *Bioinformatics*. 2013;29(13):i326–334. DOI: 10.1093/bioinformatics/btt219

[179] Chu HT, Hsiao WW, Chen JC, Yeh TJ, Tsai MH, Lin H, Liu YW, Lee SA, Chen CC, Tsao TT, Kao CY. EBARDenovo: highly accurate de novo assembly of RNASeq with efficient chimera-detection. *Bioinformatics*. 2013;29(8):1004–1010. DOI: 10.1093/bioinformatics/btt092

[180] Maretty L, Sibbesen JA, Krogh A. Bayesian transcriptome assembly. *Genome Biol*. 2014;15(10):501. DOI: 10.1186/s13059-014-0501-4

Chapter 5

Computational Analysis and Integration of MeDIP-seq Methylome Data

Gareth A. Wilson and Stephan Beck

Additional information is available at the end of the chapter

http://dx.doi.org/10.5772/61207

Abstract

The combinatorial number of possible methylomes in biological time and space is astronomical. Consequently, the computational analysis of methylomes needs to cater for a variety of data, throughput and resolution. Here, we review recent advances in 2nd generation sequencing (2GS) with a focus on the different methods used for the analysis of MeDIP-seq data. The challenges and opportunities presented by the integration of methylation data with other genomic data types are discussed as is the potential impact of emerging 3rd generation sequencing (3GS) based technologies on methylation analysis.

Keywords: DNA methylation, methylome, immuno precipitation, analysis pipeline

1. Introduction

For many years it's been widely known by scientists that, despite possessing the same DNA sequence, not all genes can be active in all cells within an organism all of the time. It is through the regulation of genes that we are able to see phenotypic differences between cells with identical genotypes. In the late 1930's, Conrad Waddington introduced the term 'epigenetic landscape' to provide a metaphor for the cellular mechanisms leading to this regulation [1]. These regulatory, or epigenetic, patterns can be seen to persistently influence gene expression levels through cell division. Hence, epigenetics involves the study of marks and mechanisms that control gene expression in a mitotically and potentially meiotically heritable manner [2].

One such mechanism is DNA methylation (or more specifically cytosine methylation), an important epigenetic modification. DNA methylation, in conjunction with histone modifications, remodeling complexes and non-coding RNAs, plays a vital role in regulating genome dynamics. In combination with these other modifications, DNA methylation can control the

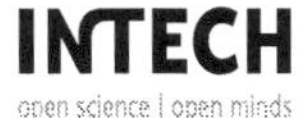

accessibility of the underlying DNA to the transcriptional machinery through the modulation of chromatin density. As a result DNA methylation is involved in a diverse range of processes including embryogenesis, genomic imprinting, cellular differentiation, DNA protein interactions and gene regulation [3].

In mammalian genomes, DNA methylation occurs almost exclusively at palindromic CpG dinucleotides. CpG dinucleotides are found throughout the genome but are significantly depleted (21% of that expected in the human genome [4]) in comparison to other dinucleotide combinations. This is due to the hypermutability of methylated cytosines [5] where spontaneous deamination to thymine occurs. However as a result of chance or potentially due to their functional importance, a minority of CpGs are maintained against this loss.

The surviving CpGs are often found at a high density in localised genomic regions termed CpG islands (CGIs) [3]. Unlike the majority of CpGs, these regions, of approximately 1kb in length (though different algorithms produce different CGI predictions [6]), are largely unmethylated and have been found to overlap the promoter regions of 60–70% of all human genes, representing all constitutively expressed genes and approximately 40% of those displaying tissue specific expression patterns [7, 8]. Unmethylated CGIs are able to recruit CpG binding proteins such as Cfp1 [9], these in turn lead to the modification of histone tails [10] and the formation of permissive chromatin domains, potentially enabling the initiation of transcription [11]. In contrast, methylated CGIs are associated with gene silencing. This silencing can occur via various routes such as inhibiting the recruitment of DNA binding proteins from their target sites [12] or alternatively through the recruitment of methyl-CpG-binding domain (MBD) proteins that in turn recruit histone modifying complexes to the methylated sites [13].

Whilst methylation changes at CGIs is perhaps the most studied region, methylation occurs in other genomic locations as well. CpG island shores represent regions of lower CpG density flanking a CGI. They are generally defined as reaching 2kb upstream and downstream of an island. It has been found that most tissue specific methylation occurs in these shore regions rather than the islands [14, 15]. Additionally, high levels of DNA methylation can be found in repetitive genomic regions. Rather than directly regulating the transcriptional potential of a gene, this methylation is seen to prevent chromosomal instability [16-18].

Although DNA methylation is largely found in the CpG dinucleotide, it has also been reported in humans and mouse at CHG and CHH sites [19, 20]. In comparison with a methylated CpG site, methylated non-CpG sites display a much lower level of methylation within a cell population [21] and show lower conservation between cell lines [22]. The mechanisms and functionality of non-CpG methylation are currently unclear but the levels appear to decrease during differentiation whilst being restored in induced pluripotent stem cells. This potentially suggests a role in the origin and maintenance of the pluripotent state [19, 23, 24].

DNA methylation changes have been associated with numerous conditions. Many cancers have shown hypomethylation at repetitive sequences thus promoting chromosomal instability. Examples include the LINE repeat L1 in a range of tumours [25] and satellite repeats ALRα and SATR1 in peripheral nerve sheath tumours [26]. Hypomethylation at specific promoters can lead to aberrant expression of oncogenes, whilst in contrast hypermethylation at specific island or shore sites can lead to transcriptional inactivation of genes involved in pathways such as DNA repair and apoptosis [2, 13]. Neurological disorders such as Alzheimer's and Multiple sclerosis have been associated with aberrant DNA methylation as have autoimmune diseases such as ICF syndrome and rheumatoid arthritis [2].

2. Methods for the study of genome-wide DNA methylation

Even within the relatively new field of second-generation (or next-generation) sequencing (2GS), a plethora of methods exist for the exploration of DNA methylation and the analysis of the ensuing data (Table 1). Such methods include the use of restriction endonucleases, or the bisulphite conversion of DNA. Here we discuss in detail the analysis of affinity enrichment techniques, specifically MeDIP-seq. For a full review of other methods see [27].

Software	Method	Summary	Publication
Batman	MeDIP-seq	Bayesian tool for methylation analysis of MeDIP profiles	[33]
Bismark	Bisulphite	Maps bisulfite treated sequencing reads through in-silico bisulfite conversion of both reads and genome. Performs methylation calling in a quick and easy-to-use fashion.	[81]
Bis-SNP	Bisulphite	Estimates methylation probabilities of different cytosine context to determine genotypes and methylation levels simultaneously.	[61]
BSMAP	Bisulphite	Mapping software for bisulphite sequencing. BSMAP aligns the Ts in the reads to both Cs and Ts in the reference by building a "seed" index of the reference genome.	[82]
BS-Seeker	Bisulphite	Accurate and fast mapping of bisulfite-treated short reads through in-silico bisulfite conversion of both reads and genome.	[83]
EpiExplorer	Various	Web tool that allows you to use large reference epigenome datasets for your own analysis without complex scripting or preprocessing.	[58]
Epigenome Browser	Various	Resource for visualizing and interacting with whole-genome datasets. The browser currently hosts Human Epigenome Atlas data produced by the Roadmap Epigenomics project.	[84]

Software	Method	Summary	Publication
MEDIPS	MeDIP-seq	Bioconductor package providing a comprehensive approach for normalizing and analyzing MeDIP-seq data	[38]
MeDUSA	MeDIP-seq	Performs a full analysis of MeDIP-seq data, including sequence alignment, QC and determination and annotation of DMRs	[40]
MeQA	MeDIP-seq	Pipeline for the pre-processing, quality assessment, read distribution and methylation estimation for MeDIP-seq datasets	[39]
MethMarker	Validation	Implements a systematic workflow for design, optimization and (computational) validation of DNA methylation biomarkers.	[85]
Methylcoder	Bisulphite	Software pipeline for bisulfite-treated sequences	[86]
MethylSeekR	Bisulphite	Accurately identifies the footprints of active regulatory regions from bisulfite-sequencing data	[87]
Metmap	Methyl-seq	Produces corrected site-specific methylation states from MethylSeq experiments and annotates unmethylated islands across the genome.	[88]
Sherman	Validation	Simulates ungapped high-throughput datasets for bisulfite sequencing. Allows for evaluation of the influence of common problems observed in many sequencing experiments.	http://tinyurl.com/bwkttgh

Table 1. Examples of software available for the analysis of 2GS methylation data.

Buoyed by the success of combining chromatin immunoprecipitation with second generation sequencing for genome-wide studies of histone modifications and transcription factor binding sites [28] (termed ChIP-seq), similar techniques were adopted for methylation. These methods generally involve either enrichment through methylcytosine-specific protein domains (e.g. MethylCap[29], MBD-seq[30]) or through antibody-mediated immunoprecipitation (e.g. MeDIP[31], MRE-seq[32]) prior to sequencing[33, 34]. Such approaches, whilst not offering the resolution of bisulphite sequence data, are both genome-wide and increasingly affordable. Concordance in methylation calls between different enrichment and bisulphite methods have been shown to be high[35, 36]. In methylated DNA immunoprecipitation (MeDIP), an antibody capable of recognizing 5mC is utilized to immunoprecipitate the methylated fraction of the genome. One issue that has been highlighted with enrichment methods such as MeDIP, is the necessity to take the sequencing to saturation in order to confirm lack of methylation at a CpG site. Such a policy would be costly and would generate a vast amount of redundant data and as such saturation has not been reached with these methods. Methylation-sensitive restriction enzymes (MRE) target unmethylated CpGs for sequencing thus one alternative suggestion is to integrate the MRE-seq method with MeDIP-seq. Such integration will have the benefit of reducing the need for saturation sequencing and will highlight regions of intermediate methylation, which would be difficult to detect using a single method. Going a step further, if coupled with single nucleotide polymorphism (SNP) profiling, it would also be possible to detect potential allele-specific epigenetic states[35].

MeDIP-seq is a popular enrichment technique for interrogating the methylation status of cytosines across entire genomes. It has been used in numerous studies including the first mammalian methylome [33] and the first cancer methylome [26]. In the next section, approaches for the analysis of MeDIP-seq data will be discussed in greater detail.

3. Computational approaches for the analysis of MeDIP-seq data

A number of computational tools have been developed for the analysis of MeDIP data (Table 1), including Batman [33], MEDME [37], MEDIPS [38], MeQA [39] and MeDUSA [40]. The method to use depends very much on the questions you want to ask of the data, and as a result the type of analysis performed can be described as analyzing absolute methylation or, alternatively, relative methylation.

3.1. Absolute methylation

The efficiency of immunoprecipitation in MeDIP is largely dependent on the density of methylated CpG sites. Therefore, it is difficult to distinguish true variation in enrichment, and hence methylation, from confounding effects caused by fluctuations in CpG density. This bias needs to be corrected for in order to perform accurate and biologically relevant comparisons of methylation states between different genomic regions.

The first method to try and correct for this bias was called Batman (Bayesian Tool for Methylation Analysis)[33]. This tool was originally written to analyse MeDIP-chip data, but can also be applied to 2GS. Batman, distributed as a suite of Java scripts, models the effect of varying densities of methylated CpGs on MeDIP enrichment, resulting in the transformation of the count of the aligned sequence read depth within a 100bp region into a quantitative measure of DNA methylation. Such data can then be used to compare global methylation scores between methylomes or between feature types (e.g. CpG islands, exons) within a methylome. Batman was used for the analysis of the first mammalian methylome[33] and also the first cancer methylome[26]. Unfortunately, Batman was disproportionately time consuming to run, even when running with multiple processors. The R BioConductor package[41] MEDIPS v1.8 [38] attempted to utilize much of the methodology used in the Batman approach whilst outperforming the computation time by orders of magnitude. By implementing MEDIPS as an R package, this method is also more approachable for the majority of users, requiring less computational knowledge to run the methods. In addition to generating genome-wide methylation scores, MEDIPS sought to provide MeDIP-seq specific quality control metrics such as calculating the degree of enrichment of CpG-rich sequenced reads relative to genomic background. Finally, MEDIPS provided a methodology for determining the location of differentially methylated regions (DMRs) between samples. Whilst MEDIPS, building on the strengths of Batman, undoubtedly provided an important step forward in the analysis of MeDIP-seq data, it also had significant issues that need to be considered both before use and when interrogating output from the program. For example, the DMR calling algorithm requires an input sample to be sequenced in addition to the immunoprecipitated sample, thus effectively doubling costs.

3.2. Relative methylation

Methods for calculating absolute methylation have proven to be useful when identifying large global changes, for example hypomethylation of satellite repeats in peripheral nerve sheath tumours[26]. Additionally, transforming MeDIP-seq data from read counts to a methylation score has assisted in validating experiments against bisulphite data[33]. However, as yet, these methods have not provided a framework for determining the location of DMRs in a statistically rigorous manner. To achieve this, relative changes in DNA methylation between cohorts can be determined, rather than absolute changes within a cohort. As such the problem has much in common with other sequencing protocols, such as identifying differential expression between RNA-seq cohorts or identifying peaks from a ChIP-seq sample. This commonality opens up an abundance of methods that can be used or adapted for MeDIP-seq sample analysis, for example peak finding using MACS[42, 43], or DMR finding using DESeq [44] or edgeR [45].

There are several hurdles to cross when analysing MeDIP-seq data, particularly during the identification of DMRs. Read counts need to be normalized to eliminate biases as a result of variability in sequencing depth between samples. Whilst global read count normalization can help address this problem, it does not account for 'competition' effects. RNA-seq provides an example of such effects, in which condition specific highly expressed genes can lead to a depressed read count in other genes and hence a bias when comparing samples[46]. An analogous situation can be found in MeDIP-seq, where sample-specific repeat methylation could potentially diminish reads in other genomic regions and introduce bias to analyses, particularly given the large amount of repetitive sequence methylated in the genome. Further, despite falling sequencing costs, MeDIP-seq experiments will often have few biological replicates. As a result, it can be difficult to obtain reliable estimates of model parameters to fit statistical models and thereby locate real differences between samples. By using methods such as DESeq that estimate variance in a local fashion, it is possible to remove potential selection biases [44]. Additionally, DESeq estimates a flexible, mean-dependent local regression rather than attempting to reliably estimate both the variance and mean parameters of the distribution from limited numbers of replicates. Typically, there is enough data available in these experiments to allow for sufficiently precise local estimation of the dispersion [44] and hence avoid bias towards certain areas of the dynamic range when identifying DMRs. Finally, accurate biological interpretation could be compromised by differences in DNA fragment size distributions between samples. Performing fragment length normalization through read subsampling to equalize the distributions can eliminate this potential bias.

Additionally, the methods developed for absolute methylation calculation are unable to take account of non-CpG methylation and, due to the models used being based on local CpG density, the presence of non-CpG methylation could adversely skew the output. In contrast, a relative methylation approach should be able to locate differences in methylation driven by asymmetric non-CpG methylation[47], taking advantage of the affinity of the MeDIP-seq antibody for methylated cytosine (rather than exclusively selecting for methylated CpGs).

The first pipeline to provide a comprehensive methodology for analyzing MeDIP-seq data, with the focus on accurate and statistically rigorous identification of DMRs, was MeDUSA (Methylated DNA Utility for Sequence Analysis) (https://www.ucl.ac.uk/cancer/medical-genomics/medusaproject) [40]. MeDUSA (v1) utilized a number of software packages to perform a complete analysis of MeDIP-seq data. This included sequence alignment, quality control (QC), and determination and annotation of DMRs. The novel aspect of MeDUSA was the approach to DMR calling. It utilized the USeq suite of tools, specifically MultipleReplicaScanSeqs (MRSS) and EnrichedRegionMaker [48]. MRSS formatted data for use in the BioConductor package DESeq [44]. DESeq determined significant differential counts between cohorts. These regions are passed to EnrichedRegionMaker to determine if multiple regions can be combined to create single larger regions. MeDUSA proceeded to provide initial annotation of these DMR regions.

More recently new versions of both MEDIPS (v1.10) and MeDUSA (v2) have been released. The MEDIPS package now incorporates methods from the edgeR [45] bioconductor package to provide a DMR calling methodology analogous to that used in MeDUSA. However, the approach and implementation employed by MEDIPS is more efficient (both time and computational) than the DMR calling method used in MeDUSA v1. As a consequence, MeDUSA (v2) now utilises MEDIPS for the DMR calling stage of the pipeline.

4. Data integration

As more studies are published and sequencing costs fall, the opportunity to integrate methylation datasets with other data types increases[49]. Whilst being able to detect changes in methylation is interesting, it is more interesting, and indeed more likely to be of functional importance, if this change associates with other detectable biological signals. For example, the potential of associating a methylation change with a corresponding change in transcription of a particular splice variant[50-52] from RNA-seq, or with an increase in binding of a specific transcription factor using ChIP-seq data[53].

In addition to the published sequence and array based datasets stored in public repositories such as GEO[54], a number of datasets are pre-loaded in public Genome Browsers. For example, the UCSC Genome Browser provides access to data from the ENCODE project[55], including expression data in the form of RNA-seq and regulatory data generated through ChIP-seq representing several different cell lines and various primary tissue types. Compressed file formats such as bigWig and bigBed[56] make it relatively simple to load and visualize multiple data types (Figure 1) whilst software such as bedTools[57] allow for quick intersections between data to be determined. EpiExplorer functions as a user-friendly web-based solution for providing initial annotations of feature sets [58], such as differentially methylated regions. It enables exploratory analysis of user-uploaded data and provides links to many external public datasets. As datasets become larger and more complex, other methods of integration may be required, for example an unsupervised clustering approach may be useful [49, 59].

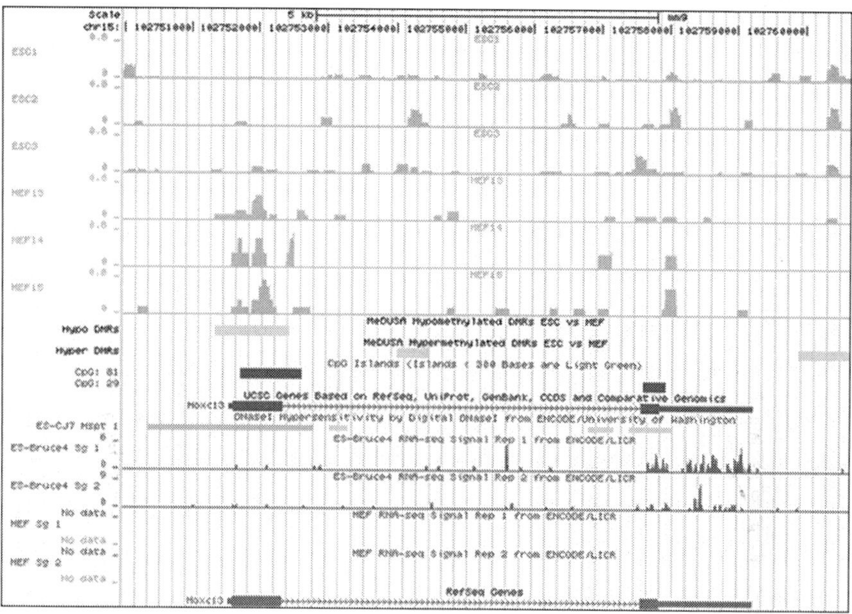

Figure 1. Visualising MeDUSA output in UCSC Genome Browser. MeDIP tracks are shown for 3 embryonic stem cell (ESC) replicates and 3 Mouse embryonic fibroblasts (MEF) replicates over the Hoxc13 gene. The CpG island in the promoter region is hypomethylated in the ESC samples, suggesting more permissible chromatin in ESCs than in MEFs. This is supported by the ES-CJ7 DNase I Hypersensitivity track. Additionally the RNA-seq tracks show transcriptional differences in this gene between ESCs and MEFs.

In addition to transcriptomic and regulatory data, it is also possible to integrate methylation data with genomic information. A perceived difference in methylation at a given CpG dinucleotide between samples could be caused by one sample possessing a methylated cytosine whilst the other sample possesses an unmethylated cytosine. Alternatively, the methylation difference could be due to the presence of a SNP, seeing the cytosine replaced with an alternative base. Therefore, the use of genotype profiling can clarify whether a methylation difference is a result of genetic or epigenetic changes. The need to consider both genetic and epigenetic changes came to the fore with the release of the Illumina Infinium HumanMethylation450 BeadChip. This chip allows for the interrogation of 485000 potential sites of methylation. However, a significant proportion of these sites are also sites of known SNPs[60]. Thus, any difference detected at these sites could be driven by epigenetic or genetic factors. Whilst this is an issue for the array analysis, tools such as Bis-SNP are able to make

SNP calls from bisulphite sequencing data, in doing so allowing for both accurate quantification of methylation levels and for identification of allele-specific epigenetic events such as imprinting [61].

A recent study utilised a combination of SNP, expression and methylation data to determine whether methylation has a passive or active role in gene regulation [62]. Three models were considered for the relationship between methylation and regulation. The first model described how a SNP would independently influence expression and methylation, for example through SNP modification of a transcription factor binding site (the impact on methylation of small changes to nucleotides constituting a TFBS have been explored in a recent tri-primate methylome study [89]). In the second model, a SNP would impact upon methylation, which, in turn, would modify expression. The final model shows a SNP affecting expression that consequently alters the methylation state. It was found that, in reality, each of these models occurs in different contexts with the frequency of the model varying according to cell type [62, 63]. Such studies underline the complexity inherent in, and the difficulty in deciphering, regulatory interactions and should serve as a warning to those seeking overly simplistic interpretations [63].

Extending the genetic effect out from a single site to an entire region, it is possible that methylation levels could be strongly influenced by the haplotypic phase[64]. Haplotype specific methylation (HSM) is a result of the cumulative methylation effect driven by the phase of a number of CpG-SNPs within the haplotype. This signal was strong enough to be identified across the 47kb FTO linkage disequilibrium block[65]. Such a finding is only possible through the integration of DNA methylation data and genome wide association study data. It is also worth remembering at this juncture that whether a measured methylation difference is due to a SNP or not, the downstream impact on the transcriptional potential of the chromosomal region in question could be the same.

5. Future perspectives

The field of epigenetics and specifically the study of DNA methylation have emerged as major areas of research in recent years. This rise can be largely attributed to the impact of emerging technologies, particularly 2GS. Projects that would have been perceived as impossible just a few years ago have been completed and more are underway. The International Human Epigenome Consortium (IHEC) (http://www.ihec-epigenomes.org/) was established to provide high-resolution reference epigenome maps to the research community by coordinating large-scale international efforts. The grand aim of which is to generate 1000 reference epigenomes. Various initiatives worldwide have joined IHEC in an attempt to complete the goal. In Europe, the BLUEPRINT Project[66] will take the IHEC goal forward and in doing so improve our understanding of the human epigenome – of which the methylome is a key constituent.

There are still many questions associated with the role of DNA methylation. Some with regards to the biology, and some the techniques used. It is important to know, for example, if using an enrichment based technique, what the specificity of your antibody is. Different antibodies appear to show differing levels of repeat enrichment when performing MeDIP[67]. It would be of benefit to standardize these analyses. Similarly, different bisulphite conversion protocols may lead to differing conversion success. Global CpG methylation levels obtained from WGBS for 3 human embryonic stem cell (HESC) lines showed surprising variability (72% - 85%)[68]. This could be due to unstable gain and loss of methylation as previously reported in embryonic stem cells (ESCs)[69, 70], but it could also be a result of pre-analysis protocol and lab specific differences in sample preparation. Equally, it will be interesting to discover more about the biological roles and genomic location of the different cytosine modifications (5-hydroxyme-thylcytosine[47], 5-Formylcytosine and 5-Carboxylcytosine[71]) and also non-CpG methylation.

New technologies with the potential for adaption for the analysis of DNA methylation are being developed constantly. For example, improved methods of methylation validation would be highly beneficial. Often hundreds or thousands of potential candidate regions are generated from a multi-sample MeDIP-seq comparison, and similar numbers could be produced by future EWAS (Epigenome-Wide Association Studies)[72]. Ideally, many of these regions would be validated using a different technology. Targeted bisulphite sequencing is often used, however this can often be laborious and time-consuming. Combining new technologies such as microdroplet-based PCR target enrichment (e.g. RainDance Technologies) with 2GS has recently been developed into a high-throughput platform termed RainDropBS-seq [73], providing an excellent option to remove the validation bottle-neck. There is also the emergence of third generation sequencing on the horizon. Third generation sequencing (3GS) theoretically promises many advantages over existing 2GS methods including higher throughput, longer read lengths, improved accuracy and requiring smaller amounts of starting material[74], indeed some companies e.g. Oxford Nanopore Technologies, are promising single molecule sequencing[75, 76]. The potential of single molecule nanopore sequencing is particularly exciting for researchers working in the field of DNA methylation. Theoretically, it should be possible to sequence complex mammalian genomes and determine any base modifications such as methylation[77], potentially including hitherto undiscovered modifications, without the need for any of the treatments or enrichments discussed above.

As the large-scale projects, such as IHEC, BLUEPRINT and increasingly clinically oriented projects such as OncoTrack progress, it is expected that many methods and tools will become standardized. This will be an important step in translating epigenomic knowledge from the bench to the clinic[78, 79]. In the future, it is hoped that a patient will be treated with drugs tailored to their particular condition – this is of particular relevance for cancer patients. Preliminary work using whole genome, exome and RNA-seq has demonstrated the potential for treating a real patient in a relatively short time period (24 days) and a relatively low cost (~$3600)[80]. Adding reliable epigenetic information, utilising the IHEC reference genomes, to this diagnostic toolbox is a logical next step. Extrapolating from these advances, it is quite clear that the bottleneck is shifting from logistics and data generation to computational analysis.

Acknowledgements

Research in the Beck lab was supported by: Wellcome Trust (99148), Royal Society Wolfson Research Merit Award (WM100023), IMI-JU OncoTrack (115234) and EU-FP7 projects, EPIGENESYS (257082) and BLUEPRINT (282510).

Author details

Gareth A. Wilson* and Stephan Beck

*Address all correspondence to: gareth.wilson@crick.ac.uk

Medical Genomics, UCL Cancer Institute, University College London, London, UK

References

[1] Waddington CH. An introduction to modern genetics. New York,: The Macmillan company; 1939. 2 p.l., 7 -441 p. p.

[2] Portela A, Esteller M. Epigenetic modifications and human disease. Nat Biotechnol. 2010;28(10):1057-68.

[3] Bird A. DNA methylation patterns and epigenetic memory. Genes Dev. 2002;16(1): 6-21.

[4] Lander ES, Linton LM, Birren B, Nusbaum C, Zody MC, Baldwin J, et al. Initial sequencing and analysis of the human genome. Nature. 2001;409(6822):860-921.

[5] Duncan BK, Miller JH. Mutagenic deamination of cytosine residues in DNA. Nature. 1980;287(5782):560-1.

[6] Illingworth RS, Bird AP. CpG islands--'a rough guide'. FEBS Lett. 2009;583(11): 1713-20.

[7] Weber M, Hellmann I, Stadler MB, Ramos L, Paabo S, Rebhan M, et al. Distribution, silencing potential and evolutionary impact of promoter DNA methylation in the human genome. Nat Genet. 2007;39(4):457-66.

[8] Saxonov S, Berg P, Brutlag DL. A genome-wide analysis of CpG dinucleotides in the human genome distinguishes two distinct classes of promoters. Proc Natl Acad Sci U S A. 2006;103(5):1412-7.

[9]   Thomson JP, Skene PJ, Selfridge J, Clouaire T, Guy J, Webb S, et al. CpG islands influence chromatin structure via the CpG-binding protein Cfp1. Nature. 2010;464(7291): 1082-6.

[10] Blackledge NP, Zhou JC, Tolstorukov MY, Farcas AM, Park PJ, Klose RJ. CpG islands recruit a histone H3 lysine 36 demethylase. Mol Cell. 2010;38(2):179-90.

[11] Blackledge NP, Klose R. CpG island chromatin: A platform for gene regulation. Epigenetics. 2011;6(2):147-52.

[12] Kuroda A, Rauch TA, Todorov I, Ku HT, Al-Abdullah IH, Kandeel F, et al. Insulin gene expression is regulated by DNA methylation. PLoS One. 2009;4(9):e6953.

[13] Esteller M. Epigenetic gene silencing in cancer: the DNA hypermethylome. Hum Mol Genet. 2007;16 Spec No 1:R50-9.

[14] Doi A, Park IH, Wen B, Murakami P, Aryee MJ, Irizarry R, et al. Differential methylation of tissue- and cancer-specific CpG island shores distinguishes human induced pluripotent stem cells, embryonic stem cells and fibroblasts. Nat Genet. 2009;41(12): 1350-3.

[15] Irizarry RA, Ladd-Acosta C, Wen B, Wu Z, Montano C, Onyango P, et al. The human colon cancer methylome shows similar hypo- and hypermethylation at conserved tissue-specific CpG island shores. Nat Genet. 2009;41(2):178-86.

[16] Esteller M. Cancer epigenomics: DNA methylomes and histone-modification maps. Nat Rev Genet. 2007;8(4):286-98.

[17] Gaudet F, Hodgson JG, Eden A, Jackson-Grusby L, Dausman J, Gray JW, et al. Induction of tumors in mice by genomic hypomethylation. Science. 2003;300(5618):489-92.

[18] Walsh CP, Chaillet JR, Bestor TH. Transcription of IAP endogenous retroviruses is constrained by cytosine methylation. Nature genetics. 1998;20(2):116-7.

[19] Lister R, Pelizzola M, Dowen RH, Hawkins RD, Hon G, Tonti-Filippini J, et al. Human DNA methylomes at base resolution show widespread epigenomic differences. Nature. 2009;462(7271):315-22.

[20] Stadler MB, Murr R, Burger L, Ivanek R, Lienert F, Scholer A, et al. DNA-binding factors shape the mouse methylome at distal regulatory regions. Nature. 2011;480(7378): 490-5.

[21] Dyachenko OV, Schevchuk TV, Kretzner L, Buryanov YI, Smith SS. Human non-CG methylation: are human stem cells plant-like? Epigenetics : official journal of the DNA Methylation Society. 2010;5(7):569-72.

[22] Chen PY, Feng S, Joo JW, Jacobsen SE, Pellegrini M. A comparative analysis of DNA methylation across human embryonic stem cell lines. Genome Biol. 2011;12(7):R62.

[23] Laurent L, Wong E, Li G, Huynh T, Tsirigos A, Ong CT, et al. Dynamic changes in the human methylome during differentiation. Genome Res. 2010;20(3):320-31.

[24] Lister R, Pelizzola M, Kida YS, Hawkins RD, Nery JR, Hon G, et al. Hotspots of aberrant epigenomic reprogramming in human induced pluripotent stem cells. Nature. 2011;471(7336):68-73.

[25] Wilson AS, Power BE, Molloy PL. DNA hypomethylation and human diseases. Biochim Biophys Acta. 2007;1775(1):138-62.

[26] Feber A, Wilson GA, Zhang L, Presneau N, Idowu B, Down TA, et al. Comparative methylome analysis of benign and malignant peripheral nerve sheath tumors. Genome research. 2011;21(4):515-24.

[27] Laird PW. Principles and challenges of genome-wide DNA methylation analysis. Nat Rev Genet. 2010;11(3):191-203.

[28] Park PJ. ChIP-seq: advantages and challenges of a maturing technology. Nature reviews Genetics. 2009;10(10):669-80.

[29] Cross SH, Charlton JA, Nan X, Bird AP. Purification of CpG islands using a methylated DNA binding column. Nature genetics. 1994;6(3):236-44.

[30] Serre D, Lee BH, Ting AH. MBD-isolated Genome Sequencing provides a high-throughput and comprehensive survey of DNA methylation in the human genome. Nucleic Acids Res. 2010;38(2):391-9.

[31] Weber M, Davies JJ, Wittig D, Oakeley EJ, Haase M, Lam WL, et al. Chromosome-wide and promoter-specific analyses identify sites of differential DNA methylation in normal and transformed human cells. Nat Genet. 2005;37(8):853-62.

[32] Maunakea AK, Nagarajan RP, Bilenky M, Ballinger TJ, D'Souza C, Fouse SD, et al. Conserved role of intragenic DNA methylation in regulating alternative promoters. Nature. 2010;466(7303):253-7.

[33] Down TA, Rakyan VK, Turner DJ, Flicek P, Li H, Kulesha E, et al. A Bayesian deconvolution strategy for immunoprecipitation-based DNA methylome analysis. Nat Biotechnol. 2008;26(7):779-85.

[34] Brinkman AB, Simmer F, Ma K, Kaan A, Zhu J, Stunnenberg HG. Whole-genome DNA methylation profiling using MethylCap-seq. Methods. 2010;52(3):232-6.

[35] Harris RA, Wang T, Coarfa C, Nagarajan RP, Hong C, Downey SL, et al. Comparison of sequencing-based methods to profile DNA methylation and identification of monoallelic epigenetic modifications. Nat Biotechnol. 2010;28(10):1097-105.

[36] Bock C, Tomazou EM, Brinkman AB, Muller F, Simmer F, Gu H, et al. Quantitative comparison of genome-wide DNA methylation mapping technologies. Nat Biotechnol. 2010;28(10):1106-14.

[37] Pelizzola M, Koga Y, Urban AE, Krauthammer M, Weissman S, Halaban R, et al. MEDME: an experimental and analytical methodology for the estimation of DNA methylation levels based on microarray derived MeDIP-enrichment. Genome research. 2008;18(10):1652-9.

[38] Chavez L, Jozefczuk J, Grimm C, Dietrich J, Timmermann B, Lehrach H, et al. Computational analysis of genome-wide DNA methylation during the differentiation of human embryonic stem cells along the endodermal lineage. Genome research. 2010;20(10):1441-50.

[39] Huang J, Renault V, Sengenes J, Touleimat N, Michel S, Lathrop M, et al. MeQA: a pipeline for MeDIP-seq data quality assessment and analysis. Bioinformatics. 2012;28(4):587-8.

[40] Wilson GA, Dhami P, Feber A, Cortazar D, Suzuki Y, Schulz R, et al. Resources for methylome analysis suitable for gene knockout studies of potential epigenome modifiers. GigaScience. 2012;1(1).

[41] Gentleman RC, Carey VJ, Bates DM, Bolstad B, Dettling M, Dudoit S, et al. Bioconductor: open software development for computational biology and bioinformatics. Genome Biol. 2004;5(10):R80.

[42] Sati S, Tanwar VS, Kumar KA, Patowary A, Jain V, Ghosh S, et al. High resolution methylome map of rat indicates role of intragenic DNA methylation in identification of coding region. PLoS One. 2012;7(2):e31621.

[43] Zhang Y, Liu T, Meyer CA, Eeckhoute J, Johnson DS, Bernstein BE, et al. Model-based analysis of ChIP-Seq (MACS). Genome Biol. 2008;9(9):R137.

[44] Anders S, Huber W. Differential expression analysis for sequence count data. Genome Biol. 2010;11(10):R106.

[45] Robinson MD, McCarthy DJ, Smyth GK. edgeR: a Bioconductor package for differential expression analysis of digital gene expression data. Bioinformatics. 2010;26(1): 139-40.

[46] Robinson MD, Oshlack A. A scaling normalization method for differential expression analysis of RNA-seq data. Genome Biol. 2010;11(3):R25.

[47] Ficz G, Branco MR, Seisenberger S, Santos F, Krueger F, Hore TA, et al. Dynamic regulation of 5-hydroxymethylcytosine in mouse ES cells and during differentiation. Nature. 2011;473(7347):398-402.

[48] Nix DA, Courdy SJ, Boucher KM. Empirical methods for controlling false positives and estimating confidence in ChIP-Seq peaks. BMC Bioinformatics. 2008;9:523.

[49] Hawkins RD, Hon GC, Ren B. Next-generation genomics: an integrative approach. Nature reviews Genetics. 2010;11(7):476-86.

[50] Chodavarapu RK, Feng S, Bernatavichute YV, Chen PY, Stroud H, Yu Y, et al. Relationship between nucleosome positioning and DNA methylation. Nature. 2010;466(7304):388-92.

[51] Hodges E, Smith AD, Kendall J, Xuan Z, Ravi K, Rooks M, et al. High definition profiling of mammalian DNA methylation by array capture and single molecule bisulfite sequencing. Genome research. 2009;19(9):1593-605.

[52] Lyko F, Foret S, Kucharski R, Wolf S, Falckenhayn C, Maleszka R. The honey bee epigenomes: differential methylation of brain DNA in queens and workers. PLoS Biol. 2010;8(11):e1000506.

[53] Shukla S, Kavak E, Gregory M, Imashimizu M, Shutinoski B, Kashlev M, et al. CTCF-promoted RNA polymerase II pausing links DNA methylation to splicing. Nature. 2011;479(7371):74-9.

[54] Barrett T, Edgar R. Gene expression omnibus: microarray data storage, submission, retrieval, and analysis. Methods Enzymol. 2006;411:352-69.

[55] A user's guide to the encyclopedia of DNA elements (ENCODE). PLoS Biol. 2011;9(4):e1001046.

[56] Kent WJ, Zweig AS, Barber G, Hinrichs AS, Karolchik D. BigWig and BigBed: enabling browsing of large distributed datasets. Bioinformatics. 2010;26(17):2204-7.

[57] Quinlan AR, Hall IM. BEDTools: a flexible suite of utilities for comparing genomic features. Bioinformatics. 2010;26(6):841-2.

[58] Halachev K, Bast H, Albrecht F, Lengauer T, Bock C. EpiExplorer: live exploration and global analysis of large epigenomic datasets. Genome Biol. 2012;13(10):R96.

[59] Wang Z, Zang C, Rosenfeld JA, Schones DE, Barski A, Cuddapah S, et al. Combinatorial patterns of histone acetylations and methylations in the human genome. Nature genetics. 2008;40(7):897-903.

[60] Wang D, Yan L, Hu Q, Sucheston LE, Higgins MJ, Ambrosone CB, et al. IMA: an R package for high-throughput analysis of Illumina's 450K Infinium methylation data. Bioinformatics. 2012;28(5):729-30.

[61] Liu Y, Siegmund KD, Laird PW, Berman BP. Bis-SNP: Combined DNA methylation and SNP calling for Bisulfite-seq data. Genome Biol. 2012;13(7):R61.

[62] Gutierrez-Arcelus M, Lappalainen T, Montgomery SB, Buil A, Ongen H, Yurovsky A, et al. Passive and active DNA methylation and the interplay with genetic variation in gene regulation. Elife. 2013;2:e00523.

[63] Muers M. Gene expression: Disentangling DNA methylation. Nature reviews Genetics. 2013;14(8):519.

[64] Bell CG. Integration of genomic and epigenomic DNA methylation data in common complex diseases by haplotype-specific methylation analysis. Personalized Medicine. 2011;8(3):243.

[65] Bell CG, Finer S, Lindgren CM, Wilson GA, Rakyan VK, Teschendorff AE, et al. Integrated Genetic and Epigenetic Analysis Identifies Haplotype-Specific Methylation in the FTO Type 2 Diabetes and Obesity Susceptibility Locus. PLoS One. 2010;5(11):e14040.

[66] Adams D, Altucci L, Antonarakis SE, Ballesteros J, Beck S, Bird A, et al. BLUEPRINT to decode the epigenetic signature written in blood. Nat Biotechnol. 2012;30(3):224-6.

[67] Matarese F, Carrillo-de Santa Pau E, Stunnenberg HG. 5-Hydroxymethylcytosine: a new kid on the epigenetic block? Mol Syst Biol. 2011;7:562.

[68] Flicek P, Amode MR, Barrell D, Beal K, Brent S, Chen Y, et al. Ensembl 2011. Nucleic Acids Res. 2011;39(Database issue):D800-6.

[69] Ooi SK, Wolf D, Hartung O, Agarwal S, Daley GQ, Goff SP, et al. Dynamic instability of genomic methylation patterns in pluripotent stem cells. Epigenetics Chromatin. 2010;3(1):17.

[70] Humpherys D, Eggan K, Akutsu H, Hochedlinger K, Rideout WM, 3rd, Biniszkiewicz D, et al. Epigenetic instability in ES cells and cloned mice. Science. 2001;293(5527):95-7.

[71] Ito S, Shen L, Dai Q, Wu SC, Collins LB, Swenberg JA, et al. Tet proteins can convert 5-methylcytosine to 5-formylcytosine and 5-carboxylcytosine. Science. 2011;333(6047):1300-3.

[72] Rakyan VK, Down TA, Balding DJ, Beck S. Epigenome-wide association studies for common human diseases. Nature reviews Genetics. 2011;12(8):529-41.

[73] Guilhamon P, Eskandarpour M, Halai D, Wilson GA, Feber A, Teschendorff AE, et al. Meta-analysis of IDH-mutant cancers identifies EBF1 as an interaction partner for TET2. Nat Commun. 2013;4:2166.

[74] Schadt EE, Turner S, Kasarskis A. A window into third-generation sequencing. Hum Mol Genet. 2010;19(R2):R227-40.

[75] Mason CE, Elemento O. Faster sequencers, larger datasets, new challenges. Genome Biol. 2012;13(3):314.

[76] Cherf GM, Lieberman KR, Rashid H, Lam CE, Karplus K, Akeson M. Automated forward and reverse ratcheting of DNA in a nanopore at 5-A precision. Nat Biotechnol. 2012;30(4):344-8.

[77] Clarke J, Wu HC, Jayasinghe L, Patel A, Reid S, Bayley H. Continuous base identification for single-molecule nanopore DNA sequencing. Nat Nanotechnol. 2009;4(4):265-70.

[78] Lyon GJ. Personalized medicine: Bring clinical standards to human-genetics research. Nature. 2012;482(7385):300-1.

[79] Scudellari M. Genomics contest underscores challenges of personalized medicine. Nat Med. 2012;18(3):326.

[80] Roychowdhury S, Iyer MK, Robinson DR, Lonigro RJ, Wu YM, Cao X, et al. Personalized oncology through integrative high-throughput sequencing: a pilot study. Sci Transl Med. 2011;3(111):111ra21.

[81] Krueger F, Andrews SR. Bismark: a flexible aligner and methylation caller for Bisulfite-Seq applications. Bioinformatics. 2011;27(11):1571-2.

[82] Xi Y, Li W. BSMAP: whole genome bisulfite sequence MAPping program. BMC Bioinformatics. 2009;10:232.

[83] Chen PY, Cokus SJ, Pellegrini M. BS Seeker: precise mapping for bisulfite sequencing. BMC Bioinformatics. 2010;11:203.

[84] Zhou X, Maricque B, Xie M, Li D, Sundaram V, Martin EA, et al. The Human Epigenome Browser at Washington University. Nat Methods. 2011;8(12):989-90.

[85] Schuffler P, Mikeska T, Waha A, Lengauer T, Bock C. MethMarker: user-friendly design and optimization of gene-specific DNA methylation assays. Genome Biol. 2009;10(10):R105.

[86] Pedersen B, Hsieh TF, Ibarra C, Fischer RL. MethylCoder: software pipeline for bisulfite-treated sequences. Bioinformatics. 2011;27(17):2435-6.

[87] Burger L, Gaidatzis D, Schubeler D, Stadler MB. Identification of active regulatory regions from DNA methylation data. Nucleic Acids Res. 2013.

[88] Singer M, Boffelli D, Dhahbi J, Schonhuth A, Schroth GP, Martin DI, et al. MetMap enables genome-scale Methyltyping for determining methylation states in populations. PLoS Comput Biol. 2010;6(8):e1000888.

[89] Wilson GA, Butcher LM, Foster HR, Feber A, Roos C, Walter L, et al. Human-specific epigenetic variation in the immunological Leukotriene B4 Receptor (LTB4R/BLT1) implicated in common inflammatory diseases. Genome medicine. 2014;6(3):19.

Next Generation Sequencing of Microorganisms

Analysis of Next-generation Sequencing Data in Virology - Opportunities and Challenges

Sunitha M. Kasibhatla, Vaishali P. Waman, Mohan M. Kale and Urmila Kulkarni-Kale

Additional information is available at the end of the chapter

http://dx.doi.org/10.5772/61610

Abstract

Viruses are the most abundant and the smallest organisms, which are relatively simple to sequence. Genome sequence data of viruses for individual species to populations outnumber that of other species. Although this offers an opportunity to study viral diversity at varying levels of taxonomic hierarchy, it also poses challenges for systematic and structured organization of data and its downstream processing. Extensive computational analyses using a number of algorithms and programs have opened exciting opportunities for virus discovery and diagnostics, apart from augmenting our understanding of the intriguing world of viruses. Unravelling evolutionary dynamics of viruses permits improved understanding of phenomena such as quasispecies diversity, role of mutations in host switching and drug resistance, which enables the tangible measurements of genotype and phenotype of viruses. Improved understanding of geno-/serotype diversity in correlation with antigenic diversity will facilitate rational design and development of efficacious vaccines against emerging and re-emerging viruses. Mathematical models developed using the genomic data could be used to predict the spread of viruses due to vector switching and the (re)emergence due to host switching and, thereby, contribute towards designing public health policies for disease management and control.

Keywords: Virus/viral evolution, population diversity, recombination, selection pressure, phylogeny and typing

1. Introduction

1.1. Viruses: Special class of organisms

Viruses form a major class of biological entities encompassing diverse environments ranging from algae in marine ecosystems to soil, plant, human and animal systems. Several metage-

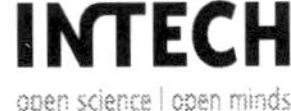

nomic studies have revealed the possibility of viruses being the dominant species of our biosphere [1]. Deep sequencing efforts have shown that viruses form 10^6–10^9 particles per millilitre of seawater [2]. It is also interesting to note that ~90% of the reads obtained from such experiments did not encode proteins, which are reported in other organisms, including viruses, that have been characterised so far. This clearly demonstrates that the actual viral diversity has not been sampled in an adequate manner so far. A crucial aspect of viral studies is the disease burden associated with them, which is known to be enormous with serious economic implications. World Health Organization documents that the global burden of communicable diseases (of which viral diseases form a major chunk) is ~15 million annually [3].

Beyond abundance aspects, study of viral evolution and genetic variations enabled the proposal of the virocentric standpoint of the evolution. Viruses gained centre stage for reasons such as being smallest replicating entities, having short generation time, large population sizes and high replication and mutation rates. Attributes such as variation in genome sizes, gene pool, shape and assembly of particles are responsible for viruses to attain pivotal role in the study of evolution [4]. It has been observed that all plausible replication and expression strategies have been employed by viruses to dynamically adapt to the ever-changing environments. Processes like complementation, recombination, reassortment, high mutation rate and existence as quasispecies enable the viruses to outgrow and outcompete the host immune system. The molecular forces driving these processes can be delineated by sequencing and the subsequent analyses.

1.2. Viral sequencing methods

The distinction of complete genome ever to be sequenced belongs to bacteriophage ΦX174 with a genome size of 5,386 bases and was achieved through the Sanger's shotgun-sequencing approach [5]. The major aim of early sequencing projects was to characterize the genomic content of an organism in terms of its coding potential. Over the last few years, the unprecedented growth in the area of sequencing technologies has had a huge impact on the way viral genomes are being addressed. The scale of generating and handling data, which was unimaginable previously, has become a reality today due to the advent of Next-Generation Sequencing (NGS) technologies. Advantages of NGS over the conventional Sanger sequencing approach are the rapid generation of sequencing data on a very massive scale and at affordable cost. NGS also provides scope for wide range of studies that include transcriptomics, gene expression and regulation (DNA–protein interaction), single-nucleotide polymorphism (SNP) and RNA profiling. Sequencing of viruses, in particular, has been important to understand the spread of epidemics, the circulating viral particles and the improvement of strains for vaccine design. Different technologies such as Roche 454 [6], Illumina [7], Ion Torrent [8] and more recently the fourth-generation sequencing methodologies popularly called single-cell sequencing, *viz.* Oxford Nanopore [9] and Pacific Biosciences [10], are available for sequencing.

Sample preparation and enrichment are the prerequisites for sequencing the viromes. Filtration and centrifugation on caesium chloride density gradient have proved to enrich the virus-like particles. A strategy like depletion of host rRNAs is also known to increase the virus fraction and has been attributed to the discovery of several novel RNA viruses [11]. In plant virology, use of CF11 cellulose spin column is routinely used for deep sequencing of dsRNA.

There exist several scenarios for sequencing viral genomes such as sequencing of individual strains or population [12]. Sequencing of individual genomes helps to catalogue the genes encoded in a particular strain and is a vital step for in-depth characterization studies. Sequencing of multiple isolates/strains/species enables understanding of the factors responsible for varying virulence using comparative genomic approaches [13]. For understanding the co-evolution of viral and host genomes, in particular, archaea and bacteria, Clustered Regularly Interspaced Short Palindromic Repeats (CRISPR) spacer sequencing is used [14]. CRISPR are found in archaea and bacteria that serve as an antiviral mechanism in which viral genomic sequences are integrated as CRISPR spacers into the host, thereby making it immune to viral infection [15]. Understanding complex dynamics of virus–host interactions in higher organisms using sequencing provides valuable insights into transmission between animal reservoirs [16]. Sequencing of 'Auxiliary metabolic genes', which are involved in processes like motility and transcriptional repression, enables to unravel the viral genes that influence host machinery in diverse ways [17].

1.3. Data assembly and annotations

Output from NGS technologies results in gigabases of raw sequence data per experiment. Extensive computational analysis using a number of algorithms and applications is required to infer biological significance. Generic steps include mapping of reads using either *de novo* approach or re-sequencing approach, identification of SNPs and detection of insertions/ deletions (indels) and further downstream processing.

The various steps involved in data preprocessing are:

i.   Removal of adaptors and low-quality sequences: This is an important step in data pre-processing, and tools such as FASTX [18] and FASTQC [19] are used for this purpose. Care should be taken in case of paired-end sequences to ensure that the reads trimmed based on the quality is reflected in both the forward and the reverse FASTQ files. In case of multiplex sequencing data, an additional step of 'de-multiplexing' based on barcodes is mandatory.

ii.   Screening host sequences: Despite the methods being available for viral enrichment, it has been observed that contamination of host/vector sequences is a routine scenario. Filtering of such data ensures that no error is propagated.

Following preprocessing, reference-based mapping or *de novo* assembly of the processed reads can be carried out.

1.3.1. Reference-mapping

Alignment with a reference genome is a method of choice for most NGS experiments. Preprocessed reads when mapped to a well-annotated reference genome ensure transfer of annotations to the query genome in a hassle-free manner with statistical confidence, especially in indel-free regions. Polymorphic regions can also be identified, which account for the isolate-specific variants that may be responsible for the observed phenotype. The algorithms generally rely on indexing of either the query reads or the reference genome using suffix tree or hashing strategy [20–22]. Indexing the reference genome has been proved to be computationally advantageous and is widely preferred. Indexing is followed by gapped or ungapped alignment based on either Smith–Waterman [23] or Needleman–Wunsch dynamic programming approaches [24]. Gaps indicate indels and are important to gain strain-/species-specific properties. The quality of the reference alignment can be improved by using large inserts available in paired-end reads as compared to single-end reads wherein forward and reverse orientation of reads cannot be calculated. Downstream processing of aligned and assembled reads involves delineating the variant regions followed by annotation. It is also important to remove polymerase chain reaction (PCR) artefacts before variant calling as the duplicated reads hamper its sensitivity. Discovery of *Schmallemberg* virus, a new member of genus *Orthobunyavirus* that causes foetal abnormalities in ruminants [25], is attributed to a reference-based assembly approach.

Delineation of variant regions: All deviations from reference genome can be delineated as variants, which include SNPs and indels. Variant regions contribute to the nucleotide diversity in virus populations and hence play a vital role in their evolution and dynamics. One of the main parameters indicative of nucleotide diversity is the comparison of synonymous to non-synonymous codon substitution. Synonymous mutations result in neutral substitution, which enable in maintaining the phenotype, as compared to non-synonymous substitutions, which lead to amino acid alteration and hence may affect phenotype. It is interesting to note that the existence of overlapping reading frames in viruses often constrains synonymous substitutions. Hence, computation of the magnitude of synonymous and non-synonymous polymorphism within viral populations will provide a handle to assess the role of neutral evolution and genetic drift in viral evolution. A more detailed discussion of the role of these substitution ratios in adaptive evolution of viruses is given in Section 4.5.

Tools like SNPgenie [26] and VirVarSeq [27] have been developed with a focus on calling SNPs from pooled viral samples by including codon information in an explicit manner and hence are more sensitive than traditional SNP callers [28, 29].

1.3.2. De novo assembly

Preprocessed reads are assembled using *de novo* approaches, when a closely related homologue is unavailable to serve as a reference. It should be mentioned that genome assembly is computationally challenging and also requires trained manpower. Sequencing depth plays a major role in determining the quality of the assembly as does the length of the reads. Popularly used assemblers are based on de Bruijin graph approach in which reads are divided into subsequences called k-mers of length k [30]. The *k*-mers form the nodes of a graph, which are linked when a *k-1*mer is shared among them. The overall process requires large amounts of computer memory (RAM) and specialized compute clusters.

The steps involved in assembly process are:

i.   Based on Overlap–Layout–Consensus principle, information stored in scattered reads are used to make contiguous regions termed 'contigs', which are generally devoid of polymorphisms.

ii.   Using insert information, 'contigs' are combined to form 'scaffolds'. Gaps between contigs are usually filled with nucleotides (*N*s).

iii.   Scaffolds in conjunction with synteny and geneorder information are used to build larger scaffolds.

Building a draft genome is an iterative process and involves parameter optimization, and it is advised that more than one type of assembler be used as each of them has been built for a definite purpose and has unique features. The final assembled genome is evaluated on the basis of N50 parameter. N50 is the median of assembled sequence lengths, in which longer sequences are given more weightage. Mis-assemblies due to wrong orientation of reads and low-complexity regions are, however, not accounted for in N50 parameter and tools like *amosvalidate*, which combines multiple validation procedures, are recommended [31].

One of the major limitations of *de novo* assembly using NGS data is its reporting of large proportion of incorrect recombinants. This arises mainly due to overlapping of short reads of varying quality and coverage, which in turn pave way for the introduction of spurious SNPs, ultimately resulting in artefacts in assembly. The *in silico* chimeras thus produced amplify diversity estimation and complicate true recombination detection. Efforts are being made to overcome this issue using probabilistic method, which assumes that true SNPs are under selection pressure and hence co-occur within a haplotype as compared to random SNPs [32]. Methods such as Iterative Virus Assembler (IVA) [33] and Paired-Read Iterative Contig Extension (PRICE) [34] have also been developed to overcome caveats associated with varying read depths and enable detection of regions with extensive genomic diversity. Assembly pipelines like VirAmp [35], VICUNA [36], SPAdes [37] offer many choices of tools and parameters for carrying out hassle-free assembly of viral genomes.

Novel approaches are also being introduced with special emphasis on viral metagenomic projects, *viz.* Progressive Filtering of Overlapping small RNAs (PFOR) [38]. PFOR is capable of identifying replicating circular RNAs by separating terminal small RNAs from internal small RNAs based on *k*-mer overlap. PFOR2, a multi-threaded version of PFOR, has recently been developed, which reduced the running time of filtering step by 90%. Novel viroids like *Hop stunt viroid* (HpSVd), *Grapevine yellow speckle viroid* (GYSVd) and *Grapevine hammerhead viroid-like RNA* (GHVd RNA) have been identified using this tool. Hence, *de novo* assembly has tremendous scope in unravelling the vast virome that has been unaddressed previously and there exists need for development of more efficient assembly algorithms, which will make it more tractable for use by larger scientific community.

2. Genome databases

Initial effort towards sequencing of viral genomes resulted in accumulation of genomic data in primary repositories such as GenBank [39], European Molecular Biology Laboratory (EMBL) [40] and DNA Data Bank of Japan (DDBJ) [41] and now continues to rise in International Nucleotide Sequence Database Collaboration (INSDC) [42]. Genome databases and resources dedicated to viruses were developed subsequently [43–47]. Lists of useful databases, resources and analysis tools have also been compiled previously [13, 48]. Most of these resources archive complete genome sequences, their annotations and derived data such as viral variations, multiple sequence alignments (MSAs) and phylogenetic trees, to name a few. Some of the viral genome resources are briefly described below.

2.1. National Center for Biotechnology Information (NCBI) viral genome resource

This reference resource is designed to catalogue publicly available genomic sequences of viruses deposited in INSDC [49]. It attempts to curate reference genome sequences and leverages on the knowledge of experts to annotate as well as to identify important viral sequences.

2.2. *ViralZone*

This resource is developed and maintained at the Swiss Institute of Bioinformatics. The objective of the resource is to link textbook knowledge, fact sheets and images to the genomic and proteomic data with an objective to facilitate the study of viral diversity [50].

2.3. Virus Pathogen Database and Analysis Resource (ViPR)

The ViPR [51] is supported under the Bioinformatics Resource Centers (BRC) programme of National Institute of Allergy and Infectious Diseases (NIAID). The database currently provides access to molecular data of viruses including complete genomes of 14 viral families. Analytical and visualization tools for metadata-driven statistical sequence analysis, data filtering, analytical workflows and utility of personal workbench are provided to the users.

In addition to these, several organism-specific resources have been developed such as HCV Database [52] for *Hepatitis C virus* and IVDB [53] for *Influenza virus* and HIV [54].

Annotation of the sequence (gene/genome/protein) records is an integral step in downstream processing of database entries. A well-curated reference record serves as template for transfer of annotation in terms of features such as gene boundaries, associated functions (molecular/ cellular/pathway) and non-coding regions [49]. Such annotations will be highly useful in subsequent analysis and model building. The challenges of managing dedicated resources for viral genomes are relatively different as compared to the genomic databases of model and other organisms. The pace of sequencing and the quantum of genomic data being generated are affecting identification of reference genomes and annotations of genomes of strains and isolates. Additionally, to study the spatio-temporal evolution and to model the viral populations, it is desirable to tag metadata such as the place and date of isolation of viruses with the corresponding genomic entries.

3. Impact of NGS technologies on virology

Molecular analysis of viruses using data generated by NGS has revolutionized virology. While understanding the sequence–structure–function relationships, it has also resulted in the development of new areas of research such as phyloinformatics and immunoinformatics, which translates raw data into information. The information generated from these independent yet interlinked areas, when put together fits as pieces of jigsaw puzzle (Figure 1), leading to an improved understanding of the viral diseases and, thereby, the development of antiviral therapies.

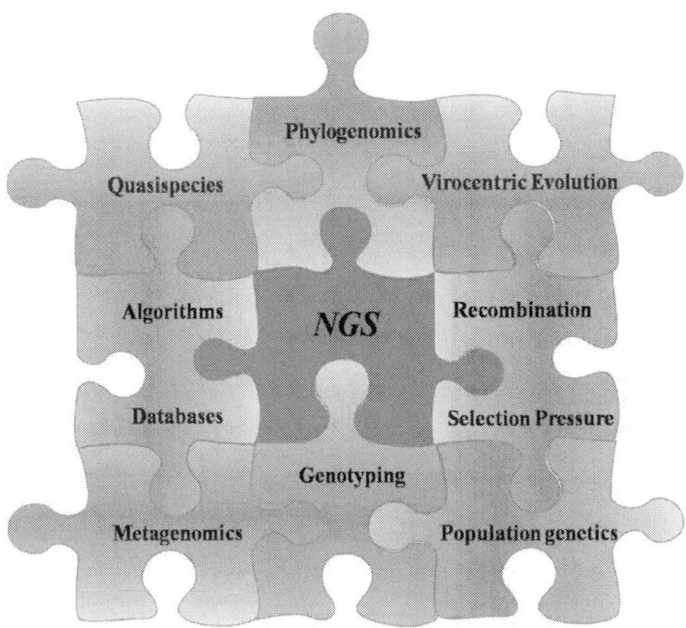

Figure 1. Scope of research in virology enabled and augmented due to availability of NGS data.

3.1. Unravelling mutational landscapes in viral quasispecies

Viral quasispecies are mutant swarms generated mainly by RNA viruses during replication, which is known to be error-prone due to the lack of proofreading activity of RNA-dependent RNA polymerase. The resulting mosaic is a dynamic distribution of non-identical but related replicons that cannot be detected using conventional sequencing approaches. Hence, quasi-species remained unexplored for a considerable time, even though the theoretical concept for quasispecies was put forth by Eigen in 1970 [55]. With the advent of NGS technologies, the generation of large genomic datasets became a reality. Due to the sequencing error issues, it was still tough to demarcate true genetic variations. Circular Sequencing (CirSeq), a novel experimental approach that creates template of tandem repeats of circularized genomic RNA fragments has been developed by Andino's group [56]. CirSeq reduces the sequencing error drastically as the repeats get sequenced in a redundant manner for every genomic fragment. A consensus reduces the theoretical error close to 10^{-11}, which enables capture of the entire mutational spectrum of RNA virus populations. CirSeq was employed to study seven serial passages of *Poliovirus* replicated in HeLa cells. Mutation frequency was computed for every passage and their fitness was determined by mapping onto the 3D structure of proteins. As expected, majority of the mutations detected were neutral substitutions, thus highlighting robustness as driving force for adaptation and evolution [56]. This study clearly delineates the viral mutations responsible for quasispecies structure and highlights the extent of genetic variation that can be maintained in a population.

Microevolution in an evolving quasispecies population is responsible for the sequence diversity in *Porcine reproductive and respiratory syndrome virus* (PRRSV). PRRSV is the causative agent of late-term reproductive failure in sows and respiratory distress in pigs and hence has large economic impact. Genomic complexity of PRRSV due to multiple circulating genotypes results in antigenic diversity, which, in turn, is responsible for lack of effective vaccine development [57]. Sanger sequencing has identified open reading frames ORF5 and ORF7 as the polymorphic regions of the virus genome, encoding major immunogenic epitopes. In order to study the genome-wide polymorphisms, deep sequencing of PRRSV was carried out and amino acid substitutions in ORFs 2–7 in PRRSV strains obtained from pigs that lack B and T cells were studied [58]. By analysing nucleotide substitutions over time followed by compa-rative genomics with non-pathogenic variants, the role of mutation and selection in preserving the pathogenesis or fitness of PRRSV was well documented in this study.

3.2. Detection of low-frequency variants

Low-frequency variants or minority quasispecies are the variants that occur with a frequency of <20–25% in a viral population [59]. Minority quasispecies refers to the memory genomes that were dominant at an earlier phase of quasispecies evolution and can play an important role in conferring drug resistance in viruses such as *Human Immunodeficiency Virus type-1* (HIV-1) and *Influenza virus*. Minority quasispecies of drug-resistant viruses can rapidly re-emerge as major populations after the reintroduction of drug pressure. In case of HIV-1, presence of such low-frequency variants has been linked with early failure to the antiretroviral therapy [59, 60]. Emergence of highly pathogenic subtype of *Avian Influenza viruses* (HPAI) has also been explained on the basis of low-frequency variants. Ultra-deep sequencing was used to study the emergence of HPAI from that of less pathogenic (Low Pathogenic Avian Influenza (LPAI)) progenitor viruses [61].

3.3. Inter- and intra-host genetic diversity

The rate of viral evolution and the effectiveness of its transmission are determined by inter- and intra-host genetic diversity. Mutation rate and selection pressure ascertain viral diversity. Factors like mixed infections and random processes such as genetic drift and population bottlenecks also contribute to the genetic diversity of viruses both within and among hosts. Transmission fitness influences the effective spread of viruses and is responsible for its stable maintenance in the environment [62].

Intra-host genetic diversity in *Zucchini yellow mosaic virus* (ZYMV), a plant RNA virus known to infect *Cucurbitaceae* plants, has been studied using NGS [63]. Population bottlenecks were investigated for this aphid-borne virus and are thought to occur during both inter-host vector transmission and systemic movement within an individual plant. ZYMV populations infecting cucumbers with and without vector were sequenced followed by *de novo* assembly and variant calling. Analysis revealed that the low-frequency mutants present in the initial population got fixed rapidly in vector-transmitted viruses, whereas the same continued to remain as minor variants in mechanically inoculated viruses. In addition, regions known to be responsible for vector transmission were conserved in all samples. It is interesting to know that previous studies using Sanger sequencing of the coat protein of ZYMV, which is involved in interaction with aphids, could not detect mutations when transmitted between or within plants. However, this study reported six mutations in coat protein with frequency of occurrence as low as ~3%. Such studies provide an insight into the complex dynamics of genetic diversity of an emerging viral infection with implications in disease management.

3.4. Viral metagenomics

NGS has revolutionized metagenomics in a major way by ensuring high data throughput and by removing the hassles of cultivation/isolation by providing cost-effective options. Metagenomics involves sequencing of samples from diverse environments spanning across the biosphere [64]. The initial attempts at characterizing the viral metagenomes were more of an enumeration nature [65] and provided a glimpse of the enormous diversity underlying the previously unculturable communities. NGS has paved way for extensive characterization of the functional role of virome in hosts harbouring them [66, 67]. Analysis of metagenomics data is challenging as it includes simultaneous assembly of multiple genomes/transcriptomes and the complex interplay between them. Two major methods based on 'sequence-similarity' and 'sequence composition' are usually used for categorization of samples in metagenomics. It has been observed that the alignment-free 'sequence composition'-based methods provide better means of classifying viral samples as 'sequence similarity'-based methods could only classify up to 30% of the reads [68].

In a major study involving analysis of dsDNA viruses from 43 ocean samples obtained from across the globe revealed several intriguing observations [69]. Genes shared across different samples were used as 'core genes' for comparison. 'Niche-differentiation' of different viral populations based on the layer of the ocean they occupy was observed. As viruses rely on the host machinery to replicate, a direct relationship was observed between the community structures of both viruses and hosts. Environmental factors like salinity also influenced the viral persistence and hence their diversity. Technological advances in viral metagenomics would help to unravel the underlying rules of viral evolution and ecology, the so-called 'Genomic rulebook of viruses' [70].

3.5. Genotype–phenotype correlation studies

3.5.1. Receptor switching

A key event during any viral infection is the interaction of viruses with the host receptors on the plasma membrane. This serves as an entry point for viruses to access resources of the host cell and is very crucial for tropism. This interaction is known to be very specific and is responsible for activation of the signalling processes that recruit cellular machinery of the host for viral replication. The specificity of receptor binding defines host range that a virus can infect and the extent of tissue tropism that a virus can display. Switching of receptors thus enables the virus to increase its host range and/or gain access to the previously unaffected cell types.

HIV-1 enters the target host cell by binding to CD4 receptor along with a co-receptor (in majority of cases, chemokine C-C motif receptor 5 (CCR5)) using its spike protein. Monitoring of the co-receptor usage using phenotype-based assays provided clues for the likely shift from CCR5 to chemokine C-X-C motif receptor 4 (CXCR4). However, due to the low resolution of these procedures, this transition could not be captured effectively. NGS of the variable loop region (V3) of the envelope gene containing determinants of co-receptor usage revealed the stepwise mutational pathway involved in the transition from CCR5 to CXCR4 [71]. The observation of the low-frequency intermediate variants provided an insight into the fitness landscape of *HIV-1* and provided clues to tackle the disease progression in a rational manner.

3.5.2. Immune escape

The *de novo* sequencing approach has helped to analyse the heterogeneity of *Influenza A virus* (strain A/Nagano/RC1-L/200 or H1N1) isolated from 2009 pandemic. The amino acid changes in haemagglutinin protein (G172E and G239N) were observed to be associated with the immune escape [72].

4. Bioinformatics methods for viral genomics

Bioinformatics approaches help to estimate and analyse population diversity by studying genetic recombination, mutation, selection and, thereby, assist in correlation of genotype to phenotype. The methods relevant to these aspects are discussed below with emphasis on the analysis of viral populations.

4.1. Methods for quasispecies reconstruction

Quasispecies reconstruction refers to the estimation of number of viral variants and their frequency. Each viral variant in a quasispecies is considered as a haplotype. Tools available for this purpose include Short Read Assembly into Haplotypes (ShoRAH) [73], Quasispecies Reconstruction algorithm (QuRe) [74] and QuasiRecomb [75].

4.1.1. Short Read Assembly into Haplotypes (ShoRAH)

Principle: This method uses Bayesian principle to estimate the genetic diversity of mixed samples obtained through NGS by incorporating subroutines for correction of sequencing errors [73]. It can detect viral haplotypes with frequencies as low as 0.1%.

Algorithm steps:

i.   Alignment: The program requires a FASTA input file of NGS reads along with a reference sequence. It performs pairwise alignment of all reads to the reference sequence and generates a multiple sequence alignment (MSA).

ii.   Error correction (local haplotype reconstruction): Using MSA as a starting point, a set of overlapping windows is analysed by employing a model-based probabilistic clustering algorithm to obtain (i) haplotype sequences, (ii) their frequencies, (iii) corrected reads and (iv) posterior probability of the reconstruction.

iii.   Global haplotype reconstruction: The set of corrected reads is analysed under parsimony principle, which results in identification of set of unique reads of maximum length.

iv.   Frequency estimation: Using maximum likelihood (ML) and expectation maximization algorithm, the frequencies of the reconstructed haplotypes are estimated.

4.1.2. Quasispecies Reconstruction algorithm (QuRe)

Principle: QuRe [74] is based on a heuristic algorithm and automatically reconstructs a set of error-free, full-gene/genome variants from a collection of long NGS reads (>100 bp).

Algorithm steps:

i.   Overlaps between the reference genome and reads are generated in terms of k-mers.

ii.   Mapping of k-mers is then carried out to obtain genomic co-ordinates.

iii.   Generates a multinomial distribution based on the alignment scores of true matches along with the matches with randomly shuffled reads.

iv.   Coverage, nucleotide content and entropy of each mapped genomic position are then calculated.

v.   Errors are corrected based on Poisson distribution model, parameterized differently for homopolymeric and non-homopolymeric regions.

vi.   Reconstruction of quasispecies is carried out using the sliding window approach by calculating maximal coverage and read diversity, which reduces the false positives, *i.e., in-silico* recombinants.

4.1.3. QuasiRecomb

Principle: It employs the jumping Hidden Markov Model (HMM)-based probabilistic statistics for inference of viral quasispecies, especially for estimating the intra-patient viral haplotype distribution [75]. This method assumes that the true genetic diversity is generated by a few sequences (called generators) through mutation and recombination, and that the observed diversity results from additional sequencing errors.

Algorithm steps:

i.   Distribution of haplotypes in a given population is modelled to account for either point mutation or recombination in the form of probability tables and jumping HMM states respectively.

ii.   Expectation maximization algorithm is used to estimate posterior probabilities associated with rare events of mutation and recombination.

4.2. Methods to study viral population genetics

Genetic structure of a population refers to the number of distinct subpopulations, identified using a characteristic set of allele frequencies [76]. A model-based population analysis can be performed using the STRUCTURE program [77] based on genomic data. The program can infer the genetic structure in haploid, diploid and polyploid species [78].

4.2.1. STRUCTURE program

Principle: This method is based on Bayesian clustering approach and employs Markov Chain Monte Carlo (MCMC) algorithm to identify genetically distinct subpopulations based on allele frequencies. It assigns individuals to subpopulations based on likelihood estimates. In case of haploids, the program assumes that the loci are in linkage equilibrium or only weakly linked [78]. The program accounts for recombination by incorporating ancestry models such as admixture and linkage models. An admixed strain is assigned with a membership score to belong to two or more subpopulations, to indicate its mixed ancestry. Linkage model is an extension of admixture model to account for weak linkage that arises as a result of admixture linkage disequilibrium (LD). Therefore, the extent of linkage equilibrium within the markers needs to be tested prior to usage of the STRUCTURE program. The relevant linkage analysis (LIAN) programs and measures are discussed in Section 4.3.

Input genotype data: A wide range of markers such as multi-locus genotype data, microsatellites, SNPs can be used as an input. In case of viruses, the polymorphic sites or more specifically the parsimony-informative (PIs) sites obtained from genome-based alignment are suitable markers for population genetic analyses. A PI site contains at least two types of nucleotide bases and at least two of which occur with a minimum frequency of two. The position of each

PI corresponds to a locus. At every locus, any of the four bases (A, T, G and C) and the gap is considered as an allele.

Algorithm steps:

i.   Carry out MSA of complete genomes and extract PI sites.

ii.   Estimate the degree of linkage equilibrium and test the null hypothesis about the same.

iii. Simulate data using burn-in and burn-length with values in the range of 10,000–1,00,000. Check the convergence of parameters and consistency of clustering results.

iv.   Estimate the appropriate number of clusters (K) using independent runs with varying values of K.

v.   Determine the best K either by comparing mean of log likelihoods [77] or based on an *ad hoc* statistic, ΔK [79].

vi.   Validate the genetic structure hypothesis using Analysis of MOlecularVAriance (AMOVA) based on Fixation index (F_{ST}) as implemented in ARLEQUIN software [80]. F_{ST} represents the extent of genetic differentiation among subpopulations and ranges between 0 (no differentiation) and 1 (complete differentiation).

Salient features of the STRUCTURE program:

i.   This method is advantageous over traditional molecular phylogenetic methods in terms of classification of recombinant strains.

ii.   User can incorporate prior information such as geographic location of samples.

Limitations:

i.   Variation in sample size may affect the clustering.

ii.   This method is not suitable for datasets having high linkage disequilibrium.

Case studies:

The ability of the admixture model to account for recombination has been used to analyse the extent of recombination and its role in determining the population structure of viruses such as *Hepatitis B virus* [81] and *Rhinoviruses* [82].

Population genomic study of *Hepatitis B virus* (HBV) was carried out using both admixture and linkage models (with burn-in of 20,000 and burn-length of 40,000). HBV is an enveloped DNA virus and belongs to the genus *Orthohepadnavirus* and family *Hepadnaviridae*. It is known to consist of eight genotypes designated as A–H, each of which has characteristic geographic distribution. This method helped to resolve the hierarchical nature of population subdivision with the presence of four major clusters (F_{ST} = 0.497, p < 0.0001) and eight sub-clusters. The extent of recombination was observed to be low [81].

Rhinoviruses represent the highly diverse members of genus *Enterovirus* and family *Picornaviridae*. They are ss (+) RNA viruses with genome of ~7,200 bases. There are three species, *viz.*

Rhinovirus A, -B and *-C,* each of which is further subdivided into distinct serotypes. The STRUCTURE-based analysis revealed a strong evidence for existence of seven genetically distinct subpopulations (with $F_{ST} = 0.45$, $p = 0$). *Rhinovirus A* and *Rhinovirus C* were subdivided into four and two subpopulations respectively, whereas *Rhinovirus B* species remain undivided. Furthermore, usage of both the admixture and the linkage models (with burn-in of 20,000 and burn-length of 40,000) helped to resolve the role of recombination in diversification of subpopulations. In case of *Rhinovirus A,* intra-species recombination was common, whereas in case of *Rhinovirus* C, intra- and inter-species recombination were observed to cause diversity [82].

4.3. Methods to compute linkage disequilibrium

Linkage equilibrium refers to the statistical independence of alleles at all loci and indicates evidence of free recombination [83]. Thus, linkage disequilibrium is a measure of the correlation between the occurrences of nucleotides at different loci of the genome. The extent to which recombination occurs can be estimated in terms of the degree of linkage disequilibrium [84] using measures made available by specialized programs such as Linkage Analysis (LIAN) [83] and DNA Sequence Polymorphism (DnaSP) [85]. The extent of linkage can be inferred based on the following parameters.

i.   **Standardized index of association, I^SA:** It is a measure of the degree of haplotype-wide linkage derived from a given dataset. I^SA is computed using a formula, $I^SA = [1/(e-1)] [(V_D/V_E)-1]$, where '$V_D$' represents the observed variance of pairwise distances between haplotypes and 'V_E' represents the expected variance when all loci are in linkage equilibrium. The term $[(V_D/V_E)-1]$ is the function of rate of recombination, which is zero in case of linkage equilibrium. The number of loci analysed is denoted by 'e'. The value of I^SA can be computed by using the program called LIAN (for Linkage Analysis), which requires haplotype data as an input. This program implements both a Monte Carlo and an algebraic method to test the null hypothesis: $V_D = V_E$.

ii. $|D'|$ **and** r^2: The $|D'|$ measure is the absolute value of the difference between the observed and the expected haplotype frequency in the absence of linkage disequilibrium, which is normalized by the maximum (or minimum) possible value of this difference. The squared value of the difference between the observed and the expected haplotype frequency normalized by the variance of the allele frequency is denoted by r^2. These measures can be computed using DnaSP program [85]. The values for these measures can range between 0 (no linkage disequilibrium) and 1 (complete linkage disequilibrium) [84, 86].

Case studies:

LD provides a good measure for analysing the extent of recombination in viruses [82, 87]. For example, in case of *Rhinoviruses,* low values for LD measures ($I^SA = 0.0666$, $p < 10^{-4}$; $|D'| = 0.5409$ and that of $r^2 = 0.0613$) were observed and correlated well with the evidence of recombination obtained using independent methods [82]. Similarly, LD analyses in serotypes of *Foot and mouth disease virus* [87] helped to reveal low values of $|D'|$ and r^2, supporting high recombination.

4.4. Methods for detection of recombination

In addition to undergoing mutations, viruses are known to generate new variants through genetic recombination. Genetic recombination refers to the exchange of genetic material between strains of the same or different species of viruses [88]. Within a host, co-infected with viruses, the recombination occurs either by homologous recombination or by reassortment [89]. Homologous recombination can occur between highly similar RNA genomes usually through the process called 'copy-choice' or 'template-switching' mechanism, whereas reassortment involves exchange of genomic regions between viruses that have segmented genomes. Presence of recombinants can hamper analyses pertaining to molecular clock [90], selection pressure, phylogenetic classification [91, 92] and thus need to be detected prior to such analyses.

4.4.1. Virus Recombination Mapper (ViReMa)

ViReMa is developed to analyse the recombinants within the viral genome data derived through NGS [93]. It can detect inter-virus or virus–host recombination. This method can also detect insertion and substitution events and multiple recombination junctions within a single read.

Algorithm steps:

i. Alignment of 5' end of each read to the reference genome(s) using seed-based approach.

ii. Dynamic generation of a new read segment: 3' end of the read that fail to align is extracted or the first nucleotide from the read is trimmed. This step is iterated until all the reads are either mapped or trimmed or a combination of both.

iii. For each read, all possible recombinations are reported.

4.4.2. Recombination Detection Program version 4 (RDP4) package

In order to detect recombination, various methods have been developed and are provided in RDP4 package [94]. It identifies the significant evidence of recombination events based on the *p-value* and identifies the potential recombinant sequences and its both parents (major and minor). The main strength of the package is that it does not need any prior knowledge pertaining to non-recombinant set of reference sequences. The starting point of analysis is MSA of genomic sequences.

Algorithm steps:

i. RDP4 package sequentially tests every combination of three sequences in MSA (a triplet) for potential evidence that one of the three is a recombinant and the other two are its parents. Various recombination detection methods, such as the Ramer–Douglas–Peucker algorithm (RDP) method [95], BOOTSCAN [96, 97], maximum Chi-square (MAXCHI) method [98, 99], CHIMAERA [99], 3'-end sequencing for expression quantification (3SEQ) [100], gene conversion method (GENECONV) [101], Sister

Scanning method (SISCAN) [102], LARD [103], Topal/Difference of Sums of Squares (DSS) [104] and DNA distance plot, are used.

ii.   Following the detection of a 'recombination signal', RDP4 determines approximate breakpoint positions using HMM and then identifies the recombinant sequence using various methods such as phylogenetic profiling (PHYLPRO) [105] and Visual Recombination Detection (VisRD) [106].

iii.   The minimum number of recombination events that are needed to account for these signals are then inferred. It involves sequential disassembly of the identified recombinant sequences into respective components and iteratively rescanning the resulting expanded dataset until no further recombination signals are evident.

Salient feature:

RDP4 package provides a unified interface for multiple methods and facilitates visualization of recombination events using genomic data (up to 2,500 sequences).

Limitations:

i.   The genomic dataset up to 200 million nucleotides can be analysed and is reported to have operational limits for large genomic datasets.

ii.   Recombination analysis is likely to fail in case of poor alignments, if recombinant sequences are used as reference and sequences having ambiguous characters are included.

4.5. Methods for selection pressure analysis

Natural selection is one of the fundamental evolutionary processes that shape the genetic structure of viral populations. The ratio of non-synonymous substitution rate (dN) to synonymous substitution rate (dS) is a useful means to infer selection pressure based on a codon alignment for a particular gene. Positive selection ($dN/dS > 1$) increases the frequency of advantageous alleles, whereas the negative selection ($dN/dS < 1$) is responsible for purging (removal) of deleterious alleles.

Broadly, the selection pressure can be classified as pervasive and episodic. Pervasive selection acts across all the lineages in a phylogenetic tree, whereas the episodic selection operates on a few lineages of a tree. Various statistical methods for analysis of pervasive and episodic selection are available at the Datamonkey web-server of Hypothesis testing using Phylogenies (HyPhy) software package [107–109].

4.5.1. Single Likelihood Ancestor Counting (SLAC)

Principle: This method belongs to a class called counting methods [110]. It is suitable for pervasive selection analysis and involves estimating the number of non-synonymous and synonymous changes that have occurred at each codon throughout the evolutionary history of the sample. It involves reconstructing the ancestral sequences using likelihood-based method [111].

Algorithm steps:

i.   Nucleotide model fit: Using maximum likelihood (ML), a nucleotide model of time-reversible class is fitted to the data and tree, to obtain branch lengths and substitution rates. If multiple segments are present in the input codon alignment, base frequencies and substitution rates are inferred jointly from the whole alignment, while branch lengths are estimated for each segment separately.

ii.   Codon model fit: To obtain a global $\omega = dN/dS$ ratio, the branch lengths and substitution rate parameters are considered constant at the values estimated in 'step i'. A codon model is obtained using a combination of MG94 model and the nucleotide model of 'step i' and then fitted to the data.

iii.   Ancestral sequence reconstruction: Based on the parameter estimates obtained using steps i and ii, codons of ancestral sequences are reconstructed site by site using maximization of the likelihood of the data at the site over all possible ancestral character states. Inferred ancestral sequences are treated as known for the next step.

iv.   Inference of selection at each site: For every variable site, four quantities, *viz.* the normalized expected (*ES* and *EN*) and the observed numbers (*NS* and *NN*) are calculated for synonymous and non-synonymous substitutions respectively. SLAC estimates $dN = NN/EN$ and $dS = NS/ES$, and if $dN < dS$, a codon is called negatively selected or if $dN > dS$, it is said to be positively selected. A p-value is derived to assess the significance. The test assumes that under neutrality, a random substitution will be synonymous with probability $p = ES/(ES + EN)$.

4.5.2. Fixed-Effect Likelihood (FEL) and Internal Fixed-Effect Likelihood (IFEL)

Principle: These belong to a class of methods called 'fixed effects'. It analyses pervasive selection and involves fitting substitution rates on a site-by-site basis by assuming that the synonymous substitution rate is the same for all sites. Thus, FEL and IFEL assume the same dN/dS (ω) ratio, which is applicable to all branches and to interior branches, respectively [111].

Algorithm steps:

i.   Nucleotide and codon model fitting procedure in these methods is similar to those of SLAC method as detailed in Section 4.5.1.

ii.   Site-by-site likelihood ratio test (LRT):

FEL method: For every site, based on the parameter estimates obtained using nucleotide- and codon-fit procedure, two rate parameters namely α and β are first fitted independently and then under the constraint of $\alpha = \beta$. Here, the parameter α represents the instantaneous synonymous site rate, while β represents the instantaneous non-synonymous site rate. Furthermore, LRT is performed to infer whether α is different from β and a p-value is computed. If the p-value is significant, the site is classified based on whether $\alpha > \beta$ (indicates negative selection) or $\alpha < \beta$ (indicates positive selection).

IFEL method: It differs from FEL in following aspects:

- The selection is only tested for internal branches of the phylogenetic tree.

- Each site has three rate parameters, α, β_I (instantaneous non-synonymous site rate for internal branches) and β_L (instantaneous non-synonymous site rate for terminal branches). Here, the null model assumes that $\alpha = \beta\_I$.

4.5.3. Mixed Effects Model of Evolution (MEME)

Principle: MEME is categorized under the 'branch-site random effects' phylogenetic methods [112]. Though this method is a generalization of FEL method, it differs from FEL and IFEL, by accounting for episodic positive selection that particularly affects a subset of lineages. MEME uniquely allows the distribution of dN/dS (ω) to vary from site to site (the fixed effect) and also from branch to branch at a site (the random effect).

Algorithm steps:

i.   The steps 'i' and 'ii' are same as that of the SLAC method (Section 4.5.1), whereas there is variation in step 'iii' as follows:

ii.   The ω ratio is modelled across lineages at an individual site, i.e., each site is treated as a fixed-effect component of the model using a two-bin random distribution with $\omega- \leq 1$ (proportion p) and $\omega+$ (unrestricted, proportion $1-p$). Thus, a proportion (p) of branches at a site evolve neutrally (or under negative selection), while the remaining $(1-p)$ may evolve under diversifying selection. To test for evidence of episodic selection, a likelihood ratio test is applied.

4.6. Methods for reconstruction of molecular phylogeny

Molecular phylogenetic analyses are the most commonly performed studies in virology with major applications in viral taxonomy, systematics and genotyping. Methods for reconstruction of phylogenetic tree are broadly classified into three main categories, *viz.* distance-based, character-based and Bayesian-based and are reviewed earlier [113, 114]. Distance-based methods use pairwise distance matrix as an input for tree building. Neighbour-joining [115], minimum evolution [116] and least square [117, 118] methods are widely used methods under this category. These methods are computationally efficient and suitable for the analysis of large datasets with low levels of sequence divergence. However, these methods do not perform equally well in case of highly divergent sequences with low levels of sequence similarity. Moreover, uncertainties can be introduced due to positioning of gaps in the MSA. Character-based methods assume each site in MSA to evolve independently. The two classical methods under this category are maximum parsimony and maximum likelihood [119], which estimate the tree score based on the minimum number of changes and the log-likelihood value respectively. However, it needs to be mentioned that alignment-based phylogenetic methods are observed to misclassify taxa with mixed ancestry and/or recombination [91, 92].

The alignment-free methods have been developed as an alternative and can be classified into four categories based on the underlying principles employed. They are k-mer/word composition, substring theory, information theory and graphical representation [120].

Whole genome-based phylogenetic trees are widely used for various viruses owing to their small genome sizes and conservation of genomic structure. Phylogenomics field has gained importance as whole genome data became available enabling the study of evolution in general and epidemiology and disease surveillance, in particular. This field when analysed in the context of spatio-temporal data helps to understand the disease spread and progression during outbreaks. The program such as Bayesian Evolutionary Analysis by Sampling Trees (BEAST) has been exclusively designed for phylogeography studies [121] and is used widely to study spatio-temporal dynamics of viruses at population scale.

BEAST software provides a Bayesian Markov chain Monte Carlo (MCMC) framework for parameter estimation and hypothesis testing of evolutionary models from molecular sequence data. It brings together a large number of evolutionary models into a single coherent frame-work for evolutionary inference. Available evolutionary models include substitution, inser-tion–deletion, demographic, tree shape priors, node calibration and relaxed clock models. This combinatorial principle is advantageous as it provides a flexible system to specify models to understand various aspects of virus evolution. BEAST uniquely incorporates the time-scale data to explicitly model the rate of molecular evolution on each branch in the tree. Under the uniform rate assumption over the entire tree, the molecular clock model becomes applicable. It is the first software to incorporate the relaxed molecular clock model that does not assume constant rate across lineages.

4.7. Methods for typing of viruses

Phylogenetic analysis, whether alignment-based or alignment-free, is routinely used for genotyping/serotyping of viruses. Such analysis is carried out using the regions that are identified as markers for the purpose of classification by the expert evolutionary virologists and the International Committee of viruses (ICTV) [122]. It has been observed that genotype information for less than 10% of the viral genomes is available as part of their sequence records. As NGS technologies are producing a large number of genomic sequences for various strains, isolates and viral species, the genotype assignment gap is ever-increasing. Several tools for genotyping have been developed using both alignment-based and alignment-free methods and are most often organism-specific. NCBI Genotyping Tool is based on the sequence similarity for identifying the genotype of recombinant and non-recombinant viral sequences [123]. Similar tools exist for *Influenza virus, viz.* FluGenom [124]. Alignment-free method for phylogeny and genotyping of viruses based on the concept of Return Time Distribution has been developed *in-house* and its applicability for genotyping of viruses such as *Mumps virus, Dengue virus* and *West Nile virus* has been demonstrated [125–127].

5. The way forward

NGS has proved to be extremely useful and has become an integral part of virus research and opened up new vistas in studying viral evolution. Ample proof of the same is the characterization of the *Ebola virus* infection in West Africa (2014 outbreak), wherein the patient samples were sequenced using NGS to trace the origin and transmission of the infection as part of the global epidemic surveillance strategy [128]. The discovery followed by the development of vaccine [129] has been made in a short time span owing to the genomics-enabled translational research. In order to harness the use of NGS in virology, care needs to be exerted to avoid misinterpretation and over-interpretation of the data. It must be noted that starting from sample collection, DNA/RNA extraction, PCR amplification, library preparation up to sequencing are prone to errors, which have been explained [130] very comprehensively. Circumventing these issues, application of NGS in virology has enabled basic and applied research to take a quantum leap. The thorough understanding of the intricacies of a quasis-pecies structure aids in tracing the mutational network operational due to selection pressures. Furthermore, characterization of intra- and inter-host viral evolution helps in understanding the role of host immune system on the genetic variability of viruses. Such data when analysed in the context of population genetics provide constructs to understand emergence of new strains/lineages. Reverse vaccinology [131] enabled via genomics is expected to accelerate the rate of vaccine discovery, thereby, reducing the virus-associated disease burden.

Acknowledgements

The authors would like to acknowledge the Department of Biotechnology (DBT), Government of India for the infrastructural facilities. Dr. Urmila Kulkarni-Kale acknowledges Centre of Excellence (CoE) Grant to the Bioinformatics Centre from the DBT. Sunitha M Kasibhatla acknowledges the support of Bioinformatics Resources and Applications Facility (BRAF), C-DAC, Pune. Vaishali P. Waman acknowledges DBT fellowship (2010–2015).

Author details

Sunitha M. Kasibhatla[1,2], Vaishali P. Waman[1], Mohan M. Kale[3] and Urmila Kulkarni-Kale[1*]

*Address all correspondence to: urmila@bioinfo.net.in; urmila.kulkarni.kale@gmail.com

1 Bioinformatics Centre, Savitribai Phule Pune University (formerly University of Pune), Ganeshkhind, Pune, Maharashtra, India

2 Bioinformatics Group, Centre for Development of Advanced Computing, Pune University Campus, Ganeshkhind, Pune, Maharashtra, India

3 Department of Statistics, Savitribai Phule Pune University (formerly University of Pune), Ganeshkhind, Pune, Maharashtra, India

References

[1] Kristensen DM, Mushegian AR, Dolja VV, Koonin EV. New dimensions of the virus world discovered through metagenomics. Trends Microbiol. 2010;18(1):11–9. DOI: 10.1016/j.tim.2009.11.003.

[2] Mizuno CM, Rodriguez-Valera F, Kimes NE, Ghai R. Expanding the marine virosphere using metagenomics. PLoS Genet. 2013;9(12):e1003987. DOI:10.1371/journal.pgen.1003987.

[3] Dye C, Mertens T, Hirnschall G, Mpanju-Shumbusho W, Newman RD, Raviglione MC, Savioli L, Nakatani H. WHO and the future of disease control programmes. Lancet. 2013;381(9864):413–8. DOI:10.1016/S0140-6736(12)61812-1.

[4] Koonin EV, Dolja VV. A virocentric perspective on the evolution of life. Curr Opin Virol. 2013;3(5):546–57. DOI:10.1016/j.coviro.2013.06.008.

[5] Sanger F, Air GM, Barrell BG, Brown NL, Coulson AR, Fiddes CA, Hutchison CA, Slocombe PM, Smith M. Nucleotide sequence of bacteriophage phi X174 DNA. Nature. 1977;265(5596):687–95. DOI:10.1038/265687a0.

[6] Roche 454. Available from: http://www.454.com/ [Accessed: 2015-08-10]

[7] Illumina. Available from: http://www.illumina.com/ [Accessed: 2015-08-10]

[8] Ion Torrent. Available from: https://www.lifetechnologies.com [Accessed: 2015-08-10]

[9] Oxford Nanopore. Available from: https://www.nanoporetech.com/ [Accessed: 2015-08-10]

[10] Pacific Biosciences. Available from: http://www.pacificbiosciences.com/ [Accessed: 2015-08-10]

[11] Marston DA, McElhinney LM, Ellis RJ, Horton DL, Wise EL, Leech SL, David D, de Lamballerie X, Fooks AR. Next generation sequencing of viral RNA genomes. BMC Genomics. 2013;14(1):444. DOI:10.1186/1471-2164-14-444.

[12] Quiñones-Mateu ME, Avila S, Reyes-Teran G, Martinez MA. Deep sequencing: becoming a critical tool in clinical virology. J Clin Virol. 2014;61(1):9–19. DOI:10.1016/j.jcv.2014.06.013.

[13] Kulkarni-Kale U, Waman V, Raskar S, Mehta S, Saxena S. Genome to vaccinome: role of bioinformatics, immunoinformatics & comparative genomics. Curr Bioinform. 2012;7(4):454–66. DOI:10.2174/15748936113089990014.

[14] Anderson RE, Brazelton WJ, Baross JA. Using CRISPRs as a metagenomic tool to identify microbial hosts of a diffuse flow hydrothermal vent viral assemblage. FEMS Microbiol Ecol. 2011;77(1):120–33. DOI:10.1111/j.1574-6941.2011.01090.x.

[15] Horvath P, Barrangou R. CRISPR/Cas, the immune system of bacteria and archaea. Science. 2010;327(5962):167–70. DOI:10.1126/science.1179555.

[16] Wylie KM, Weinstock GM, Storch GA. Virome genomics: a tool for defining the human virome. Curr Opin Microbiol. 2013;16(4):479–84. DOI:10.1016/j.mib.2013.04.006.

[17] Sharon I, Battchikova N, Aro EM, Giglione C, Meinnel T, Glaser F, Pinter RY, Breitbart M, Rohwer F, Béjà O. Comparative metagenomics of microbial traits within oceanic viral communities. ISME J. 2011;5(7):1178–90. DOI:10.1038/ismej.2011.2.

[18] FastX toolkit. Available from: http://hannonlab.cshl.edu/fastx_toolkit/index.html [Accessed: 2015-08-10]

[19] FastQC. Available from: http://www.bioinformatics.babraham.ac.uk/projects/fastqc/ [Accessed: 2015-08-10]

[20] Li H, Durbin R. Fast and accurate long-read alignment with Burrows-Wheeler transform. Bioinformatics. 2010;26(5):589–95. DOI:10.1093/bioinformatics/btp698.

[21] Li H, Durbin R. Fast and accurate short read alignment with Burrows-Wheeler transform. Bioinformatics. 2009;25(14):1754–60. DOI:10.1093/bioinformatics/btp324.

[22] Langmead B, Trapnell C, Pop M, Salzberg SL. Ultrafast and memory-efficient alignment of short DNA sequences to the human genome. Genome Biol. 2009;10(3):R25. DOI:10.1186/gb-2009-10-3-r25.

[23] Smith TF, Waterman MS. Identification of common molecular subsequences. J Mol Biol. 1981;147(1):195–7.

[24] Needleman SB, Wunsch CD. A general method applicable to the search for similarities in the amino acid sequence of two proteins. J Mol Biol. 1970;48(3):443–53.

[25] Rosseel T, Scheuch M, Höper D, De Regge N, Caij AB, Vandenbussche F, Van Borm S. DNase SISPA-next generation sequencing confirms Schmallenberg virus in Belgian field samples and identifies genetic variation in Europe. PLoS One. 2012;7(7):e41967. DOI:10.1371/journal.pone.0041967.

[26] Nelson CW, Moncla LH, Hughes AL. SNPGenie: estimating evolutionary parameters to detect natural selection using pooled next-generation sequencing data. Bioinformatics. 2015. pii: btv449.

[27] Verbist BM, Thys K, Reumers J, Wetzels Y, Van der Borght K, Talloen W, Aerssens J, Clement L, Thas O. VirVarSeq: a low-frequency virus variant detection pipeline for Illumina sequencing using adaptive base-calling accuracy filtering. Bioinformatics. 2015;31(1):94–101. DOI:10.1093/bioinformatics/btu587.

[28] Li H. A statistical framework for SNP calling, mutation discovery, association mapping and population genetical parameter estimation from sequencing data. Bioinformatics. 2011;27(21):2987–93. DOI:10.1093/bioinformatics/btr509.

[29] DePristo MA, Banks E, Poplin R, Garimella KV, Maguire JR, Hartl C, Philippakis AA, del Angel G, Rivas MA, Hanna M, McKenna A, Fennell TJ, Kernytsky AM, Sivachenko AY, Cibulskis K, Gabriel SB, Altshuler D, Daly MJ. A framework for variation discovery and genotyping using next-generation DNA sequencing data. Nat Genet. 2011;43(5):491–8. DOI:10.1038/ng.806.

[30] Zerbino DR, Birney E. Velvet: algorithms for de novo short read assembly using de Bruijn graphs. Genome Res. 2008 May;18(5):821–9. DOI:10.1101/gr.074492.107.

[31] Phillippy AM, Schatz MC, Pop M. Genome assembly forensics: finding the elusive mis-assembly. Genome Biol. 2008;9(3):R55. DOI:10.1186/gb-2008-9-3-r55.

[32] Yang X, Charlebois P, Macalalad A, Henn MR, Zody MC. V-Phaser 2: variant inference for viral populations. BMC Genomics. 2013;14(1):674. DOI: 10.1186/1471-2164-14-674.

[33] Hunt M, Gall A, Ong SH, Brener J, Ferns B, Goulder P, Nastouli E, Keane JA, Kellam P, Otto TD. IVA: accurate de novo assembly of RNA virus genomes. Bioinformatics. 2015;31(14):2374–6. DOI:10.1093/bioinformatics/btv120.

[34] Ruby JG, Bellare P, Derisi JL. PRICE: software for the targeted assembly of components of (Meta) genomic sequence data. G3 (Bethesda). 2013;3(5):865–80. DOI: 10.1534/g3.113.005967.

[35] Wan Y, Renner DW, Albert I, Szpara ML. VirAmp: a galaxy-based viral genome assembly pipeline. Gigascience. 2015;4(1):19. DOI:10.1186/s13742-015-0060-y.eCollection 2015.

[36] Yang X, Charlebois P, Gnerre S, Coole MG, Lennon NJ, Levin JZ, Qu J, Ryan EM, Zody MC, Henn MR. De novo assembly of highly diverse viral populations. BMC Genomics. 2012;13(1):475. DOI:10.1186/1471-2164-13-475.

[37] Bankevich A, Nurk S, Antipov D, Gurevich AA, Dvorkin M, Kulikov AS, Lesin VM, Nikolenko SI, Pham S, Prjibelski AD, Pyshkin AV, Sirotkin AV, Vyahhi N, Tesler G, Alekseyev MA, Pevzner PA. SPAdes: a new genome assembly algorithm and its applications to single-cell sequencing. J Comput Biol. 2012;19(5):455–77. DOI:10.1089/cmb.2012.0021.

[38] Zhang Z, Qi S, Tang N, Zhang X, Chen S, Zhu P, Ma L, Cheng J, Xu Y, Lu M, Wang H, Ding SW, Li S, Wu Q. Discovery of replicating circular RNAs by RNA-seq and computational algorithms. PLoS Pathog. 2014;10(12):e1004553. DOI:10.1371/journal.ppat.1004553.

[39] Benson DA, Cavanaugh M, Clark K, Karsch-Mizrachi I, Lipman DJ, Ostell J, Sayers EW. GenBank. Nucleic Acids Res. 2013;41(Database issue):D36–42. DOI:10.1093/nar/gks1195.

[40] Cochrane G, Alako B, Amid C, Bower L, Cerdeño-Tárraga A, Cleland I, Gibson R, Goodgame N, Jang M, Kay S, Leinonen R, Lin X, Lopez R, McWilliam H, Oisel A,

Pakseresht N, Pallreddy S, Park Y, Plaister S, Radhakrishnan R, Rivière S, Rossello M, Senf A, Silvester N, Smirnov D, Ten Hoopen P, Toribio A, Vaughan D, Zalunin V. Facing growth in the European Nucleotide Archive. Nucleic Acids Res. 2013;41(Database issue):D30–5. DOI:10.1093/nar/gks1175.

[41] Kodama Y, Mashima J, Kosuge T, Katayama T, Fujisawa T, Kaminuma E, Ogasawara O, Okubo K, Takagi T, Nakamura Y. The DDBJ Japanese Genotype-phenotype Archive for genetic and phenotypic human data. Nucleic Acids Res. 2015;43(Database issue):D18–22. DOI:10.1093/nar/gku1120.

[42] INSDC. Available from: http://www.insdc.org/ [Accessed: 2015-08-10]

[43] Hiscock D, Upton C. Viral Genome DataBase: storing and analyzing genes and proteins from complete viral genomes. Bioinformatics. 2000;16(5):484–5.

[44] Albà MM, Lee D, Pearl FM, Shepherd AJ, Martin N, Orengo CA, Kellam P. VIDA: a virus database system for the organization of animal virus genome open reading frames. Nucleic Acids Res. 2001;29(1):133–6. DOI:10.1093/bioinformatics/16.5.484.

[45] Kulkarni-Kale U, Bhosle S, Manjari GS, Kolaskar AS. VirGen: a comprehensive viral genome resource. Nucleic Acids Res. 2004;32(Database issue):D289–92.

[46] Hirahata M, Abe T, Tanaka N, Kuwana Y, Shigemoto Y, Miyazaki S, Suzuki Y, Sugawara H. Genome Information Broker for Viruses (GIB-V): database for comparative analysis of virus genomes. Nucleic Acids Res. 2007;35(Database issue):D339–42. DOI: 10.1093/nar/gkl1004.

[47] Chang S, Zhang J, Liao X, Zhu X, Wang D, Zhu J, Feng T, Zhu B, Gao GF, Wang J, Yang H, Yu J, Wang J. Influenza Virus Database (IVDB): an integrated information resource and analysis platform for influenza virus research. Nucleic Acids Res. 2007;35(Database issue):D376–80.

[48] Sharma D, Priyadarshini P, Vrati S. Unraveling the web of viroinformatics: computational tools and databases in virus research. J Virol. 2015;89(3):1489–501. DOI:10.1128/JVI.02027-14.

[49] Brister JR, Ako-Adjei D, Bao Y, Blinkova O. NCBI viral genomes resource. Nucleic Acids Res. 2015;43(Database issue):D571–7. DOI:10.1093/nar/gku1207.

[50] Hulo C, de Castro E, Masson P, Bougueleret L, Bairoch A, Xenarios I, Le Mercier P. ViralZone: a knowledge resource to understand virus diversity. Nucleic Acids Res. 2011;39(Database issue):D576–82. DOI:10.1093/nar/gkq901.

[51] Pickett BE, Greer DS, Zhang Y, Stewart L, Zhou L, Sun G, Gu Z, Kumar S, Zaremba S, Larsen CN, Jen W, Klem EB, Scheuermann RH. Virus pathogen database and analysis resource (ViPR): a comprehensive bioinformatics database and analysis resource for the coronavirus research community. Viruses. 2012;4(11):3209–26. DOI:10.3390/v4113209.

[52] Kuiken C, Hraber P, Thurmond J, Yusim K. The hepatitis C sequence database in Los Alamos. Nucleic Acids Res. 2008;36(Database issue):D512–6. DOI:10.1093/nar/gkm962.

[53] Chang S, Zhang J, Liao X, Zhu X, Wang D, Zhu J, Feng T, Zhu B, Gao GF, Wang J, Yang H, Yu J, Wang J. Influenza Virus Database (IVDB): an integrated information resource and analysis platform for influenza virus research. Nucleic Acids Res. 2007;35(Database issue):D376–80. DOI:10.1093/nar/gkl779.

[54] HIV Sequence databases. Available from: http://www.hiv.lanl.gov [Accessed: 2015-08-10]

[55] Eigen M. Self organization of matter and the evolution of biological macromolecules. Naturwissenschaften. 1971;58(10):465–523.

[56] Acevedo A, Brodsky L, Andino R. Mutational and fitness landscapes of an RNA virus revealed through population sequencing. Nature. 2014;505(7485):686–90. DOI: 10.1038/nature12861.

[57] Lu ZH, Archibald AL, Ait-Ali T. Beyond the whole genome consensus: unravelling of PRRSV phylogenomics using next generation sequencing technologies. Virus Res. 2014;194(Pt 2):167–74. DOI:10.1016/j.virusres.2014.10.004.

[58] Chen N, Dekkers JC, Ewen CL, Rowland RR. Porcine reproductive and respiratory syndrome virus replication and quasispecies evolution in pigs that lack adaptive immunity. Virus Res. 2015;195(2):246–9. DOI:10.1016/j.virusres.2014.10.006.

[59] Metzner K. The significance of minority drug-resistant quasispecies. In: Geretti AM, editor. Antiretroviral resistance in clinical practice. London: Mediscript; 2006. Chapter 11.

[60] Li JZ, Paredes R, Ribaudo HJ, Svarovskaia ES, Metzner KJ, Kozal MJ, Hullsiek KH, Balduin M, Jakobsen MR, Geretti AM. Low-frequency HIV-1 drug resistance mutations and risk of NNRTI-based antiretroviral treatment failure: a systematic review and pooled analysis. JAMA. 2011;305(13):1327–35. DOI:10.1001/jama.2011.375.

[61] Monne I, Fusaro A, Nelson MI, Bonfanti L, Mulatti P, Hughes J, Murcia PR, Schivo A, Valastro V, Moreno A. Emergence of a highly pathogenic avian influenza virus from a low-pathogenic progenitor. J Virol. 2014;88(8):4375–88. DOI:10.1128/JVI.03181-13.

[62] Rodpothong P, Auewarakul P. Viral evolution and transmission effectiveness. World J Virol. 2012;1(5):131–4. DOI:10.5501/wjv.v1.i5.131.

[63] Simmons HE, Dunham JP, Stack JC, Dickins BJ, Pagán I, Holmes EC, Stephenson AG. Deep sequencing reveals persistence of intra- and inter-host genetic diversity in natural and greenhouse populations of zucchini yellow mosaic virus. J Gen Virol. 2012;93(Pt 8):1831–40. DOI:10.1099/vir.0.042622-0.

[64] Rosario K, Breitbart M. Exploring the viral world through metagenomics. Curr Opin Virol. 2011;1(4):289–97. DOI:10.1016/j.coviro.2011.06.004.

[65] Yang J, Yang F, Ren L, Xiong Z, Wu Z, Dong J, Sun L, Zhang T, Hu Y, Du J, Wang J, Jin Q. Unbiased parallel detection of viral pathogens in clinical samples by use of a metagenomic approach. J Clin Microbiol. 2011;49(10):3463–9. DOI:10.1128/JCM.00273-11.

[66] Lecuit M, Eloit M. The human virome: new tools and concepts. Trends Microbiol. 2013;21(10):510–5. DOI:10.1016/j.tim.2013.07.001.

[67] Stobbe AH, Roossinck MJ. Plant virus metagenomics: what we know and why we need to know more. Front Plant Sci. 2014;5:150. DOI:10.3389/fpls.2014.00150.

[68] Soueidan H, Schmitt LA, Candresse T, Nikolski M. Finding and identifying the viral needle in the metagenomic haystack: trends and challenges. Front Microbiol. 2015;5(29):739. DOI:10.3389/fmicb.2014.00739.

[69] Brum JR, Ignacio-Espinoza JC, Roux S, Doulcier G, Acinas SG, AlbertiA,Chaffron S, Cruaud C, de Vargas C, Gasol JM, Gorsky G, Gregory AC, Guidi L, Hingamp P, Iudicone D, Not F, Ogata H, Pesant S, Poulos BT, Schwenck SM, Speich S, Dimier C, Kandels-Lewis S, Picheral M, Searson S; Tara Oceans Coordinators, Bork P, Bowler C, Sunagawa S, Wincker P, Karsenti E, Sullivan MB. Ocean plankton. Patterns and ecological drivers of ocean viral communities. Science. 2015;348(6237):1261498. DOI:10.1126/science.1261498.

[70] Wommack KE, Nasko DJ, Chopyk J, Sakowski EG. Counts and sequences, observations that continue to change our understanding of viruses in nature. J Microbiol. 2015;53(3):181–92. DOI:10.1007/s12275-015-5068-6.

[71] Bunnik EM, Swenson LC, Edo-Matas D, Huang W, Dong W, Frantzell A, Petropoulos CJ, Coakley E, Schuitemaker H, Harrigan PR, van 't Wout AB. Detection of inferred CCR5- and CXCR4-using HIV-1 variants and evolutionary intermediates using ultra deep pyrosequencing. PLoS Pathog. 2011;7(6):e1002106.

[72] Kuroda M, Katano H, Nakajima N, Tobiume M, Ainai A, Sekizuka T, Hasegawa H, Tashiro M, Sasaki Y, Arakawa Y. Characterization of quasispecies of pandemic 2009 influenza A virus (A/H1N1/2009) by de novo sequencing using a next-generation DNA sequencer. PLoS One. 2010;5(4):e10256. DOI:10.1371/journal.pone.0010256.

[73] Zagordi O, Bhattacharya A, Eriksson N, Beerenwinkel N. ShoRAH: estimating the genetic diversity of a mixed sample from next-generation sequencing data. BMC Bioinform. 2011;12:119. DOI:10.1186/1471-2105-12-119.

[74] Prosperi MC, Salemi M. QuRe: software for viral quasispecies reconstruction from next-generation sequencing data. Bioinformatics. 2012;28(1):132–3.

[75] Töpfer A, Zagordi O, Prabhakaran S, Roth V, Halperin E, Beerenwinkel N. Probabilistic inference of viral quasispecies subject to recombination. J Comput Biol. 2013;20(2):113–23. DOI:10.1093/bioinformatics/btr627.

[76] Chakraborty R. Analysis of genetic structure of populations: meaning, methods, and implications. In: Majumder P, editor. Human population genetics. New York: Springer 1993. p. 189–206. DOI:10.1007/978-1-4615-2970-5_14.

[77] Pritchard JK, Stephens M, Donnelly P. Inference of population structure using multilocus genotype data. Genetics. 2000;155(2):945–59.

[78] Falush D, Stephens M, Pritchard JK. Inference of population structure using multilocus genotype data: linked loci and correlated allele frequencies. Genetics. 2003;164(4): 1567–87.

[79] Evanno G, Regnaut S, Goudet J. Detecting the number of clusters of individuals using the software STRUCTURE: a simulation study. Mol Ecol. 2005;14(8):2611–20. DOI:10.1111/j.1365-294X.2005.02553.x.

[80] Excoffier L, Laval G, Schneider S. Arlequin (version 3.0): an integrated software package for population genetics data analysis. Evol Bioinform Online. 2005;1:47.

[81] Szmaragd C, Balloux F. The population genomics of hepatitis B virus. Mol Ecol. 2007;16(22):4747–58. DOI:10.1111/j.1365-294X.2007.03564.x.

[82] Waman VP, Kolekar PS, Kale MM, Kulkarni-Kale U. Population structure and evolution of rhinoviruses. PloS One. 2014;9(2):e88981. DOI:10.1371/journal.pone.0088981.

[83] Haubold B, Hudson RR. LIAN 3.0: detecting linkage disequilibrium in multilocus data. Bioinformatics. 2000;16(9):847–9.

[84] Slatkin M. Linkage disequilibrium understanding the evolutionary past and mapping the medical future. Nat Rev Genet. 2008;9(6):477–85. DOI:10.1038/nrg2361.

[85] Librado P, Rozas J. DnaSP v5: a software for comprehensive analysis of DNA polymorphism data. Bioinformatics. 2009;25(11):1451–2. DOI:10.1093/bioinformatics/btp187.

[86] Devlin B, Risch N. A comparison of linkage disequilibrium measures for fine-scale mapping. Genomics. 1995;29(2):311–22.

[87] Haydon DT, Bastos AD, Awadalla P. Low linkage disequilibrium indicative of recombination in foot-and-mouth disease virus gene sequence alignments. J Gen Virol. 2004;85(Pt 5):1095–100. DOI:10.1099/vir.0.19588-0.

[88] Alejska M, Kurzyńska-Kokorniak A, Broda M, Kierzek R, Figlerowicz M. How RNA viruses exchange their genetic material. Acta Biochem Pol. 2001;48(2):391–408.

[89] Simon-Loriere E, Holmes EC. Why do RNA viruses recombine? Nat Rev Microbiol. 2011;9(8):617–26. DOI:10.1038/nrmicro2614.

[90] Schierup MH, Hein J. Recombination and the molecular clock. Mol Biol Evol. 2000;17(10):1578–9.

[91] Posada D, Crandall KA. The effect of recombination on the accuracy of phylogeny estimation. J Mol Evol. 2002;54(3):396–402.

[92] Martin DP, Lemey P, Posada D. Analysing recombination in nucleotide sequences. Mol Ecol Resour. 2011;11(6):943–55. DOI:10.1111/j.1755-0998.2011.03026.x.

[93] Routh A, Johnson JE. Discovery of functional genomic motifs in viruses with ViReMa–a Virus Recombination Mapper–for analysis of next-generation sequencing data. Nucleic Acids Res. 2014;42(2):e11–e11. DOI:10.1093/nar/gkt916.

[94] Martin DP, Lemey P, Lott M, Moulton V, Posada D, Lefeuvre P. RDP3: a flexible and fast computer program for analyzing recombination. Bioinformatics. 2010;26(1):2462–3. DOI:10.1093/bioinformatics/btq467.

[95] Martin D, Rybicki E. RDP: detection of recombination amongst aligned sequences. Bioinformatics. 2000;16(6):562–3. DOI:10.1093/bioinformatics/16.6.562.

[96] Salminen MO, Carr JK, Burke DS, McCutchan FE. Identification of breakpoints in intergenotypic recombinants of HIV type 1 by bootscanning. AIDS Res Hum Retroviruses. 1995;11(11):1423. DOI:10.1089/aid.1995.11.1423.

[97] Martin D, Posada D, Crandall K, Williamson C. A modified bootscan algorithm for automated identification of recombinant sequences and recombination breakpoints. AIDS Res Hum Retroviruses. 2005;21(1):98–102. DOI:10.1089/aid.2005.21.98.

[98] Smith JM. Analyzing the mosaic structure of genes. J Mol Evol. 1992;34(2):126–9.

[99] Posada D, Crandall KA. Evaluation of methods for detecting recombination from DNA sequences: computer simulations. Proc Natl Acad Sci. 2001;98(24):13757–62. DOI:10.1073/pnas.241370698.

[100] Boni MF, Posada D, Feldman MW. An exact nonparametric method for inferring mosaic structure in sequence triplets. Genetics. 2007;176(2):1035–47. DOI:10.1534/genetics.106.068874.

[101] Padidam M, Sawyer S, Fauquet CM. Possible emergence of new geminiviruses by frequent recombination. Virology. 1999;265(2):218–25. DOI:10.1006/viro.1999.0056.

[102] Gibbs MJ, Armstrong JS, Gibbs AJ. Sister-scanning: a Monte Carlo procedure for assessing signals in recombinant sequences. Bioinformatics. 2000;16(7):573–82. DOI:10.1093/bioinformatics/16.7.573.

[103] Holmes EC, Worobey M, Rambaut A. Phylogenetic evidence for recombination in dengue virus. Mol Biol Evol. 1999;16(3):405–9.

[104] McGuire G, Wright F. TOPAL 2.0: improved detection of mosaic sequences within multiple alignments. Bioinformatics. 2000;16(2):130–4. DOI:10.1093/bioinformatics/16.2.130.

[105] Weiller GF. Phylogenetic profiles: a graphical method for detecting genetic recombinations in homologous sequences. Mol Biol Evol. 1998;15(3):326–35.

[106] Lemey P, Lott M, Martin DP, Moulton V. Identifying recombinants in human and primate immunodeficiency virus sequence alignments using quartet scanning. BMC Bioinform. 2009;10(1):126.

[107] Delport W, Poon AF, Frost SD, Pond SLK. Datamonkey 2010: a suite of phylogenetic analysis tools for evolutionary biology. Bioinformatics. 2010;26(19):2455–7. DOI: 10.1093/bioinformatics/btq429.

[108] Pond SLK, Frost SD. Datamonkey: rapid detection of selective pressure on individual sites of codon alignments. Bioinformatics. 2005;21(10):2531–3. DOI:10.1093/bioinformatics/bti320.

[109] Pond SLK, Muse SV. HyPhy: hypothesis testing using phylogenies. In: Nielsen R, editor. Statistical methods in molecular evolution. New York: Springer; 2005. p. 125–181. DOI:10.1093/bioinformatics/bti079.

[110] Suzuki Y, Gojobori T. A method for detecting positive selection at single amino acid sites. Mol Biol Evol. 1999;16(10):1315–28.

[111] Pond SLK, Frost SD. Not so different after all: a comparison of methods for detecting amino acid sites under selection. Mol Biol Evol. 2005;22(5):1208–22.

[112] Murrell B, Wertheim JO, Moola S, Weighill T, Scheffler K, Pond SK. Detecting individual sites subject to episodic diversifying selection. PLoS Genet. 2012;8(7):e1002764. DOI:10.1093/molbev/msi105.

[113] Kolekar P, Kale M, Kulkarni-Kale U. In: Lopes H, editor. Molecular evolution & phylogeny: what, when, why & how? Croatia: InTech Open Access Publisher; 2011. DOI: 10.5772/20225.

[114] Yang Z, Rannala B. Molecular phylogenetics: principles and practice. Nat Rev Genet. 2012;13(5):303–14. DOI:10.1038/nrg3186.

[115] Saitou N, Nei M. The neighbor-joining method: a new method for reconstructing phylogenetic trees. Mol Biol Evol. 1987;4(4):406–25.

[116] Cavalli-Sforza LL, Edwards AW. Phylogenetic analysis. Models and estimation procedures. Am J Hum Genet. 1967;19(3):233.

[117] Fitch WM, Margoliash E. Construction of phylogenetic trees. Science. 1967;155(3760): 279–84.

[118] Desper R, Gascuel O. Fast and accurate phylogeny reconstruction algorithms based on the minimum-evolution principle. J Comput Biol. 2002;9(5):687–705. DOI: 10.1089/106652702761034136.

[119] Felsenstein, J. Evolutionary trees from DNA sequences: a maximum likelihood approach. J Mol Evol. 1981;17(6):368–76.

[120] Cheng J, Cao F, Liu Z. AGP: a multimethods web server for alignment-free genome phylogeny. Mol Biol Evol. 2013;30(5):1032–7. DOI:10.1093/molbev/mst021.

[121] Drummond AJ, Suchard MA, Xie D, Rambaut A. Bayesian phylogenetics with BEAUti and the BEAST 1.7. Mol Biol Evol. 2012;29(8):1969–73. DOI:10.1093/molbev/mss075.

[122] Kolekar PS, Kale MM, Kulkarni-Kale U. Genotyping of Mumps viruses based on SH gene: Development of a server using alignment-free and alignment-based methods. Immunome Res. 2011;7(3):1–7.

[123] Kolekar P, Kale M, Kulkarni-Kale U. Alignment-free distance measure based on return time distribution for sequence analysis: applications to clustering, molecular phylogeny and subtyping. Mol Phylogenet Evol. 2012;65(2):510–22. DOI:10.1016/j.ympev.2012.07.003.

[124] Kolekar P, Hake N, Kale M, Kulkarni-Kale U. WNV Typer: a server for genotyping of West Nile viruses using an alignment-free method based on a return time distribution. J Virol Methods. 2014;198(1):41–55. DOI:10.1016/j.jviromet.2013.12.012.

[125] King AMQ, Adams MJ, Carstens EB, Lefkowitz EJ, editors. Virus taxonomy: classification and nomenclature of viruses: Ninth Report of the International Committee on Taxonomy of Viruses. San Diego: Elsevier Academic Press; 2012.

[126] Rozanov M, Plikat U, Chappey C, Kochergin A, Tatusova T. A web-based genotyping resource for viral sequences. Nucleic Acids Res. 2004;32(Web Server issue):W654–9.

[127] Lu G, Rowley T, Garten R, Donis RO. FluGenome: a web tool for genotyping influenza A virus. Nucleic Acids Res. 2007;35(Web Server issue):W275–9.

[128] Gire SK, Goba A, Andersen KG, Sealfon RS, Park DJ, Kanneh L, Jalloh S, Momoh M, Fullah M, Dudas G, Wohl S, Moses LM, Yozwiak NL, Winnicki S, Matranga CB, Malboeuf CM, Qu J, Gladden AD, Schaffner SF, Yang X, Jiang PP, Nekoui M, Colubri A, Coomber MR, Fonnie M, Moigboi A, Gbakie M, Kamara FK, Tucker V, Konuwa E, Saffa S, Sellu J, Jalloh AA, Kovoma A, Koninga J, Mustapha I, Kargbo K, Foday M, Yillah M, Kanneh F, Robert W, Massally JL, Chapman SB, Bochicchio J, Murphy C, Nusbaum C, Young S, Birren BW, Grant DS, Scheiffelin JS, Lander ES, Happi C, Gevao SM, Gnirke A, Rambaut A, Garry RF, Khan SH, Sabeti PC. Genomic surveillance elucidates Ebola virus origin and transmission during the 2014 outbreak. Science. 2014;345(6202):1369–72. DOI:10.1126/science.1259657.

[129] Huttner A, Dayer JA, Yerly S, Combescure C, Auderset F, Desmeules J, Eickmann M, Finckh A, Goncalves AR, Hooper JW, Kaya G, Krähling V, Kwilas S, Lemaître B, Matthey A, Silvera P, Becker S, Fast PE, Moorthy V, Kieny MP, Kaiser L, Siegrist CA; VSV-Ebola Consortium. The effect of dose on the safety and immunogenicity of the VSV Ebola candidate vaccine: a randomised double-blind, placebo-controlled phase 1/2 trial. Lancet Infect Dis. 2015; 15(10): 1156 - 1166. DOI:10.1016/S1473-3099(15)00154-1.

[130] McElroy K, Thomas T, Luciani F. Deep sequencing of evolving pathogen populations: applications, errors, and bioinformatic solutions. Microb Inform Exp. 2014;4(1): 1. DOI:10.1186/2042-5783-4-1.

[131] Rappuoli R. Vaccines, emerging viruses, and how to avoid disaster. BMC Biol. 2014;12(1):100. DOI:10.1186/s12915-014-0100-6.

Chapter 7

RNA-seq – Revealing Biological Insights in Bacteria

Mariana P. Santana, Flavia F. Aburjaile, Mariana T.D. Parise, Sandeep Tiwari, Artur Silva, Vasco Azevedo and Anne Cybele Pinto

Additional information is available at the end of the chapter

http://dx.doi.org/10.5772/61669

Abstract

New technologies are constantly being released and the improvements therein bring advances not only to transcriptome, the focus of this chapter, but also to diverse areas of biological research. Since the announcement and application of the RNA-seq approach, discoveries are being made in this field, but when we consider bacterial species, this progress proceeded a few years behind. However, with the application of RNA-seq derivative approaches, we can gain biological insights into the bacterial world and aspire to uncover the mysteries involving gene expression, organization and other functional genomic features.

Keywords: RNA-seq, bacteria, transcriptomics, bioinformatics analysis workflow

1. Introduction

RNA-seq technology has driven advances in gene expression analysis through new-generation sequencing platforms, as they are versatile, powerful and ensure quality results with accuracy and reproducibility never reached before. This technology generates information that provides meaning to the set of transcripts (transcriptome), opening up possibilities for understanding cell behavior in different environments. RNA is an important component within the cell, since it plays different roles as a messenger regulatory molecule and carrier; and, it is also essential for the maintenance of housekeeping genes [1].

In 2005, the first new generation of sequencing technology was released and has been evolving rapidly [2]. After starting the process of gene expression analysis in bacteria [3, 4] at a more accessible cost, shorter experimental time and without probes, the technology took off and today overlaps other tools used for this purpose, such as microarray technology, until now extremely useful for this type of analysis.

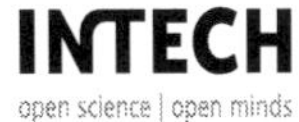

2. Applications of RNA-seq

Understanding the transcriptome is essential to knowledge of the functional genomics of an organism. The development of next-generation sequencing (NGS) impacts different areas, such as medical and industrial, and has gone through a revolutionary process. Different approaches, among them the RNA-seq technique, have emerged in the fields of microbiology and molecular biology in order to aid in understanding and bring solutions to bacterial domain investigations. In this section, we will detail some applications that are part of our current context.

2.1. The medical field

The applications of these NGS technologies in medicine have allowed expansion in the fields of diagnosis, treatment and prevention, especially concerning bacterial diseases. One of their major applications has been the quantification of expression levels of each transcript under different conditions that simulate the intracellular environment. Such work has been done by Pinto et al. (2014) to understand the host–pathogen relationship [5]. Westermann et al. (2012) demonstrated the validity of this technique, with the transcriptome of the pathogenic bacteria as their host, using the dual RNA-seq that simultaneously analyzed the gene expressions of the pathogen and host [6]. This gives us better understanding of the systems biology involving bacteria and their hosts, helping scientists to develop drugs and vaccines.

Another field that has been explored extensively involves metatranscriptome, as scientists have sought to comprehend the composition and regulation of microbial ecosystems [7, 8]. To pursue this, they have used the RNA-seq technique to generate, and allow the interpretation of, a large volume of very reliable data. Leimena et al. (2013) also validated the RNA-seq technique using the microbiota of a human small intestine with ileostomy. Their aim was to understand the interactions involved in this microbial ecosystem and how these relationships can be associated with disease [8]. Transcriptome analysis pipelines (see Section 5) can be used with different experimental designs and applied to many bacteria in addition to those in the medical field.

2.2. The industrial field

Industrial applications have been developed in recent years, mainly in the probiotic industry, since it benefits the world economy. Bisanz et al. (2014) used the RNA-seq technique [9] to show the metatranscriptome of probiotic yogurt, seeking to understand the metabolic activities that allow the survival of this organism in the products. Their results show the adaptive capacity of this bacterium, as well as the variation in differential gene expression, yielding the taste or storage life of the product [9]. Studies such as these are important because they enrich the knowledge of the industrial field and open new possibilities for an attractive area in the marketplace, which results in improvement in the quality of the product that is ultimately delivered to the consumer.

In addition to the probiotic market, another important area is the bacterial production and synthesis of biomolecules. Wiegand et al. (2013) used the RNA-seq technique to understand the regulatory RNAs in the fermentation of *Bacillus licheniformis*. Their study identified active genomic regions which, in turn, contribute to the efficiency and optimization of the fermentation process, which can promote the industrial production of exoenzymes and antibiotics [10].

Microorganisms produce antioxidant molecules that can be used in the pharmaceutical and cosmetic industries. They also produce other compounds, such as propionate, that are applicable in the production of chemical aids and are produced by *Propionibacterium freudenreichii ssp. shermanii*, which one is considered valuable in the food industry [11]. In this area, the RNA-seq technology is very promising and its application can bring advances in these studies.

3. RNA-seq and derivative techniques

3.1. RNA-seq

The RNA-seq technology is able to identify all RNAs directly and quantitatively: coding and non-coding, rare and abundant, smaller and larger. This method provides information about the transcription start site (TSS), untranslated regions (UTRs), detection of unknown open reading frames (ORFs), improved quality in genomic annotation [12], and also allows the distinction between primary and processed transcripts (dRNA-seq) [13].

The major constraint is to ensure representatives for rare transcripts. In this case, the recommendation is either to increase the representation of reads per library [14] or to enhance these transcripts, eliminating the ribosomal (rRNA) and transfer (tRNA) RNAs that are in abundance in the cells representing about 95% of total RNA [15].

Despite RNA-seq generally being considered the gold standard for gene expression analysis, some researchers nevertheless find it complicated to define this technology as the gold standard. It is a method that is available in different platforms and address different strategies, showing advantages and disadvantages. However, the superiority of this technology, compared to others in the past, is not questioned [16].

Despite the technological superiority, the need for biological replicates and depth of sequencing remains. Hence, the results may achieve greater reliability and reproducibility [17]. Differentially expressed genes are better appraised when there are samples with more biological replicates, as compared to enhanced depth with fewer replicates [18].

Transcriptomics studies have contributed a revolution in the study of the bacterial environment. Different bacterial species have been targeted for RNA-seq studies [5, 13, 19, 20], and gene expression-based discovery has transformed the scientific paradigm of these organisms. The detection of an unexpected amount of coding genes in *Helicobacter pylori* has demonstrated that, despite having a small compact genome, the transcriptome of this bacterium is extremely complex [13].

A surprising result was the detection of a large number of transcription start sites (TSS). This has never been achieved before using any technology aside from derivative RNA-seq technology, like the differential RNA-seq (dRNA-seq), which differentiated primary transcripts that exhibit triphosphate ends from processed transcripts that present monophosphate ends, such as rRNAs and tRNAs. In this case, to enrich mRNA, the strategy was to treat all the RNA samples with exonuclease enzymes that degrade nucleotide monophosphate. This strategy identified 5'UTR ends, operons and antisense transcription, thus providing a new perception of the organization of the bacterial transcriptome and a new model for the analysis of individual genes [13].

The results obtained allow the inference of a role of 5'UTR regions. A correlation between size and cell function was proposed by the researchers, who found that larger size is related to pathogenicity [13]. These results show how little knowledge there is regarding microorganisms, believed to be the simplest form of life, yet which nevertheless prove to be more complex than previously anticipated. This leaves a lot to be discovered.

An RNA-seq application that has been widely used in bacterial genomes is found in studies focused on identifying small RNAs (sRNA). These elements are regulators of various biological processes and were initially studied primarily in *Escherichia coli* [21]. However, with the advances in technology, it has been possible to identify and characterize small RNAs in a variety of bacterial species [13, 22, 23]. Yan et al. (2013) identified an expression profile of sRNA in the *Yersinia pestis*, both *in vitro* and *in vivo*. This has allowed the identification of new sRNAs and the recognition of gene expression modulation during the infection process, thus improving the understanding of the transcription regulation mechanisms of this organism [24]. The importance of studies involving sRNA also includes assistance in research related to antibiotics therapies, a study in initial development despite a lot of knowledge to be better exploited [25].

RNA-seq has been used in different areas and situations. Advanced studies using this technology can detect details in cell expression [26]. Even with the difficulties in separating eukaryotic and prokaryotic materials, it was possible to distinguish the simultaneous expression profiles between the host–pathogen responses through dual transcriptome studies. This work allowed to disclosure the host response against the bacterial infection and virulence factors, enabling the infectious process determination [27]. These studies contribute to the research in the field of biological infection by examining diverse pathogens with different life cycles and methods of infection and providing crucial knowledge for studies of diagnostics and vaccines, such as metatranscriptomics study.

After a relatively short time on the market, RNA-seq can accurately reveal structural and functional elements of bacteria. The mapping of transcripts in the genome can refine the annotation or even identify new regions, improve the quality of the studied genome compared to regions previously annotated by predictors or assembled using an *ab initio* approach [28, 29], and can even check the abundance of transcript expression.

Data coming from a quality genome tends to provide more promising results, responding to the biological question being investigated by researchers. In search of a quality genome, *ab initio* transcripts assembly or even a hybrid approach, which uses both the reference genome and *ab initio* assembly, become an auspicious endeavour to solve many problems encountered in the genome and complicated to adjust [28].

Pinto et al. (2012) conducted a study of *Corynebacterium pseudotuberculosis* adopting *ab initio* assembly and, therefore, were able to identify differences in the expression of active genes under different environmental conditions. This allowed them to detect new possible virulence factors involved in pathogenicity, making them targets for vaccine development, diagnosis or treatment against caseous lymphadenitis disease caused by this bacterium [30].

These results suggest the importance of this technology and the possibility of going further with a tool that aims to improve, and probably will expand, the field of analysis. This could bring the results increasingly closer to bacterial molecular reality.

3.2. tagRNA-seq

Bacterial RNA can be divided in two groups: primary and processed transcripts. Primary transcripts are represented by the presence of 5′-triphosphate (5′PPP), which includes messenger RNA (mRNA) and small RNAs (sRNA). Processed transcripts are those carrying 5′-monophosphate (5′P), such as mature ribosomal RNA (rRNA) and transfer RNA (tRNA).

Transcriptome represents approximately 95% of the total bacterial transcriptome [15]. A recently developed approach called dRNA-seq [13] revolutionized the study of the primary transcripts by considering the 5′ difference between the primary and the processed groups, as mentioned previously (see Section 3.1).

RNAs are very stable and during preparation, considering the "wet-lab" experiments, some transcripts are partially or totally degraded. 5′PPP and 5′P are two of the mechanisms of protection against exonucleases and the first degraded portion of the transcripts. During that process, information is lost and some primary transcripts end up with 5′P and are treated as processed transcripts. Consequently, they are eliminated by the dRNA-seq technique. A new methodology was created to overcome this problem by tagging and clustering the two groups together in an RNA-seq-derived approach named tagRNA-seq [31]. This technique also considers the difference between processed and primary transcripts, but instead of degrading the processed ones, two different ligation reactions are implemented with two different markers: PSS-tag (processed start site) and TSS-tag (transcription start site). They differ in their nucleotide sequence. Figure 1 exhibits briefly the methodology, considering the three main steps: (1) the first reaction tags (PSS-tag) on the processed transcripts; (2) treatment with tobacco alkaline phosphatase (TAP), where the 5′PPP loses two phosphates, which allows the third step; (3) the second ligation reaction (TSS-tag) on the primary transcripts. After those steps are completed, the transcripts are sequenced and, due to the different markers, they can be distinguished and compared [31].

This methodology was first described for *Enterococcus faecalis* [31] and was based on another technique, 5′tagRACE [32], a 5′RACE derived method. The results provided by tagRNA-seq improved the annotation of the *E. faecalis* genome by having identified or corrected several genome portions, including both non-coding and coding regions. This study also compared different libraries to prove the effectiveness of this innovative approach. With this, it provided

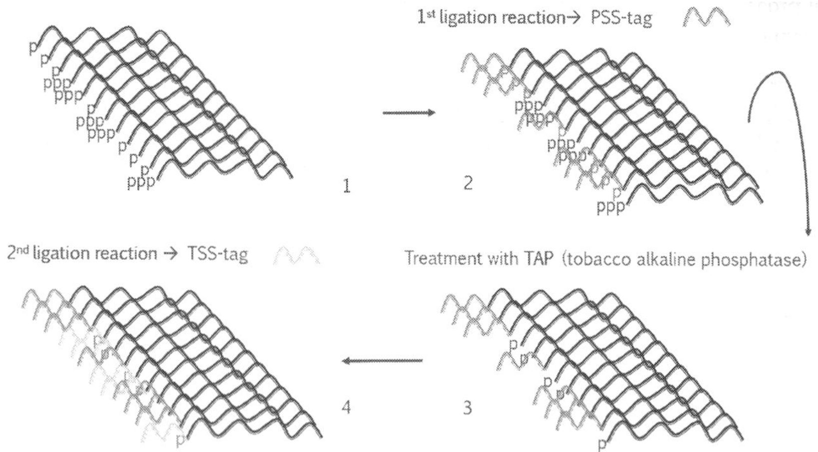

Figure 1. The three main steps of the tagRNA-seq approach. (1) The first ligation reaction, during which the attachment of the PSS-tag (blue) to the processed transcripts (5′P) occurs. (2) Treatment with tobacco alkaline phosphatase (TAP), turning triphosphate to monophosphate groups. (3) The second ligation, corresponding to the TSS-tag (yellow) marker on the previously 5′PPP group (primary transcripts). The different markers allow the differentiation of the triphosphate and monophosphate groups after sequencing.

a new method capable of differentiating primary and processed RNAs and was suited to better comprehending of the genetic information of bacteria as other groups [31].

dRNA-seq and tagRNA-seq are approaches that enable a new view of the transcriptome by selecting the primary transcripts for sequencing or by differentiating the primary from the processed transcripts, for a broader insight into the transcriptome. These state-of-the-art techniques promise a better understanding of RNA structures like TSS, 5′UTR, promoters, among others, besides the knowledge of non-annotated genes and small RNAs.

3.3. FRT-seq (flowcell reverse transcription sequencing)

Flowcell reverse transcription sequencing (FRT-seq) is a new and improved methodology, derived from the RNA-seq technology that was created for Illumina sequencers. Unlike RNA-seq, FRT-seq does not require amplification by PCR, a step that usually introduces bias into the results by displaying an erroneous view of the quantity of some RNA species [33]. Other important features of the Illumina sequencing methodology are the ability to generate strand-specific information, the use of pair-end libraries and the need for a considerable initial amount of RNA template. PCR-free amplification is a major step towards a more comprehensive library, akin to the original one, but without the formation of intermolecular priming artefacts among other errors. It will probably become a fairly useful technique in the near future [33, 34]. Third-generation sequencing platforms, like Nanopore and PacBio, also use amplification-free approaches. However, neither is currently being broadly used since they still exhibit sequencing errors.

FRT-seq comprises the fragmentation of the template (e.g., mRNA) followed by ligation of adapters in both the 3′ and the 5′ ends, which are responsible for the hybridization of the template with oligonucleotides on the flowcell surface. The next steps performed are quantification, reverse transcription and then sequence reaction [33, 34].

This approach can be applied to both eukaryotes and prokaryotes, although the number of published papers involving eukaryotes is more substantial. From the bacterial world, we can quote papers involving *Salmonella enterica* [23] and *Shigella fleneri* [35] in which FRT-seq was applied as a complementary approach to describe the transcriptional landscape of the species. In both cases, FRT-seq showed greater sensitivity and excellent concordance when compared to other approaches and replicates.

The *S. enterica* paper [23] shows that FRT-seq is as efficient as the RNA-seq and dRNA-seq techniques (Figure 2) (Table 1). Figure 2 compares nine different RNA libraries: TEX (1, 2, 3), RNA-seq (1, 2, 3, *) and FRT-seq (depleted and not depleted). TEX (libraries treated with terminator exonuclease) is a dRNA-seq methodology (see Sections 3.1 and 3.2) that, together with the first three RNA-seq biological replicates, was sequenced using a 454 (1 and 2) or an Illumina GAII (3 and FRT-seq) sequencer and the RNA-seq* (library enriched for small RNA species) was sequenced using Illumina HiSeq. The charts relate the percentages of different RNA species and show that the FRT-seq libraries provide similar or better results than the other approaches. The data presented in Table 2 also support this claim, especially considering both the total number of reads and the uniquely mapped reads achieved using the FRT-seq libraries.

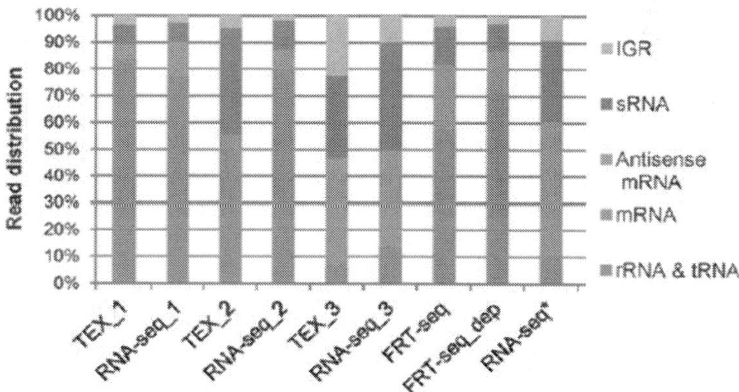

Figure 2. Sequencing methodology comparison. Adapted from [23]. IGR – Intergenic region; TEX – libraries treated with terminator exonuclease; RNA-seq* – library enriched for small RNA species (sRNA).

Library	Sequencing technology	Description	Total number	Number of reads (not mapped)	Number of reads (uniquely mapped)	Percent uniquely mapped reads [%]	Minimum fold coverage[#]
TEX_1	454	dRNA-seq library biological replicate 1	161,031	72,623	88,408	54.90	1.11
RNA-seq_1	454	RNA-seq library biological replicate 1	248,993	83,030	165,963	66.65	2.03
TEX_2	454	dRNA-seq library biological replicate 2	111,462	10,785	100,677	90.32	2.16
RNA-seq_2	454	RNA-seq library biological replicate 2	93,337	38,577	54,760	58.67	0.61
TEX_3	Illumina GAII	dRNA-seq library biological replicate 3	1,738,867	122,058	1,211,426	69.67	20.99
RNA-seq_3	Illumina GAII	RNA-seq library biological replicate 3	2,148,563	136,871	1,360,113	63.30	21.16
RNA-seq*	Illumina HiSeq	RNA-seq library biological replicate 4	3,750,797	164,658	2,596,010	69.21	25.11
FRT-seq	**Illumina GAII**	**FRT-seq library biological replicate 5**	**18,563,218**	**4,203,715**	**2,456,792**	**13.23**	**16.42**
FRT-seq dep	**Illumina GAII**	**FRT-seq library biological replicate 5 rRNA depleted**	**24,585,564**	**9,652,397**	**4,093,744**	**16.65**	**27.77**

Table 1. Sequencing statistics. Adapted from [23]

The *S. fleneri* paper [35] also reports a favourable result concerning FRT-seq. In fact, this approach revealed a larger gene repertoire than the RNA-seq (Table 2).

	RNA-seq		FRT-seq	
	Condition A	Condition B	Condition A	Condition B
Total number of mapped reads	20,099,597	22,736,494	49,925,286	47,605,241
Total number of reads mapping to genes	1,525,782	2,271,423	3,037,954	2,585,600
Reads mapping genes in sense	1,195,446	1,958,533	2,469,828	2,129,951
Reads mapping genes in antisense	330,336	312,890	568,126	455,649

Table 2. Sequencing statistics. Adapted from [31].

The data presented in this topic demonstrate the quality of this recently published methodology and, according to the authors [33, 34], new updates are still being developed. This will probably provide an even better approach for users. The fact that this technique is only applicable for Illumina sequencers is a drawback; but, since this sequencing platform is available worldwide, this disadvantage can easily be fixed. Perhaps, in the near future, it can be extended to work in other sequencing platforms. Another particularity of this technique is its efficiency with AT-rich genomes, which does not constrain its application with AT-poor genomes. This is due to the PCR-free amplification, which raises a question for other sequencers like Nanopore and PacBio. Despite these issues, this technology has a bright future and is a great advance over the conventional RNA-seq.

3.4. Chromatin immunoprecipitation followed by sequencing (ChIP-seq)

Chromatin immunoprecipitation followed by sequencing (ChIP-Seq) is a technique for the genome-wide profiling of DNA-binding proteins, histone modifications or nucleosomes [36]. ChIP-Seq has become an essential tool for studying gene regulation and epigenetic mechanisms. It offers higher resolution, less noise and greater coverage than its array-based predecessor, the ChIP-chip [37, 38]. This approach has six main steps: (1) it is initiated with cell cultures that are grown under defined conditions; and, when the cultures reach the desired stage of development, they are treated with formaldehyde for the cross-linking of proteins and DNA; (2) the chromatin is sheared by sonication into small fragments (200–600 bp); (3) an antibody specific to the protein is used to immunoprecipitate the DNA–protein complex; (4) the cross-links are reversed by heating; (5) the released DNA is subjected to high-throughput sequencing and (6) in silico analysis is carried out in which the resulting sequencing reads are studied for quality and then cropped, based on the quality of the reads [38–40]. The cropped reads are then aligned to a reference genome. Afterwards, areas of enrichment in the ChIP-seq data are identified and those areas, usually called peaks, represent where the transcription factors (TF) bind throughout the genome. CisGenome, MOSAiCs and MACS are some known algorithms that have been utilized in bacterial ChIP-seq analysis [38, 41]. After peaks are associated with genes downstream, a number of bioinformatics analyses can be carried out, including identification and analysis of motifs, differential analysis and association with expression data for deep understanding of bacterial regulon. This is shown in Figure 3 [36].

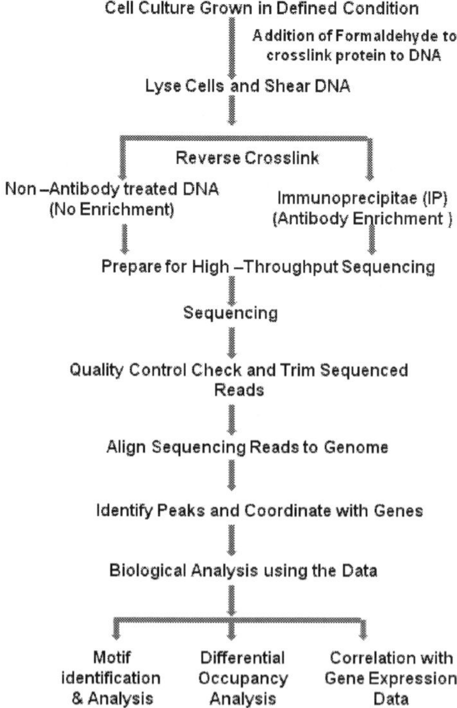

Figure 3. ChIP-seq sample preparation and analysis. Adapted from [36].

As whole-genome transcription profiling cannot reveal whether the influence of the transcription factors (TF) on RNA levels is direct or indirect, this requires identification of transcription factors binding within the appropriate promoter region. ChIP-seq provides information about where the TF are bound. Thus, by integrating ChIP methods and transcription profiling, it is possible to identify all direct regulatory targets of a TF for a given condition. For example, work carried out by Stringer et al. (2014) on the *araC* gene of *Escherichia coli* and *Salmonella enterica* has identified direct regulatory targets of AraC, including five novel target genes: *ytfQ*, *ydeN*, *ydeM*, *ygeA* and *polB* [42]. Although ChIP-seq has been used only in moderation to study bacterial systems in a few bacterial species, such as *Vibrio harveyi*, *V. cholerae*, *Rhodobacter sphaeroides*, *Mycobacterium tuberculosis*, *S. enterica* and *Caulobacter crescentus* [36, 37, 43–45], it is used to identify novel regulatory interactions, even for well-studied proteins [46, 47].

ChIP-seq, in combination with RNA-seq, could be an efficient tool to get detailed information about bacterial transcription regulation and how bacteria respond to different external conditions.

3.5. RNA immunoprecipitation sequencing (RIP-seq)

RNA immunoprecipitation (RIP) is the study of intracellular RNA and protein binding; it is a tool for understanding the dynamic process of post-transcriptional regulatory networks. With this technique, an antibody is used against a protein of interest to recover the RNA species bound to the protein. Since the sequence information of the RNA species bound to a specific protein is often desired, an approach combining RNA immunoprecipitation with sequencing technology (RIP-seq) was created [48]. The main challenge of RIP-seq is the cross-linking step, which is relatively inefficient and only a small amount of RNA is available to construct the library [48, 49]. After that step, treatment with endonuclease elucidates the specific binding sites within the RNA, as they will be protected from digestion. This is followed by purification of the RNA–protein complexes using electrophoresis and high-throughput sequencing [48, 50]. Finally, the data obtained from the sequencer are analyzed using bioinformatics tools. The first study using the RIP-seq-based technique was carried out on *Salmonella* by Sittka et al. (2008) [51]. They used the RNA-binding property of the Hfq protein in their analysis and, as a result, many new sRNA were discovered [52]. Thus, RIP-Seq could be an efficient tool for the identification of bacterial non-coding RNAs.

3.6. LEA-seq (low error amplicon sequencing)

The LEA-seq technique (low error amplicon sequencing) emerged in 2013 and was developed and patented by Gordon and Faith (2014) [53]. This method was created to improve the quality and depth of sequencing runs, since the massive amount of data produced by NGS has caused a high error rate in the sequencing, due to problems with the algorithms or platform reading lengths [53].

LEA-seq is a nucleic acid sequencing technique that identifies events that occur at low frequency, seeking to understand mutation events. The three basic steps for implementing this technique are: (1) linear PCR, (2) exponential PCR and (3) sequencing. This technique is performed based on bacterial 16S sequencing in which PCR carries numerous times and each amplified PCR uses specific primers for each linear molecule [53].

The LEA-seq technique is a quantitative method that has the advantages of generating and reading. This permits the formation of a consensus and the elimination of errors for each molecule. Currently, the available techniques do not support error detection in sequencing or identification of whether there is a real variation in the sequence of that microorganism. The multiple sequencing, using the LEA-seq technique, supports better quality and precision about the organism.

The study by Faith et al. (2013) aimed to identify the composition of the faecal microbiota of adults and to understand the role of these bacterial species and their therapeutic potential for intestinal diseases. This technique allowed them to work with a large number of samples (over 500 isolates), as well as to achieve a fast and accurate analysis of the data [54].

Researchers have a continuing interest in improving this technique, since it can be used for clinical investigation due to its high accuracy: for example, in patients with genetic mutations or somatic mutations. LEA-seq can assist in the search for knowledge about intestinal microbiota, as it may reveal their composition, opening up prospects for the diagnosis, treatment and prevention of gastrointestinal tract diseases.

3.7. CRISPR (clustered regularly interspaced short palindromic repeats)

Ishino et al. (1987) were the first to describe CRISPR [55]. This system has been identified in 40% of bacterial genomes so far [56] and they are defined as short repetitions of grouped bases. The determination of the CRISPR locus and the characterization of adjacent genes, known as *cas* genes, responsible for the function of CRISPR, only occurred in 2002 [57]. The CRISPR/Cas system uses small non-coding RNAs in association with Cas proteins. Cas9 is a nuclease which cleaves DNA in the selected region, so that the CRISPR system/Cas9 can be used to edit genomes.

CRISPR/Cas activity involves three main mechanisms: (1) acquisition, the step in which the DNA fragment is inserted into the CRISPR locus in the genome of interest; (2) transcription, in which the CRISPR locus is transcribed and processed; (3) interference, in which the ejection of nucleic acids occurs. All those mechanisms contribute to bacterial persistence in the environment [58, 59]. Furthermore, CRISPR provides mechanisms to limit the spread of antibiotic resistance or virulence factors. However, Gophna et al. (2015) demonstrated that, even though there are different measurements to evaluate horizontal gene transfer, it is not possible to identify a correlation between the CRISPR/Cas system and the evolution of the species. Changes occur only at the population level [60].

RNA-seq helped in the annotation transcription of regions, mainly non-coding, and also enabled the identification of CRISPR elements in prokaryotes [61]. The CRISPR system can also be used as a tool in studies centered on gene regulation, since this system is able to activate or repress genes.

Zoephel and Randau (2013) discuss how the structure of CRISPR can affect the maturation of RNA and, thus, influence the functionality of the CRISPR/Cas system [62]. The RNA-seq approach was used to evaluate differential gene expression in *S. aureus*, a pathogen of major importance. It was able to identify the CRISPR in these strains and helped in investigating their possible role, since these regions show an adaptive response to infection [63]. Thus, we see the importance of the use of the RNA-seq approach in the magnification of knowledge about function in prokaryotes.

4. RNA Sequencing Platforms

The RNA-seq approach can be applied to different next-generation sequencing platforms and the results obtained by them are proportional to the machine capability. In Table 3, a comparison is made with some of the platforms currently most employed [64].

Company Name	Instrument	Version	Run Time (Hours)	Read Lengths (Mean)	Reads Per Run (Millions)	Applications
Illumina	HiSeq 2000	High Output	132	50	6,000	Gene expression, Splice junction detection, variant calling, fusion
Illumina	HiSeq 2500	High Output	132	50	6,000	Gene expression, Splice junction detection, variant calling, fusion
Illumina	MiSeq	v2 kit	39	250	30	Splice junction detection, variant calling,
Life Technologies	PGM	318 Chip	7.3	176	6	Splice junction detection, variant calling
Life Technologies	Proton	Proton I chip	2-4	81	70	Gene expression, Splice junction detection, variant calling
Pacific Biosciences	RS	RS	0.5-2	1,289	0.03	Splice junction detection, variant calling, full-length gene coverage
Roche	454	GS FLX+	20	686	1	Splice junction detection

Table 3. Different Next Generations sequencing platforms in the study of RNA-seq. Adopted and modified from [64].

5. Bioinformatics Analysis

Experimental investigations in prokaryotes have been facilitated, extended and complemented using computational approaches [65]. Large amounts of data have been generated from RNA-seq experiments which need to be stored and analyzed using computational techniques and tools [66]. This amount has become a bottleneck to bioinformatics analysis and to biologists, since today's transcriptome analysis consists of experiments and data evaluation [65]. Extracting biological information from RNA-seq datasets requires bioinformatics knowledge and tools, making the software choice an important issue for successful RNA-seq analysis [65, 67].

According to Chierico et al. (2015) [68] and Pinto et al. (2011) [67], RNA-seq can be understood as a five-step process: (1) isolation of the total RNA of the organism; (2) mRNA enrichment; (3) synthesis of cDNA; (4) NGS sequencing, which returns raw data to the (5) bioinformatics analysis [67]. A flowchart of this process can be seen in Figure 4.

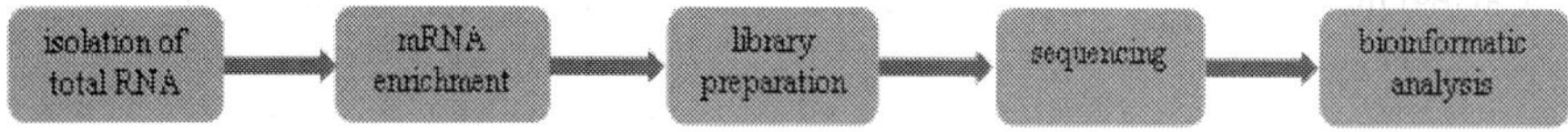

Figure 4. RNA-seq five-step process.

This session focuses on bioinformatics analysis and the computational tools available. Based on a literature review [29, 65, 67–69], bioinformatics analysis can be comprehended as the extraction and classification/division of biological information gleaned from the sequencing of raw data (Figure 5).

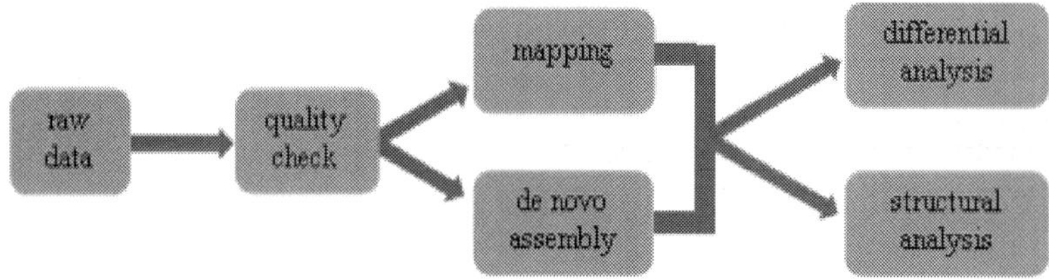

Figure 5. Bioinformatics analysis workflow

5.1. Bioinformatics workflow

The quality check step aims to increase the accuracy of the results by removing sequences that may contain errors [70]; trimming sequences introduced in the library preparation step, such as adapters and poly(A)-tails [71]; and, removing reads with low phred quality. However, in that regard, the use of poor-quality databases can lead to less precise results [72]; considering this, the quality check can affect the next steps drastically.

Some RNA-Seq pipelines, like ReaDemption [71], implement quality checking which performs quality trimming, removes adapters and poly(A) tails and discards reads shorter than a given cut-off (the default cut-off is 12 nucleotides (nt)). Quality assessment [72] evaluates the quality based on quality-graph analysis and estimated coverage. According to Backofen et al. (2014) [65], FastQC (http://www.bioinformatics.babraham.ac.uk/projects/ fastq c/) is a tool commonly used to check read quality and to determine the quality profile of the reads. Software suites can also be used for this purpose, FASTX-Toolkit (http://hannonlab.cshl.edu/fastx_toolkit/) provides tools to remove sequences attached in previous steps and to perform other pre-processing strategies on raw data.

After the quality check, if a reference genome is available, then a mapping step will be done; otherwise, *de novo* assembly. Mapping consists of producing the transcriptome map by aligning reads to a reference genome [67]. This aims to detect the right position of the reads and to distinguish between sequencing errors and genetic variations [73]. Abundant mapping software has been released, differing in their algorithms, memory management, velocity and computational cost [65]. This makes the choice of a mapping tool a challenge. McClure et al.

(2013) [69] made a comparison between SOAP2, BWA, Bowtie and Bowtie2 aligners using 75 RNA-seq experiment data. The comparison of mapping algorithms applied to IonTorrent data can be seen in [73]. After mapping quality is evaluated, ReadXplorer software offers quality classification of read mapping in order to provide information about the quality and quantity of each single read mapping [74]. This approach is recommended when a high-quality genome is available as a reference. If one is unavailable, transcripts should be assembled *de novo* [29].

De novo assembly can be used when investigating poorly studied organisms [14], complex microbial communities or uncultivable organisms [29]. Both DNA and RNA must be assembled, but transcriptome assembly is significantly different than genome assembly [75]; thus, it is important to use RNA assemblers. Tjaden (2015) [29] affirms that assemblers should be specifically designed to prokaryotes, owing to the different challenges of eukaryotic and prokaryotic transcriptomes. Bacterial genomes are often denser than eukaryotic genomes, considering the proximity of the genes. Neighbouring bacterial transcripts can overlap, making it difficult to identify transcript boundaries appropriately. Non-coding eukaryotic RNA models are not appropriate for detecting bacterial small regulatory RNAs [29]. An assembly comparison of three different software titles (Trinity, SOAPdenovo2 and Rockhooper 2), using data from nine different bacteria, can be seen in [29].

When reference mapping or *de novo* assembly is done, data can be analyzed structurally and differentially. The main purpose of differential analysis is to determine the differences in expression among different growth conditions or treatments [76]. Several software titles have been released for this purpose, but there is no consensus about best practices, which makes it difficult to select a tool or method. Seyednasrollah et al. (2013) [76] compared eight differential expression software packages using two real, publicly available datasets. Software that analyzes differential expression can be based on the Poisson method (DEGseq and Myrna), negative binomial method (edgeR and DEseq) or other methods [67, 76]. Pinto et al. (2011) [67] recommends using DEseq or edgeR when analyzing replicates.

Transcriptome annotation and classification can be based on structural analysis, evaluating transcripts regarding the genomic region with which they have been associated and in which they have been classified: protein-coding, non-coding and intergenic regions [65]. Aiming to predict ncRNA transcripts, several computational methods have been developed. Herbig and Nieselt (2011) [77] highlight the SIPHT, sRNAFinder, sRNAscanner, NOCORNAr and sRNAPredict software. NOCORNAr distinguishes itself as it is useful for predicting and characterizing ncRNAs in bacteria [77].

Assessing transcripts concerning genomic regions rely on transcript annotation. The computational approach is convenient to use due to its velocity and precision, compared to manual annotation. However, human supervision of the results is considered important in order to avoid false-positives or missing features [1]. With this technique, some main structures must be detected: 5' transcript ends, 3' transcript ends, TSS and operon [1, 65].

a.   Transcript boundaries identification

Annotation of transcript boundaries is important for operon identification and regulatory analyses [1]. Identifying 5' UTR is not always possible; a significant number of transcripts lacking 5' UTR were found in bacteria and called leaderless transcripts. In this situation, the transcript translation start site and the transcription start site remain in almost the same position [65]. Annotation of 3' UTR is important in order to obtain the entire analytical value of the RNA-seq data. Creecy and Conway (2014) [1] affirm that the current best method for detecting 3' ends is to search for correlations between replicates data. They highlight that the software package TransTermHP can find intrinsic terminators successfully.

b.   TSS identification

TSS annotation can assist in ncRNA annotation and polycistronic transcripts [65]. According to Creecy and Conway (2013) [1], it is essential to discover unknown transcripts and to analyze operon, 5' UTR and promoters architecture. Although there are no well-established strategies for TSS identification, owing to scarce knowledge about transcription start sites in bacteria, with computational developments in both computational analyses and "wet-lab" experiments, TSS annotation has become more feasible [65]. TSSAR is a dRNA-seq data-based tool for rapid annotation of TSS that considers dRNA-seq library statistics [78]. According to Backofen et al. (2014) [65], the main advantage is in the statistical analysis presented as an easy-to-use web service. The TSSpredator tool provides automated TSS detection and classification from RNA-seq data, performing a genome-wide comparative prediction of TSS [79]. A comparison among manual annotation, TSSpredator and TSSAR annotation can be seen in [78].

c.   Operon identification

The operon represents clusters of co-transcribed genes regulated by the same regulatory sequence and co-transcribed into a single mRNA. This structure has immense biological importance, improving functional gene annotation and giving important information to studies of drug targeting, functional analyses and antibiotic resistance [80]. To handle operon occurrence complexity, the occurrence should be detected using operon architecture (i.e., 5' ends and 3' ends) and have sufficient read coverage to connect promoters and terminators. A strong indication that an operon is real is that at least 90% of the bases of the reads is covered [1]. Chuang et al. (2012) [80] classify computational methods to predict operons and they evaluate 15 algorithms with respect to accuracy, specificity and sensitivity.

5.2. RNA-seq pipeline tools

Not all pipeline tools feature the complete RNA-seq workflow described earlier. To help with tool selection, a software functionalities comparison was developed and is shown in Table 4. To provide additional support, important issues about each software are described, below.

Rockhopper is a system designed specifically for bacterial transcriptome RNA-seq data analysis. A novel approach to mapping transcripts is implemented in this software (similar to the Bowtie2 approach). Mapping normalization is performed followed by transcripts assembly, identification of transcript boundaries, quantification of transcript abundance, testing for differential gene expression and operon prediction. Analysis results are presented using Integrative Genome Viewer, which allows different experiments to be viewed simultaneously [69].

Tool	Quality Check	Mapping	*De novo* assembly	Differential analyses
Rockhopper [69]	-	x	x	x
Rockhopper 2 [29]	-	-	x	x
RNA-Rocket [81]	x	x	-	x
READemption [71]	x	x	-	x
ReadXplorer [74]	x	-	-	x

Table 4. Software comparison.

Rockhopper 2 is a comprehensive system focused on *de novo* assembly that supports differential analysis and transcripts abundance quantification. According to Tjaden (2015) [29], it does not require high-performance computers and can run on personal computers. Rockhopper 2 implements a novel *de novo* assembly algorithm for bacterial transcriptomes. The algorithm works in two stages: (1) candidate transcripts are assembled using a found k-mer and (2) sequencing reads are mapped to candidate transcripts aimed at filtering candidate transcripts to high-quality final transcripts. Concerning differential analysis, Rockhopper 2 first normalizes each RNA-seq dataset, enabling it to compare different experiments or samples [29].

RNA-Rocket aims to simplify the process of aligning RNA-seq data to a reference genome and to generate quantitative transcript profiles. It is built on Galaxy, to provide the tools and services necessary to process RNA-seq data. Some of its benefits are: the possibility of sharing results across research groups; the support of batch analysis for multiple samples; and, the integration of tools and projects, integrating data from the PATRIC platform [81].

READemption pipeline aims to integrate individual RNA-seq analysis tasks and provides a user-friendly tool with a command line interface. This tool was primarily developed to analyze bacterial transcriptome. In order to use the full capacity of modern computers and reduce run time, READemption offers parallel data processing. First, it performs quality trimming of polyA and adapters followed by mapping, coverage calculation, gene expression quantification, differential gene expression analysis and plotting. The software is able to analyze RNA-seq data from Illumina and 454 platforms.

ReadXplorer offers straightforward visualization and analysis functions built around its unique read mapping classification. Analyses such as TSS and operon detection, differential expression, RPKM value and read count calculations are available in ReadXplorer and can be exported to Microsoft Excel files. Read mapping classification sorts read mappings into three different classes: perfect match, best match and common match. These classifications are incorporated in all analyses functions.

5.3. Bioinformatics challenges

Through bibliographic research [29, 66, 69, 71, 82, 83], it has been concluded that bioinformatics has many challenges related to computational issues. RNA-seq experiments generate large amounts of data that must be computationally processed, analyzed, stored and retrieved using a great deal of computational power. In addition to the computational issues, it is important to take into account that not all bioinformatic researchers have extensive computational experience: this makes the lack of user-friendly tools a problem for some users and an important issue for developers. However, great computers, excellent bioinformatic researchers and user-friendly tools do not guarantee successful analysis. The software selected must be appropriate to each biological question and to the organisms studied. Even with all questions presented here, RNA-seq analysis has been very successful in recent years. This success can lead us to imagine the wonderful possibilities for RNA-seq bioinformatic analyses in the future.

Author details

Mariana P. Santana[1], Flavia F. Aburjaile[1], Mariana T.D. Parise[1], Sandeep Tiwari[1], Artur Silva[2], Vasco Azevedo[1*] and Anne Cybele Pinto[1]

*Address all correspondence to: vasco@icb.ufmg.br

1 Instituto de Ciências Biológicas-ICB/UFMG, Departamento de Biologia Geral, Pampulha, Belo Horizonte, Minas Gerais, Brasil

2 Centro de Ciências Biológicas, Departamento de Genética. Universidade Federal do Pará, Campus do Guamá, Guamá. Belém, Pará, Brasil

References

[1] Creecy JP, Conway T. Quantitative bacterial transcriptomics with RNA-seq. Curr Opin Microbiol 2015;23:133–40.

[2] Margulies M, Egholm M, Altman WE, Attiya S, Bader JS, Bemben LA, et al. Genome sequencing in microfabricated high-density picolitre reactors. Nature 2005 Sep 15;437(7057):376–80.

[3] Perkins TT, Kingsley RA, Fookes MC, Gardner PP, James KD, Yu L, et al. A strand-specific RNA-Seq analysis of the transcriptome of the typhoid bacillus Salmonella typhi. PLoS Genet 2009 Jul;5(7):e1000569.

[4] Passalacqua KD, Varadarajan A, Ondov BD, Okou DT, Zwick ME, Bergman NH. Structure and complexity of a bacterial transcriptome. J Bacteriol 2009 May 15;191(10):3203–11.

[5] Pinto AC, Sá PHCG de, Ramos RTJ, Barbosa S, Barbosa HPM, Ribeiro AC, et al. Differential transcriptional profile of Corynebacterium pseudotuberculosis in response to abiotic stresses. BMC Genomics 2014 Jan 9;15(1):14.

[6] Westermann AJ, Gorski, SA and Vogel J. Dual RNA-seq of pathogen and host. Nat Rev Microbiol 2012;10:618–30.

[7] Macklaim JM, Fernandes AD, Bella JMD, Hammond J-A, Reid G, Gloor GB. Comparative meta-RNA-seq of the vaginal microbiota and differential expression by Lactobacillus iners in health and dysbiosis. Microbiome 2013 Apr 12;1(1):12.

[8] Leimena MM, Ramiro-Garcia J, Davids M, van den Bogert B, Smidt H, Smid EJ, et al. A comprehensive metatranscriptome analysis pipeline and its validation using human small intestine microbiota datasets. BMC Genomics 2013;14:530.

[9] Bisanz JE, Macklaim JM, Gloor GB, Reid G. Bacterial metatranscriptome analysis of a probiotic yogurt using an RNA-Seq approach. Int Dairy J 2014;39(2):284–92.

[10] Wiegand S, Dietrich S, Hertel R, Bongaerts J, Evers S, Volland S, et al. RNA-Seq of Bacillus licheniformis: active regulatory RNA features expressed within a productive fermentation. BMC Genomics 2013;14(1):667.

[11] Wang Z, Yang S-T. Propionic acid production in glycerol/glucose co-fermentation by Propionibacterium freudenreichii subsp. shermanii. Bioresour Technol 2013;137:116–23.

[12] Sorek R, Cossart P. Prokaryotic transcriptomics: a new view on regulation, physiology and pathogenicity. Nat Rev Genet 2010 Jan;11(1):9–16.

[13] Sharma CM, Hoffmann S, Darfeuille F, Reignier J, Findeiß S, Sittka A, et al. The primary transcriptome of the major human pathogen Helicobacter pylori. Nature. 2010 Mar 11;464(7286):250–5.

[14] Haas BJ, Chin M, Nusbaum C, Birren BW, Livny J. How deep is deep enough for RNA-Seq profiling of bacterial transcriptomes? BMC Genomics 2012 Dec 27;13(1):734.

[15] Bischler T, Siew Tan H, Nieselt K, Sharma CM. Differential RNA-seq (dRNA-seq) for annotation of transcriptional start sites and small RNAs in Helicobacter pylori. Methods [Internet]. 2015 Jul 6 [cited 2015 Jul 6]; Available from: http://www.sciencedirect.com/science/article/pii/S1046202315002546

[16] Kratz A, Carninci P. The devil in the details of RNA-seq. Nat Biotechnol 2014 Sep;32(9):882–4.

[17] Sendler E, Johnson GD, Krawetz SA. Local and global factors affecting RNA sequencing analysis. Anal Biochem 2011;419(2):317–22.

[18] Liu Y, Zhou J, White KP. RNA-seq differential expression studies: more sequence or more replication? Bioinformatics 2014 Feb 1;30(3):301–4.

[19] Isabella VM, Clark VL. Deep sequencing-based analysis of the anaerobic stimulon in Neisseria gonorrhoeae. BMC Genomics 2011 Jan 20;12(1):51.

[20] Patenge N, Pappesch R, Khani A, Kreikemeyer B. Genome-wide analyses of small non-coding RNAs in streptococci. Front Genet 2015;6:189.

[21] Gottesman S, Storz G. Bacterial small RNA regulators: versatile roles and rapidly evolving variations. Cold Spring Harb Perspect Biol [Internet]. 2011 Dec [cited 2015 Jul 2];3(12). Available from: http://www.ncbi.nlm.nih.gov/pmc/articles/PMC3225950/

[22] Papenfort K, Vogel J. Regulatory RNA in bacterial pathogens. Cell Host Microbe 2010 Jul 22;8(1):116–27.

[23] Kröger C, Dillon SC, Cameron ADS, Papenfort K, Sivasankaran SK, Hokamp K, et al. The transcriptional landscape and small RNAs of Salmonella enterica serovar Typhimurium. Proc Natl Acad Sci 2012 May 15;109(20):E1277–86.

[24] Yan Y, Su S, Meng X, Ji X, Qu Y, Liu Z, et al. Determination of sRNA expressions by RNA-seq in Yersinia pestis grown in vitro and during infection. PLoS ONE 2013 Sep 11;8(9):e74495.

[25] Storz G, Vogel J, Wassarman KM. Regulation by small RNAs in bacteria: expanding frontiers. Mol Cell 2011 Sep 16;43(6):880–91.

[26] Van Dijk EL, Auger H, Jaszczyszyn Y, Thermes C. Ten years of next-generation sequencing technology. Trends Genet 2014;30(9):418–26.

[27] Humphrys MS, Creasy T, Sun Y, Shetty AC, Chibucos MC, Drabek EF, et al. Simultaneous transcriptional profiling of bacteria and their host cells. PLoS ONE 2013 Dec 4;8(12):e80597.

[28] Martin JA, Wang Z. Next-generation transcriptome assembly. Nat Rev Genet 2011 Sep 7;12(10):671–82.

[29] Tjaden B. De novo assembly of bacterial transcriptomes from RNA-seq data. Genome Biol 2015;16(1):1.

[30] Pinto AC, Ramos RTJ, Silva WM, Rocha FS, Barbosa S, Miyoshi A, et al. The core stimulon of Corynebacterium pseudotuberculosis strain 1002 identified using ab initio methodologies. Integr Biol 2012;4(7):789.

[31] Innocenti N, Golumbeanu M, d' Hérouël AF, Lacoux C, Bonnin RA, Kennedy SP, et al. Whole genome mapping of 5'RNA ends in bacteria by tagged sequencing: a comprehensive view in Enterococcus faecalis. ArXiv Prepr ArXiv14101925 [Internet]. 2014 [cited 2014 Dec 15]; Available from: http://arxiv.org/abs/1410.1925

[32] Fouquier d'Herouel A, Wessner F, Halpern D, Ly-Vu J, Kennedy SP, Serror P, et al. A simple and efficient method to search for selected primary transcripts: non-coding and antisense RNAs in the human pathogen Enterococcus faecalis. Nucleic Acids Res 2011 Apr 1;39(7):e46–e46.

[33] Mamanova L, Turner DJ. Low-bias, strand-specific transcriptome Illumina sequencing by on-flowcell reverse transcription (FRT-seq). Nat Protoc 2011 Nov;6(11):1736–47.

[34] Mamanova L, Andrews RM, James KD, Sheridan EM, Ellis PD, Langford CF, et al. FRT-seq: amplification-free, strand-specific transcriptome sequencing. Nat Methods 2010 Feb;7(2):130–2.

[35] Vergara-Irigaray M, Fookes MC, Thomson NR, Tang CM. RNA-seq analysis of the influence of anaerobiosis and FNR on Shigella flexneri. BMC Genomics 2014 Jun 6;15(1):438.

[36] Myers KS, Park DM, Beauchene NA, Kiley PJ. Defining bacterial regulons using ChIP-seq methods. Methods [Internet]. 2015 [cited 2015 Jul 17]; Available from: http://www.sciencedirect.com/science/article/pii/S1046202315002285

[37] Myers KS, Yan H, Ong IM, Chung D, Liang K, Tran F, et al. Genome-scale analysis of Escherichia coli FNR reveals complex features of transcription factor binding. PLoS Genet 2013;9(6):e1003565.

[38] Park PJ. ChIP–seq: advantages and challenges of a maturing technology. Nat Rev Genet 2009;10(10):669–80.

[39] Johnson DS, Mortazavi A, Myers RM, Wold B. Genome-wide mapping of in vivo protein-DNA interactions. Science 2007;316(5830):1497–502.

[40] Robertson G, Hirst M, Bainbridge M, Bilenky M, Zhao Y, Zeng T, et al. Genome-wide profiles of STAT1 DNA association using chromatin immunoprecipitation and massively parallel sequencing. Nat Methods 2007;4(8):651–7.

[41] Gentleman RC, Carey VJ, Bates DM, Bolstad B, Dettling M, Dudoit S, et al. Bioconductor: open software development for computational biology and bioinformatics. Genome Biol 2004;5(10):R80.

[42] Stringer AM, Currenti S, Bonocora RP, Baranowski C, Petrone BL, Palumbo MJ, et al. Genome-scale analyses of Escherichia coli and Salmonella enterica AraC reveal non-canonical targets and an expanded core regulon. J Bacteriol 2014;196(3):660–71.

[43] Haycocks JRJ, Sharma P, Stringer AM, Wade JT, Grainger DC. The molecular basis for control of ETEC enterotoxin expression in response to environment and host. PLoS Pathog 2015 Jan 8;11(1):e1004605.

[44] Singh SS, Singh N, Bonocora RP, Fitzgerald DM, Wade JT, Grainger DC. Widespread suppression of intragenic transcription initiation by H-NS. Genes Dev 2014 Feb 1;28(3):214–9.

[45] Kahramanoglou C, Seshasayee ASN, Prieto AI, Ibberson D, Schmidt S, Zimmermann J, et al. Direct and indirect effects of H-NS and Fis on global gene expression control in Escherichia coli. Nucleic Acids Res 2011 Mar 1;39(6):2073–91.

[46] Wade JT, Struhl K, Busby SJ, Grainger DC. Genomic analysis of protein–DNA interactions in bacteria: insights into transcription and chromosome organization. Mol Microbiol 2007;65(1):21–6.

[47] Grainger DC, Aiba H, Hurd D, Browning DF, Busby SJW. Transcription factor distribution in Escherichia coli: studies with FNR protein. Nucleic Acids Res 2007 Jan 1;35(1):269–78.

[48] Chu Y, Corey DR. RNA sequencing: platform selection, experimental design, and data interpretation. Nucleic Acid Ther 2012;22(4):271–4.

[49] Hafner M, Landthaler M, Burger L, Khorshid M, Hausser J, Berninger P, et al. Transcriptome-wide identification of RNA-binding protein and microRNA target sites by PAR-CLIP. Cell 2010;141(1):129–41.

[50] Chi SW, Zang JB, Mele A, Darnell RB. Argonaute HITS-CLIP decodes microRNA–mRNA interaction maps. Nature 2009;460(7254):479–86.

[51] Sittka A, Lucchini S, Papenfort K, Sharma CM, Rolle K, Binnewies TT, et al. Deep sequencing analysis of small noncoding RNA and mRNA targets of the global post-transcriptional regulator, Hfq. PLoS Genet 2008;4(8):e1000163.

[52] Cho S, Cho Y, Lee S, Kim J, Yum H, Kim SC, et al. Current challenges in bacterial transcriptomics. Genomics Inform 2013;11(2):76.

[53] Gordon JI, Faith JJ. Methods of low error amplicon sequencing (LEA-Seq) and the use thereof [Internet]. Google Patents; 2014 [cited 2015 Jul 14]. Available from: https://www.google.com/patents/US20140357499

[54] Faith JJ, Guruge JL, Charbonneau M, Subramanian S, Seedorf H, Goodman AL, et al. The long-term stability of the human gut microbiota. Science 2013;341(6141):1237439.

[55] Ishino Y, Shinagawa H, Makino K, Amemura M, Nakata A. Nucleotide sequence of the iap gene, responsible for alkaline phosphatase isozyme conversion in Escherichia coli, and identification of the gene product. J Bacteriol 1987;169(12):5429–33.

[56] Kunin V, Sorek R, Hugenholtz P. Evolutionary conservation of sequence and secondary structures in CRISPR repeats. Genome Biol 2007;8(4):R61.

[57] Jansen R, Embden J, Gaastra W, Schouls L, others. Identification of genes that are associated with DNA repeats in prokaryotes. Mol Microbiol 2002;43(6):1565–75.

[58] Gasiunas G, Barrangou R, Horvath P, Siksnys V. Cas9–crRNA ribonucleoprotein complex mediates specific DNA cleavage for adaptive immunity in bacteria. Proc Natl Acad Sci 2012;109(39):E2579–86.

[59] Jinek M, Chylinski K, Fonfara I, Hauer M, Doudna JA, Charpentier E. A programmable dual-RNA–guided DNA endonuclease in adaptive bacterial immunity. Science 2012;337(6096):816–21.

[60] Gophna U, Ron EZ. Virulence and the heat shock response. Int J Med Microbiol IJMM 2003 Feb;292(7-8):453–61.

[61] Heidrich N, Dugar G, Vogel J, Sharma CM. Investigating CRISPR RNA biogenesis and function using RNA-seq. CRISPR Methods Protoc 2015;1–21.

[62] Zoephel J, Randau L. RNA-Seq analyses reveal CRISPR RNA processing and regulation patterns. Biochem Soc Trans 2013 Dec;41(6):1459–63.

[63] Osmundson J, Dewell S, Darst SA. RNA-Seq reveals differential gene expression in Staphylococcus aureus with single-nucleotide resolution. PLoS ONE 2013 Oct 7;8(10):e76572.

[64] Li S, Tighe SW, Nicolet CM, Grove D, Levy S, Farmerie W, et al. Multi-platform assessment of transcriptome profiling using RNA-seq in the ABRF next-generation sequencing study. Nat Biotechnol 2014 Aug 24;32(9):915–25.

[65] Backofen R, Amman F, Costa F, Findei S, Richter AS, Stadler PF. Bioinformatics of prokaryotic RNAs. RNA Biol 2014;11(5):470–83.

[66] McGettigan PA. Transcriptomics in the RNA-seq era. Curr Opin Chem Biol 2013 Feb; 17(1):4–11.

[67] Pinto AC, Melo-Barbosa HP, Miyoshi A, Silva A, Azevedo V. Review application of RNA-seq to reveal the transcript profile in bacteria. Genet Mol Res 2011;10(3):1707–18.

[68] Del Chierico F, Ancora M, Marcacci M, Camma C, Putignani L, Conti S. Choice of next-generation sequencing pipelines. Bacterial Pangenomics [Internet]. Springer; 2015 [cited 2015 Jul 14]. p. 31–47. Available from: http://link.springer.com/protocol/ 10.1007/978-1-4939-1720-4_3

[69] McClure R, Balasubramanian D, Sun Y, Bobrovskyy M, Sumby P, Genco CA, et al. Computational analysis of bacterial RNA-Seq data. Nucleic Acids Res 2013 Aug 1;41(14):e140–e140.

[70] De Sá PH, Veras AA, Carneiro AR, Pinheiro KC, Pinto AC, Soares SC, et al. The impact of quality filter for RNA-Seq. Gene 2015;563(2):165–71.

[71] Förstner KU, Vogel J, Sharma CM. READemption–A tool for the computational analysis of deep-sequencing-based transcriptome data. Bioinformatics 2014;btu533.

[72] Ramos RT, Carneiro AR, Baumbach J, Azevedo V, Schneider MP, Silva A. Analysis of quality raw data of second generation sequencers with Quality Assessment Software. BMC Res Notes 2011 Apr 18;4(1):130.

[73] Caboche S, Audebert C, Lemoine Y, Hot D. Comparison of mapping algorithms used in high-throughput sequencing: application to Ion Torrent data. BMC Genomics 2014;15(1):264.

[74] Hilker R, Stadermann KB, Doppmeier D, Kalinowski J, Stoye J, Straube J, et al. Read-Xplorer—visualization and analysis of mapped sequences. Bioinformatics 2014;btu205.

[75] Haas BJ, Papanicolaou A, Yassour M, Grabherr M, Blood PD, Bowden J, et al. De novo transcript sequence reconstruction from RNA-seq using the Trinity platform for reference generation and analysis. Nat Protoc 2013;8(8):1494–512.

[76] Seyednasrollah F, Laiho A, Elo LL. Comparison of software packages for detecting differential expression in RNA-seq studies. Brief Bioinform [Internet]. 2013 Dec 2 [cited 2014 Apr 30]; Available from: http://bib.oxfordjournals.org/cgi/doi/10.1093/bib/bbt086

[77] Herbig A, Nieselt K. nocoRNAc: characterization of non-coding RNAs in prokaryotes. BMC Bioinformatics 2011;12(1):40.

[78] Amman F, Wolfinger MT, Lorenz R, Hofacker IL, Stadler PF, Findei S. TSSAR: TSS annotation regime for dRNA-seq data. BMC Bioinformatics 2014;15(1):89.

[79] Dugar G, Herbig A, Förstner KU, Heidrich N, Reinhardt R, Nieselt K, et al. High-resolution transcriptome maps reveal strain-specific regulatory features of multiple Campylobacter jejuni isolates. 2013 [cited 2015 Jul 14]; Available from: http://dx.plos.org/10.1371/journal.pgen.1003495

[80] Chuang L-Y, Chang H-W, Tsai J-H, Yang C-H. Features for computational operon prediction in prokaryotes. Brief Funct Genomics 2012;els024.

[81] Warren AS, Aurrecoechea C, Brunk B, Desai P, Emrich S, Giraldo-Calderón GI, et al. RNA-Rocket: an RNA-Seq analysis resource for infectious disease research. Bioinformatics 2015;btv002.

[82] Van Verk MC, Hickman R, Pieterse CM, Van Wees SC. RNA-Seq: revelation of the messengers. Trends Plant Sci 2013;18(4):175–9.

[83] Dai L, Gao X, Guo Y, Xiao J, Zhang Z, others. Bioinformatics clouds for big data manipulation. Biol Direct 2012;7(1):43.

Chapter 8

Dealing with the Data Deluge – New Strategies in Prokaryotic Genome Analysis

Leonid Zaslavsky, Stacy Ciufo, Boris Fedorov, Boris Kiryutin, Igor Tolstoy and Tatiana Tatusova

Additional information is available at the end of the chapter

http://dx.doi.org/10.5772/62125

Abstract

Recent technological innovations have ignited an explosion in microbial genome sequencing that has fundamentally changed our understanding of biology of microbes and profoundly impacted public health policy. This huge increase in DNA sequence data presents new challenges for the annotation, analysis, and visualization bioinformatics tools. New strategies have been designed to bring an order to this genome sequence shockwave and improve the usability of associated data. Genomes are organized in a hierarchical distance tree using single-copy ribosomal protein marker distances for distance calculation. Protein distance measures dissimilarity between markers of the same type and the subsequent genomic distance averages over the majority of marker-distances, ignoring the outliers. More than 30,000 genomes from public archives have been organized in a marker distance tree resulting in 6,438 species-level clades representing 7,597 taxonomic species. This computational infrastructure provides a foundation for prokaryotic gene and genome analysis, allowing easy access to pre-calculated genome groups at various distance levels. One of the most challenging problems in the current data deluge is the presentation of the relevant data at an appropriate resolution for each application, eliminating data redundancy but keeping biologically interesting variations.

Keywords: Genome analysis, clusters, proteins, bacteria, prokaryotes

1. Introduction

Prokaryotes are probably the largest and the most diverse group of cellular organisms.

The number of described species is now about 12,000, and the number of species on earth is estimated in the millions [1]. Recent rapid advances in sequencing technologies provided a

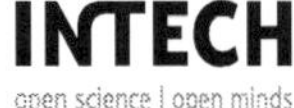

relatively cheap and fast way of studying the diversity of microbial species by discovering representatives of novel divisions or even phyla [2] and analyzing the variation within the species by sequencing closely related genomes from the ecological microbial populations or clinical studies of pathogenic bacteria.

Historically, prokaryotic organisms were organized by classical taxonomic ranking system (species, genus, family, order, and phylum). Delineation of prokaryotic species was originally based on phenotypic information, pathogenicity, and environmental observations. Due to the high mutation level, fast replication rate, and efficient DNA exchange mechanisms, microbial organisms can easily adapt to their habitats. Genomic studies have shown that different species living in similar ecological environments show similarity at the genomic level (e.g., congruent evolution of water-living bacteria from various taxonomic origins [3]) while same pathogenic species (or symbionts) rapidly adapting to the new hosts become quite different at genomic level (e.g., *Buchnera aphidicola* [4], *Serratia symbiotica* [5]).

Next-generation sequencing technologies provide new insights into the life of microbes and their interactions with the host, but they do not classify the organisms in a traditional way. Many novel species are described as "candidatus" or "<genus> sp."

The genomes of uncharacterized isolates of the Candidatus Arthromitus, host-specific intestinal symbionts, comprise a distinct clade within the Clostridiaceae [6].

http://www.ncbi.nlm.nih.gov/genome/13597

The number of uncharacterized species is rapidly growing in public genome collections. As of November 2014, almost half of bacterial and archaeal species in NCBI Refseq data set remain uncharacterized. (Bacteria: 3,559 uncharacterized, 7,597 total; Archaea: 162 uncharacterized, 399 total.)

The need for different approaches to the identification of microbial species that can take into account the advantages of the growing massive volume of genomic sequence data is being actively discussed in the research community.

Scientists from different disciplines (taxonomists, ecologists, and evolutionary biologists) have different interpretations of species defined by the framework of their needs and the tools they use for identification. A recent review [7] describes the history and present state of various methods of description of prokaryotic species. The authors suggest the concept of species as "a category that circumscribes monophyletic, and genomically and phenotypically coherent populations of individuals that can be clearly discriminated from other such entities by means of standardized parameters."

Comparative analysis requires a target: a coherent group of isolates with some degree of similarity defined by the goal of the study (the analysis of pathogen outbreak performed at the species level or below, while biodiversity studies use broader group such as families or phyla). Several groups have attempted to delineate the taxonomy of Archaea and Bacteria using the methods based on single-copy universally conserved markers [8-13]. Other methods are discussed in recent reviews [14].

Different species vary dramatically in terms of the sampling density and data quality. Clinical and epidemiological studies produce large data sets of closely related (clonal) genomes (Table 1), while other species are sampled very coarsely. Genomic and proteomic structure of a densely sampled group of related strains is commonly described by the concept of pan-genome [15] species.

The complexity of the data is challenging to the analysis, representation, and visualization of the data sets. One of the challenges is the amount of the resources required for a brute-force processing approach (e.g., BLAST all-to-all of 35 million proteins will take five days on 1,000 processors). Another big problem is data heterogeneity and redundancy: the closest-neighbor results will often contain long list of nearly identical objects, making it difficult to identify more distant neighbors.

Here we describe a combined approach that provides a robust, fast, and scalable method of defining the sequence similarity genome groups that can be used for comparative genome analysis and resolve some known issues with the delineation of species in traditional taxonomy.

2. Materials and methods

The genomes are organized in hierarchical groups calculated with different methods. The universal ribosomal markers approach is used to build a distance tree and to define species and superspecies-level clades (genome groups). The species-level clades are further refined by using whole-genome alignments and creating tight (clonal) genome groups.

2.1. NCBI hardware and software

The hardware available at NCBI includes a Univa Grid Engine (UGE) Grid-Engine-based computer farm and PanFS scalable storage system connected through a powerful router. The most recent version UGE 8.2.1 includes support for Linux GROUPs, support for Window server execution nodes, and a beta version of DRMMA2 (Distributed Resource Management and Application API 2). A large weakly coupled distributed computer system like this requires coarse-grained parallelization approaches with minimal communication between the processes. Many processing steps, such as computing BLAST hits, are naturally parallel.

2.2. Data snapshot

A given data snapshot represents a collection of genome (and protein) sequences and metadata available at the time. Navigating through millions of nucleotide sequences in public archives to find a set that comprises a whole-genome collection can be sometimes challenging. GenBank release 207 contains 182,188,746 sequences, and 189,739,230,107 nucleotides. The traditional NCBI sequence repository was designed for GenBank records in the early 1990s. It is organized as a collection of single-nucleotide sequence records with annotated sequences stored as nucleotide–protein sets. By GenBank requirements, each sequence record should be associated with the organisms registered in the NCBI Taxonomy Database. For the first 10 years of microbial genome sequencing, each species has a unique genome representation in public sequence archives. When sequencing costs decreased, researchers began to explore microbial population structure and the intraspecies differences. NCBI Taxonomy group began assigning Taxonomy ID for strain level nodes as proxies of unique genome identifiers. More recently, next-generation sequencing and rapid pathogen detection approaches have shifted the paradigm from a single isolate representing an organism to multiisolate projects often representing almost identical isolates from the outbreak analysis. These closely related genomes differ by metadata only: patient information, date, and place of sample collection. NCBI has created new resources that capture the sequence data and metadata information: BioProject, BioSample, and Assembly [16]. A triplet of these identifiers uniquely defines a genome with the metadata that can be used for further comparative analysis.

NCBI internal database UniCol is used to store collections of the nucleotide and protein sequence data associated with every BioProject, BioSample, Assembly triplet. The database provides a tracking history for a given snapshot with the sequence assembly and metadata available at the time.

Clade_id	Name	Genomes	Clonal groups	Taxonomy
19988	*Staphylococcus aureus*	4182	118	species
19668	*Escherichia, Shigella*	2479	986	multiple
20829	*Mycobacterium tuberculosis*	1844	11	species
19669	*Salmonella*	971	139	genus
19507	*Acinetobacter*	846	306	genus
19252	*Helicobacter pylori*	432	258	species
20104	*Streptococcus*	394	154	genus
19672	*Enterobacter, Klebsiella*	384	149	multiple
20137	*Enterococcus*	354	161	genus
19921	*Brucella*	335	9	genus

Table 1. Calculated clades may include a single species, a single genus, or multiple genera for closely related species.

2.3. Genome quality assessment

There are several criteria that are used to evaluate the quality of genome assembly.

The N50/L50 metrics are automatically calculated for each genome. Acceptable values are dependent on genome size, and genomes which do not meet the criteria are not processed for Refseq. For known clades, the genome size is expected to fall within 2 standard deviations from the mean for clades, which have at least 10 members. This standard allows for the identification of partial genomes and unusually large genomes, which may indicate a bad assembly or contamination.

Some genomes submitted to GenBank represent an assembly from a mixed culture (accession # AKNF01000000 is a mixed culture of *Shigella flexneri* 1235-66 and an unknown *Shigella* species) or a hybrid of different species or a chimera genome (accession # AP012495 chimera genome constructed by cloning the whole genome of *Synechocystis* strain PCC6803 into the *Bacillus subtilis* 168 genome). Partial and "anomalous" assemblies are clearly flagged in NCBI assembly database and not included in clade analysis.

2.4. Marker to genome alignment

Genome distance is defined as an average of pairwise protein distances of universally conserved single-copy proteins as defined in [8] (Table 2).

Genomic markers (E.coli K12 accessions)	Genomic markers
NP_417801	ribosomal protein S12
NP_417800	ribosomal protein S7
NP_414564	ribosomal protein S2
NP_418410	ribosomal protein L11
NP_418411	ribosomal protein L1
NP_417779	ribosomal protein L3
NP_417774	ribosomal protein L22
NP_417773	ribosomal protein S3
NP_417769	ribosomal protein L14
NP_417767	ribosomal protein L5
NP_417765	ribosomal protein S8
NP_417100	ribosomal protein l6p/L9E
NP_417762	ribosomal protein S5
NP_417757	ribosomal protein S13
NP_417756	ribosomal protein S11
NP_417698	ribosomal protein L13
NP_417697	ribosomal protein S9
NP_417634	ribosomal protein S15P/S13E
NP_417770	ribosomal protein S17
NP_417772	ribosomal protein L16/L10E
NP_417760	ribosomal protein L15
NP_417763	ribosomal protein L18
NP_417755	ribosomal protein S4

Table 2. List of genomic markers used in genomic analysis. Escherichia coli K-12 accessions are given as an example. Each marker has a corresponding protein cluster which is used in the analysis.

2.5. Genome distance

Protein marker distances and genomic distance are designed to be robust while remaining appropriately sensitive. Protein distance measuring dissimilarity between markers of the same type is designed to ignore differences in protein lengths and tuned to measure dissimilarity in internal parts of the sequences. The subsequent genomic distance averages over the majority of marker-distances, ignoring the outliers.

2.5.1. Protein distances

Consider proteins i and j, having the best aggregated BLAST alignment of length L_{ij} with aggregated score S_{ij}. Assume that the proteins have lengths L_i and L_j and self-scores S_{ii} and S_{jj}. Define normalized scores: $s_{ij} = S_{ij} / L_{ij}$, $s_{ii} = S_{ii} / L_i$, $s_{jj} = S_{jj} / L_j$.

Then define protein distances:

$$d_{ij} = 1 - \min\left(1, \frac{s_{ij}}{\min\left(s_{ii}, s_{jj}\right)}\right) \tag{1}$$

Distance (1) is an identity-like characteristic calculated from the aggregated BLAST [17] scores (using positives based on BLOSUM62 matrix [22]). For full-length alignment, it can be reduced to $1 - \frac{s_{ij}}{\min(S_{ii}, S_{jj})}$. However, when lengths are different; distance (1) avoids penalizing nonaligned ends of the proteins, taking into account only mutation events.

2.5.2. Genomic distances

Suppose that genomes i and j have N_{ij}^a types of markers found in both genomes, with N_{ij}^h of them having acceptable BLAST hits.

Define the offset $\Delta_{ij} = \max\left(3, \frac{N_{ij}^h}{4}, 1 + N_{ij}^a - N_{ij}^h\right)$. Order marker distances in the ascending order: $d_{ij}^{(0)} \le d_{ij}^{(1)} \le ... \le d_{ij}^{\left(N_{ij}^h - 1\right)}$. Then robust genomic distance is defined by the formula:

$$D_{ij} = \frac{\sum_{p=\Delta_{ij}}^{p=N_{ij}^h - \Delta_{ij} - 1} d_{ij}^{(p)} l_{ij}^{(p)}}{\sum_{p=\Delta_{ij}}^{p=N_{ij}^h - \Delta_{ij} - 1} l_{ij}^{(p)}}, \tag{2}$$

where $l_{ij}^{(p)}$ are corresponding alignment length. The marker-protein distances are weighted by alignment lengths $l_{ij}^{(p)}$ in order to provide where possible results similar to the original method in [8] based on concatenation of proteins. However, the use of offset Δ_{ij} allows filtering out outliers since the averaging in (2) is performed over $N_{ij}^h - 2\Delta_{ij}$ distances in the middle. For each phylum level group, an agglomerative hierarchical clustering tree is built using the complete linkage clustering algorithm [19, 20].

2.6. Genome clustering pipeline

The pipeline for calculating genome clades consists of three major components (see Figure 1). The first is the collection of the input data from NCBI main sequence repositories. The genomic data are dynamic: hundreds of new genomes and assembly updates are submitted to NCBI each day. We create a snapshot of all live genome assemblies and their nucleotide sequence components (chromosomes, scaffolds, and contigs) and store them in an internal relational database: UniCol. The genome data set is organized into large groups (phyla and superphyla defined by NCBI Taxonomy). The assemblies are then filtered by quality and passed to the processing script. Ribosomal protein markers are predicted in every genome to overcome problems with the genome annotations (missing and/or incorrect annotations) and to normalize markers' data set. Marker predictions are performed by aligning reference protein markers against full genome assemblies. Assemblies with at least 17 markers are passed to the next step. Genome distance is calculated as an average of pairwise protein distances of markers shared in a pair of genomes. Finally, agglomerative hierarchical clustering trees are built within phylum-level groups. Clades at the species level are calculated using species-aware algorithm. Superclade trees are constructed by sectioning the trees at the distance of 0.25.

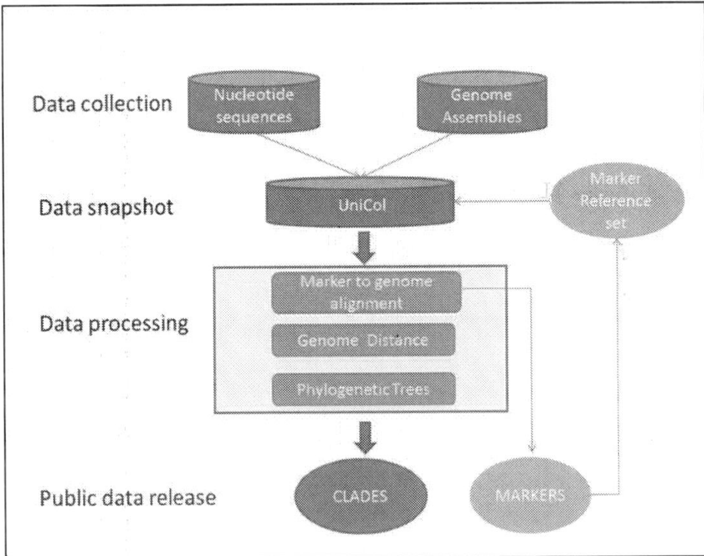

Figure 1. Dataflow of ribosomal-marker-based clade (genome group) processing. Ribosomal markers (in green) are maintained outside of the main pipeline (in blue). Clades and markers are available on NCBI FTP site: ftp:// ftp.ncbi.nlm.nih.gov/genomes/GENOME_REPORTS/CLADES/   ftp://ftp.ncbi.nlm.nih.gov/genomes/ GENOME_REPORTS/MARKERS/

2.7. Clades and superclades

Due to biological, historical, and sampling reasons, microbial organisms have very different levels of strain variation within species. Using the genome data available in public archives we have calculated the diameter of the species defined by NCBI Taxonomy (see Figure 2).

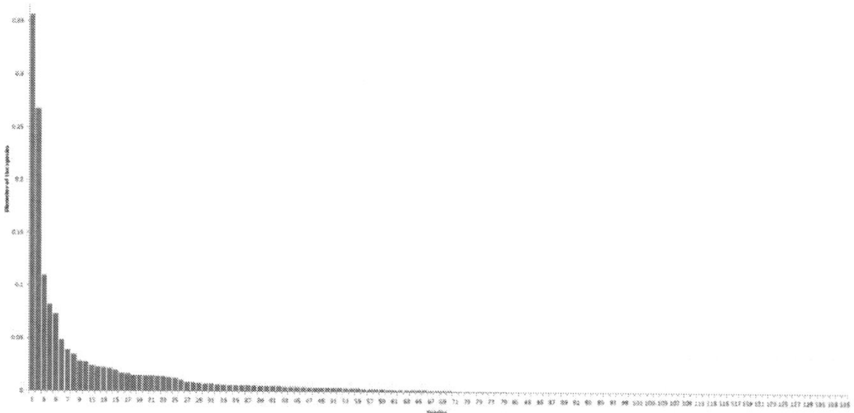

Figure 2. Distribution of Taxonomy-defined species diameter. Y axes – diameter of species, X axes – species numbered in the descending diameter order.

Instead of using one fixed threshold, we utilize a taxonomy-aware algorithm that allows increasing the size of a genomic group in certain circumstances. Two distance threshold, the lower threshold d_lower and the upper threshold d_upper, are established (currently, we use values d_lower = 0.015 and d_upper = 0.025). Genomes with the lowest common ancestor with height d_lower or below are always in the same group, while genomes with the lowest common ancestor with height above d_upper are never placed together. In between d_lower and d_upper, taxonomic information is used: two subgroups are merged in a larger group if any pair of species in a group is already together in one of two subgroups (i.e., there are no new merges of species). Species are defined according to the NCBI taxonomic records [16].

Phylum-level trees are not practical for presentation and evaluation of closely related genomes. However, it is important to see the relationships (distance) between close clades (see Figure 3).

2.8. Genome groups

Species-level clades are further refined by whole-genome alignments using megablast with default parameters [18]. The genome groups are defined by clustering the genomes at 95% identity and 90% coverage. An example of genome groups for *Klebsiella pneumonia* clade is shown in Figure 4. For each group a representative genome with the highest level of assembly and annotation quality is selected.

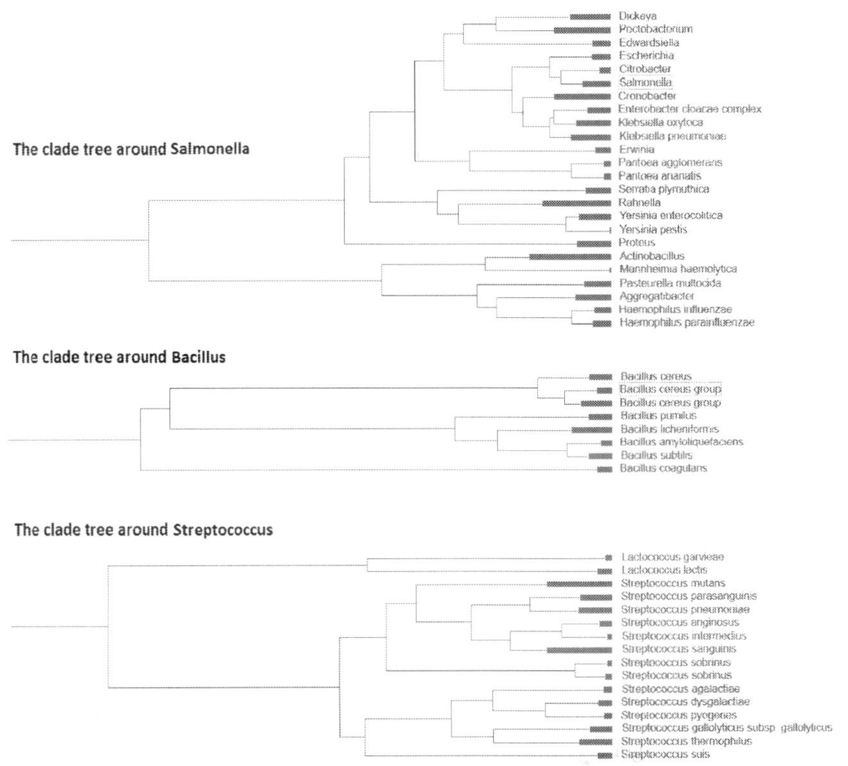

Figure 3. Superclade tree for three abundant groups: A – Salmonella, B – Bacillus, C – Streptococcus. Green boxes represent clades; box size is proportional to the number of genome in a clade.

3. Results and discussion

Large clades obtain additional members in each subsequent snapshot (see Figure 5). The process assigns related genomes to the same clade consistently. There is also a large growth in singleton clades, reflecting an increasing interest in sequencing taxonomically distinct organisms.

We have developed an infrastructure for grouping all whole-genome sequence assemblies at various proximity levels. By using universally conserved ribosomal genes we define the species-level groups. We propose a set of 23 single-copy marker gene families that have consistent evolutionary histories. The proposed ribosomal protein-marker distance and genomic distance are tailored to achieve robustness, while remaining appropriately sensitive.

The major objective of our approach is to generate and actively maintain the target sets for pan-genome analysis. These ribosomal-marker-based groups (clades) roughly correspond to

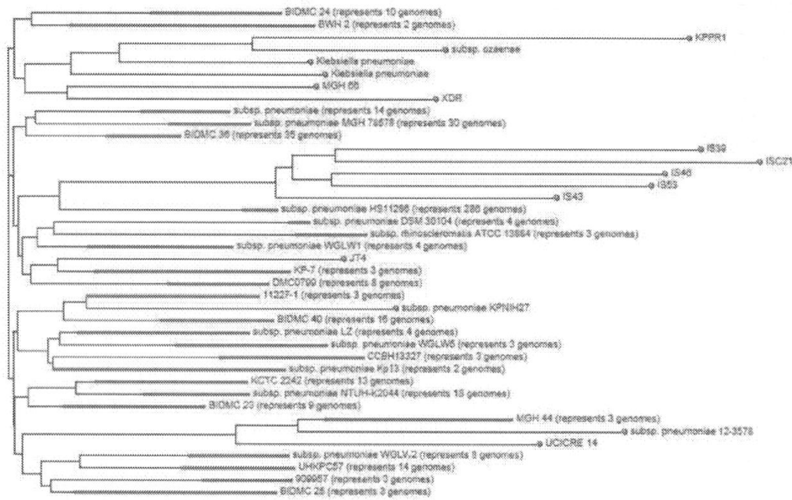

Figure 4. *Klebsiella pneumonia* clade contains 534 full genome assemblies organized in 25 closely related genomic groups. Blue circles at the end of the branch represent a single genome; green boxes represent a group of genomes with the box size proportional to the number of genomes.

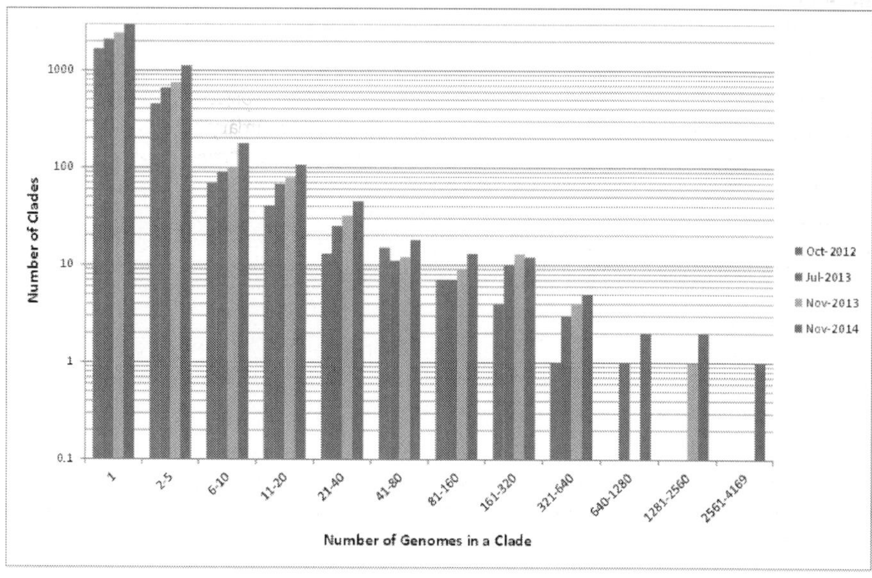

Figure 5. Clade growth in four sequential snapshots.

the species level as defined by NCBI Taxonomy. The subclades are calculated to show the closeness of the groups at the higher level. The relationship within the species-level group is further refined with whole pairwise genome alignment performed by megablast [18]. Tight genomic groups are defined at the level of 95% identity over the 95% genome coverage. By using the representative genomes from the tight groups, we can reduce the redundancy in comparative genomic studies. Other targets can be used for more refined population variation studies within species or SNP analysis for pathogen outbreak detection. These target sets require more accurate distance measure such as whole genomic alignments, K-mer distance [21].

3.1. Clades and species

Using a taxonomy-aware clustering algorithm does not completely solve the discrepancies between the species-level clades and traditional species. Genome sequences provide great opportunity to refine the classical taxonomic description of prokaryotes [23]. All cases of discrepancy were manually evaluated; most of them have been resolved by literature support. Some examples are described below.

3.1.1. Different species merged into a single clade

Escherichia coli and some *Shigella* species are combined in a single clade by ribosomal marker distance. *Shigella,* which is recognized as a genus with four species in most situations, taxonomically belongs to the diverse *E. coli* group, but the genus-level distinction has been retained due to historical recognition of its medical significance. *Shigella* has adapted to higher primates as the only natural hosts.

The genus *Brucella* consists of 10 classically recognized species [http://icsp.org/subcommittee/brucella/] based on antigenic/biochemical characteristics and primary host species: *Brucella abortus*(cattle); *Brucella canis* (dogs); *Brucella ceti* (marine mammals); *Brucella inopinata; Brucella melitensis* (sheep and goats); *Brucella microti; Brucella neotomae* (rodents); *Brucella ovis* (sheep); *Brucella pinnipedialis* (marine mammals); *Brucella suis* (swine, cattle, rodents, wild ungulates), and recently described in [24] *Brucella papionis* isolated from baboons (*Pappio* spp.). The wave of Next-Generation Sequencing brought in almost a hundred new isolates from a population of *Brucella,* which are clearly distinct from currently recognized species that are tentatively designated at the species level. These unnamed isolates have not yet been characterized using traditional methods, or the species name has not yet been validly published. *Brucella* genus–level clade is shown in Figure 6.

Single species represented by multiple clades

Prochlorococcus and marine *Synechococcus* organisms are small marine cyanobacteria, their genomes are characterized by small size and an evolutionary trend toward low GC content [25]. Whereas many shared derived characters define *Prochlorococcus* as a clade, many genome-based analyses recover them as paraphyletic. The single species, *Prochlorococcus marinus,* comprises six named ecotypes. Our ribosomal marker analysis and whole-genome alignment (described above in section on Methods) analysis suggests that this species should be repre-

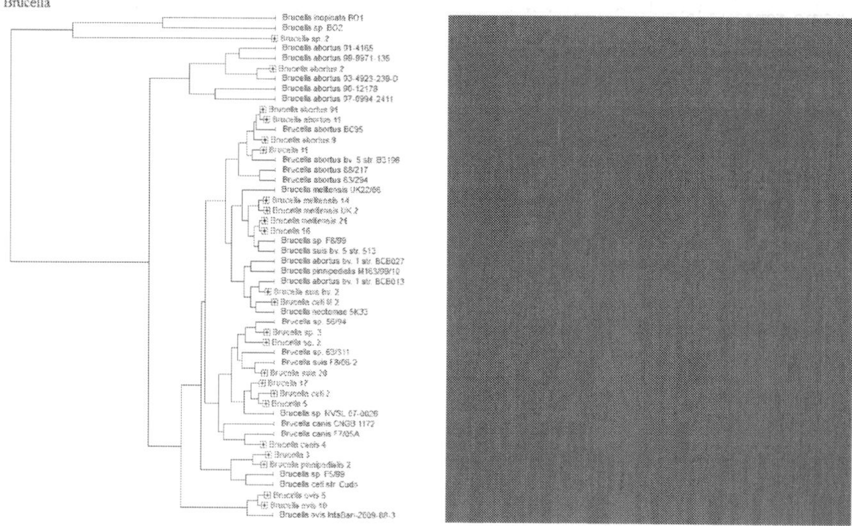

Figure 6. Ribosomal-marker-based clade comprises various species of Brucella. The pairwise genome distance is defined by the number of shared proteins in the core set of Brucella pan-genome. Green dots – proteins present in CORE set; red dots – proteins absent in CORE set.

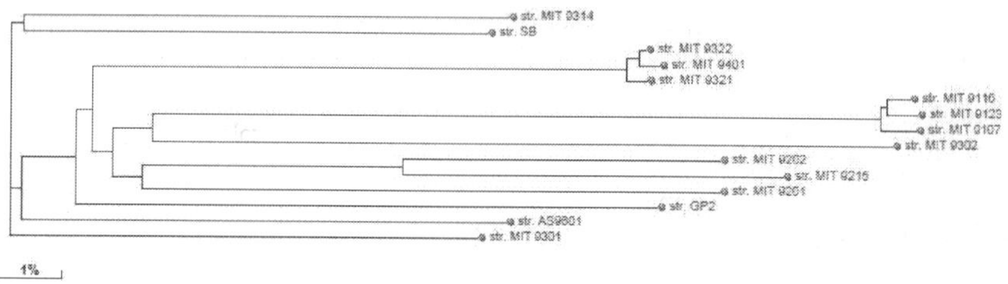

Figure 7. *Prochlorococcus marinus* interspecies diversity. The dendrogram is calculated using blast genome alignment score (%identity). The leaf nodes displayed as circles represent genomes of individual isolates/strains.

sented by 11 different clades (see Figure 7.) These results are supported by recent genomic analysis of the genus of *Prochlorococcus* [26].

Novel species from noncultured not-isolated single cell and metagenome assemblies and new unclassified isolates (<genus> sp.) from clinical and epidemiological studies can be organized in hierarchical groups by genome sequence comparison methods. These groups can be used for downstream analysis: 1) pan-genome by clades not species; 2) groups of closely related genomes below species that can be calculated by nucleotide whole-genome comparison like K-mer or BLAST; 3) classification validation; 4) visualization of large data sets by selecting the genome representatives. Some of the applications marker-based clades and tight genome groups have been previously briefly described in [27,28].

4. Conclusions

No matter how impressive the numbers of genome sequencing projects are, they represent a miniscule fraction of the total number of bacterial species. The future genomic analysis tools will have to take into consideration the uncertain origin of the DNA sequences during analysis. Making sense of genomic data is one of the goals that are aided by the genome clustering procedure. The hierarchical infrastructure provides the foundation for further development of genome analysis and visualization tools.

Acknowledgements

This research was supported by the Intramural Research Program of the NIH, National Library of Medicine. The authors are thankful to David J. Lipman, James Ostell, Scott Federhen, Michael Galperin, Eugene Koonin, Yury I. Wolf for productive discussions and to Vyacheslav Brover for the database support.

Author details

Leonid Zaslavsky, Stacy Ciufo, Boris Fedorov, Boris Kiryutin, Igor Tolstoy and Tatiana Tatusova*

*Address all correspondence to: tatiana@ncbi.nlm.nih.gov

National Center for Biotechnology Information, National Library of Medicine, National Institutes of Health, Bethesda, MD, USA

References

[1] Yarza P, Yilmaz P, Pruesse E, Glöckner FO, Ludwig W, Schleifer KH, Whitman WB, Euzéby J, Amann R, Rosselló-Móra R. Uniting the classification of cultured and uncultured bacteria and archaea using 16S rRNA gene sequences. *Nat Rev Microbiol.* 2014;12(9):635-45.

[2] Rinke C, Schwientek P, Sczyrba A, Ivanova NN, et al. Insights into the phylogeny and coding potential of microbial dark matter. *Nature.* 2013;499(7459):431-7.

[3]   Audic S, Robert C, Campagna B, Parinello H, Claverie JM, Raoult D, Drancourt M. Genome analysis of Minibacterium massiliensis highlights the convergent evolution of water-living bacteria. *PLoS Genet.* 2007;3(8):138.

[4]   MacDonald SJ, Thomas GH, Douglas AE. Genetic and metabolic determinants of nutritional phenotype in an insect-bacterial symbiosis. *Mol Ecology.* 2011;20(10):2073-84.

[5]   Manzano-Marín A, Latorre A. Settling down: the genome of Serratia symbiotica from the aphid Cinara tujafilina zooms in on the process of accommodation to a cooperative intracellular life. *Genome Biol Evol.* 2014;6(7):1683-98.

[6]   Pamp SJ, Harrington ED, Quake SR, Relman DA, Blainey PC.. Single-cell sequencing provides clues about the host interactions of segmented filamentous bacteria (SFB). *Genome Res.* 2012;22(6):1107-19.

[7]   Rosselló-Móra R, Amann R. Past and future species definitions for Bacteria and Archaea. *Syst Appl Microbiol.* 2015;Feb 20:22-3.

[8]   Ciccarelli FD, Doerks T, von Mering C, et al. Toward automatic reconstruction of a highly resolved tree of life. *Science.* 2006;311(5765):1283-7.

[9]   Mende DR, Sunagawa S, Zeller G, Bork P. Accurate and universal delineation of prokaryotic species. *Nat Methods.* 2013;10(9):881-4.

[10] Lang JM, Darling AE, Eisen JA. Phylogeny of bacterial and archaeal genomes using conserved genes: supertrees and supermatrices. *PLoS One.* 2013;8(4):{PT PageRange}e62510{/PageRange PT}.

[11] Wu D, Jospin G, Eisen JA. Systematic identification of gene families for use as "markers" for phylogenetic and phylogeny-driven ecological studies of bacteria and archaea and their major subgroups. *PLoS One.* 2013;8(10):{PT PageRange}e77033{/PageRange PT}.

[12] Darling AE, Jospin G, Lowe E, Matsen FA IV, Bik HM, Eisen JA. PhyloSift: phylogenetic analysis of genomes and metagenomes. *PeerJ.* 2014;2:e243.

[13] Tanabe AS, Toju H. *PLoS One.* 2013;8:e76910.

[14] Larsen MV, Cosentino S, Lukjancenko O, Saputra D, Rasmussen S, Hasman H, Sicheritz-Pontén T, Aarestrup FM, Ussery DW, Lund O. Benchmarking of methods for genomic taxonomy. *J Clin Microbiol.* 2014;52(5):1529-39.

[15] Vernikos G, Medini D, Riley DR, Tettelin H. Ten years of pan-genome analyses. *Curr Opin Microbiol.* 2015;Feb(23):148-54.

[16] NCBI Resource Coordinators. Database resources of the National Center for Biotechnology Information. *Nucleic Acids Res.* 2014;42(Database issue):D7-17.

[17] Altschul SF, Gish W, Miller W, Myers EW, Lipman DJ. Basic local alignment search tool. *J Mol Biol.* 1990;215:403-10.

[18] McGinnis S, Madden TL. BLAST: at the core of a powerful and diverse set of sequence analysis tools. *Nucleic Acids Res*. 2004;32(Web Server Issue):W20-5.

[19] Everitt BS, Landau S, Leese M, Stahl D. Cluster Analysis. 5th ed. Wiley; 2011.

[20] Felsenstein J. *Inferring Phylogenies*. 2nd ed. Sinauer Associates; 2004.

[21] Compeau P, Pevzner P, Teslar G. How to apply de Bruijn graphs to genome assembly. *Nature Biotechnol*. 2011;29(11):987-91.

[22] Henikoff S, Henikoff JG. Amino acid substitution matrices from protein blocks. *Proc Natl Acad Sci USA*. 1992;89(22):10915-19.

[23] Whitman WB. Genome sequences as the type material for taxonomic descriptions of prokaryotes. *Syst Appl Microbiol*. 2015;Feb 20:24-7.

[24] Whatmore AM, Davison N, Cloeckaert A, Al Dahouk S., Zygmunt MS, Brew S D, Perrett LL, Koylass MS, Vergnaud G, Quance C, Scholz HC, Dick, EJ, Hubbard G, Schlabritz-Loutsevitch NE. Brucella papionis sp. nov., isolated from baboons (Papio spp.). *Int J Sys Evolution Microbiol*. 2014;64:4120-28.

[25] Olga Zhaxybayeva, W. Ford Doolittle, R. Thane Papke†, J. Peter Gogarten. Intertwined evolutionary histories of marine Synechococcus and Prochlorococcus marinus. *Genome Biol Evol*. 2009;1:325-339.

[26] Thompson CC, Silva GG, Vieira NM, Edwards R, Vicente AC, Thompson FL. Genomic taxonomy of the genus prochlorococcus. *Microb Evol*. 2013;66(4):752-62.

[27] Zaslavsky L, Tatusova TA. Clustering analysis of proteins from microbial genomes at multiple levels of resolution. *Lect Notes Comp Sci*. 2015;9096:438-9.

[28] Tatusova T, Ciufo S, Federhen S, Fedorov B, McVeigh R, O'Neill K, Tolstoy I, Zaslavsky L. Update on RefSeq microbial genomes resources. *Nucleic Acids Res*. 2015;43(Database Issue):D599-605.

Next Generation Sequencing of Agricultural Plants

Reaping the Benefits of Next-generation Sequencing Technologies for Crop Improvement — Solanaceae

Sushil Satish Chhapekar, Rashmi Gaur, Ajay Kumar and Nirala Ramchiary

Additional information is available at the end of the chapter

http://dx.doi.org/10.5772/61656

Abstract

Next-generation sequencing (NGS) technologies make possible the sequencing of the whole genome of a species decoding a complete gene catalogue and transcriptome to allow the study of expression pattern of entire genes. The huge data generated through whole genome and transcriptome sequencing not only provide a basis to study variation at gene sequence (such as single-nucleotide polymorphism and InDels) and expression level but also help to understand the evolutionary relationship between different crop species. Furthermore, NGS technologies have made possible the quick correlations of phenotypes with genotypes in different crop species, thereby increasing the precision of crop improvement. The Solanaceae family represents the third most economically important family after grasses and legumes due to high nutritional components. The current advances in NGS technology and their application in Solanaceae crops made several progresses in the identification of genes responsible for economically important traits, development of molecular markers, and understanding the genome organization and evolution in Solanaceae crops. The combination of high-throughput NGS technologies with conventional crop breeding has been shown to be promising in the Solanaceae translational genomics research. As a result, NGS technologies has been seen to be adopted in a large scale to study the molecular basis of fruit and tuber development, disease resistance, and increasing quantity and quality of crop production.

Keywords: Solanaceae, NGS, capsicum, eggplant, tomato, potato

1. Introduction

In developing countries, "population" and "food security" are the two major issues. These problems get worse with the sudden climate changes that hamper production, yield, and quality of food crops. Therefore, to keep in mind the food security for billions of peoples, an initiative is required for improving the quality and yield of important crops. Several traditional

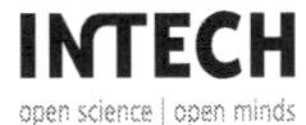

plant-breeding practices have been carried out for producing new varieties that can withstand with such changing climatic conditions besides increasing the productivity. These time-consuming practices could make considerable progress in crop improvement using selective germplasm, however, resulted in loss of biodiversity in the process. The recent advances in crop genomics, particularly the use of high throughput next-generation sequencing (NGS) technologies, look promising to identify causal genetic factors at genome by sequencing the whole genome and transcriptome of a species. As a result, the complete gene catalogue of a crop species and functional genes in different tissues could be identified besides allowing studying the genetic pathways involved in growth and development and biochemical pathways that eventually could be correlated with the crop phenotypes [1, 2]. Furthermore, the sequence data generated in vast amount provide a basis of genetic variation such as single-nucleotide polymorphisms (SNPs), which ultimately provide a relationship between genotype and phenotype in different species.

The Solanaceae family comprises approximately 2500 flowering plant species under 102 genera. The family represents the third most economically important family after grasses and legumes. Among the most important plants of this family are the potato (*Solanum tuberosum*), eggplant (*Solanum melongena*), tomato (*Solanum lycopersicun*), and capsicum or pepper (*Capsicum annuum*). They serve as important food crops and consumed worldwide due to their high nutritional components. Solanaceae crops have high nutritional value due to the presence of quality proteins, mineral salts, starch, vitamins, and antioxidants. Tomato majorly contrib-utes to dietary nutrition globally with beneficial effects to human health mainly attributed to antioxidant compounds in the fruit such as lycopene and several other compounds such as carotenoids, zeaxanthin, and vitamin C. Capsicum fruits are rich source of metabolites that are beneficial for human health, such as carotenoids (provitamin A), vitamin C, vitamin A (which destroy free radicals), vitamin E, flavonoids, and capsaicinoids (anticancer agent). Although these compounds function as antioxidants and nutrients, they are used in traditional medicine also due to their enormous medicinal properties. Eggplant serves as an excellent source of antioxidants such as anthocyanins and several phenolics. Apart from this, it has a significant effect in reducing blood and liver cholesterol rates in humans. Worldwide, potato tubers are the principal source of starch along with proteins, vitamins, and antioxidants.

Here in this chapter, an attempt has been made to compile current research progress made based on NGS technology in four most important Solanaceae crop plants: tomato, potato, eggplant, and pepper. Furthermore, the application of NGS technology on those four crops toward translational research has been discussed.

2. Next-generation sequencing technologies

Knowing the genome sequence of a species has an advantage in crop breeding. This became possible with the revolution of DNA sequencing technologies. The Sanger method [3] was the first-generation sequencing method based on DNA chain termination method of the single-pass sequencing of one clone at a time. With the advent of NGS technologies, the sequencing of complete genome or transcriptome of a species/genotype has become possible within a few hours. Utilizing various NGS platforms that are based on diverse chemistry and detection methods, several crop genomes, including major Solanaceae crops have been sequenced [4–7]. Among the various NGS technologies, three widely utilized platforms are Roche/454, Illumina Genome Analyzer (GA), and ABI SOLiD. The Roche/454 GSFLX chemistry is based on pyrosequencing and can produce up to 1 million reads of 600 bp to 1 kb [8]. The ABI SOLiD chemistry is based on emulsion polymerase chain reaction and sequencing by ligation technology, which can sequence up to 100 million reads of 50 bp in size [9]. The Illumina/Solexa GA based on sequencing by synthesis method produces 320 to 640 million reads of 100–150 bp [10].

The third- and the fourth-generation sequencing technologies are being developed, the majority of which allow the detection of single molecules with real-time sequencing. The popular third-generation sequencing platforms are Ion Torrents/Life Technologies, Heli-Scope™/Helicos Biosciences, and PacBio RS/Pacific Biosciences. The fourth generation is nanopore sequencing technology (Roche/IBM and Oxford). Ion Torrent company introduced a very different approach in 2010 as "Personal Genomic Machine," which was later commercialized by Life Technology. The chemistry is based on the real-time detection of the pH change (release of hydrogen ions), with the incorporation of a nucleotide into a growing DNA strand by a silicon detector [11]. The technology provides an average read length of ~ 200 bp. The HeliScope introduced by Helicos BioSciences was the first commercially available single-molecule sequencing (SMS) platform [12]. The technology is based on highly sensitive fluorescence detection system with the incorporation of each nucleotide carrying fluorescent dye in the growing strand. The read length obtained ranges from 30 to 35 bp. PacBio RS, a single-molecule real-time (SMRT) sequencing technology, is based on the DNA sequencing by synthesis method and contains the provision of the real-time imaging of fluorescently tagged nucleotides for studying the sequence and structure of nucleic acid [13]. This technology not only can produce a comparatively longer DNA sequence (average read lengths of 5500–8500 bp) but also has wider application in epigenetics research as the technology is able to detect DNA methylation such as 4-methylctosine (mC), 5-mC, and 6-methyladenine (mA) [14].

The development of nanopore sequencing technology [15] begins an era of fourth-generation sequencing technology and has promised a cheap and fast method of sequencing. The principle involves threading a single-stranded DNA/RNA molecule electrophoretically through a nanopore that causes altering the pore's electrical properties and thereby modulating the ionic current through the nanopore. Braha et al. [16] designed a biosensor using "α-hemolysin," a toxin isolated from *Staphylococcus aureus*. The first commercial sequencing device was announced by Oxford Nanopore Technologies in 2012. Later, the technology was adapted and commercialized by other companies like Roche with IBM, Electronic BioSciences, and NABsys [17, 18]. This technology has advantage as sample preparation is not needed and the trans-duction and recognition occur in real time, on a molecule-by-molecule basis. The technology produces very long reads (up to 10 kb), which could be are capable of inexpensive *de novo* sequencing.

3. Application of NGS technology in Solanaceae genetics and genomics studies

NGS technologies have numerous potential applications in plant genetics and genomics, which include generation of genomic resources, complete decoding of a species genome, differential gene expression studies, whole genome association studies (WGAS), genomics assisted breeding (GAB), etc. (Figure 1).

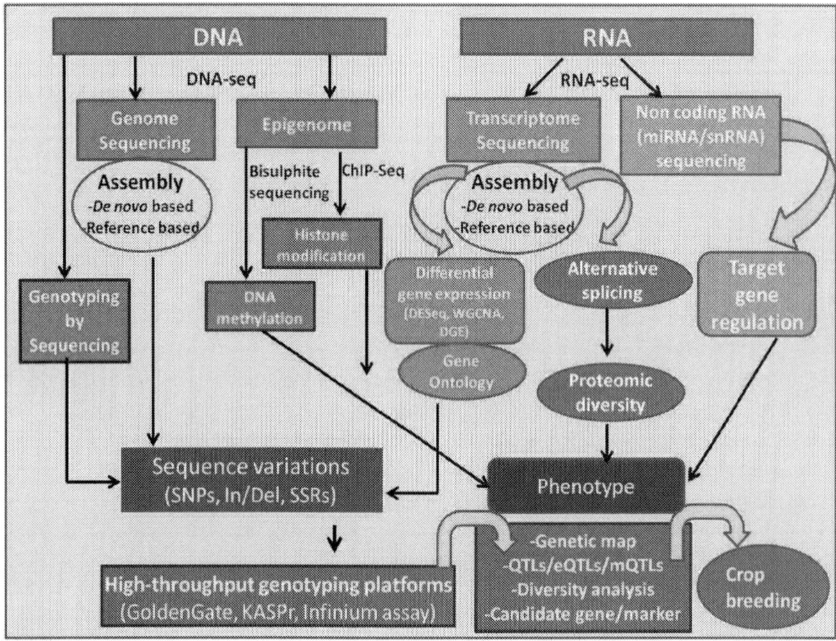

Figure 1. Overview of NGS applications in plant genetics and genomics

3.1. Transcriptome profiling of Solanaceae

Transcriptome sequencing of a species is the first step to access the functionally active genes. The transcriptome sequencing either by first-generation Sanger sequencing or by high throughput NGS approaches provides an insight into the expression of genes in a particular tissue/or different developmental stages of a species. The vast amount of sequencing data serve as a useful resource for the identification of sequence variations for the development of various markers, which would enable the mapping of candidate genes/QTLs for important traits. These applications have been discussed below in four important Solanaceae crops.

3.1.1. Potato

Potato (*S. tuberosum*) is the world's fourth largest crop after maize, rice, and wheat. It has a number of ploidy levels ranging from diploid ($2n$ = 24) to triploids, tetraploids, pentaploids, and hexaploids. Most of the cultivated varieties are autotetraploid ($4n$ = 48). Potato is the world's most important food crops that have edible tuber produced from stolons under favorable environmental conditions. It is accepted worldwide as a cheap source of dietary starch, protein, vitamins, and antioxidants, especially to feed large populations in developing countries. To date, only 4,20,074 ESTs are available in NCBI database (http://www.ncbi.nlm.nih.gov/nucest/?term=potato) that served as a valuable resource in various studies of gene discovery and expression analysis in potato germplasm [19–22]. In 2011, Massa et al. [23] reported a transcriptome sequence of *S. tuberosum* group Phureja clone DM1-3 516R44 using Illumina GAII platform. In this study, a total of 22,704 transcripts were identified, and 83% of these were of known function. The expression analysis was performed in a set of 32 tissues at various developmental stages and revealed that more than twenty thousand genes were found to be expressed in normal potato tissue and of these, some showed tissue-specific expression. In another study, using the weighted gene correlation network analysis (WGCNA), 18 gene co-expression modules were identified that comprised of a total of 5400 genes [24]. These modules were classified according to the high correlated expression profiles of genes in particular developmental stages. Two modules contained mainly transcription factors that showed co-expression in fruit development (e.g., Leafy Cotyledon 1 and transcriptional factor B3 domains) and tuber-tissue-specific expression (e.g., APETALA and WRKY). In another study, using digital gene expression (DGE) profiling, five genes encoding for DOF protein, a blue light receptor, a lectin, a syntaxin-like protein, and a protein with unknown function were found to be specifically associated with photoperiodic tuberization [25]. Hamilton et al. [26] published transcriptome sequencing of three potato cultivars and identified a total of 55,340 SNPs using the Maq SNP filter. In 2013, a whole-genome transcript analysis of the pollen mRNA of *Solanumtuberosum*, *S. demissum*, and their reciprocal F_1 hybrids was performed using Illumina GAII platform [27]. A total of 12.6 billion bases were obtained and were assembled into 13,020 transcripts. They identified the transcriptional differences between these samples and also identified nuclear genes that contributed to the differences observed in reciprocal crosses. Very recently, a comparative transcriptome analysis of white and purple potato was reported using Illumina HiSeq 2000 platform [28]. *De novo* assembly of the reads was performed for each cultivar using Trinity version r20131110 (http://trinityrnaseq.sourceforge.net/). A total of 209 million paired-end reads were assembled into 60,930 transcripts. They identified candidate genes encoding transcription factors involved in anthocyanin biosynthesis. In a very interesting study, Aulakh et al. [29] reported global gene expression comparisons between wild-type (Bintje) and an activation-tagged mutant *underperformer* (*up*) using RNA-seq and identified approximately 1600 genes that were differentially expressed between them, thereby suggesting the modification of various biological pathways in the mutant variety.

3.1.2. Tomato

Tomato is an important vegetable crop that supplies vitamins and nutrients and consumed in different forms around the world. Whole transcriptome sequencing of six tomato accessions

Solanum pimpinellifolium was performed by sequencing by synthesis method of Illumina GAII [30]. This resulted in the generation of 17 Gb of sequence data with 291,915,037 high-quality reads and represented an average of 32.5 Mb of transcriptomic sequence per accession. By using these data, a large number of SNPs were identified to analyze genetic variation in cultivated and wild populations. A leaf transcriptome sequence data of tomato cv. Hongtaiyang 903 were generated using Illumina RNA-seq, which resulted in 50,616 transcripts [31]. Eighty-four percent of these transcripts were functionally annotated in the NCBI nr database and 94.5% in the tomato reference genome [24]. Of these, 14,371 transcripts were found to be involved in 310 pathways. An expression analysis revealed that 2787 transcripts showed significant expression after exogenous ABA treatment. These transcripts were related to ABA signaling pathway, various transcription factors, heat shock proteins, and pathogen resistance. The RNA-seq of one cultivated (*Solanum lycopersicum* M82) and five wild species with two red-fruited (*Solanumpimpinellifolium* and *Solanum galapagense*) and three green-fruited (*Solanum habrochaites*, *Solanum chmielewski*, and *Solanum pennellii*) varieties of tomato was performed to study the changes in gene expression and diversity in DNA sequence of these six species [32]. From this analysis, they identified several distinguishable polymorphic positions between cultivated and wild genotypes. Further, to examine the effect of the fungal symbiosis of tomato root on tomato fruit metabolism, Zouari et al. [33] performed an RNA-Seq of *S. lycopersicum* cv. Moneymaker using Illumina GA and studied transcriptome profiling during fruit maturation. A total of 712 differentially expressed genes in fruits from mycorrhizal and control plants were identified. The majority of the regulated genes were involved in various functions such as photosynthesis, stress response, transport, amino acid synthesis, and carbohydrate metabolism. Further, it was found that AM fungi can serve as a replacement of exogenous fertilizer for the growth of tomato plant with nutrient rich fruits. In addition, to examine the hormonal response in tomato roots, Gupta et al. [34] published a transcriptome atlas of tomato root using Illumina RNA-Seq method. By mapping the 165 million reads onto the tomato reference genome (*S. lycopersicum*), they identified differential expression pattern after various hormonal treatments. To look into regulatory and metabolic pathways specific to fruit tissues, Matas et al. [35] reported a transcriptome study coupled with laser capture microdissection. Five fruit pericarp tissues were sequenced by the pyrosequencing method of GSFLX platform (Roche) and identified 20,976 high-quality expressed unigenes, which included genes that showed expression specific to particular cell type and tissue. Very recently, Mou et al. [36] performed a global analysis of transcriptome of cherry tomato (*Lycopersicon esculentum* var. *cerasiforme* "XinTaiyang") fruit after exogenous treatment of ABA and nordihydroguaiaretic acid (an inhibitor of ABA biosynthesis) to study their effect on fruit ripening process. Of the total 25,728 genes, 10,388 were found to be differentially expressed. The data also revealed the upregulation and downregulation of pigment-related genes after exogenous ABA and NDGA treatment, respectively. Moreover, they also suggested the transcriptional abundance of candidate genes involved in photosynthesis during inhibition of endogenous ABA, which highlighted the significance of ABA in the regulation of ripening process in tomato fruit. Further, to utilize the large amount of transcriptome data for tomato for studying gene expression analysis, Bostan and Chiusano [37] recently presented a web-based platform, i.e., NexGenEx-Tom, that contain collection of high quality transcriptome data of several tissue at various stages of the development of different tomato genotypes and serve as a useful approach for analysis of gene expression profiling and comparisons in various tissues/ genotypes.

3.1.3. Pepper (Capsicum)

The capsicum is a diploid, $2x = 2n = 12$, and self-pollinating plant. Capsicum is closely related to other members of the Solanaceae family, such as potato, tomato, and tobacco, that originated in the New World. The genus contains 39 species of which only six species are cultivated, such as *C. annuum, C. baccatum, C. frutescence, C. chinense, C. pubescens,* and *C. assamicum* [38, 39]. These Capsicum species are grouped as pungent (hot/spicy) and nonpungent (sweet) pepper based on the presence and absence of capsaicinoid compounds, respectively, and therefore used as a major ingredient in various cuisines around the world. The fruit contains beneficial metabolites such as carotenoids (provitamin A), vitamins C and E, flavonoids, and capsaici-noids. It is also used as a coloring agent in food and also have several medicinal properties and thus used in making of traditional medicine. Moreover, several studies have suggested an effective role of capsaicinoids in inhibiting the growth of cancer [40–42], the painkiller in arthritis, reducing appetite, and weight management [43–45]. For chili pepper, a large number of varieties are available that are well adapted in diverse climate conditions around the world [46]. Many studies were targeted toward various aspects, including the development of genetic and genomic resources for crop improvement [39]. A *Capsicum* transcriptome database (DB, http://www.bioingenios.ira.cinvestav.mx:81/Joomla/) was developed by the sequencing of *C. annuum* transcriptome from different tissues [47]. They have obtained 1,324,516 raw reads from which 32,314 high-quality contigs, and 51,118 singletons were assembled. Functional annota-tion of the 75% of the contigs was done resulting in 7481 novel sequences. Further, using 454 GS-FLX pyrosequencing platform, the transcriptome analysis of red pepper (*C. annuum* L. TF68) was carried out [48]. They obtained approximately 30.63 Mb of EST data with 9818 contigs and 23,712 singletons. In another study, Nicolai et al. [49] performed transcriptome analysis using Roche 454 pyrosequencing, and this consists of 23,748 contigs and 60,370 singletons. Using the data, they identified a total of 11,849 SNPs and 853 SSRs. However, in a separate study, Ashrafi et al. [50] used three chili genotypes, namely, Maor, Early Jalapeno, and Criollo de Morelos-334 (CM334) for transcriptome sequencing. From the first assembly, they identified a total of 4236 SNPs and 2489 SSRs, while the second transcriptome assembly based on Illumina GAII resulted in 22,000 high-quality putative SNPs and 10,398 SSRs. Recently, the Pepper GeneChip array from Affymetrix in *Capsicum* for polymorphism detec-tion and expression analysis was reported [51]. Further, the hybridization of genomic DNA from 40 diverse *C. annuum* lines and few lines from other cultivated species such as *C. frutescens, C. chinense,* and *C. pubescens* resulted in generation of 33,401 single-position marker (SPP) from 13,323 unigenes. Liu et al. [52] constructed *de novo* transcriptome assembly in *C. frutescens* and obtained 54,045 high-quality unigenes in which a total of 4072 SSRs were identified, including three candidate genes i.e., dihydroxyacid dehydratase (DHAD), Thr deaminase (TD), and prephenate aminotransferase (PAT) involved in the capsaicinoid biosynthesis pathway. Additionally, a total of 9150 putative SNPs in 3349 contigs were identified between *C. frutescens* and *C. annuum.* In another study, a high-throughput transcriptome profiling in two *C. annuum* varieties resulted in 279,221 and 316,357 sequenced reads with a total of 120.44 and 142.54 Mb of sequence data. A total of 9701 and 12,741 potential SNPs were identified [53].

3.1.4. Eggplant

Eggplant or brinjal (*S. melongena* L.), an autogamous diploid ($2n = 2x = 24$), is the third most important vegetable crop from the genus *Solanum* after potato (*S. tuberosum*) and tomato (*S. lycopersicum*). The eggplant is widely grown in Asia, the Middle and Near East, Southern Europe, and Africa [54]. The eggplant fruit serves as an excellent source of antioxidants like anthocyanin and phenolics [55, 56] and the tolerance to abiotic and biotic stresses [57]. Therefore, several genetic studies have been carried out from the last two decades targeting various fruit traits such as size/shape and color. Moreover, the different origin of eggplant from other Solanaceae spp. makes it an important crop for comparative and evolutionary studies. In this regard, various aspects have been focused by researchers such as the development of genetic resources like molecular markers and genetic map that have been utilized for comparative analysis with other spp. of the Solanaceae family. The eggplant belongs to the *Leptostemonum* clade, which is far lagged behind the potato and tomato (potato clade) in terms of the development of genomic resources as only a total of 226,664 nucleotide sequences were available in NCBI database, of which majority (98,086) were obtained from ESTs generated by Fukuoka et al. [58]. These 98,086 ESTs were assembled into 16,245 unigenes that covered only a limited portion of eggplant transcriptome. Later, transcriptome sequencing was carried out using Illumina sequencing and reads were assembled into contigs using Trinity program [59]. Of these, 80% (27,393) of unigenes showed matches with the sequences available in NCBI nr database. A total of 29,717 genes were functionally annotated. A comparison of eggplant with 11 plant proteomes resulted in 276 high-confidence single-copy orthologous groups and revealed that eggplant and its wild *Leptostemonum* clade relative "turkey berry" split ~6.66 million years ago in the late Miocene and the *Leptostemonum* split ~15.75 Mya from the potato clade in the middle Miocene.

3.2. Whole genome and transcriptome sequencing of Solanaceae spp.

Whole genome sequencing of a species reveals the structural organization of genome, including a number of protein-coding and non-protein-coding genes and repetitive elements and serves as the basis for finding genome-wide analysis of genetic variation, QTL mapping, diversity analysis, association mapping of agronomically important traits for crop improvement, and comparative study of genome evolution between different species.

3.2.1. Potato genome

The draft sequence of 844 Mb genome of a homozygous double-monoploid genotype named DM (DM1-3 516R44) was sequenced using three methods, namely, Sanger method, Roche/454 Pyrosequencing, and Illumina sequencing-by-synthesis method and assembled using the SOAPdenovo assembly algorithm (PGSC; The Potato Genome Sequencing Consortium, 2011) [6]. A heterozygous diploid line, i.e., RH (RH89-039-16) was also sequenced using shotgun sequencing of BACs and WGS, and its reads were mapped to the reference assembly of DM genome (http://potatogenome.net). About 86% of the genome was anchored and assembled into pseudomolecules. A total of 39,031 protein-coding genes were obtained; of them, 90% were located on 12 pseudomolecules. To overcome the problem of heterozygosity and inbreeding depression, which is the major drawback in potato improvement using traditional breeding practices, the researchers selected a homozygous, double-monoploid form, referred as DM for sequencing and integrated with sequence data of heterozygous diploid line RH. The potato genome was the first among the asterid species to be sequenced, and a total of 2642 high-confidence asterid-specific and 3372 potato lineage-specific genes were identified and also found the collinearity with 97.5% identity between DM and RH genome. Furthermore, they identified 3.67 million SNPs and 275 gene-specific presence/absence variations and concluded that the homozygous alleles were the reason for the reduced level of vigor in DM line. They also studied the evolution of tuber development, which revealed that about 15,235 genes were found to be expressed in developing tubers.

3.2.2. Tomato genome

In the year 2012, the Tomato Genome Consortium (TGC, 2012) [5] reported the draft genome sequence of inbred cultivar of tomato "Heinz 1706" using a combination of NGS technologies (454/Roche GS FLX, Illumina Genome Analyser, and SOLiD sequencing). They predicted the genome size of 900 Mb, which were assembled in 91 scaffolds aligned to 12 chromosomes. The data revealed only 0.6% nucleotide divergence (in two tomato genotypes) compared to 8% divergence with potato. The alignment of tomato–potato orthologous regions confirmed nine large inversions during evolution. They predicted about 34,727 (in tomato) and 35,004 (in potato) protein-coding genes. The analysis suggested that the genome triplications could have added new gene family members such as RIN (ripening-inhibitor), CNR (colorless nonripening), ACS (associated with ethylene biosynthesis), PHYB1/PHYB2 for red light photoreceptors, and PSY1/PSY2 (phytoene synthase) for lycopene biosynthesis that mediate important fruit-specific functions such as fleshiness and color. Further, the study reported the presence of noncoding RNAs (ncRNA) with the identification of 96 miRNA genes in tomato and 120 miRNA genes in potato genome. In another study, Aflitos et al. [60] performed the resequencing of 84 tomato accessions and explored the genetic variability present among those cultivated tomato and its wild progenitor. They identified more than 10 million SNPs in wild species, signifying the dramatic genetic erosion of tomato. Furthermore, through comparative sequence alignment, group-, species-, and accession-specific polymorphism was observed, which may be linked to agronomically important fruit traits. Such information may be easily used by recent high-throughput genotyping methods for the detection of genetic variability across extensive populations. The genomic information provided by these projects could be used for comparative genetic and genomic studies and in-depth sequence analysis in Solanaceae.

3.2.3. Pepper genome

The recent advancement in the sequencing and development of NGS technologies has accelerated the genetics and genomics studies of capsicum. Recently, a draft genome sequence of a diploid hot pepper, i.e., "*C. annum* cv 'CM334'" (Criollo de Morelos 334), was published [7]. The variety CM334 has been utilized in breeding practices as it showed resistance against *Phytophthora capsici*, pepper mottle virus, and root-knot nematodes. The authors reported sequencing a total of 650.2 Gb pepper genome, which is approximately equal to 186.6× genome coverage of 3.48 Gb estimated *C. annuum* genome by utilizing Illumina platform. Filtered reads were assembled into 37,989 scaffolds using SOAPdenovo and SPACE (total 3.06 Gb). Anchoring of those contigs on high-density genetic map could assembled 86% of the (2.63 Gb; 1357 scaffolds) scaffolds onto 12 pseudomolecules of capsicum genome. A total of 34,903 protein-coding genes were identified using the PGA annotation pipeline. The comparative analysis showed a high level of conservation with its closest relative, i.e., tomato, as 17,397 orthologous gene sets were identified, and their expression studies revealed that 8.8% of them showed expression in leaf tissue and 46.4% were found to be expressed in pericarp tissue. As the pepper genome is four times larger than tomato, the genome size increment seen is mainly due to the presence of a large number of repetitive elements such as LTR retrotransposons. Of the reported retrotransposons, the Gypsy family was found to present 12-fold more than the Copia family when compared to another genome such as tomato, maize, and barley. Moreover, the expression analysis of different capsaicinoid pathway genes showed that all genes were expressed at 16 DPA, 25 DPA, and mature green stages of pepper fruit, but their orthologous genes hardly showed any expression in tomato and potato fruits. This study confirms the specificity of capsaicinoid pathway in the development of pungent flavor in pepper fruit.

To provide a better understanding of evolution and domestication of capsicum, Qin et al. [61] reported two reference genome sequences of cultivated Zunla-1 (*C. annuum* L.) and wild Chiltepin (*C. annuum* var. glabriusculum) pepper. They estimated the genome size of 3.26 Gb and 3.07 Gb, respectively. The reads were assembled in scaffolds comprising 3.48 and 3.35 Gb, respectively. They found different transposable elements (TEs) that covered ~2.7 Gb (81%) of the genome and estimated that the pepper genome expanded ~0.3 Mya. Approximately 79% of 3.48 Gb scaffolds contained 34,476 protein-coding genes that were anchored to chromosomes by a high-density genetic map. Using an in-house-generated program, they identified 6527 long noncoding RNAs (lncRNAs), which comprised 5976 intergenic and 222 intron-overlapping lncRNAs. In addition, the sequencing of small RNAs from five different tissues allowed the identification of 5581 phased siRNAs. Based on plant micro-RNAs (miRNAs) miRBase database, a total of 176 miRNAs were discovered of which 35 were found to be specific to pepper. They also predicted 1104 target genes that have putative functions such as dihydrolipoamide dehydrogenase (*Capana12g000245*) and α-CT (*Capana09g001602*) genes from capsaicinoid biosynthetic pathway, suggesting the regulation of capsaicinoid biosynthesis by miRNAs. Further, they identified 31% constitutively expressed genes and also 3670 genes that were showing tissue-specific expression. The annotation of these genes resulted in the identification of candidate genes for various traits. By a comparison of cultivated and wild pepper genomes with data of 20 resequencing accessions, they identified genes for domestication, which revealed molecular footprints of artificial selection. Moreover, they identified 51 gene families involved in capsaicinoid biosynthesis, and based on the phylogenetic analysis, they concluded that independent pepper-specific duplications in 13 gene families had occurred compared with tomato, potato, and *Arabidopsis*.

3.2.4. Eggplant genome

To elucidate the genome structure and complexity, a draft genome sequence of eggplant has recently been published in which the whole genome shotgun sequencing of eggplant variety named as "Nakate-Shinkuro" was carried out using HiSeq 2000 sequencer (Illumina) [62]. The high-quality reads were assembled using SOAPdenovo v1.05 into 1,321,157 scaffolds and presented a draft genome assembly "SME_r2.5.1" that spanned approximately 74% (833.1 Mb) of the total 1127 Mb of the eggplant genome. Also, transcriptome sequencing of "AE-P03" and "LS1934" was carried out using Roche/454 FLX sequencer (Roche Diagnostics, Basel, Switzerland). By merging the two data sets, a hybrid assembly was produced using PCAP.rep that constituted 81,273 hybrid scaffolds of a total of 836.8 Mb in size. They predicted about 42,035 protein-coding genes in SME_r2.5.1 by Augustus 2.7. A total of 16,573 genes were located on superscaffolds and showed an orthologous relationship with tomato.

3.3. Sequence-based molecular marker discovery and genetic mapping

Sequence-based molecular markers have been used in many comparative and functional genomics studies because of their preferable features like genome-wide distribution, chromosome-specific location, co-dominant inheritance, and reproducibility. The high-throughput NGS technologies produce a huge amount of data, which is highly suitable for the identification of a large number of sequence variations in genome or transcriptome. For SNP identification, various SNP calling programs such as SOAPsnp [63], MAQ [64], Atlas-SNP2 [65], SAMtools [66], and GATK [67, 68] have been used commonly [69].

In tomato, Sim et al. [70] developed the first large-scale SNP genotyping array using 8784 SNPs based on NGS-derived transcriptome sequences of six different genotypes [71]. They constructed three high-density linkage maps using interspecific F_2 populations (with various accessions of S. lycopersicum and S. pennellii). The physical positions of about 7666 SNPs were identified relative to the draft tomato genome sequence and found that the genetic and the physical distances were persistent. Such maps help to provide details of genetic order and recombination, also to improve gene assemblies and to dissect the complex traits. In another study, the genome-wide SNP genotyping was carried out with 7617 SNPs in 40 tomato lines and identified 6474 polymorphic SNPs [72]. Further, the effect of SNPs on protein function was studied, which revealed that the function of about 200 genes was altered by the substitutions phenomenon.

In eggplant, Barchi et al. [73] mapped QTLs associated with anthocyanin pigmentation using inter- and intraspecific linkage maps. They used a combination of the restriction site-associated DNA (RAD) strategy with high throughput sequencing (Illumina) to generate SNPs. A total of 415 of the 431 markers were assembled into twelve major and one minor linkage group, covering 1390 cM distance.

Very recently, in pepper, Devran et al. [74] developed molecular markers tightly linked to potyvirus resistance 4 (Pvr4) by sequencing the parental lines and progenies using Illumina Hi-Seq2500 in combination with bulked segregant analysis (BSA) approach. By comparative analysis, they identified the syntenic regions between resistant and susceptible progenies, and more than 5000 single-nucleotide variants (SNVs) were identified that were converted into CAPS markers and used to map *Pvr4* locus using F_2 mapping populations. In a separate study, intron-targeting (IT) markers were developed from the NGS (5500xl SOLiD)-derived transcripts in tetraploid potato cv. White lady [75]. These markers were tested on various potato genotypes and in other *Solanum* species. A detailed list of reports of NGS-based molecular marker is given in Table 1.

S. No.	Type of study	Population/species	Number of SSRs	Number of SNPs/ InDels	NGS platform	Reference
	Capsicum					
1	Transcriptome profiling	TF68 (*Capsicum annuum*)	751	1536 SNPs 101 InDels	454 GS-FLX	[39]
2	Transcriptome profiling	Yolo Wonder and Criollo de Morelos 334 (both *C. annuum*)	853	11,849	454 GS-FLX and Illumina	[40]
3	Transcriptome profiling	Bukang (*C. annuum*) First assembly	2,489	4,236	Illumina	[41]
		Second assembly	10,398	22,000	Illumina	
4	Transcriptome profiling	Xiaomila (*Capsicum frutescens*)	4,072	9,150	Illumina	[43]
5	Transcriptome profiling	Mandarin (*C. annuum*)	–	1025	454 GS-FLX	[44]
		Blackcluster (*C. annuum*)	–	1059		
6	Whole genome re-sequencing	BA3 (*C. annuum*)	–	154,519 InDels	Illumina	[76]
		BA07 (*C. annuum*)	–	149,755 InDels		
7	Genome sequencing with BSA	SR231 and Criollo de Morelos334 (*C. annuum* L.)	–	5,000 SNV	Illumina HiSeq 2500	[74]
	Tomato					
1	Whole genome re-sequencing	Ailsa Craig, Furikoma, M82, Tomato Chuukanbonhon Nou 11, Ponderosa and Regina (All are inbred lines of *Solanum lycopersicum*)	–	1536 SNPs were selected for genotyping of which 1293 successfully genotyped and 1248 found polymorphic	Re-sequencing with ABI SOLiD and Genotyping by Illumina GoldenGate Assay	[77]
2	Whole transcriptome sequencing	8 accessions of (*S. lycopersicum*) and 1 of (*Solanum pimpinellifolium*)	–	62,576 non redundant putative SNPs	Illumina	[30]

S. No.	Type of study	Population/species	Number of SSRs	Number of SNPs/ InDels	NGS platform	Reference
	Capsicum					
3	Whole genome re-sequencing and transcriptome re-sequencing	Several accessions of *S. lycopersicum* and *S. pimpinellifolium*	–	4,812,432 non-redundant SNPs	Illumina and 454 GS-FLX	[78]
4	Whole genome sequencing	*S. pimpinellifolium*	–	4,680,647	Illumina and 454 GS-FLX	[78]
5	Whole genome re-sequencing	'Micro-Tom' and 'Heinz 1706' of *S. lycopersicum*	–	1,231,191	Illumina and 454	[79]
6	Genome sequencing and transcriptome sequencing	*S. lycopersicum* accessions	–	6,000 (identified) 5528 (validated)	Illumina and 454	[80]
	Eggplant					
1	Genome sequencing	accessions of *Solanum melongena* and *Solanum aethiopicum*	2,000 putative SSRs	10,089 SNPs 874 (InDels)	Illumina	[81]
	Potato					
1	Transcriptome sequencing	*Solanum tuberosum*	–	575,340 SNPs	Illumina	[26]
2	Genome sequencing	*S. tuberosum*	–	111,212 SNPs 13,094 InDels	Illumina	[82]

Note: SNP—single-nucleotide polymorphism, SNV—single-nucleotide variant, SSR—simple sequence repeat, InDels—insertion/deletion.

Table 1. List of transcriptome and whole genome sequencing using NGS technologies for development of genomic resources in Solanaceae crop plants

3.4. Epigenomics during the age of next-generation sequencing technologies

Molecular breeding has a crucial role in the improvement of crops. Although conventional breeding program brought a substantial increment of food production, however, with rapid population growth worldwide, crop improvement should be accelerated so that climate resilient, biotic stress-resistant, high-nutritional, and high-productivity cultivars could be developed. The advent of NGS made it possible to study phenotypic variations caused by genetic and epigenetic modification to facilitates crop improvement. The term epigenotype was first introduced by Conrad H. Waddington to demonstrate the sum of interrelated developmental pathways that enable one genome to give rise to multiple epigenomes and consequently to multiple cell types that make up the whole organism. Nowadays, the term epigenetics is commonly referred to all kinds of heritable changes that are not caused by changes in the alteration of DNA sequences but are triggered by chemical modifications on the DNA (cytosine methylation) or on histone modifications (e.g., acetylation, methylation) bringing about modulation of chromatin structure and function [83]. In recent years, small RNAs have been emerged as key players in controlling epigenetic changes throughout the plant genome.

3.4.1. DNA methylation

DNA methylation refers to the covalent addition of methyl group to the cytosine base at position 5 by the action of DNA methyl transferases. In mammals, cytosine methylation occurs mostly at CG sites and rarely at non-CG sites, while in plants, cytosine methylation can occur in both CG and non-CG contexts. Non-CG methylation involves both symmetrical and asymmetrical sites, CHG and CHH, respectively (H = A, T, or C). Much of our knowledge with respect to DNA methylation is based on the studies performed on model plant *Arabidopsis thaliana*. DNA methylation in plants is being catalyzed principally by three different enzymes. The maintenance of symmetrical CG methylation during DNA replication is carried out by *Methyltransferase1* (*MET1*) (homolog of animal DNA methyltransferase DNMT1), while CHG methylation is catalyzed by the plant-specific *chromomethylase 3* (CMT3) and asymmetric CHH methylation is mediated by *domains rearranged methyltransferase 2* (*DRM2*) (similar to the mammalian *DNMT3* family) activity, which works through RNA-directed DNA methylation (RdDM) pathway [83, 84].

The first ever single-base resolution methylomes of tomato fruits were established, which revealed that fruit epigenome is not static, and the changes occur continuously during different stages of fruit development. The whole genome bisulfite sequencing was employed to study four different stages of fruit development. This study identified 52,095 differentially methylated regions of the 90% of the genome covered in this analysis in wild-type tomato fruits. Comparative analysis of fruits from two nonripening mutants of tomato viz ripening-inhibitor (rin) and Colorless nonripening (Cnr) demonstrated the changes in the methylation patterns in the wild type and the mutants [85]. The *Cnr* mutation in tomato restricts normal ripening process in tomato resulted in a colorless fruits develop a colorless pericarp [86]. Silencing of the *SlCMT3* gene in tomato resulted in the increased expression of *LeSPL-CNR* that encodes for SBP-box transcription factor, which was located in the *Cnr* locus that ultimately triggers *Cnr* fruits to ripen normally. These studies revealed that the induced ripening of *Cnr* fruits is associated with a reduction of methylation at CHG sites of the *LeSPL-CNR* promoter, while a decrease of DNA methylation in differentially methylated regions associated with the *LeMADS-RIN* binding sites [87, 88].

3.4.2. Histone modifications

The interaction between DNA and proteins has a crucial role in the regulation of gene expression. Chromatin immunoprecipitation (ChIP) can be employed to study such interactions. These interactions can be explored using a technique called ChIP, microarray platforms (ChIP-on-chip or ChIP-chip) [89, 90]. More recently, NGS-based techniques are being used for studying histone modifications where ChIP-Seq combines ChIP with massively parallel direct sequencing. ChIP-enriched DNA is sequenced directly, using the Solexa/Illumina platform, and the readings were mapped to the reference genome. Histone modification phenomenon includes methylation, acetylation, phosphorylation, ubiquitination, sumoylation, and ADP-ribosylation. These modifications bring changes directly and cause structural changes to the chromatin or indirectly through the mediator proteins. All histone modifications are reversible and provide versatile ways for regulating gene expression during plant development and their responses to environmental stimuli. The study found that the reversible acetylation and deacetylation of specific *Lys* residues on core histone N-terminal tails catalyzed by histone acetyltransferases (HDA) and histone deacetylases (HDAC), respectively [91, 92]. The action of both enzymes regulates biological processes like transcriptional regulation. It was found that generally, hyperacetylated histones are associated with gene activation, whereas hypoacetylated histones were involved in gene inactivation. ChIP-seq was employed to identify the targets of *ASR1* starting out with the purification of *ASR1*, by using the high-quality anti-*ASR1* antibody. ChIP-seq data generated through this helped in identifying the genes encoding aquaporins and those associated with the cell wall; these genes were associated with drought stress response [93]. There are several studies reported where ChIP-seq along with ChIP-chip methods were used to search genomes for locations associated with binding of several transcription factors (TFs) such as *RIN* and *fruitful* homologs (FUL1/FUL2) [85, 94, 95]. The investigation of genome-wide targets for the main regulators of fruit ripening viz. *RIN*, *FUL1*, and *FUL2* by combining RNA-Seq with ChIP-chip assay identified a total of 292, 860, and 878 target ripening-associated genes in tomato [85, 95]. Therefore, a combination of ChIP-seq and RNA-Seq with ChIP-chip are imperative tools nowadays and can be employed for better understanding of transcriptional networks underlying tomato development.

3.5. Noncoding RNA (ncRNAs) in crop improvement

Recent advances in next-generation genome and transcriptome sequencing with thorough bioinformatics and computational analysis laid to the discovery of numerous RNA types. The ncRNAs are one of the great examples of such techniques. The ncRNAs has emerged as a key product of eukaryotic transcriptionary machinery with a critical role in the regulatory mechanism. The ncRNAs are being classified as housekeeping ncRNAs and regulatory ncRNAs [96]. The rRNAs, tRNAs, small nuclear RNAs (snRNAs), and small nucleolar RNAs (snoRNAs) are under the "housekeeping" ncRNAs, whereas the "regulatory" ncRNAs are known as small ncRNAs (such as miRNAs and siRNAs) and long noncoding RNA (lncRNAs) [96, 97].

3.5.1. Role of long noncoding RNAs in Solanaceae

The lncRNAs are defined as a non-protein-coding functional RNAs of more than 200 bp in length with regulatory function and principally transcribed by RNA polymerase II. The identification of lncRNA in plants and especially in Solanaceae is still at infancy as compared with the human/animal genome. The application of high-throughput NGS technologies toward identification and the characterizations of lncRNAs are being reported. Recently, by analyzing around 200 *A. thaliana* transcriptome data sets, about 6480 lncRNAs were identified in the intergenic regions of the genome [98]. Further, 439 lncRNAs were identified in maize [99], and in a more comprehensive way by integrating all available data sets for maize transcriptome, high confidence 1704 lncRNAs were identified [100]. However, a systemic study on lncRNAs in Solanaceae has not been done except some few reports. In pepper, a total of 5976 long intergenic ncRNAs (lincRNAs), 222 intronic overlapping lncRNAs, and 329 bidirectional overlapping lncRNAs were identified from RNA-seq data of unopened flower buds [44]. Recently, a genome-wide identification of lncRNAs in tomato was reported [101]. The study identified a total of about 3679 lncRNAs from wild-type AC tomato and mutant ripening fruit (*rin*). The analysis further reported that out of 3530 and 3679 lncRNAs identified in wild-type and *rin* mutant tomatoes, only 23 and 126 lncRNAs were transcribed specifically in wild-type and *rin* mutant tomatoes, respectively. Most of the lncRNAs are derived from intergenic regions. It was also found that 490 lncRNAs were upregulated in ripening mutant fruits, while 187 lncRNAs were downregulated, suggesting the involvement of lncRNAs in the regulation of fruit ripening. However, the function of lncRNAs has not been fully understood and studied. In a more conclusive study, the role of lncRNAs known as *COOLAIR* (cool-assisted intronic noncoding RNA) and *COLDAIR* (cold-assisted intronic noncoding RNA) during vernalization was investigated. These lncRNAs are involved in the epigenetic silencing of *FLC* gene that subsequently promotes flowering [102]. The identification and the characterization of novel lncRNAs have enormous potential to open new windows for crop improvement. Therefore, databases of lncRNAs named as PLncDB (plant long noncoding RNA database) [103] and PNRD (plant ncRNA Database) [104] have been developed which provide information about the functions and role of lncRNAs in plants.

3.5.2. Role of miRNAs in regulation of gene expression

MicroRNAs (miRNAs) are approximately 21 nucleotides long in length, and they are a class of noncoding RNAs that play an important role in regulating gene expression in plants [105–107]. Plant miRNAs mostly exert their effects by cleavage of target mRNA with full complementarity, and their target sites are mostly found in coding regions thus altering the gene expression [105–107]. Recent studies have shown that plant miRNAs also repress translation via a slicer-independent mechanism and, therefore, mediates the expression of the genes posttranscriptionally [108, 109].

There are mainly two major approaches for identifying miRNAs in plants: (1) experimental and (2) bioinformatic approaches. An experimental approach includes forward genetics, direct cloning, and next-generation high-throughput sequencing. High-throughput sequencing technology showed significant progress in small RNA identification and has become commonly available and affordable tool nowadays. A large number of miRNAs have been identified by means of high-throughput sequencing and available in online database (http://www.mirbase.org, accessed June 21, 2014), which currently holds 35,828 mature miRNA products from 223 species. The majority of miRNAs identified so far have been obtained from only a few model plant species, such as *A. thaliana*, *Oryza sativa*, *Glycine max*, and *Medicago truncatula*. Despite the largest family in the plant kingdom, the annotated miRNAs are still very limited in Solanaceae [110–113]. It is necessary to understand the function of miRNAs in Solanaceae. The study of the miRNAs in pepper has been reported based on identification using an *in silico* approach [114]. However, there is a need to employ high-throughput sequencing approaches on the pepper to discover miRNAs. Recently high-throughput sequencing technologies have been employed to identify miRNAs in pepper from ten different tissues such as leaf, stem, root, flower, and six developmental stages of fruits. Based on a bioinformatics pipeline, the researchers successfully identified 29 and 35 families of conserved and novel miRNAs, respectively. Moreover, their miRNA targets were also predicted computationally, many of which were experimentally validated using 5' rapid amplification of cDNA ends (RACE) analysis. Among them, one of the confirmed novel targets of miR-396 was a domain-rearranged *methyltransferase*, the major *de novo* methylation enzyme responsible for RNA-directed DNA methylation in plants. These studies carried out using NGS technologies provide a basis for understanding the functional roles of miRNAs in pepper that can be explored for the crop improvement [115].

Kim et al. [114] identified miRNAs and their target genes by analyzing expressed sequence tag (EST) data from five different species of Solanaceae, wherein they revealed the presence of at least 11 miRNAs and 54 target genes in pepper (*C. annuum* L.) and 22 miRNAs with 221 target genes in potato (*S. tuberosum* L.). Apart from this, they identified a total of 12 miRNAs with 417 target genes in tomato, 46 miRNAs with 60 target genes in tobacco (*Nicotiana tabacum* L.), and 7 miRNAs with 28 target genes in *Nicotiana benthamiana*. Further, the identified miRNAs with their target genes were submitted to the SolmiRNA database, (http://gene-pool.kribb.re.kr/SolmiRNA). They showed the presence of both conserved and specific miRNAs, which may play crucial roles in the growth and development of Solanaceae plants. In addition, 12 miRNAs were randomly selected from a differentially expressed conserved miRNA family and subjected to qRT-PCR validation. Of these, the expression level of nta-miR167d was highly enriched in the leaf tissue, whereas the expression level of nta-miR319a and nta-miR160c were specifically found in stem and root tissues, respectively. The target prediction showed that most of the targets genes were those which codes for transcription factors involved in cellular and metabolic processes [116]. Similar study was performed where deep sequencing of leaf, stem, and root, and four early developmental stages of tubers were performed [117]. The study revealed a total of 89 conserved miRNAs belonging to 33 families and 147 novel miRNAs with 112 candidate potato-specific miRNAs. Digital expression profiling based on TPM (transcripts per million) and qRT-PCR analysis of conserved and potato-specific miRNAs revealed that some of the miRNAs showed tissue-specific expression (leaf, stem, and root), while a few demonstrated tuber-specific expressions. Further, targets were predicted for the identified conserved and potato-specific miRNAs. The predicted targets of four conserved miRNAs are as follows, *ARF16* (*auxin response factor* 16) for miR160, NAM (*no apical meristem*) for miR164, RAP1 (relative to *Apetala2* 1) for miR172, and HAM (*hairy meristem*) for miR171. Later they were experimentally validated using 5' RLM-RACE (RNA ligase mediated rapid amplification of cDNA ends). The list of databases for miRNA identification is presented as Table 2.

Database	Description	Link	Reference
miRBase	Database of published miRNA sequences and their annotation	http://www.mirbase.org/	[118–122]
deepBase	A platform for annotating and discovering small and long ncRNAs (microRNAs, siRNAs, and piRNAs) from next generation sequencing data	http://deepbase.sysu.edu.cn/	[123]
miRanda-microRNA.org	Database for predicted microRNA targets, target downregulation scores and experimentally observed expression patterns	http://www.microrna.org/microrna/home.do	[124]
DIANA-mirGen 2.0	Database of miRNA genomic information and regulation	http://diana.cslab.ece.ntua.gr/mirgen/	[125]
miRNAMap	miRNAMap Genomic maps of miRNA genes and their target genes in human, mouse, rat, and other metazoan genomes	http://mirnamap.mbc.nctu.edu.tw/	[126, 127]
PMRD	Plant miRNA database with large information of plant microRNAs data, consisting of microRNA sequence and their target genes, secondary dimension structure, expression profiling, genome browser, etc.	http://bioinformatics.cau.edu.cn/PMRD/	[128]

Table 2. List of databases for miRNA identification

3.5.3. miRNAs in plant growth and development

To investigate the role of miRNAs in ovary and fruit development of tomatoes, transgenic plants were generated by overexpressing MIR167. The transgenic plants showed a reduction in leaf size and internode length as well as shortened petals, stamens, and styles. The RNA-Seq analysis identified many genes with altered expression patterns in tomato. Of these, *SpARF6* and *SpARF8* genes involved in flower maturation in *Arabidopsis* have been found to be significantly down regulated [129]. In a separate study, it was found that transgenic tomato plants harboring AtMIR156b (*A. thaliana* miRNA 156b family) precursor resulted in abnormal flower and fruit morphology; in addition, the fruits were characterized by the growth of extra carpels and ectopic structures [130]. Moreover, these transgenic lines also displayed increased the expression of genes, which are involved in maintenance of meristem and formation of new organs such as *LeT6/TKN2* (a KNOX-like class I gene) and *GOBLET* (a NAM/CUC-like gene). Overall, these observations suggest that the miR156 is involved in the maintenance of the meristematic activity of ovary tissues and participates in the normal fleshy fruit development.

Several miRNAs have been identified in the fruit tissue. However, no miRNA has been experimentally validated to be involved in fruit ripening. Recently, *SlymiR157* and *SlymiR156* have been shown to regulate ripening and softening of tomato fruits. SlymiR157 governs the expression of key ripening gene *LeSPL-CNR* by miRNA-induced mRNA degradation and by translational repression. Furthermore, qRT-PCR profiling of key ripening-related genes reveals that the SlymiR157-target LeSPL-CNR may also affect the expression of *LeMADS-RIN*, *LeHB1*, *SlAP2a*, and *SlTAGL1* [131]. Table 3 contains the list of databases for miRNA target gene prediction.

Database	Description	Link	References
starBase	Interaction Networks of lncRNAs, miRNAs, competing endogenous RNAs (ceRNAs), RNA-binding proteins (RBPs), and mRNAs from large-scale CLIP-Seq (HITS-CLIP, PAR-CLIP, iCLIP, and CLASH) data	http://starbase.sysu.edu.cn/	[132, 133]
miRwalk 2.0	Database with collection of predicted and experimentally verified miRNA–target interactions with various novel and unique feature	http://zmf.umm.uniheidelberg.de/ apps/zmf/mirwalk2/index.html	[134]
targetScan	Database and Webserver for predicted miRNA targets in animals	http://www.targetscan.org/	[135–137]
DIANA-TarBase v7.0	DIANA-TarBase v7.0 provides for the first time hundreds of thousands of high quality manually curated experimentally validated miRNA–gene interactions	http:// diana.imis.athenainnovation.gr/ DianaTools/index.php?r=tarbase/ index	[138, 139]
DIANA -microT v3.0	Accurate microRNA target prediction database	http://diana.cslab.ece.ntua.gr/microT/	[140, 141]
miRecords	Manually curated database of experimentally validated miRNA–target interactions	http://c1.accurascience.com/ miRecords/prediction_query.php	[142]
picTar	PicTar: a computational method for identifying common targets of microRNAs	http://pictar.mdc-berlin.de/	[143]
RNA22	Web based browser to identity miRNA targets	https://cm.jefferson.edu/rna22/ Interactive/	[144]
micTarBase	miRTarBase has accumulated more than fifty thousand miRNA–target interactions (MTIs)	http://mirtarbase.mbc.nctu.edu.tw/	[126, 127]

Database	Description	Link	References
RNALogo	Database with novel graphical representation of the patterns in an aligned RNA sequences with a consensus structure	http://rnalogo.mbc.nctu.edu.tw/	[145]
miRGator	Database with microRNA diversity, expression profiles, and target relationships	http://mirgator.kobic.re.kr/	[146–148]
miRNAMap	miRNAMap Genomic maps of miRNA genes and their target genes in human, mouse, rat, and other metazoan genomes	http://mirnamap.mbc.nctu.edu.tw/	[112]
miRDB	Webserver for miRNA target prediction and functional annotation	http://mirdb.org/miRDB/	[149]
RNA hybrid	This tool is primarily meant as a means for microRNA target prediction	http://bibiserv.techfak.uni-bielefeld.de/rnahybrid/	[150]
miRU, psRNAtarget	A Plant Small RNA Target Analysis Server	http://plantgrn.noble.org/psRNATarget/	[151]
miRNEST	miRNEST is an integrative collection of animal, plant and virus microRNA data	http://rhesus.amu.edu.pl/mirnest/copy/browse.php	[152]
PMTED	Plant MicroRNA Target Expression Database	http://pmted.agrinome.org/by_mirna.jsp	[153]
MIREX	A platform for comparative exploration of plant pri-miRNA expression data	http://www.comgen.pl/mirex2/	[154]
TAPIR	Target prediction for plant microRNAs	http://bioinformatics.psb.ugent.be/webtools/tapir/	[155]
PASmiR	A database for miRNA molecular regulation in plant abiotic stress	http://pcsb.ahau.edu.cn:8080/PASmiR/	[156]

Table 3. List of databases for miRNA target gene prediction

3.5.4. miRNAs in biotic stress

miRNAs have been identified in many plants with their diverse regulatory roles in biotic stresses. miRNA sequencing was used to investigate the miRNA expression difference between the tomatoes treated with and without *Phytophthora infestans*. Using high-throughput sequencing technologies, they could identify a total of 207 known miRNAs and 67 novel miRNAs. In addition to this, a total of 70 miRNAs were differentially regulated in the plants treated with *P. infestans*; of these, 50 were downregulated and 20 were upregulated. Also, a total of 73 target genes were identified for 28 differentially expressed miRNAs by using psRNATarget analysis [157].

The fungus *Fusarium oxysporum* f. sp. *lycopersici* causes vascular wilt disease in tomato. A comparative miRNA profiling of susceptible (Moneymaker) and resistant (Motelle) tomato cultivars were performed to explore the role of miRNAs in tomato defense against *F. oxysporum*. *SlmiR482f* and *SlmiR5300* were repressed during infection of Motelle with *F. oxysporum*. Four predicted mRNA targets, two each of slmiR482f and slmiR5300, displayed increased expression in resistant Motelle. This was further confirmed by co-expression analysis in *N. benthamiana*. Silencing of the targets in the resistant Motelle cultivar compromised the resistance to *F. oxysporum* and confirmed the role of these genes in fungal resistance [158].

3.5.5. miRNAs in abiotic stress

Abiotic stress (such as salt, drought, and heat) is becoming a major constraint to crop production due to the climate change. miRNAs have been found to play a significant role in tolerance to these stresses. For example, in tomato, transgenic lines were generated by the overexpression of miR169 family member: Sly-miR169c that displayed reduced stomatal opening, decreased transpiration rate, reduced water loss, and enhanced drought tolerance [159]. In eggplant, the high-throughput sequencing of salt tolerant species was performed and identified 98 conserved miRNAs from 37 families [160]. Some of them were found to be expressed under salt stress. These studies provide a better understanding about the regulation of gene expression under abiotic stresses for genetic improvement of crops.

4. High-throughput genotyping technologies

With the development of various NGS platforms, thousands to millions of SNPs have been identified from whole genome and transcriptome sequence data. Therefore, various high-throughput genotyping platforms were developed simultaneously for large-scale genotyping of SNPs in a large set of individuals. These platforms are the GoldenGate Genotyping Technology (GGGT; Illumina, San Diego, CA, USA) [161], BeadChip-based Infinium assay (Illumina) [162], SNPStream (Beckman Coulter, USA) [163], GeneChip (Affymetrix, USA) [164], and competitive allele-specific PCR, KASPar (KBioscience, UK) [165].

4.1. GoldenGate Genotyping Technology (GGGT)

The Illumina GGGT is a custom-based platform that covers construction of 96-1536 SNPs assay. The method is based on BeadArray technology, which includes immobilization of genomic DNA on avidin-coated particle. A further step is annealing of two allele-specific oligonucleotides and a locus-specific oligonucleotide for each SNP, later allele-specific primer extension for generating allele-specific products followed by PCR amplification with universal primers. It is a custom-based genotyping platform that allows screening of a vast number of samples (up to 3072 SNPs) using a single multiplexed assay. Shirasawa et al. [77] utilized 1536-plex SNP genotyping in tomato, of which 1293 were genotyped successfully. Moreover, 1248 SNPs showed clear polymorphism in 663 accessions. For eggplant, Barchi et al. [73] identified >10,000 potential SNPs. Of these, 384 highest quality SNPs were used to genotype 23 diverse eggplant germplasm with respect to fruit shape and color, and observed polymorphic information content values ranged from 0.29 to 0.5 with a mean value of 0.43.

4.2. BeadChip-based Infinium assay (Illumina)

It includes whole genome amplification followed by hybridization to oligonucleotide probe attached to a bead, extension, and detection of fluorescence by iScan Reader. The assay considers up to four million SNPs in a single sample run, or even up to several hundred thousand multiple samples in the same array. The chemistry involves incubation of samples on bead chip where they anneal to locus-specific 50-mers covalently linked to beads followed by allele-specific single-base extension, fluorescent staining, signal amplification, scanning in a dual-color channel reader, and analysis. This technology is advantageous as one can use a premade array that is easily available commercially for selected species. Hamilton et al. [26] identified 69,011 high confidence SNPs from six potato cultivars and used for genotyping with the Infinium platform. A total of 96 of these SNPs were used to assess allelic diversity in 248 germplasms and found 82 informative SNPs for subsequent analyses. In 2012, Felcher et al. [166] reported "Infinium 8303 Potato Array" comprising of 8303 functional markers which includes 3018 from candidate genes of interest by utilizing the transcriptome data from Hamilton et al. [26]. These were used for the genotyping and development of linkage maps. In tomato, a large-scale SNP genotyping array using 8784 SNPs were obtained from transcriptome sequencing [30] and later used for construction of a high-density linkage map of tomato [70].

4.3. SNPStream (Beckman coulter)

This method involves a single-base extension assay and tag array technology. It starts with a multiplexed SNP-specific PCR followed by a primer extension reaction using tagged primers and fluorescent-labeled nucleotide terminators, i.e., ddNTPs. The products are captured on a tag array, which is then scanned to detect the hybridized extension primers and produce calls. It allows the processing of up to three million genotypes in 384 samples at a time. This genotyping system combines solid-phase primer extension assay and universal tags for SNP genotyping. The instrument allows processing of 4,600–3,000,000 genotypes per day [167].

4.4. GeneChip (Affymetrix, USA)

The GeneChip assays are based on allelic discrimination by the direct hybridization of genomic DNA to arrays containing locus- and allele-specific oligonucleotides (25 mers). Genomic DNA is digested with a restriction endonuclease and ligated to adaptors, which are then amplified by PCR using a single universal primer thereby creating a reduced representation of the genome [168]. These PCR amplicons are fragmented, end-labeled, and hybridized. The fluorescence signal is recorded by the GeneChip 3000 scanner (Affymetrix). The hybridization scanning is evaluated as positive and negative signals. Hill et al. [42] developed a GeneChip® array for analysis of polymorphism and expression in Capsicum. The array was designed from 30,815 unigenes, and hybridization was performed using genomic DNA of 40 diverse lines of *C. annum*. They detected 33,401 single-position polymorphisms within 13,323 unigenes. A total of 251 highly informative markers across these *C. annuum* lines were found. Also, a region of 8.7 cM was detected around Pun1 locus in nonpungent line that showed no polymorphism.

In tomato, an oligonucleotide array was developed with 22,821 probe sets, which correspond to 22,714 unigenes [169]. Genomic DNA isolated from three *S. lycopersicum* varieties, i.e., FL7600 (fresh-market), OH9242 (processing), and PI114490 (var. cerasiformae), were used to hybridize with that array. They identified 189 putative single feature polymorphisms, and a subset of these was utilized for validation which resulted in the identification of 279 SNPs and 27 InDels in 111 loci. Moreover, a subset of validated SNPs was used for analysis of genetic diversity in 92 tomato varieties and accessions.

4.5. KASPar (KBioscience, UK)

The KBioscience-competitive allele-specific PCR (KASPar) is a simple, cost-effective, and flexible way for determining both SNP and InDel in genotypes. It is a custom-based technology that covers 96-1536-well plate formats like Illumina's GGGT. It relies on the discrimination power of a novel form of competitive allele-specific PCR to determine the alleles at a specific locus. The improvement has been made by incorporating a 5′–3′ exonuclease cleaved *Taq* DNA polymerase (the engineered *Taq* increases its discrimination power) and a homogeneous fluorescence resonance energy transfer (FRET) detection system, which makes this technology more competent among the genotyping platforms. From the pepper transcriptome sequence data, Ashrafi et al. [41] identified a large number of SNPs. A subset of them was validated by KASPar assay and identified 78 polymorphic SNPs.

5. Genotyping By Sequencing (GBS)

This technology is comparatively new in which genomic DNAs from large mapping populations are sequenced followed by SNP identification. This allows a rapid way for dissecting QTLs for economically important traits in large mapping populations besides allowing genetic diversity and the phylogenetic study between large numbers of accessions/genotypes. This approach is based on reduced representation sequencing, which involves the digestion of genomic DNA with appropriate restriction enzyme to capture a targeted portion of the genome followed by adapter (DNA-barcoded) ligation, PCR amplification, and sequencing of multiplexed libraries [170, 171]. For sequencing, the Illumina's GAII and HiSeq and latest with the Torrent PGM and Proton (Life Technologies) are used. To analyze the large sequencing data, several automated pipelines are being developed, including TASSEL, UNEAK, and IGST. Besides *de novo* SNP discovery, it offers the greatest advantage for those crops in which the solid reference genome sequence is absent. GBS has emerged as a high-throughput, robust, and cost-effective tool for genome-wide association studies and genomics-assisted breeding in numbers of plant and animal species, in particular for those having a complex genome. The utility of GBS has been demonstrated very well for discovery and genotyping of large number of SNPs, genetic mapping, diversity analysis, and population structure [172]. Among Solanaceae family, in potato, a high-quality sequence data of 12.4 Gb was obtained from which 129,156 sequence variants have been identified and mapped to 2.1 Mb of the potato reference genome with average read depth of 636 per cultivar [173].

6. Genome-Wide Association Study (GWAS)

The advent of NGS technologies provides a large number of sequence variants (mainly SNPs) within a shorter period. These sequence variants can be utilized for QTL mapping, GWAS, and germplasm characterization. The establishment of an association between genotype and phenotype is a very challenging task. For crop improvement, it is necessary to determine the genetic basis of the agronomic trait. GWAS is a powerful technique for detecting natural variation and fine mapping of QTL underlying complex traits [174]. It requires a collection of individuals or a population of diverse genotypes and highly polymorphic markers that showed genome-wide distribution. This is a very robust method, in comparison to biparental cross-mapping, to map multiple traits simultaneously. In tomato, Shirasawa et al. [77] reported the whole genome resequencing of six tomato cultivars and detected 1.5 million SNPs by mapping the reads onto the reference genome (SL2.40). They utilized Illumina GoldenGate assay for genotyping of 1536 SNPs in 663 tomato accessions. There was no population structure observed when analyzing the genetic relationship using the STRUCTURE software. Further, they identified a total of nine SNP loci that were found to be associated with eight morpho-logical traits. To overcome the low polymorphism in cultivated tomato (*S. lycopersicum*), they used genome admixture of the cultivated and its wild ancestor (*S. pimpinellifolium*) for association mapping in tomato [175].

7. Next-generation sequencing toward translational research

7.1. Fruit traits (size, shape, ripening, and development)

The transcriptome studies in Solanaceae crops such as potato revealed the identification of transcription factors associated with fruit development. A total of 632 lineage-specific genes were identified, of which 289 genes were asterid specific and 343 were potato specific [23]. They identified 290 genes, including *pectin esterase, lipoxygenase,* and *malate synthase. Leafy Cotyledon 1 (LEC 1)* and transcriptional factor *B3* were found to be co-expressed in fruit tissues. These TFs are consistently found to be involved in plant embryo development.

In tomato, using NGS technologies, several SNPs successfully differentiating between cherry type and round/beef type tomatoes were identified [80]. The SNP data revealed that cherry tomatoes share more SNPs with *S. pimpinellifolium*, a wild relative of the tomato. This revealed a close phylogenetic relationship of cherry tomato with the wild type. Several SNPs belonged to the chromosomal region that harbors genes/QTLs related to fruit weight, size, shape, and color, indicating that the SNPs may be used to explore the other fruit traits. In a miRNA study, it was observed that the transgenic tomato plants harboring AtMIR156b precursor resulted in abnormal flower and fruit morphology [130], indicating that mir156b plays crucial role in ovary and normal fleshy fruit development.

7.2. Tuber

The transcriptome of tuber tissue showed the presence of several transcripts that are specific for tuber. Around 90 genes were co-expressed in tuber, including the genes involved in starch biosynthesis pathway such as *glucose 6-phosphate/phosphate translocator* and storage proteins such as *patatin* [23]. The *APETALA* and *WRKY* transcription factors were specifically found to be expressed in tubers. Further, using DGE profiling, the photoperiodic tuberization-specific genes were identified and suggested that the potato tuberization may be controlled by the genes associated with flowering time in other plant species [25]. These data contribute toward the development of powerful resources that could be used in candidate gene mining for important agricultural traits.

7.3. Pungency

Pungency is a special and economically important quality trait only found in pepper fruits, and it has been studied extensively [7, 43]. NGS technology has a wide scope to explore this trait and provides insights into the capsaicinoid pathway revealing the genes/loci associated with pungency. The transcriptome profiling of *C. frutescens* revealed the identification of three structural genes, namely, dihydroxyacid dehydratase (DHAD), Thr deaminase (TD), and prephenate aminotransferase (PAT) involved in the capsaicinoid biosynthesis pathway [43]. They claimed the identification of several new candidate genes involved in the capsaicinoid pathway. The comparative transcriptomic study of pepper with potato and tomato showed that the different capsaicinoid pathway genes were expressed during placenta development at 16 DPA, 25DPA, and mature green stages of pepper fruits, but their orthologous genes hardly showed any expression in tomato and potato fruit [7]. The study confirmed the specificity of capsaicinoid pathway in the development of pungency in pepper fruit.

7.4. Disease resistance

Using NGS technology, single-nucleotide variants (SNVs) were identified in resistant and susceptible pepper population for potato virus Y and pepper mottle virus. The comparative genomic tools were used to align the SNVs with syntenic region/loci of tomato. Later, the SNVs were converted into PCR-based CAPS (cleaved amplified polymorphic site) marker to map *potyvirus resistance 4* (*pvr4*) locus. These molecular markers could be used in large-scale marker assisted selection (MAS) programs [74].

7.5. Hormone and stress

Global transcriptome profiling of exogenously applied ABA tomato seedling revealed the identification of a large number of genes related to various stress responses [31]. These included several transcription factors, heat shock proteins, and pathogen resistance. Apart from this, salicylic acid, jasmonic acid, and ethylene signaling pathways were upregulated by exogenous ABA. The study suggested the role of ABA in improving pathogen resistance and abiotic stress tolerance. Moreover, the tomato transgenic lines were developed with the overexpression of Sly-miR169c, a miR169 family member. The transgenic plants displayed reduced stomatal opening, decreased transpiration rate, reduced water loss, and enhanced drought tolerance [159].

8. Conclusion and future direction

As the sequencing technologies are advancing at a rapid rate, enormous genomic information is being generated for Solanaceae crop plants. The question at present is how to utilize this enormous NGS-generated information for Solanaceae translational research. The large-scale phenotyping and transcriptome and whole genome resequencing of diverse genotypes from each species and their correlation will help in the identification of genetic region and eventually of candidate genes in the genomes. The integration of classical genetics, QTL mapping, and whole genome and transcriptome sequencing would be helpful in accelerating the Solanaceae translational research. Consideration of noncoding RNAs and epigenetics mechanism while designing breeding strategies would expedite the manipulation of mechanisms underlying various developmental aspects of plant biology in Solanaceae. Furthermore, the use of NGS technology provides an opportunity to investigate and understand the structure and evolution of complex Solanaceae genomes.

Author details

Sushil Satish Chhapekar, Rashmi Gaur, Ajay Kumar and Nirala Ramchiary*

*Address all correspondence to: nrudsc@gmail.com

School of Life Sciences, Jawaharlal Nehru University, New Delhi, India

References

[1] Schmidt MA, Barbazuk WB, Sandford M, et al. Silencing of soybean seed storage proteins results in a rebalanced protein composition preserving seed protein content without major collateral changes in the metabolome and transcriptome. Plant Physiol. 2011;156:330–345. doi:10.1104/pp.111.173807.

[2] Suzuki T, Igarashi K, Dohra H, et al. A new omics data resource of *Pleurocybella porrigens* for gene discovery. PLoS One. 2013;8(7):e69681. doi:10.1371/journal.pone.0069681.

[3] Sanger F, Nicklen S, Coulson AR. DNA sequencing with chain-terminating inhibitors. Proc Natl Acad Sci USA. 1977;74(12):5463–5467.

[4] Metzke ML. Sequencing technologies: the next generation. Nat Rev Genet. 2010;11:31–46. doi:10.1038/nrg2626.

[5] The Tomato Genome Consortium. The tomato genome sequence provides insights into fleshy fruit evolution. Nature. 2012;485(7400):635–641. doi:10.1038/nature11119.

[6]   Potato Genome Sequencing Consortium. Genome sequence and analysis of the tuber crop potato. Nature. 2011;475(7355):189–195. doi:10.1038/nature10158.

[7]   Kim S, Park M, Yeom SI, et al. Genome sequence of the hot pepper provides insights into the evolution of pungency in *Capsicum* species. Nat Genet. 2014;46(3):270–278. doi:10.1038/ng.2877.

[8]   Margulies M, Egholm M, Altman WE, et al. Genome sequencing in microfabricated high-density picolitre reactors. Nature. 2005;437 (7057):376–80. doi:10.1038/nature03959.

[9]   Valouev A, Ichikawa J, Tonthat T, et al. A high-resolution, nucleosome position map of *C. elegans* reveals a lack of universal sequence-dictated positioning. Genome Res. 2008;18 (7):1051–1063. doi:10.1101/gr.076463.108

[10] Bentley DR. Whole-genome re-sequencing. Curr Opin Genet Dev. 2006;16(6):545–552. doi:10.1016/j.gde.2006.10.009.

[11] Rothberg JM, Hinz W, Rearick TM, et al. An integrated semiconductor device enabling non-optical genome sequencing. Nature. 2011;475:348–52. doi:10.1038/nature10242.

[12] Harris, TD, Buzby PR, Babcock H, et al. Single-molecule DNA sequencing of a viral genome. Science. 2008;320:106–109. doi:10.1126/science.1150427.

[13] Eid J, Fehr A, Gray J, et al. Real-time DNA sequencing from single polymerase molecules. Science. 2009;323:133–138. doi:10.1126/science.

[14] Flusberg BA, Webster DR, Lee JH, et al. Direct detection of DNA methylation during single-molecule, real-time sequencing. Nat Methods. 2010;7:461–465. doi:10.1038/nmeth.1459.

[15] Kasianowicz, JJ, Brandin E, Branton D, Deamer DW. Characterization of individual polynucleotide molecules using a membrane channel. Proc Natl Acad Sci U S A. 1996;93:13770–13773.

[16] Braha, O. et al. Designed protein pores as components for biosensors. Chem Biol. 1997;4:497–505.

[17] Branton D, Deamer DW, Marziali A, et al. The potential and challenges of nanopore sequencing. Nat Biotechnol. 2008;26:1146–1153. doi:10.1038/nbt.1495.

[18] Maitra RD, Kim J, Dunbar WB. Recent advances in nanopore sequencing. Electrophoresis. 2012;33(23):3418–3428. doi:10.1002/elps.201200272.

[19] Flinn B, Rothwell C, Griffiths R, et al. Potato expressed sequence tag generation and analysis using standard and unique cDNA libraries. Plant Mol Biol. 2005;59:407–433. doi:10.1007/s11103-005-0185-y.

[20] Ronning CM, Stegalkina SS, Ascenzi RA, et al. Comparative analyses of potato expressed sequence tag libraries. Plant Physiol. 2003;131:419–429. doi:http://dx.doi.org/10.1104/pp.013581.

[21] Rensink W, Hart A, Liu J, Ouyang S, Zismann V, Buell CR. Analyzing the potato abiotic stress transcriptome using expressed sequence tags. Genome. 2005;48:598–605.

[22] Li X, Griffiths R, Lague M, et al. EST sequencing and analysis from cold-stored and reconditioned potato tubers. Acta Hortic. 2007;745:491–493.

[23] Massa AN, Childs KL, Lin H, Bryan GJ, Giuliano G, Robin Buell C. The transcriptome of the reference potato genome *Solanum tuberosum* group Phureja clone DM1-3 516R44. PLoS One. 2011;6(10). doi:10.1371/journal.pone.0026801.

[24] Zhang B, Horvath S. A general framework for weighted gene co-expression network analysis. Stat Appl Genet Mol Biol. 2015;4(1):1544–6115, doi:10.2202/1544-6115.1128.

[25] Shan J, Song W, Zhou J. Transcriptome analysis reveals novel genes potentially involved in photoperiodic tuberization in potato. Genomics. 2013;102(4):388–396. doi:10.1016/j.ygeno.2013.07.001.

[26] Hamilton JP, Hansey CN, Whitty BR, et al. Single nucleotide polymorphism discovery in elite North American potato germplasm. BMC Genomics. 2011;12(1):302. doi:10.1186/1471-2164-12-302

[27] Sanetomo R, Hosaka K. Pollen transcriptome analysis of *Solanum tuberosum* ($2n=4x=48$), *S. demissum* (2n=6x=72), and their reciprocal F1 hybrids. Plant Cell Rep. 2013;32:623–636. doi:10.1007/s00299-013-1395-4.

[28] Liu Y, Lin-Wang K, Deng C, et al. Comparative transcriptome analysis of white and purple potato to identify genes involved in anthocyanin biosynthesis. PLoS One. 2015;10(6):e0129148. doi:10.1371/journal.pone.0129148.

[29] Aulakh SS, Veilleux RE, Dickerman AW, Tang GZ, Flinn BS. Characterization and RNA-seq analysis of underperformer, an activation-tagged potato mutant. Plant Mol Biol. 2014;84(6):635–658. DOI 10.1007/s11103-013-0159-4.

[30] Hamilton JP, Sim SC, Stoffel K, Van Deynze A, Buell CR, Francis DM. Single nucleotide polymorphism discovery in cultivated tomato via sequencing by synthesis. Plant Genome. 2012;5(1):17–29. doi:10.3835/plantgenome2011.12.0033.

[31] Wang Y, Tao X, Tang XM, et al. Comparative transcriptome analysis of tomato (*Solanum lycopersicum*) in response to exogenous abscisic acid. BMC Genomics. 2013.14:81. doi:10.1186/1471-2164-14-841.

[32] Koenig D, Jiménez-Gómez JM, Kimura S, et al. Comparative transcriptomics reveals patterns of selection in domesticated and wild tomato. Proc Natl Acad Sci USA. 2013;110:E2655–E2662. doi:10.1073/pnas.1309606110.

[33] Zouari I, Salvioli A, Chialva M, et al. From root to fruit: RNA-Seq analysis shows that arbuscular mycorrhizal symbiosis may affect tomato fruit metabolism. BMC Genomics. 2014;15:221. doi:10.1186/1471-2164-15-221.

[34] Gupta S, Shi X, Lindquist IE, Devitt N, Mudge J, Rashotte AM. Transcriptome profiling of cytokinin and auxin regulation in tomato root. J Exp Bot. 2013;64(2):695–704. doi:10.1093/jxb/ers365

[35] Matas AJ, Yeats TH, Buda GJ, et al. Tissue and cell-type specific transcriptome profiling of expanding tomato fruit provides insights into metabolic and regulatory specialization and cuticle formation. Plant Cell. 2011;23:3893–3910. doi:http://dx.doi.org/10.1105/tpc.111.091173

[36] Mou W, Li D, Luo Z, Mao L, Ying T. Transcriptomic analysis reveals possible influences of ABA on secondary metabolism of pigments, flavonoids and antioxidants in tomato fruit during ripening. PLoS One. 2015;10(6):e0129598. doi:10.1371/journal.pone.0129598.

[37] Bostan H, Chiusano ML. NexGenEx-Tom: a gene expression platform to investigate the functionalities of the tomato genome. BMC Plant Biol. 2015;15:48. doi 10.1186/s12870-014-0412-2.

[38] Reifschneider FJB. Capsicum. Pimentas e pimentões no Brasil. Embrapa Comunicação para Transferência de Tecnologia, Brasilia, 2000;113pp.

[39] Ramchiary N, Kehei M, Brahma V, Kumaria S, Tandon P. Application of genetics and genomics towards Capsicum translational research. Plant Biotechnol Rep. 2014;8:101–123. doi:10.1007/s11816-013-0306-z.

[40] Surh YJ. Cancer chemoprevention with dietary phytochemicals. Nat Rev Cancer. 2003;3:768–780. doi:10.1038/nrc1189.

[41] Ito K, Nakazato T, Yamato K, et al. Induction of apoptosis in leukemic cells by homovanillic acid derivative, capsaicin, through oxidative stress: implication of phosphorylation of p53 at Ser-15 residue by reactive oxygen species. Cancer Res. 2004;64:1071–1078. doi:10.1158/0008-5472.CAN-03-1670.

[42] Mori A, Lehmann S, O'Kelly J, et al. Capsaicin, a component of red peppers, inhibits the growth of androgen-independent, p53 mutant prostate cancer cells. Cancer Res. 2006;66:3222–3229 doi:10.1158/0008-5472.CAN-05-0087.

[43] Lejeune MP, Kovacs EM, Westerterp-Plantenga MS. Effect of capsaicin on substrate oxidation and weight maintenance after modest body-weight loss in human subjects. Br J Nutr. 2003;90:651–659. doi:http://dx.doi.org/10.1079/BJN2003938.

[44] Westerterp-Plantenga MS, Smeets A, Lejeune MP. Sensory and gastrointestinal satiety effects of capsaicin on food intake. Int J Obesity. 2005;29:682–688. doi:10.1038/sj.ijo.0802862.

[45] Ludy MJ, Moore GE, Mattes RD. The effects of capsaicin and capsiate on energy balance. Critical review and meta-analyses of studies in humans. Chem Senses. 2012;37:103–121. doi:10.1093/chemse/bjr100.

[46] Lannes SD, Finger FL, Schuelter AR, Casali VWD. Growth and quality of Brazilian accessions of *Capsicum chinense* fruits. Sci Hortic. 2007;112:266–270. doi:10.1016/j.scienta.2006.12.029.

[47] Góngora-Castillo E, Fajardo-Jaime R, Fernández-Cortes A, et al. The capsicum transcriptome DB: a "hot" tool for genomic research. Bioinformation. 2012;8:043–047.

[48] Lu FH, Cho MC, Park YJ. Transcriptome profiling and molecular marker discovery in red pepper, *Capsicum annuum* L. TF68. Mol Biol Rep. 2012;39:3327–3335. doi: 10.1007/s11033-011-1102-x.

[49] Nicolai M, Pisani C, Bouchet JP, Vuylsteke M, Palloix A. Discovery of a large set of SNP and SSR genetic markers by high-throughput sequencing of pepper (*Capsicum annuum*). Genet Mol Res. 2012;11: 2295–2300. doi:10.4238/(2012).

[50] Ashrafi H, Hill T, Stoffel K, et al. De novo assembly of the pepper transcriptome (*Capsicum annuum*): a benchmark for in silico discovery of SNPs, SSRs and candidate genes. BMC Genomics. 2012;13:571. doi:10.1186/1471-2164-13-571.

[51] Hill TA, Ashrafi H, Reyes-Chin-Wo S, et al. Characterization of *Capsicum annuum* genetic diversity and population structure based on parallel polymorphism discovery with a 30K unigene pepper GeneChip. PLoS One. 2013;8: e56200. doi:10.1371/journal.pone.0056200.

[52] Liu S, Li W, Wu Y, Chen C, Lei J. *De novo* transcriptome assembly in chili pepper (*Capsicum frutescens*) to identify genes involved in the biosynthesis of capsaicinoids. PLoS One. 2013;8:e48156. doi:10.1371/journal.pone.0048156.

[53] Ahn YK, Tripathi S, Kim JH, et al. Transcriptome analysis of *Capsicum annuum* varieties Mandarin and Blackcluster: assembly, annotation and molecular marker discovery. Gene. 2013;533:494–499. doi:10.1016/j.gene.2013.09.095.

[54] Daunay MC, Lester RN. The usefulness of taxonomy for Solanaceae breeders, with special reference to the genus *Solanum* and to *Solanum melongena* L. (eggplant). Capsicum Newslett. 1998;7:70–79

[55] Azuma K, Ohyama A, Ippoushi K, et al. Structures and antioxidant activity of anthocyanins in many accessions of eggplant and its related species. J Agric Food Chem. 2008;56:10154–10159. doi:10.1021/jf801322m.

[56] Stommel JR. Whitaker BD. Phenolic acid content and composition of eggplant fruit in a germplasm core subset. J Am Soc Hort Sci. 2003;128:704–710.

[57] Sakata Y, Monma S, Narikawa T, Komochi S. Evaluation of resistance to bacterial wilt and Verticillium wilt in eggplants (*Solanum melongena* L.) collected in Malaysia. J Jpn Soc Hort Sci. 1996;65:81–88. doi:http://doi.org/10.2503/jjshs.65.81.

[58] Fukuoka H, Yamaguchi H, Nunome T, Negoro S, Miyatake K, Ohyama A. Accumulation, functional annotation, and comparative analysis of expressed sequence tags in

eggplant (*Solanum melongena* L.), the third pole of the genus *Solanum* species after tomato and potato. Gene. 2010;450:76–84. doi:10.1016/j.gene.2009.10.006.

[59] Yang X, Cheng YF, Deng C, Ma Y, Wang ZW, Chen XH, Xue LB. Comparative transcriptome analysis of eggplant (*Solanum melongena* L) and turkey berry (*Solanum torvum* Sw): phylogenomics and disease resistance analysis. BMC Genomics. 2014;15:412. doi:10.1186/1471-2164-15-412.

[60] Aflitos S, Schijlen E, Jong H, et al. Exploring genetic variation in the tomato (Solanum section Lycopersicon) clade by whole-genome sequencing. Plant J. 2014;80(1):136–148. doi:10.1111/tpj.12616.

[61] Qin C, Yu C, Shen Y, Fang X, Chen L, Min J, et al. Whole-genome sequencing of cultivated and wild peppers provides insights into *Capsicum* domestication and specialization. Proc Natl Acad Sci. 2014;111(14):5135–5140. doi:10.1073/pnas.1400975111.

[62] Hirakawa H, Shirasawa K, Miyatake K, et al. Draft genome sequence of eggplant (*Solanum melongena* L.): the representative *Solanum* species indigenous to the Old World. DNA Res. 2014;21:649–60. doi:10.1093/dnares/dsu027.

[63] Li R, Li Y, Fang X, Yang H, Wang J, Kristiansen K. SNP detection for massively parallel whole-genome resequencing. Genome Res. 2009;19(6):1124–1132.

[64] Li H, Ruan J, Durbin R. Mapping short DNA sequencing reads and calling variants using mapping quality scores. Genome Res. 2008;18:1851–1858. doi:10.1101/gr.078212.108.

[65] Shen Y, Wan Z, Coarfa C, et al. A SNP discovery method to assess variant allele probability from next-generation resequencing data. Genome Res. 2010;20(2):273–280. doi:10.1101/gr.096388.109.

[66] Li H, Handsaker B, Wysoker A, et al. The sequence alignment/map format and SAMtools. Bioinformatics. 2009. 25(16):2078–2079. doi:10.1093/bioinformatics/btp352.

[67] McKenna A, Hanna M, Banks E. The genome analysis toolkit: a MapReduce framework for analyzing next-generation DNA sequencing data. Genome Res. 2010;20:1297–1303. doi:10.1101/gr.107524.110.

[68] DePristo MA, Banks E, Poplin R, et al. A framework for variation discovery and genotyping using next-generation DNA sequencing data. Nat Genet. 2011;43(5):491–498. doi:10.1038/ng.806.

[69] Pabinger S, Dander A, Fischer M, et al. A survey of tools for variant analysis of next-generation genome sequencing data. Brief Bioinform. 2013;15(2):256–78. doi: 10.1093/bib/bbs086

[70] Sim S-C, Durstewitz G, Plieske J, et al. Development of a large snp genotyping array and generation of high-density genetic maps in tomato. PLoS One. 2012;7(7):e40563. doi:10.1371/journal.pone.0040563

[71] Hamilton JP, Sim S, Stoffel K, et al. Single nucleotide polymorphism discovery in cultivated tomato via sequencing by synthesis. Plant Genome. 2012;5:17–29. doi:10.3835/plantgenome2011.12.0033.

[72] Hirakawa H, Shirasawa K, Ohyama A, et al. Genome-wide SNP genotyping to infer the effects on gene functions in tomato. DNA Res. 2013;20(3):221–233. doi:10.1093/dnares/dst005.

[73] Barchi L, Lanteri S, Portis E, et al. A RAD tag derived marker based eggplant linkage map and the location of QTLs determining anthocyanin pigmentation. PLoS One. 2012;7(8):e43740. doi:10.1371/journal.pone.0043740.

[74] Devran Z, Kahveci E, Ozkaynak E, Studholme DJ, Tor M. Development of molecular markers tightly linked to Pvr4 gene in pepper using next-generation sequencing. Mol Breed. 2015;35(4):101. doi:10.1007/s11032-015-0294-5.

[75] Ahmadvand R, Poczai P, Hajianfar R, et al. Next generation sequencing based development of intron-targeting markers in tetraploid potato and their transferability to other Solanum species. Gene. 2014;540(1):117–121. doi:10.1016/j.gene.2014.02.045.

[76] Li W, Cheng J, Wu Z, et al. An InDel-based linkage map of hot pepper (*Capsicum annuum*). Molecular Breeding. 2015;35(1), 1–10. doi:10.1007/s11032-015-0219-3.

[77] Shirasawa K, Fukuoka H, Matsunaga H, et al. Genome-wide association studies using single nucleotide polymorphism markers developed by re-sequencing of the genomes of cultivated tomato. DNA Res. 2013;20(6), 593–603. doi:10.1093/dnares/dst033.

[78] Kim JE, Oh SK, Lee JH, Lee BM, Jo SH. Genome-wide SNP calling using next generation sequencing data in tomato. Mol Cells. 2014;37(1),36. doi:10.14348/molcells.2014.2241.

[79] Kobayashi M, Nagasaki H, Garcia V, et al. Genome-wide analysis of intraspecific DNA polymorphism in 'Micro-Tom', a model cultivar of tomato (*Solanum lycopersicum*). Plant Cell Physiol. 2014;55(2):445–454. doi:10.1093/pcp/pct181.

[80] Víquez-Zamora M, Vosman B, Van de Geest H, et al. Tomato breeding in the genomics era: insights from a SNP array. BMC Genomics. 2013;14:354. doi:10.1186/1471-2164-14-354.

[81] Barchi L, Lanteri S, Portis E, et al. Identification of SNP and SSR markers in eggplant using RAD tag sequencing. BMC Genomics. 2011;12:304. doi:10.1186/1471-2164-12-304.

[82] Uitdewilligen JG, Wolters AMA, Bjorn B, et al. A next-generation sequencing method for genotyping-by-sequencing of highly heterozygous autotetraploid potato. PLoS One. 2013;8(5), e62355. doi:10.1371/journal.pone.0062355.

[83] Law JA, Jacobsen SE. Establishing, maintaining and modifying DNA methylation patterns in plants and animals. Nat Rev Genet. 2010;11:204–20. doi:10.1038/nrg2719.

[84] Zemach A, Kim MY, Hsieh P-H, Coleman-Derr D, et al. The *Arabidopsis* nucleosome remodeler DDM1 allows DNA methyltransferases to access H1-containing hetero-chromatin. Cell. 2013;153:193–205. doi:10.1016/j.cell.2013.02.033.

[85] Zhong S, Fei Z, Chen YR, et al. Single-base resolution methylomes of tomato fruit development reveal epigenome modifications associated with ripening. Nat Biotechnol 2013;31:154–159. doi:10.1038/nbt.2462.

[86] Thompson A, Tor M, Barry C, et al. Molecular and genetic characterization of a novel pleiotropic tomato-ripening mutant. Plant Physiol. 1999;120:383–90.

[87] Manning K, Tor M, Poole M, et al. A naturally occurring epigenetic mutation in a gene encoding an SBP-box transcription factor inhibits tomato fruit ripening. Nat Genet 2006;38:948–52. doi:10.1038/ng1841.

[88] Chen W, Kong J, Qin C, et al. Requirement of CHROMOMETHYLASE3 for somatic inheritance of the spontaneous tomato epimutation colourless non-ripening. Sci Rep. 2015b;5:9192. doi:10.1038/srep09192.

[89] Solomon MJ, Larsen PL, Varshavsky A. Mapping protein–DNA interactions in vivo with formaldehyde: evidence that histone H4 is retained on a highly transcribed gene. Cell. 1988;53:937–47. doi:10.1016/S0092-8674(88)90469-2.

[90] Kaufmann K, Muino JM, Jauregui R, et al. Target genes of the MADS transcription factor SEPALLATA3: integration of developmental and hormonal pathways in the *Arabidopsis* flower. PLoS Biol. 2009;7:e1000090. doi:10.1371/journal.pbio.1000090.

[91] Pandey R, Muller A, Napoli CA, et al. Analysis of histone acetyltransferase and histone deacetylase families of *Arabidopsis thaliana* suggests functional diversification of chromatin modification among multicellular eukaryotes. Nucleic Acids Res. 2002;30:5036–5055.

[92] Chen ZJ, Tian L. Roles of dynamic and reversible histone acetylation in plant development and polyploidy. Biochim Biophys Acta. 2007;1769:295–307. doi:10.1016/j.bbaexp.2007.04.007.

[93] Ricardi MM, González RM, Zhong S, et al. Genome-wide data (ChIP-seq) enabled identification of cell wall-related and aquaporin genes as targets of tomato ASR1, a drought stress-responsive transcription factor. BMC Plant Biol. 2014;14:29. doi: 10.1186/1471-2229-14-29.

[94] Fujisawa M, Nakano T, Ito Y. Identification of potential target genes for the tomato fruit-ripening regulator RIN by chromatin immunoprecipitation. BMC Plant Biol. 2011;11:26. doi:10.1186/1471-2229-11-26.

[95] Fujisawa M, Shima Y, Nakagawa H, et al. Transcriptional regulation of fruit ripening by tomato FRUITFULL homologs and associated MADS box proteins. Plant Cell. 2014;26(1):89–101. doi:10.1105/tpc.113.119453.

[96] Kim ED, Sung S. Long noncoding RNA: unveiling hidden layer of gene regulatory networks. Trends Plant Sci. 2012;17:16–21. doi:10.1016/j.tplants.2011.10.008.

[97] Zhu QH, Wang MB. Molecular functions of long non-coding RNAs in plants. Genes (Basel). 2012;3:176–190. doi:10.3390/genes3010176.

[98] Liu J, Jung C, Xu J, et al. Genome-wide analysis uncovers regulation of long intergenic noncoding RNAs in *Arabidopsis*. Plant Cell. 2012;24(11):4333–4345. doi:10.1105/tpc. 112.102855.

[99] Boerner S, McGinnis KM. Computational identification and functional predictions of long noncoding RNA in *Zea mays*. PLoS One. 2012;7(8):e43047. doi:10.1371/journal.pone.0043047.

[100] Li L, Eichten SR, Shimizu R, Petsch K, Yeh CT, Wu W, Muehlbauer GJ. Genome-wide discovery and characterization of maize long non-coding RNAs. Genome Biol. 2014;15(2):R40. doi:10.1186/gb-2014-15-2-r40.

[101] Zhu B, Yang Y, Li R, et al. RNA sequencing and functional analysis implicate the regulatory role of long non-coding RNAs in tomato fruit ripening. J Exp Bot. 2015;66(15): 4483–4495. DOI:10.1093/jxb/erv203.

[102] Song J, Angel A, Howard M, Dean C. Vernalization—a cold-induced epigenetic switch. J Cell Science. 2012;125(16):3723–3731. doi:10.1242/jcs.084764.

[103] Jin J, Liu J, Wang H, Wong L, Chua NH. PLncDB: plant long noncoding RNA database. Bioinformatics. 2013;29(8):1068–1071. doi:10.1093/bioinformatics/btt107.

[104] Yi X, Zhang Z, Ling Y, Xu W, Su Z. PNRD: a plant non-coding RNA database. Nucleic Acids Res. 2015;43(D1):D982–D989. doi:10.1093/nar/gku1162.

[105] Jones-Rhoades MW, Bartel DP, Bartel B. MicroRNA and their regulatory roles in plants. Annu Rev Plant Biol. 2006;57:19–53. doi:10.1146/annurev.arplant. 57.032905.105218.

[106] Zhang B, Pan X, Cobb GP, Anderson TA. Plant microRNA: a small regulatory molecule with big impact. Dev Biol. 2006;289:3–16. doi:10.1016/j.ydbio.2005.10.036.

[107] Voinnet O. Origin, biogenesis, and activity of plant microRNAs. Cell. 2009;136:669–687. doi:10.1016/j.cell.2009.01.046.

[108] Brodersen P, Sakvarelidze-Achard L, Bruun-Rasmussen M, et al. Widespread translational inhibition by plant miRNAs and siRNAs. Science. 2008;320:1185–90. doi: 10.1126/science.1159151.

[109] Lanet E, Delannoy E, Sormani R, et al. Biochemical evidence for translational repression by *Arabidopsis* microRNAs. Plant Cell. 2009;21:1762–8. doi:10.1105/tpc. 108.063412.

[110] Itaya A, Bundschuh R, Archual AJ, et al. Small RNAs in tomato fruit and leaf development. Biochim Biophys Acta. 2008;1779:99–107. doi:10.1016/j.bbagrm.2007.09.003.

[111] Moxon S, Jing R, Szittya G, et al. Deep sequencing of tomato short RNAs identifies microRNAs targeting genes involved in fruit ripening. Genome Res. 2008;18:1602–9. doi:10.1101/gr.080127.108.

[112] Zhang J, Zeng R, Chen J, Liu X, Liao Q. Identification of conserved microRNAs and their targets from *Solanum lycopersicum* Mill. Gene. 2008;423:1–7. doi:10.1016/j.gene. 2008.05.023.

[113] Knapp S. Tobacco to tomatoes: a phylogenetic perspective on fruit diversity in the Solanaceae. J Exp Bot. 2002;53:2001–2022. doi:10.1093/jxb/erf068.

[114] Kim HJ, Baek KH, Lee BW, Choi D, Hur CG. In silico identification and characterization of microRNAs and their putative target genes in Solanaceae plants. Genome. 2011;54:91–98. doi:10.1139/G10-104.

[115] Hwang D-G, Park JH, Lim JY, et al. The hot pepper (*Capsicum annuum*) microRNA transcriptome reveals novel and conserved targets: a foundation for understanding MicroRNA functional roles in hot pepper. PLoS One. 2013;8:e64238. doi:10.1371/journal.pone.0064238.

[116] Gao J, Yin F, Liu M, et al. Identification and characterization of tobacco microRNA transcriptome using high-throughput sequencing. Plant Biol. 2014;17(3):591–598. doi: 10.1111/plb.12275.

[117] Lakhotia N, Joshi G, Bhardwaj AR, et al. Identification and characterization of miRNAome in root, stem, leaf and tuber developmental stages of potato (*Solanum tuberosum* L.) by high-throughput sequencing. BMC Plant Biol. 2014;14:6. doi: 10.1186/1471-2229-14-6.

[118] Griffiths-Jones S. The microRNA registry. Nucleic Acids Res. 2004;32:D109–11. doi: 10.1093/nar/gkh023.

[119] Griffiths-Jones S, Grocock RJ, van Dongen S, Bateman A, Enright AJ. miRBase: microRNA sequences, targets and gene nomenclature. Nucleic Acids Res. 2006;34:D140–4. doi:10.1093/nar/gkj112.

[120] Griffiths-Jones S, Saini HK, van Dongen S, Enright AJ. miRBase: tools for microRNA genomics. Nucleic Acids Res. 2008;36:D154–8. doi:10.1093/nar/gkm952.

[121] Kozomara A, Griffiths-Jones S. miRBase: integrating microRNA annotation and deep-sequencing data. Nucleic Acids Res. 2011;39:D152–7. doi:10.1093/nar/gkq1027.

[122] Kozomara A, Griffiths-Jones S. miRBase: annotating high confidence microRNAs using deep sequencing data. Nucleic Acids Res. 2014;42:D68–73. doi:10.1093/nar/gkt1181.

[123] Yang JH, Shao P, Zhou H, Chen YQ, Qu LH. DeepBase: a database for deeply annotating and mining deep sequencing data. Nucleic Acids Res. 2009;38:D123–D130. doi:10.1093/nar/gkp943.

[124] Betel D, Wilson M, Gabow A, Marks DS, Sander C. The microRNA.org resource: targets and expression. Nucleic Acids Res. 2008;36:D149–53.doi:10.1093/nar/gkm995.

[125] Alexiou P, Vergoulis T, Gleditzsch M, et al. miRGen 2.0: a database of microRNA genomic information and regulation. Nucleic Acids Res. 2010;38:D137–41. doi:10.1093/nar/gkp888.

[126] Hsu SD, Chu CH, Tsou AP, Chen SJ, Chen HC, Hsu PWC, Wong YH, Chen YH, Chen GH, Huang HD. miRNAMap 2.0: genomic maps of microRNAs in metazoan genomes. Nucleic Acids Res. 2008;36:D165–9. doi:10.1093/nar/gkm1012.

[127] Hsu SD, Tseng YT, Shrestha S, et al. miRTarBase update (2014): an information resource for experimentally validated miRNA-target interactions. Nucleic Acids Res. 2014;42:D78–85. doi:10.1093/nar/gkt1266.

[128] Zhang Z, Yu J, Li D, et al. PMRD: plant microRNA database. Nucleic Acids Res. 2010;38:D806–13. DOI:10.1093/nar/gkp818.

[129] Liu N, Wu S, Van Houten J, et al. Down-regulation of AUXIN RESPONSE FACTORS 6 and 8 by microRNA 167 leads to floral development defects and female sterility in tomato. J Exp Bot. 2014;65:2507–2520. doi:10.1093/jxb/eru141.

[130] Ferreira e Silva GF, Silva EM, Azevedo M da S, et al. microRNA156-targeted SPL/SBP box transcription factors regulate tomato ovary and fruit development. Plant J. 2014;78:604–18. doi:10.1111/tpj.12493.

[131] Chen W, Kong J, Lai T, et al. Tuning LeSPL-CNR expression by SlymiR157 affects tomato fruit ripening. Sci Rep. 2015;5:7852. doi:10.1038/srep07852.

[132] Yang JH, Li JH, Shao P, Zhou H, Chen YQ, Qu LH. starBase: a database for exploring microRNA-mRNA interaction maps from Argonaute CLIP-Seq and Degradome-Seq data. Nucleic Acids Res. 2011;39:D202–9. doi:10.1093/nar/gkq1056.

[133] Li JH, Liu S, Zhou H, Qu LH, Yang JH. starBase v2.0: decoding miRNA-ceRNA, miRNA-ncRNA and protein-RNA interaction networks from large-scale CLIP-Seq data. Nucleic Acids Res. 2014;42:D92–7. doi:10.1093/nar/gkt1248.

[134] Dweep H, Sticht C, Pandey P, Gretz N. miRWalk-database: prediction of possible miRNA binding sites by 'walking' the genes of three genomes. J Biomedical Informatics. 2011;44:839–847. doi:10.1016/j.jbi.2011.05.002.

[135] Lewis BP, Burge CB, Bartel DP. Conserved seed pairing, often flanked by adenosines, indicates that thousands of human genes are microRNA targets. Cell. 2005;120:15–20. doi:10.1016/j.cell.2004.12.035.

[136] Grimson A, Farh KK-H, Johnston WK, Garrett-Engele P, Lim LP, Bartel DP. MicroRNA targeting specificity in mammals: determinants beyond seed pairing. Mol Cell. 2007;27:91–105. doi:10.1016/j.molcel.2007.06.017.

[137] Friedman RC, Farh KK-H, Burge CB, Bartel DP. Most mammalian mRNAs are conserved targets of microRNAs. Genome Res. 2009;19:92–105. doi:10.1101/gr. 082701.108.

[138] Sethupathy P, Corda B, Hatzigeorgiou AG. TarBase: a comprehensive database of experimentally supported animal microRNA targets. RNA. 2006;12:192–7. doi:10.1261/ rna.2239606.

[139] Vlachos IS, Paraskevopoulou MD, Karagkouni D, et al. DIANA-TarBase v7.0: indexing more than half a million experimentally supported miRNA:mRNA interactions. Nucleic Acids Res. 2015;43:D153–9. doi:10.1093/nar/gku1215.

[140] Maragkakis M, Alexiou P, Papadopoulos GL, et al. Accurate microRNA target prediction correlates with protein repression levels. BMC Bioinformatics. 2009;10:295. doi:10.1186/1471-2105-10-295.

[141] Maragkakis M, Reczko M, Simossis VA, et al. DIANA-microT web server: elucidating microRNA functions through target prediction. Nucleic Acids Res. 2009;37:W273–6. doi:10.1093/nar/gkp292.

[142] Xiao F, Zuo Z, Cai G, Kang S, Gao X, Li T. miRecords: an integrated resource for microRNA-target interactions. Nucleic Acids Res. 2009;37:D105–10. doi:10.1093/nar/ gkn851.

[143] Krek A, Grün D, Poy MN, et al. Combinatorial microRNA target predictions. Nat Genet. 2005;37:495–500. doi:10.1038/ng1536.

[144] Loher P, Rigoutsos I. Interactive exploration of RNA22 microRNA target predictions. Bioinformatics. 2012;28:3322–3. doi:10.1093/bioinformatics/bts615.

[145] Chang TH, Horng JT, Huang HD. RNALogo: a new approach to display structural RNA alignment. Nucleic Acid Res. 2008;36:W91–6. doi:10.1093/nar/gkn258.

[146] Nam S, Kim B, Shin S, Lee S. miRGator: an integrated system for functional annotation of microRNAs. Nucleic Acids Res. 2008;36:D159–64. doi:10.1093/nar/gkm829.

[147] Cho S, Jun Y, Lee S, et al. miRGator v2.0: an integrated system for functional investigation of microRNAs. Nucleic Acids Res. 2011;39:D158–62. doi:10.1093/nar/gkq1094.

[148] Cho S, Jang I, Jun Y, et al. MiRGator v3.0: a microRNA portal for deep sequencing, expression profiling and mRNA targeting. Nucleic Acids Res. 2013;41:D252–7. doi: 10.1093/nar/gks1168.

[149] Wong N, Wang X. miRDB: an online resource for microRNA target prediction and functional annotations. Nucleic Acids Res. 2015;43:D146–52. doi:10.1093/nar/gku1104.

[150] Rehmsmeier M, Steffen P, Hochsmann M, Giegerich R. Fast and effective prediction of microRNA/target duplexes. RNA. 2004;10:1507–17. doi:10.1261/rna.5248604.

[151] Dai X, Zhao PX. psRNATarget: a plant small RNA target analysis server. Nucleic Acids Res. 2011;39:W155–9. doi:10.1093/nar/gkr319.

[152] Szczesniak MW, Makalowska I. miRNEST 2.0: a database of plant and animal micro-RNAs. Nucleic Acid Res. 2014;42:D74–7. doi:10.1093/nar/gkt1156.

[153] Sun X, Dong B, Yin L, et al. PMTED: a plant microRNA target expression database. BMC Bioinformatics. 2013;14:174. doi:10.1186/1471-2105-14-174.

[154] Bielewicz D, Dolata J, Zielezinski A, et al. mirEX: a platform for comparative exploration of plant pri-miRNA expression data. Nucleic Acid Res. 2012;40:D191–7. doi:10.1093/nar/gkr878.

[155] Bonnet E, He Y, Billiau K, Van de Peer Y. TAPIR, a web server for the prediction of plant microRNA targets, including target mimics. Bioinformatics. 2010;26:1566–1568. doi:10.1093/bioinformatics/btq233.

[156] Zhang S, Yue Y, Sheng L, et al. PASmiR: a literature-curated database for miRNA molecular regulation in plant response to abiotic stress. BMC Plant Biol. 2013;13:33. doi:10.1186/1471-2229-13-33.

[157] Luan Y, Cui J, Zhai J, Li J, Han L, Meng J. High-throughput sequencing reveals differential expression of miRNAs in tomato inoculated with *Phytophthora infestans*. Planta. 2015;1:1405–1416. doi:10.1007/s00425-015-2267-7.

[158] Ouyang S, Park G, Atamian HS, et al. MicroRNAs suppress NB domain genes in tomato that confer resistance to *Fusarium oxysporum*. PLoS Pathogens. 2014;10:e1004464. doi:10.1371/journal.ppat.1004464.

[159] Zhang X, Zou Z, Gong P, et al. Over-expression of microRNA169 confers enhanced drought tolerance to tomato. Biotechnology Letters. 2011;33:403–409. doi:10.1007/s10529-010-0436-0.

[160] Zhuang Y, Zhou XH, Liu J. Conserved miRNAs and their response to salt stress in wild eggplant *Solanum linnaeanum* roots. Int J Mol Sci. 2014;15:839–849. doi:10.3390/ijms15010839.

[161] Fan JB, Oliphant A, Shen R, et al. Highly parallel SNP genotyping. Cold Spring Harb. Symp Quant Biol. 2003;68:69–78

[162] Oliphant A, Barker DL, Stuelpnagel JR, Chee MS. BeadArray technology: enabling an accurate, cost-effective approach to high-throughput genotyping. Biotechniques. 2002;32:S56

[163] Bell PA, Chaturvedi S, Gelfand CA, et al. SNPstream UHT: ultra-high throughput SNP genotyping for pharmacogenomics and drug discovery. Biotechniques. 2002;32:S70–77

[164] Matsuzaki H, Loi H, Dong S, et al. Parallel genotyping of over 10,000 SNPs using a one-primer assay on a high-density oligonucleotide array. Genome Res. 2004;14:414–25. doi: 10.1101/gr.2014904

[165] Nijman IJ, Kuipers S, Verheul M, Guryev V, Cuppen E. A genome-wide SNP panel for mapping and association studies in the rat. BMC Genomics. 2008;9:95. doi: 10.1186/1471-2164-9-95

[166] Felcher KJ, Coombs JJ, Massa AN, et al. Integration of two diploid potato linkage maps with the potato genome sequence. PLoS One. 2012;7:e36347. doi:10.1371/journal.pone.0036347

[167] Gupta PK, Rustgi S, Mir RR. Array-based high-throughput DNA markers for crop improvement. Heredity. 2008;101:5–18. doi:10.1038/hdy.2008.35.

[168] Kennedy GC, Matsuzaki H, Dong S, et al. Large-scale genotyping of complex DNA. Nature Biotechnol. 2003;21:1233–1237. doi:10.1038/nbt869.

[169] Sim SC, Robbins MD, Chilcott C, Zhu T, Francis DM. Oligonucleotide array discovery of polymorphisms in cultivated tomato (*Solanum lycopersicum* L.) reveals patterns of SNP variation associated with breeding. BMC Genomics. 2009;10:10. doi: 10.1186/1471-2164-10-466.

[170] Elshire RJ, Glaubitz JC, Sun Q, et al. A robust, simple genotyping-by-sequencing (GBS) approach for high diversity species. PLoS One. 2011;6:e19379. doi:10.1371/journal.pone.0019379.

[171] Poland JA, Brown PJ, Sorrells ME, Jannink JL. Development of high-density genetic maps for barley and wheat using a novel two-enzyme genotyping-by-sequencing approach. PLoS One. 2012;7:e32253. doi:10.1371/journal.pone.0032253.

[172] Mascher M, Wu S, Amand PS, Stein N, Poland J. Application of genotyping-by-sequencing on semiconductor sequencing platforms: a comparison of genetic and reference-based marker ordering in barley. PLoS One. 2013;8:e76925. doi:10.1371/journal.pone.0076925.

[173] Uitdewilligen JG, Wolters AM, D'hoop BB, et al. A next-generation sequencing method for genotyping-by-sequencing of highly heterozygous autotetraploid potato. PLoS One. 2013;8:e62355. doi:10.1371/journal.pone.0062355.

[174] Rafalski JA. Association genetics in crop improvement. Curr Opin Plant Biol. 2010;13:174–180. doi:10.1016/j.pbi.2009.12.004.

[175] Ranc N, Munos S, Xu J, et al. Genome-wide association mapping in tomato (*Solanum lycopersicum*) is possible using genome admixture of *Solanum lycope*rsicum var. cerasiforme. G3 (Bethesda). 2012;2:853–864. doi:10.1534/g3.112.002667.

Chapter 10

Perspectives on the Application of Next-generation Sequencing to the Improvement of Africa's Staple Food Crops

Melaku Gedil, Morag Ferguson, Gezahegn Girma, Andreas Gisel, Livia Stavolone and Ismail Rabbi

Additional information is available at the end of the chapter

http://dx.doi.org/10.5772/61665

Abstract

The persistent challenge of insufficient food, unbalanced nutrition, and deteriorating natural resources in the most vulnerable nations, characterized by fast population growth, calls for utilization of innovative technologies to curb constraints of crop production. Enhancing genetic gain by using a multipronged approach that combines conventional and genomic technologies for the development of stress-tolerant varieties with high yield and nutritional quality is necessary. The advent of next-generation sequencing (NGS) technologies holds the potential to dramatically impact the crop improvement process. NGS enables whole-genome sequencing (WGS) and re-sequencing, transcriptome sequencing, metagenomics, as well as high-throughput genotyping, which can be applied for genome selection (GS). It can also be applied to diversity analysis, genetic and epigenetic characterization of germplasm and pathogen detection, identification, and elimination. High-throughput phenotyping, integrated data management, and decision support tools form the necessary support-ing environment for effective utilization of genome sequence information. It is important that these opportunities for mainstreaming innovative breeding strategies, enabled by cutting-edge "Omics" technologies, are seized in Africa; however, several constraints must be addressed before the benefit of NGS can be fully realized. African breeding programs must have access to high-throughput genotyping facilities, capacity in the application of genome selection and marker-assisted breeding must be built and supported by capacity in genomic analysis and bioinformatics. This chapter demonstrates how interventions with NGS-enabled innovative strategies can be applied to increase genetic gain with insights from the Consortium of International

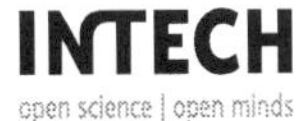

Agricultural Research (CGIAR) in general and the International Institute of Tropical Agriculture (IITA) in particular.

Keywords: Next-generation sequencing, genotype by sequencing, genome selection, plant breeding, genetic gain, developing countries

1. Introduction

Africa is the region with the highest prevalence of hunger and malnourishment. The persistent challenge of insufficient food, unbalanced nutrition, and deteriorating natural resources in the most vulnerable nations, characterized by fast population growth, calls for utilization of innovative technologies to curb constraints of crop production. Major revitalization of agricultural research in Africa is needed to underpin necessary increases in sustainable productivity in anticipation of the increase in population and changes in climate. Since many of the clonally propagated crops grown in Africa, such as cassava, yams, bananas, and plantains, and seed crops, such as cowpea, tef, sorghum, and millet, are not commonly consumed as food outside of the region, researchers in Africa have the responsibility to devise innovative breeding strategies for these crops. African agriculture is characterized by subsistence farming by smallholder farmers growing various locally adapted crops, many of which are considered understudied or "orphan" crops. These crops are vital for providing nutrition and income to resource-poor farmers, particularly in the face of confounding climatic and soil constraints. A regular supply of high-yielding nutritional varieties that respond to the changing biotic and abiotic stress environment is required. Conventional plant breeding has contributed tremendously to increased crop yields; however, the rate of genetic gain over the past few decades has been relatively slow for a number of reasons, including the lengthy breeding cycle, a characteristic of many clonally propagated crops [1]. Enhancing genetic gain entails a multifaceted approach of combining conventional and new technological advances [2,3].

The Consortium of International Agricultural Research, abbreviated as CGIAR, in collaboration with partners, is spearheading agricultural biotechnology research in Africa [4]. Several consortium research programs (CRP) are performing collaborative research on more than a dozen staple food crops of developing countries, including vegetatively propagated root, tuber, and banana (RTB), about seven grain legumes, and four dryland cereals. These crops support the livelihood of hundreds of millions of resource-limited farmers and traders in developing nations. The vegetatively propagated RTB crops (cassava, yam, potato, sweet potato, banana, and plantain) share many breeding challenges, including pathogen transmission from one generation to the next, polyploidy, low fertility and multiplication rates, and long breeding cycles. These can best be addressed by exploiting synergies across crops and technologies to increase genetic gain per unit time. Furthermore, the attainable yield potential of extensively studied crops such as rice, maize, wheat, and soybean are considerably lower in developing countries owing to unique production constraints in Africa calling for unique intervention, including genomics. Declining costs of DNA sequencing have triggered a surge in research on crops of local or regional importance and, with time, should translate into increased yields and yield stability, thus reducing the reliance on a smaller number of major crops [2,5–7].

This chapter initially outlines current and prospective genomic resources pertaining to Africa's staple crops, and then discusses how genomics strategies in the era of high-throughput next-generation sequencing technologies are being applied to increase genetic gain in developing countries with insights from CGIAR in general, and IITA in particular.

2. NGS-based omics resources: Current and prospective

2.1. Whole-genome sequencing

Knowledge of a crop genome sequence is fundamental for understanding biochemical and physiological processes that govern plant traits and the way in which they respond to environments- and biotic and abiotic stresses. The rapid evolution of genome sequencing technologies [8] has resulted in an explosion of genomic information, the sequencing of a vast number of plant genomes, and opportunities to apply this to crop improvement, e.g., through the development of genome-wide marker assays [9,10]. In the rapidly changing landscape of life science technologies, a number of new disciplines have emerged, particularly for deciphering gene function and metabolic pathways; these include transcriptomics, proteomics, metabolomics, small RNAomics, epigenomics, interactomics, together with the corresponding development of bioinformatics tools and databases to support these. It is important to ensure that, as our understanding of biological processes increases, this is translated into enhanced agricultural productivity through research for development (R4D).

The genome sequences of many major world crops have been completed in the past decade, as well as a few crops of specific importance to the developing world, including cassava, yam, tef, pigeon pea, and peanut, while many still remain to be sequenced [11–13]. A drive to sequence more crop plants, particularly orphan crops of Africa, is in progress. A recent public and private sector initiative called African Orphan Crops Consortium (AOCC, http://africa-norphancrops.org/) aims to sequence, assemble, and annotate the genomes of 100 traditional African food crops.

The cost of DNA sequencing per raw million bases fell from $8,000 to $0.1 between 2001 and 2013 according to Wetterstrand, K.A. (http://www.genome.gov/sequencingcosts/) cited in [8]. With the advent of the third-generation sequencing technologies, the cost is expected to reduce still further while the speed, quality, and throughput increase exponentially. Currently, most of the staple food crops that IITA is working on have been sequenced or are being sequenced (Table 1). The focus is thus on post-genomics analysis such as genome annotation and describing gene functions as applied to crop breeding. With a fledging bioinformatics capacity, and a network of partners in advanced laboratories as well as collaboration in the CRP of CGIAR, the breeding programs in IITA are moving toward molecular breeding for enhanced genetic gain with the aim to transfer these innovative genomics-assisted breeding schemes to our partners in the national agricultural research systems (NARS).

Species	Subspecies/ genotype	Family	Genome size (Mbp)	No. of predicted genes	Chromosome no. (2n)	Reference
Maize	*Zea mays ssp mays* B73	Poaceae	2,300	39,656	10	[15]
Soybean	*Glycine max,* variety Williams	Fabaceae	1,115	46,430	20	[16]
Cowpea	*Vigna unguiculata*	Fabaceae	620	5,888 GSRs	22	[17]
Cassava	*Manihot esculenta*	Euphorbiaceae	770	30,666	18	[18,19];
Banana	*Musa acuminata* (ssp. *malaccensis*)	Musaceae	523	36,542	22	[20]
Yam*	*Dioscorea rotundata*	Dioscoreaceae	594	21,882	20	[21]
Cacao	*Theobroma cacao* cv. *Matina*	Malvaceae	430	28,798	20	[22]

*At the time of the writing, manuscript is in preparation. Preliminary results were presented at an international conference.

Table 1. Current status of whole-genome sequences of IITA mandate crops

2.2. NGS-based genotyping and marker analysis

Massively parallel sequencing technology enabled high-throughput genotyping at an unprecedented scale. Whole-genome sequencing and re-sequencing of genome and transcriptome have yielded hundreds of thousands of single-nucleotide polymorphism (SNP) markers in several crop plants, including orphan crops. In recent years, diverse next-generation-based reduced representation protocols have been developed for the simultaneous discovery and generation of massive, genome-wide SNP data that have been applied to linkage mapping, quantitative trait locus (QTL) analysis, diversity studies, genome selection, and population genetics [14]. Protocols for reduced representation can be optimized to any species with or without a reference genome sequence [15]. The most widely used strategies for complexity reduction genotyping are restriction-site-associated DNA (RAD) [16] and genotyping by sequencing (GBS) [17], and diversity array technology (DArT)-seq, which combine complexity reduction methods and utilize a microarray platform [18]. All have been optimized for multiple plant species.

GBS protocols allow for a high level of multiplexing of up to 384 samples in one sequencing reaction, making it presently the most inexpensive and scalable assay with a library construction less complicated than RAD [19,20]. Researchers in developing countries presently focus on multiplex genotyping platforms such as GBS for genotyping cassava, yam, banana, maize, and cowpea for diversity analysis and molecular breeding. However, the deployment of such SNP markers in forward breeding, where only a few specific markers are tracked, entails the selection of suitable, cost-effective assays from a wide array of genotyping platforms such as fixed arrays or flexible singleplex assays [21]. Conversion of SNPs of interest into one of the above platforms requires bioinformatics analysis pipeline to design and optimize an assay. In the CGIAR systems, the Kompetitive Allele-Specific PCR (KASP) genotyping assay is widely applied (e.g., [22]). New initiatives are being developed to establish a cost-effective genotyping hub aiming to reduce the cost of data points by fivefold. Multiplex genotyping assays such as GBS, RAD, and DArT have been successfully used to identify SNP markers associated with the trait of interest in understudied crops. Examples include disease resistance in lupin [23], pepper [24], cassava [25,26], and beans [27].

Reduced representation sequencing (RRS)-based genotyping methods have the drawback of missing mutations at the recognition site of the restriction enzymes used [19]. The use of other enzyme combinations could circumvent this problem by altering the library construction [20, 28]. In addition, the accuracy of base calling in complex polyploids and heterozygous individuals, of which there are several examples within the root and tuber staple crops of Africa, can also be problematic. Given the rapid pace of advances in both the chemistry of sequencing such as the advent of the third-generation sequencing with longer read length and shorter assay time [29] and informatics pipelines (viz. imputation), the cost and accuracy of sequence-based genotyping are anticipated to decline in the foreseeable future.

2.3. NGS-based gene expression analysis

Transcriptomics is the study of the complete set of transcripts in a cell, and their quantity, for a specific developmental stage or physiological condition [30]. The transcriptome includes all RNA molecules, including mRNA, rRNA, tRNA, small RNAs, and other noncoding transcribed RNA and can vary with external environmental conditions. Transcriptomics studies often try to catalog these transcripts, as well as determining the transcriptional structure of genes, in terms of their start sites, 5′ and 3′ ends, splicing patterns, and other posttranscriptional modifications. By quantifying the expression levels of specific transcripts under different conditions or development stages, transcriptomics can help to understand the functional elements of the genome, including cellular processes and biochemical signaling pathways. Two main approaches have been used: based on hybridization and sequencing. Cassava is one of the very few African staple food crop to which microarrays have been applied [31–36].

Although hybridization approaches are relatively high throughput and inexpensive compared to the alternative expression assays, they do have technical limitations and require a priori knowledge of gene transcripts. NGS with its advantages of exceptional throughput and relative affordability has now enabled sufficient depth of sequencing for the study of whole transcriptome in a comprehensive manner. This method, termed RNA-Seq (RNA sequencing), has clear advantages over other existing approaches and is fast becoming the most popular method for analysis of eukaryotic transcriptome [30]. RNA-Seq also provides a far more precise measurement of levels of transcripts and their isoforms than other methods. To date, the majority of applications of RNASeq to Africa's staple crops have focused on understanding natural host responses to plant viruses. RNA sequencing was used to identify 700 uniquely overexpressed genes in the cassava brown streak disease (CBSD) resistant variety under cassava brown streak virus (CBSV) infection [37]. Although none of the overexpressed genes corresponded to known resistant gene orthologs, some belonged to hormone signaling pathways and secondary metabolites, both of which are linked to plant resistance. Similarly, the transcriptome of South African cassava mosaic virus-infected susceptible and tolerant landraces of cassava (12, 32, and 67 days post infection) was investigated [38]. Significantly, they found that susceptibility was mediated by transcriptome repression, rather than induction, and many R-gene homologues were repressed throughout infection in the susceptible individuals. In another study, NGS was deployed to investigate the role of miRNAs in plant growth and starch biosynthesis [39,40]. IITA and partners have completed an RNA-seq study in yam for the purpose of assembling the whole-genome sequence of *Dioscorea rotundata* and annotating predicted genes [41]. In addition, RNA-seq-based transcriptome has revealed rice genes involved in the signaling pathway for resistance to Striga [42] that may in turn shed light on the mechanism of resistance in other African crops that are vulnerable to Striga (e.g., maize, sorghum, and cowpea). Illumina-based sequencing of transcriptome from four underutilized leguminous crops has led to the development of markers for phylogenetics and comparative mapping [43]. NGS was used in modified bulk segregant RNA-seq (BSR-seq) method to clone a mutant gene in maize [44].

In addition, RNA-seq has been used successfully to address several production constraints of orphan crops [45–47], and it is envisaged that this will be a popular approach in the future. Other areas of interest for application of this technique are to understand the mechanism of Striga tolerance in maize and cowpea, yam anthracnose resistance, flowering and sex determination in yam, and drought tolerance in several crops (maize, cassava, cowpea). A single RNA-seq experiment involves taking samples at different stages of growth, tissue, and replicates. Multiplying the aforementioned factors by the number of crops and the number of traits per crops results in numerous libraries, which implies high assay cost. In this light, having in-house capacity to construct the libraries will significantly lower the cost and allow proper control of the experiment.

2.4. Bioinformatics and database

The field of bioinformatics has faced an unprecedented challenge, as a result of the new high-throughput technologies, particularly NGS, which has redefined the last decade of research in biology [48]. However, these technologies would never have made such progress without the attendant advances in the field of bioinformatics. Sequencing DNA and RNA has become so cheap and so vast that NGS is now a basic technology for many fields of research in medicine, basic research, as well as research in agriculture. In agricultural research, NGS is applied in whole-genome sequencing (WGS), whole-genome re-sequencing (WGRS), transcriptomics, metagenomics, and reduced representation sequencing for high-throughput SNP genotyping [15,21,28,29,49]. A genome sequence becomes only useful for biological applications when the genome is annotated and genes are described and their functions revealed [50]. Besides the functionality of genes, the variability of the genome of different varieties of a species is important to understand the different properties a species can demonstrate [13,51]. This last point together with the functionality information is a very important opportunity to support and improve breeding activities in crops of economic importance [52].

An extensive review of NGS data analysis is beyond the scope of this chapter. An insight into the status of NGS analytical tools and cross-references (articles, books, and dedicated issues of journals) are provided in a recent review [8]. The authors classified the NGS software tools into four general categories – alignment of sequence reads, base calling, and/or polymorphism detection, de novo, and genome browsing and annotation – and cited that a gamut of packages have been developed for each category by Barba et al. [8]. Of course, as the sequencing technology evolves, the bioinformatics software tools and algorithms have to be developed to keep pace with them. Likewise, workflow and various analysis strategies and challenges have been described for metagenomics [53–55].

The focus of this chapter is the application of NGS to the improvement of crops that are the mainstay of hundreds of millions of people in the developing world. Presently, the major application of NGS is genotyping by GBS and RNA-seq in crops such as cassava, yam, maize, banana, and cowpea, among others. Using these technologies necessitated the establishment of a moderate bioinformatics platform at IITA not only to serve basic bioinformatics needs but also to support the genotyping efforts in the aforementioned crops. The platform hosts the basic bioinformatics tools such as alignment and basic sequence analysis tools. For the data analysis of NGS data, the server is equipped with tools for de novo assembly [56] and mapping [57] as well as specific needs such as genotyping by sequencing [17], transcriptomics [58], noncoding RNA (ncRNA) [59,60], DNA methylation [61,62], and metagenomics [63] as new horizons to accelerate genetic gain.

It is worthwhile to describe some applications that are routinely run in IITA to support the research activities of IITA because, ultimately, the technologies are transferred to partner national research programs. GBS is a very cost-efficient genotyping approach by reducing the complexity of the genome and increasing the number of genotypes per sequencing round. There exist several bioinformatics pipelines to clean and analyze such data. IITA installed Tassel5 [64] and GATK [65] as the most useful tools. The Tassel plug-ins are assembled to a full automatic workflow to produce a filtered variant call format (VCF) file [66]. With Tassel, the bioinformatics server of IITA is able to easily analyze more than 5,500 genotypes in parallel having approximately 1.2 TB compressed sequencing data available. The analysis runs over 2 days using at most 250 GB RAM. The analysis picks about 350,000 SNPs, which get reduced by filtering to about 170,000 high-quality SNPs, which are a reasonable number for down-stream analyses such as population genetics and clustering as well as QTL analysis. The same workflow for genotyping is now applicable for different plant species, and analyses have been performed for cassava, *Dioscorea*, maize, and planned for *Musa*.

A workflow using Picard Tools and GATK is under construction and will be available for any kind of DNA sequencing data. IITA is also in the process of establishing a pipeline for the analysis of RNA-seq data using several available Illumina RNA sequencing data sets from contrasting genotypes. As a reference sequence was available, three different analyses were performed: a de novo sequence assembly to discover new unannotated genes or new alternative splice variants; mapping on the reference genome to elaborate the expression level of known, annotated genes; and the differential expression of selected genes between different genotypes. Such studies will become increasingly important for modern breeding programs since especially biotic and abiotic stresses are clearly regulated by different mechanisms other than purely genetic variations.

First experiments were conducted to study the DNA methylation profile on the model plant *Arabidopsis* to study epigenetic changes upon biotic stresses. A whole set of tools were installed and in-house scripts developed to analyze data derived from whole-genome bisulfide (BS) transformation [67]. The BS transformation converts non-methylated cysteine into a uracil and later, after polymerase chain reaction (PCR) amplification, into a thymine, whereas the methylated cysteine remains a cysteine. Since this technique is looking for single-nucleotide events and since the genomic code is "falsified," there is the need for a high-quality reference and specialized mapping strategies and statistics for the methylation calling [68]. The availability of a good-quality reference genome sequence of cassava and whole-genome re-sequencing of several clones of interest prompted DNA methylation profiling for some relevant cassava varieties. In this pilot study at IITA, currently in progress, the aim is to reveal dynamic methylation events under biotic and abiotic stresses to gain information on possible epigenetic markers for the next-generation breeding programs.

With the development of NGS noncoding RNA (ncRNA), especially the smaller species became very easy to detect, and many studies demonstrated that these ncRNAs are important players in gene regulation, regulation of DNA and histone methylation, and defense mechanisms in plants. ncRNA profiles are also important for diagnosing and characterizing virus infections in plants [69]. The virus infection triggers a defense reaction where a cascade of host ncRNA are involved, but also small interfering RNAs (siRNAs) corresponding to the viral genome are found in the plant extract. These endogenous ncRNA and the viral small RNA fragments can easily be detected by NGS. At IITA, we have the expertise and software suite of tools to search and analyze any plant ncRNAs or virus siRNAs. Again biotic and abiotic stresses in plants have a specific profile of expression of different species of ncRNA, and at IITA, we study this phenomenon to create information and tools to improve the breeding programs.

2.5. Genome editing

Genetics relies on the analysis of mutations and the phenotypic variation they cause to correlate precise sequence changes to particular genes of interest. With the help of genetic engineering techniques, desired traits can also be introduced into plants not expressing them naturally. However, the use of genetically modified crops is hindered by health, environmental, and ethical concerns. Genome editing with site-specific nucleases is the most advanced technology for precise and effective genome engineering, which promises to revolutionize applied research for crop improvement [70,71]. It involves the insertion, elimination, or replacement of a fragment of DNA at desired locations in the genome, by using engineered nucleases that create specific double-strand breaks (DSBs) and stimulate cellular DNA repair mechanisms. There are currently four classes of targetable nucleases discovered and bioengineered that are used to create site-specific DSB: zinc finger nucleases (ZFNs), transcription activator–like effector nucleases (TALENs), clustered regularly interspaced short palindromic repeat (CRISPR)/CRISPR-associated (Cas) RNA-guided nucleases (RGNs), and engineered meganuclease, also known as homing endonucleases [72–75].

Over the past few years, all of the above nucleases have been used to create target-specific mutations in model and crop plants, albeit with some limitations. In all cases, a continuing issue is the delivery of all the reagents efficiently and functionally to the cells or organisms under study. The CRISPR/CRISPR-associated protein 9 (Cas9) tool seems to overcome some of the shortcomings of the other methods [76,77]. Successful examples of targetable nucleases application are reported for *Arabidopsis*, tobacco, rice, maize, soybean, barley, cabbage, and bunchgrass by using different delivery technologies, including T-DNA plasmid from Agrobacterium, protoplasts and embryonic callus manipulation, and subsequent plant regeneration [70,78–82].

Targetable nucleases are attractive alternative biotechnological tools for trait manipulation and breeding in crop plants. By means of targetable nucleases, mutations can be produced in a very specific manner, and known mutations can be transferred between cultivars or breeding lines without disrupting a favorable genetic background. Although genome editing approaches are relatively new and not yet widely applied, their advantage in terms of safety, robustness, speed, and precision over the classical mutagenesis and breeding is undisputable [75]. Targeted genome editing using artificial nucleases, combined with accurate gene expression analyses, has the potential to accelerate plant breeding by providing the means to modify genomes rapidly in a precise and predictable manner [71] and to restore lost traits through reverse breeding [83]. Although genome editing has not yet been applied to African staple crop species, there is no doubt that this technology will assume a great importance particularly for genetic improvement of asexually propagated crops with limited flowering ability [71].

Furthermore, technologies based on targetable nucleases offer the opportunity to overcome the major concerns of the general public about transgenic crops since the organism with the edited gene do not contain the foreign DNA. In particular, the absence of extra copies of DNAs upon nonhomologous end joining (NHEJ)-mediated gene knockout makes the final plant comparable with those arising from natural mutations. However, the development of dedicated international legislations is required to effectively promote a wide application of genome editing technologies for crop improvement [70,84]. As knowledge is gained about plant genome organization and gene functions are revealed, the potential of genome editing could be mainstreamed to broaden the genetic base of crops.

2.6. Targeting Induced Local Lesions in Genomes (TILLING) and NGS-based mutation detection

One of the factors contributing to slow genetic gain in breeding of vegetatively propagated crops is the narrow genetic base of the source population. This is a result of clonal propagation as opposed to sexual reproduction, which limits recombination. TILLING (Targeting Induced Local Lesions in Genomes) [85,86] provides an alternative approach for creating novel variation in these crops [87,88]. Rare alleles harbored in germplasm collections and wild species can be accessed by TILLING and EcoTILLING by sequencing. TILLING may lead to the development of functional markers for screening-associated traits through marker-assisted selection (MAS). The technique of TILLING using high-throughput mutation discovery has already been applied successfully to more than 20 plant species [89].

A wide spectrum of mutation detection assays, ranging from heteroduplex analysis with high-pressure liquid chromatography (HPLC), screening with labeled primers, electrophoresis, microarray, the use of fluorescent dye-labeled primers assayed on ABI genetic analyzer have been used. However, these methods are generally slow, costly, and labor intensive. Application of NGS has been shown to be a cost-effective mutation detection system by re-sequencing the gene of interest in mutagenized plants [90,91]. The availability of genome sequence enables the use of reverse genetic approaches to identify mutations in specific target genes, thereby accelerating the generation of novel phenotypes. Comparative genome analysis methods offer the opportunity to select target genes involved in biosynthetic pathways and networks of traits/phenotypes of economic importance. The use of multidimensional pooling of DNA samples enables screening of DNA pools for multiple independent mutations in any target gene using NGS, which provides a cost-effective assay. This has led to the discovery of rare mutations in rice and wheat, termed TILLING by sequencing [92], tef [93], and in animals [94]. Different sample pooling schemes for NGS, which further enhance the power of NGS in processing multiple samples in parallel have been developed [95]. In light of the rapidly evolving sequencing technology together with a plethora of sample pooling schemes, combined with bar coding, it is feasible and imperative to apply TILLING by sequencing to understudied crops of Africa. A direct application of NGS to detect mutant regions in a segregating population of rice has been demonstrated in a method called MutMap [96].

2.7. QTL identification

This section discusses how NGS can be used to enhance QTL analysis. Following the advent of first-generation molecular markers such as restriction fragment length polymorphism (RFLP), random amplified polymorphic DNA (RAPD), and amplified fragment length polymorphism (AFLP), numerous studies in many crop species were launched to identify QTL, but for quantitative traits, affected by polygenes with small effects, limited success was attained in terms of application [97]. One of the explanations [98] for the limited exploitation of QTLs is the issues associated with the acquisition and summarizing of plethora of QTL information.

The rapid advance in next-generation sequencing technologies and the wide array of ultrahigh-throughput and cost-effective genotyping platforms have created a multitude of new possibilities for QTL mapping using large early-generation populations and high-density markers. Variants of NGS-based QTL identification methods, such as X-QTL, MutMap, QTL-seq, SHOREmap, and NGM, have been reviewed elsewhere [99]. Among the various NGS-based QTL mapping approaches, QTL-seq, the whole genome re-sequencing-based mapping of QTL [100], can successfully be applied to dissect key quantitative traits underlying biotic and abiotic stresses in major African staple food crops such as cassava, yam, tef, and legumes. One of the essential requirements for QTL-seq is the availability of a quality reference genome and mapping populations. The technique has been applied to rice where the whole genomes of two pooled rice DNA samples with contrasting phenotypes each in F2 and recombinant inbred line (RIL) populations were re-sequenced, after which the short reads were aligned to the reference sequence to calculate an SNP index. QTL were declared at positions where the SNP were different from the reference and had an SNP index value of 1. The analysis uses careful filtering of spurious SNPs. Conventional QTL mapping verified the candidate QTLs detected by the QTL-seq, and the method was validated by simulation analysis. QTL-seq has also been used in cucumber to map a QTL involved in flowering trait [101]. Likewise, the deployment of QTL-seq for rapid identification and fine mapping of QTLs was reported in chickpea [102] and sorghum [103].

In IITA, there are ongoing projects aiming to apply this technique to mapping of QTLs controlling disease resistance (e.g., anthracnose and yam mosaic virus), as well as root quality traits such as starch content. In cassava, the approach of genome-wide association study (GWAS) and conventional QTL mapping in F1 populations is being pursued to identify markers associated with key traits, including yield, dry matter, quality, and resistance to disease.

2.8. Metagenomics

Metagenomics is the direct genetic analysis of genomes contained within an entire community of organisms such as a microbial community, and makes use of NGS technologies and bioinformatics tools [104]. The advent of metagenomics has revolutionized the study of microbial ecology, evolution, and diversity. In plant pathology and virology, metagenomics has contributed to the sequencing of genomes within infected plants and has led to the detection of many RNA and DNA viruses and/or viroids. Other areas of application include ecology and epidemiology as well as functional genomics of pathogens, and the culture-independent analysis of a mixture of microbial genomes [8,105,106].

The application of metagenomics in crop improvement is discussed below in the disease diagnostics section as the majority of plant metagenomics studies, as applied to agriculture, relate to virology. However, there are substantial shotgun metagenome sequencing studies that investigate microbial communities in soil and plants and other environmental samples [105,107–109]. The challenges of analysis are being addressed gradually [55,104]. The analysis pipeline for metagenomics follows major steps such as raw data quality checking, filtering, assembly, taxonomic classification, abundance estimation, and relative quantification of taxons [53,54].

With growing experience in NGS data analysis and a fledging bioinformatics critical mass, IITA and partners are moving toward the application of meta-omics (-genomics, -transcriptomics, and -proteomics). In the context of African agriculture, the rapidly evolving field of metagenomics will have a significant impact in revealing the diversity of microorganisms, and in describing the relationship between host-associated microbial communities and host phenotype. The declining cost of sequencing and the associated analytical tools will likely create the opportunity to develop cost-effective and efficient diagnostic kits to address the challenge of multiple infections (pathogenic races and strains) in the major crops such as cassava [110], banana [111], and yams [112]. Survey of the incidence and distribution of viruses infecting these crops makes it one of the important tools for understanding the microbial genetics, physiology, and community ecology. The benefit of metagenomics extends to agriculturally important microbes, both disease causing and beneficial, in plant and animal production.

3. Application to crop improvement

3.1. Molecular breeding

The role of molecular markers in facilitating selection has substantially increased in the past three decades. The rapid accumulation of genomic resources provides researchers with an unprecedented wealth of information to access and manipulate genetic variation that is useful for crop improvement [113]. Genomics-assisted breeding is expected to enhance the accuracy and efficiency of breeding programs to deliver superior cultivars for sustainable agriculture. The ultrahigh throughput and decreasing cost of genotyping have elicited concepts such as genomics-assisted breeding [52] and breeding-assisted genomics [114]. Currently, the new paradigm among the Consortium of International Agricultural Research Centers (www.cgiar.org) is to mobilize "Omics" and bioinformatics-enabled interventions to assess the level of available genetic variation, to broaden the genetic bases by creating new intra- and inter-species variations, to construct new cultivars with combinations of desirable and novel traits in more efficient and effective selection schemes. The ultimate goal is to accelerate genetic gain, which will contribute to improved food and nutritional security, in an environmentally sustainable way, in low-income countries.

The unprecedented scientific and technological progress in the fields of genomics and bioinformatics can successfully be harnessed to benefit smallholder farmers in developing countries. In the face of limited agricultural inputs in developing countries, genetic improvement can play a crucial role in raising crop productivity in an environmentally sustainable way. Spurred by steadily declining costs of genotyping and unparalleled progress in computational abilities, modern genomic tools and processes are being used to devise an efficient and effective breeding strategy. The prominent constraints to breeding progress are slow genetic gain, complex traits, and genotype by environment interaction. Besides these generic constraints, neglected crops of Africa were affected by a paucity of genomic information until the dawn of NGS.

It is now feasible to access genome-wide nucleotide variation by re-sequencing the whole genome of thousands of accessions or by deploying one of the complexity reduction methods to generate high-density, genome-wide SNP markers associated with key agronomic traits attributed to quality, resilience to climate change, and biotic stresses. These technological advances led to the design of experimental populations involving multiple parents, in addition to the classical genetic mapping within specific biparental crosses. An overview of IITA's (and CGIAR's) activities in addressing crop productivity and other agricultural problems has been documented [4].

Evidence is emerging that the massive availability and accessibility of genomic resources and data management tools are paving the way for the deployment of innovative technologies to accelerate genetic gain. A number of recent reviews analyze the potential benefit of the Omics technologies to agricultural productivity and highlight various limitations that need to be addressed [19,27,52,115].

The two major approaches in the new paradigm of molecular breeding are (1) MAS for highly heritable traits and (2) GS for complex traits. These approaches involve the genotypic screening of large numbers of individuals at an early stage, selection at the seedling stage, and extensive phenotypic evaluation of fewer materials at a later stage. This reduced breeding cycles and the cost of multi-environment testing. Strategies such as GS also allow simultaneous selection for multiple traits through a selection index [52,116–119].

Broadly, there are two approaches to exploit QTLs. The first application is to detect large-effect QTLs with linkage or association analysis, whereas approaches such as GS utilize the computation of an individual breeding value based on genome-wide marker genotype, without taking into consideration the single small-effect QTLs in the prediction model.

Numerous reviews, opinion articles, and research papers have addressed the benefit, challenges, and prospect of GS crystallized in a recent review [113]. The salient features of GS include benefits such as increased gain from selection, reduced breeding cycles, and thus reducing cultivar development costs. Other advantages include utilization of genome-wide markers, afforded by ultrahigh-throughput NGS assays (compared to predecessor approaches to estimate breeding values), as well as the ability to target multiple traits for multiple environments. In clonally propagated crops, an additional advantage is the use of historical phenotype data to refine the prediction model.

Given the long cycle of breeding, African staple crops such as cassava are set to benefit from GS approaches [117,118,120], where preliminary results have indicated reduced time of breeding cycle and reasonable prediction accuracy in some traits. Various ways of refining the prediction models via repeated phenotypic evaluations are being considered. Fig. 1 depicts a 1-year GS-based breeding cycle that is underway at IITA, Nigeria. The challenge in this breeding scheme is, however, the situation of erratic flowering in some lines, which hinders recombination of selected clones due to failure to flower. Addressing the biology of flowering using genomics tools is imperative. In cereals, current studies are investigating at least two key applications of GS in maize and wheat breeding programs – predicting the genotypic values of individuals for potential release as cultivars and predicting the breeding value of candidates in rapid cycle populations. Prediction accuracy is affected by genetic relatedness of the populations and the heritability of the trait, where the prediction accuracy is lower in complex traits [121].

Utilization of molecular technologies that have revolutionized commercial crop breeding can be used as a proof of concept for adoption of such genomics-based prediction methodologies [122,123] to improve trait performance in other less-studied crops [115,116]. These approaches are being adopted in crops of importance in developing countries such as in maize and wheat [121], rice [124], pulses (legumes) [11], cassava [118,120], cowpea [125], lentil [126], soybean

[127,128], and pigeon pea [129]. With respect to the best practice for GS, various models are being put forward [113]. Below is the rapid cycling breeding scheme for cassava, a long cycle clonally propagated crop (Figure 1).

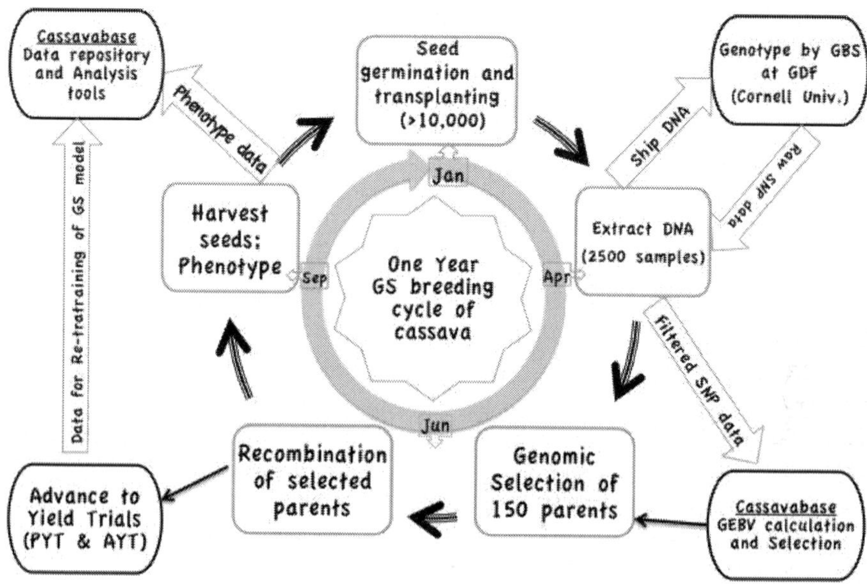

Figure 1. An overview of genomic selection-based annual breeding cycle implemented for cassava at the International Institute of Tropical Agriculture (IITA) in Nigeria. In June, crossing blocks are planted with parents selected using genomic selection and crosses made between September and November. Mature seeds are germinated and transplanted in January under irrigation. DNA is extracted from seedlings in March for genotyping by sequencing at the Genomic Diversity Facility (GDF). Raw SNP data are released to "Cassavabase" for further processing. Genomic-estimated breeding values (GEBVs) are then calculated and used to select candidate parents for the next recombination cycle. The remaining clones are also evaluated in clonal evaluation yield trials for variety development as well as for re-training the GS prediction model. **Cassavabase** (www.cassavabase.org): A bioinformatics infrastructure that integrates phenotypic data from field trials, genotypic data, as well as statistical tools in a single, user-friendly, web-based, and reliable database [130]. Breeders can use the intuitive web-based interphase to calculate genomic-estimated breeding values (GEBVs) of individuals by selecting a training population for modeling and estimating genomic-estimated breeding values of selection candidates (http://cassavabase.org/solgs). **GDF:** Genomic Diversity Facility (http://www.biotech.cornell.edu/brc/genomic-diversity-facility) provides expertise and state-of-the-art support for genotyping by sequencing (GBS) projects, including project optimization, library production, DNA sequencing, and data analysis.

It has now become evident that with advances in genotyping, fueled by NGS, phenotyping has become the rate-limiting step in genomics-enabled breeding. Concomitant development in phenotyping speed and precision is pivotal to associate genome with phenome [131] and to enable routine cost-effective high-throughput precision phenotyping. Approaches to increase throughput and quality of phenotyping range from automated and mechanized field experiment management, digital data capture, improved sample tracking methods, to deployment of ground-based and aerial advanced technologies in imaging and remote sensing [132–135].

Precision phenotyping has led to accelerated genetic gain by increasing heritability, mainly through reducing environmental variation [116,131], and reduced cost of trait measurement. Furthermore, robust and standardized screening protocols and the establishment of phenotyping hubs for abiotic (drought, nutrient use efficiency) and biotic (pest and disease hotspots) stresses are key elements for precision phenotyping to dissect the genetics of quantitative traits.

Leveraging existing data management and decision support tools to accommodate new data types and analytical tools, including digitized data collection (e.g., personal digital assistant (PDA), electronic field books) and sample tracking using bar codes, will be keys to the ultimate success of genomics breeding in developing countries.

3.2. Genetic resource management and utilization

Genebanks play an important role in safeguarding crop genetic diversity against the ongoing loss. They provide genetic variation for breeding for continued adaptation to changing environmental conditions and consumer demands [136,137]. The recent progress in DNA sequencing technologies that require less investment for generating large data is an opportunity to further investigate genetic variation maintained in the large germplasm collections held in trust by the CGIAR and increase the efficiency of genebanks. The 11 genebanks of the CGIAR conserve over 666,000 accessions of mainly food crops [138]. The International Institute of Tropical Agriculture (IITA) maintains over 28,000 accessions of major food crops of Africa, namely cowpea (*Vigna unguiculata*), cassava (*Manihot esculenta*), yam (*Dioscorea* spp.), soybean (*Glycine max*), bambara groundnut (*Vigna subterranea*), maize (*Zea mays*), and plantain and banana (*Musa* spp.). The aforementioned, including other important crops in developing countries [e.g., finger millet (*Eleusine coracana*), tef (*Eragrostis tef*), enset (*Ensete ventricosum*), grass pea (*Lathyrus sativus*) and their wild relatives], were considered understudied [2]. Large-scale characterization of all accessions and other genetic stocks is imperative to stimulate their utilization in breeding programs [139,140].

Traditionally, genebanks have used morphological descriptors for germplasm characterization; however, these are highly influenced by environmental conditions and different stages of plant development [141]. Moreover, the number of descriptors can be quite limited, thus greatly reducing the power to distinguish consanguineous varieties [142]. Molecular marker technologies have been widely applied for characterization and utilization of germplasm in genebanks [143]. However, the marker systems used prior to the advent of NGS, which sample a subset of the genome, have restricted applications mainly because of their limited abundance in the genome. NGS has enabled marker analysis at a much higher density. NGS-based genotyping, such as GBS, has been used for genetic diversity assessment of cultivated yam and its wild relatives [144] and cocoa [145], as well as other crop species. Breeding programs in the public and private sector deploy whole-genome fingerprinting of inbreds, to get an insight into the haplotype-level genetic diversity [116,140,146].

The advance in sequencing technologies is an advantage for efficient sequencing of large collections that include poorly studied species in genebanks with larger analytical power than the conventional molecular marker systems. Diversity assessments per se have huge utility in terms of germplasm utilization, such as definition of heterotic groups that enable breeders to make decisions in planning crosses for the population development. In addition to diversity assessment, NGS-based technologies are likely to impact further analysis of genetic variation, in terms of characterization of functional genetic diversity [148] and can be applied to pre-breeding activities to boost utilization of genetic resources in breeding programs [29,52,147].

NGS can also be applied to enhance management aspects of the genebanks, including identifying duplicates and identification of mislabeled accessions, both of which are common challenges in genebanks [148]. Diversity assessments using NGS could help guide the need for further targeted germplasm collection and improve the development of subsets of the collection, also referred to as core or minicore or diversity research sets, that would further improve the efficient utilization of germplasm for cultivar development.

A strong genomics and bioinformatics platform will greatly facilitate essential elements of genebank management, particularly the verification of accession identity, characterization of duplicates in the collection, and diversity analysis. Furthermore, rapid genotyping methods (e.g., GBS and WGS) will be essential for allele mining and large-scale association of genotype–phenotype, which are taken together with methods of developing trait-specific subsets, also referred to as core or mini core or diversity research sets, to greatly enhance the value of the collections for breeding and research. In particular gene pool, enhancement (pre-breeding) will be strengthened in terms of both base broadening within a species and use of crop wild relatives for the integration of key traits. Such approaches can be applied not only to staple crops but also to obtain rapid advances in the improvement of underutilized and under-researched but important crops such as cocoyam, winged bean, and African yam bean.

3.3. Breeding data management

The adoption of new Omics technologies by breeding programs in developing countries can contribute to the enhancement of breeding efficiency. There is a growing effort to harness advances in bio-computational methods and information and communication technology (ICT) to successfully utilize diverse phenotypic, environmental, genomic, and other metadata to provide decision support tools at various stages of the breeding pipeline. Modern breeding schemes such as GS and MAS involve a deluge of genotype data such as GBS-derived SNP markers, advanced statistical analysis to compute GEBV, and large amounts of high-throughput phenotype information, all of which require efficient informatics tools, automated data analysis pipelines, and decision-making tools for analysis and integration. Efficient utilization of such unprecedented volumes of genotypic, phenotypic, and other data entails development of informatics, database, and decision support tools.

Access to affordable genotyping platform by scientists in developing countries has been realized through various bilateral research-for-development projects. However, it is inconceivable to make progress without modern breeding tools and management processes that will facilitate the integration, analysis, and decision-making tools. One initiative that aims at providing some of these tools is the breeding management system (BMS) developed and promoted by the integrated breeding platform (IBP) (https://www.integrated-breeding.net/breeding-management-system). The service of BMS is delivered by IBP regional hubs that are strategically located throughout developing countries and hosted by partner research institutions such as IITA in Nigeria. The hubs provide support for adoption, customization, and use of BMS and related services, mainly through capacity building, technical support, and crop-specific expertise. Presently, IBP comprises ready-to-use information and tools for over 10 crops, including diagnostic markers and trait dictionaries.

In today's Omics era, web-based, peer-reviewed molecular databases and web servers abound [149]. An annual issue of the journal "Nucleic Acid Research" is dedicated to databases and web servers and documents a wide spectrum of databases, including a substantial number on plant databases. A comprehensive list of genomic resources (platforms and databases) relevant to genomics-enabled crop improvement, including genome sequences of crop plants, has been published recently [12]. Table 2 provides a partial list of deployed or planned breeding-relevant technology and tools currently in use. The Kazusa marker database [150] features genomics and genetics information for 10 plant species, whereas SolGenomics is a portal for several solanaceous plant species [130]. These and other breeders' toolboxes such as Soybase and MaizeGDB can serve as a starting point for comparative analysis of orphan crops with limited genomic resources.

Developments of several other similar and complementary custom-made breeding toolboxes are underway in various projects implemented in developing countries. A concerted effort by multidisciplinary teams, galvanized by various consortium research programs (CRPs), including national programs, are diligently working on development of pipelines for connecting diverse types of data to appropriate analytical tools and for processing imaging and remote sensing phenotype data.

The multidisciplinary nature of modern plant breeding/genetic research is underpinned by acquisition, analysis, and utilization of "big data" not only from field trials but also from laboratory analyses. Laboratory analysis includes analytical chemistry for profiling nutritional content and other metabolites, which entails efficient data management system. Moreover, high-density genome-wide marker data generated from next-generation sequencing for marker–trait associations as well as whole-genome expression profiling are increasingly being utilized for crop improvement pipelines. A comprehensive open-access database comprising phenotype and marker data, trial design, and analysis pipeline is a must-have to aid in streamlined integration of various data from plant breeding, including phenotypes recorded from field trials; genotypic data, gene expression, and analytical chemistry requires reliable and user-friendly database. Such a database must also have inbuilt quantitative genetics analysis tools/pipelines that would allow breeders to not only store and retrieve raw data but also calculate breeding values and selection index, design crosses, as well as field trials.

Moreover, discovery research such as QTL mapping can be done on the database through implementation of genetic mapping methods.

Project/Host	Database/Tool	Purpose	URL	Remark/ Reference
Integrated breeding platform	Breeding management system (BMS*)	Tools for Crop information management Nursery and trial management Statistical analysis Marker-assisted breeding	https:// www.integratedbreedi ng.net/	Current regional hubs: 4 in Africa, 3 in Asia
Cassavabase	NextGen cassava breeding project; Boyce Thompson Institute for Plant Research	Breeders toolbox; maps and markers; genes; phenotypes; genome sequences	http:// www.cassavabase.org/	Implemented based on SolGenomics
SolGenomics	Sol Genomics Network, Boyce Thompson Institute for Plant Research	Tomato, pepper, potato, coffee, Nicotiana, Petunia, and other solanaceous plants	http://solgenomics.net/	[159]
Soybase	USDA, Soybean Genetics Database Iowa State University	Soybean breeder's toolbox and database including genome sequences, maps, markers, genetic stocks (including mutants)	http:// www.soybase.org/	[160]
MaizeGDB	USDA funded maize genetics and genomics database	Community-oriented informatics service featuring genome browser, maps, locus, gene, QTL, diversity, metabolic pathways and others	http://maizegdb.org/	[161]
Phytozome	Department of Energy's Joint Genome Institute	The Plant Comparative Genomics portal for sequenced and annotated green plant genomes and phylogenetics	http:// phytozome.jgi.doe.gov/ pz/portal.html	[162]
Kazusa	Kazusa DNA Research Institute	SSR markers and linkage maps for 10 plant species	http:// marker.kazusa.or.jp	[158]

*BMS, hosted by IITA as a regional hub for integrated breeding platform (IBP), is a suite of interconnected software specifically designed to help breeders manage their day-to-day activities through all phases of their breeding programs.

Note: Other CGIAR-driven initiatives include Genomic and Open-source Breeding Informatics Initiative (GOBII), Integrated Genotyping Service and Support at Biosciences eastern and central Africa (BECA)/International Livestock Research Institute (ILRI), and Shared Industrial-Scale High-Throughput Genotyping Facility for delivering high-density genomics breeder's tools and low-cost genotyping services.

Table 2. Partial list of crop- or project-specific databases and breeder's toolboxes relevant to breeders in developing nations that are in use or in progress.

4. Disease diagnostics and monitoring

Plant diseases are caused by a wide array of pathogens, including viruses, bacteria, and fungi. A combination of techniques, including microscopy, serological [e.g., enzyme-linked immunosorbent assay (ELISA)], and molecular (e.g., PCR) techniques, are used in detection and identification of pathogens associated with major diseases of African food staples. Conventional methods of virus diagnostics, using antibodies and PCR, often lack the sensitivity to detect viruses that exist in low abundance and emerging viruses with unknown genomes. Therefore, next-generation deep sequencing approaches and bioinformatics analysis can be used for de novo assembly of virus and viroid genomes, to perform reliable characterization and diagnostics of known and unknown viruses and viroids [112,154,155]. In the wake of NGS technologies, powerful and high-throughput novel approaches, such as metagenomics, have been developed and widely used to analyze nucleotide sequence of microbial populations in plant samples (see section 2.8) [8,105,156]. In particular, deep sequencing of small RNA families such as short interfering RNAs (siRNAs) can be used to identify and reconstruct any DNA or RNA virus genome and its microvariants with the help of bioinformatics tools [155,157]. Furthermore, the application of NGS can be extended to insect vectors for discovery and characterization of insect viruses [109].

The potential use of NGS technologies for diagnostic programs in quarantine and certification of some fruits have been demonstrated (reviewed in [8]). Existing diagnostics tools that are deployed in several clonally propagated crops (cassava, yam, banana) for quarantine monitoring during exchange of planting material can be enhanced using NGS. In IITA, diagnostic tools have been combined with digital data capture tools for real-time surveillance and rapid diagnosis. This has been put to use for monitoring pathogens of cassava and banana in East Africa.

5. Conclusions: Prospects and perspectives

The productivity of staple food crops of hundreds of millions of people in developing countries is stagnating or diminishing as natural resources are depleted as a result of overcultivation and poor resource management, among other factors. Genetic improvement is heralded as the best option to enhance crop productivity, resilience to climate effects, and nutritional quality. The effective and efficient application of advanced biosciences tools and products holds substantial promise for enhanced agricultural productivity, improved livelihoods, and better prospects for food and nutrition security in Africa, where less-studied crops are grown as staples [114,115,158]. Genomics-enabled breeding will enable scientists to more effectively tap into the wealth of genetic variation in landraces and wild relatives for novel traits.

Next-generation sequencing has evolved to the third generation of sequencing technology and boasts even longer read length, shorter run time, and lower cost per unit data [21]. Applications of NGS are broadening at a remarkable pace from whole-genome sequencing and re-sequencing to transcript sequencing, metagenomics, and methylome sequencing. Thus, the application of NGS in agriculture is now vital to breeding, diagnosis, evolution, ecology, and basic functional genomics. SNP markers are already becoming the predominant marker types in modern breeding strategies [21,29]. Additional outcomes include the dissection of biochemical and genetic mechanisms or metabolic pathways underlying agronomically important traits, leading to a better understanding of how the genome and phenome are related [114].

The ultrahigh-throughput capacity of NGS platforms and the commercial scale of automated pipelines make it cheaper to outsource genotyping services such as GBS and RAD. Capital investment in state-of-the-art genomics facilities in all laboratories is not prudent for several reasons. However, establishment of shared resources at regional and subregional center of excellence, such as BECA, is fully recognized by stakeholders. The West Africa Biotechnology Initiative (WABI), copromoted by IITA and subregional organizations such as CORAF/WECARD (West and Central African Council for Agricultural Research and Development), is promoting such an idea and mobilizing resources toward this goal. This is likely to reduce turnaround times for GBS samples, and raise the quality of cDNA libraries.

Mainstreaming this highly promising but complex and rapidly evolving next-generation breeding scheme entails continuous training and effective information sharing. Although recent scientific progress heralded the era of molecular breeding, most public sector researchers in Africa are far from harvesting the fruit of the technological advances.

Reasons for this range from limited awareness of the technological advances to lack of adequate infrastructure, knowledge, and limited resources that are required to make use of markers in crop breeding. In recent times, that trend is changing as research institutions operating in Africa (international, regional, and national systems) strive relentlessly to accelerate the adoption and application of advanced biosciences tools in support of the region's agricultural transformation. WABI is striving to establish a center of excellence to promote the adoption of biotechnology to enable innovative approaches, resulting in increased crop yield. Availability of training and service platforms in various subregions of Africa (e.g., West and Central, East and South) will not only make it more affordable and accessible to the users and trainees in the continent but also focus more on the needs that are specific to the region's research.

Developing in-house capacity for GBS data analysis pipeline, NGS library construction, and automated DNA extraction is fundamental for routine applications of GS/MAS in breeding programs. The spectacular diffusion of ICT throughout Africa, particularly mobile phone technology and smart devices, paves the way for access to web-based education and genomic resources. Given the poor connectivity in developing countries, however, developing Internet-free databases and tools is necessary in the interim.

Efficient data management systems are a prerequisite for applying genomic information by international, national, and private sectors involved in improving the rate of genetic gain in crops. WGS and assembly require advanced instruments, skilled personnel, and strong computational capacities. It also requires improvement of assembly and continual annotation of genes as more and more information is generated by whole-genome re-sequencing or functional genomics. Integration of genomics information with other phenotypic and environment data also requires strong skill in programming and database development. Moreover, processing of big data requires basic programming skills in order to automate routine data manipulation and processing needs. Thorough knowledge in bioinformatics will afford the ability to apply comparative genomics with the aim of extending the power of genomics to orphan crops with little DNA sequence information.

The bioinformatics infrastructure at IITA can serve as a model for similar start-up bioinformatics units at the national program. Such platform hosts most of the standard bioinformatics tools to deal with any kind of sequence analysis, including shotgun and targeted DNA/RNA sequences. Importantly, analysis pipeline for GBS data is very essential for routine application of genomics in selection schemes.

Such an effort demands full engagement and transformation in the policy of national programs and other stakeholders. As expressed in previous views [52,159], relevant short-term and long-term training and institutional capacity building should be intensified. Academic institutions need to revise their curricula to develop expertise in NGS data analysis and bioinformatics. The participation of the fledging private sector also needs to be boosted.

It is clear that certain activities such as efficient DNA extraction and associated databases and decision-making breeding tools may need to operate at local levels; other activities such as GBS, SNP genotyping for forward breeding, NGS, and training may need to operate at regional levels; and curation of whole crop databases and development of analysis tools may operate at global levels. It is vital that communication occurs at all of these levels and across levels, including international institutes, NARS, and universities, and that the system remains responsive to the rapidly changing scientific environment, if NGS is to close the yield gap of staple crops in Africa.

6. Acronyms

AOCC; African Orphan Crops Consortium

BMS; Breeding management system

BS; Bisulfide

Cas9; CRISPR-associated protein 9

CBSD; Cassava brown streak disease

CBSV; Cassava brown streak virus

CGIAR; The Consortium of International Agricultural Research

CORAF/

WECARD; West and Central African Council for Agricultural Research and Development

CRISPR; Clustered regularly interspaced short palindromic repeat

CRP; Consortium research programs

DArT; Diversity Array Technology

DSB; Double-strand breaks

GBS; Genotyping by sequencing

GDF; Genomic Diversity Facility

GEBV; Genomic-estimated breeding value

GS; Genome selection

GWAS; Genome-wide association study

IBP; Integrated breeding platform

ICT; Information and communication technology

IITA; International Institute of Tropical Agriculture

KASP; Kompetitive Allele-Specific PCR

MAS; Marker-assisted selection

NARS; National agricultural research systems

ncRNA; Noncoding RNA

NGS; Next-generation sequencing

NHEJ; Nonhomologous end joining

PDA; Personal digital assistant

QTL; Quantitative trait loci

R4D; Research for development

RAD; Restriction-site-associated DNA

RGN; RNA-guided nucleases

RRS; Reduced representation sequencing

RTB; Root, tuber, and banana

siRNA; small interfering RNA

SNP; Single nucleotide polymorphism

TALENs; Transcription activator–like effector nucleases

TILLING; Targeting Induced Local Lesions in Genomes

WGS; Whole-genome sequencing

ZFN; Zinc finger nuclease

WABI; The West Africa Biotechnology Initiative (WABI),

Author details

Melaku Gedil[1*], Morag Ferguson[1], Gezahegn Girma[1], Andreas Gisel[1,2], Livia Stavolone[1,3] and Ismail Rabbi[1]

*Address all correspondence to: m.gedil@cgiar.org

1 International Institute of Tropical Agriculture, Ibadan, Nigeria

2 Institute for Biomedical Technologies – CNR, Bari, Italy

3 Institute for Sustainable Plant Protection – CNR, Bari, Italy

References

[1] Gedil M, Sartie AM. Perspectives on molecular breeding of Africa's main staple food crops – cassava and yam. Asp Appl Biol 2010;96:123–36.

[2] Varshney RK, Glaszmann J-CC, Leung H, Ribaut J-MM. More genomic resources for less-studied crops. Trends Biotechnol 2010;28:452–60. doi:10.1016/j.tibtech. 2010.06.007.

[3] Ribaut J-M, de Vicente MC, Delannay X. Molecular breeding in developing countries: challenges and perspectives. Curr Opin Plant Biol 2010;13:213–18.

[4] Gedil M, Tripathi L, Ghislain M, Ferguson M, Ndjiondjop M, Kumar PL, et al. Biotechnology success stories by the Consultative Group on International Agriculture Research (CGIAR) system. In: Wambugu F, Kamanga D, editors. Biotechnology in Africa: Emergence, Initiative and Future. Springer, Heidelberg. 2014, p. 95-114.

[5] Armstead I, Huang L, Ravagnani A, Robson P, Ougham H. Bioinformatics in the orphan crops. Brief Bioinform 2009;10:645–53.

[6] Varshney RK, Ribaut J-MM, Buckler ES, Tuberosa R, Rafalski JA, Langridge P. Can genomics boost productivity of orphan crops? Nat Biotechnol 2012;30:1172–76.

[7] Tadele Z, Esfeld K, Plaza S. Applications of high-throughput techniques to the understudied crops of Africa. Asp Appl Biol 2010;96:233–40.

[8] Barba M, Czosnek H, Hadidi A. Historical perspective, development and applications of next-generation sequencing in plant virology. Viruses 2014;6:106–36. doi: 10.3390/v6010106.

[9] Rius M, Bourne S, Hornsby HG, Chapman MA. Applications of next-generation sequencing to the study of biological invasions. Curr Zool 2015;61:488–504.

[10] Nybom H, Weising K, Rotter B. DNA fingerprinting in botany: past, present, future. Investig Genet 2014;5:1-35. doi:10.1186/2041-2223-5-1.

[11] Bohra A, Pandey MK, Jha UC, Singh B, Singh IP, Datta D, et al. Genomics-assisted breeding in four major pulse crops of developing countries: present status and prospects. Theor Appl Genet 2014;127:1263–91. doi:10.1007/s00122-014-2301-3.

[12] Dhanapal AP, Govindaraj M. Unlimited thirst for genome sequencing, data interpretation, and database usage in genomic era: the road towards fast-track crop plant improvement. Genet Res Int 2015;2015:1–15.

[13] Michael TP, Vanburen R. Progress, challenges and the future of crop genomes. Curr Opin Plant Biol 2015;24:71-81.

[14] Rowe HC, Renaut S, Guggisberg A. RAD in the realm of next-generation sequencing technologies. Mol Ecol 2011. 20:3499-3502. doi:10.1111/j.1365-294X.2011.05197.x.

[15] Leggett RM, MacLean D. Reference-free SNP detection: dealing with the data deluge. BMC Genomics 2014;15:S10. doi:10.1186/1471-2164-15-S4-S10.

[16] Baird NA, Etter PD, Atwood TS, Currey MC, Shiver AL, Lewis ZA, et al. Rapid SNP discovery and genetic mapping using sequenced RAD markers. PLoS One 2008;3:1–7. doi:10.1371/journal.pone.0003376.

[17] Elshire RJ, Glaubitz JC, Sun Q, Poland JA, Kawamoto K, Buckler ES, et al. A robust, simple genotyping-by-sequencing (GBS) approach for high diversity species. PLoS One 2011;6:1–10. doi:10.1371/journal.pone.0019379.

[18] Kilian A, Wenzl P, Huttner E, Carling J, Xia L, Blois H, et al. Diversity arrays technology: a generic genome profiling technology on open platforms. Methods Mol Biol 2012;888:67–89. doi:10.1007/978-1-61779-870-2_5.

[19] He J, Zhao X, Laroche A, Lu Z, Liu H, Li Z. Genotyping-by-sequencing (GBS), an ultimate marker-assisted selection (MAS) tool to accelerate plant breeding 2014;5:1–8. doi:10.3389/fpls.2014.00484.

[20] Hamblin MT, Rabbi IY. The effects of restriction-enzyme choice on properties of genotyping-by-sequencing libraries: a study in cassava (*Manihot esculenta*). Crop Sci 2014;54:2603–08. doi:10.2135/cropsci2014.02.0160.

[21] Thomson MJ. High-throughput SNP genotyping to accelerate crop improvement. Plant Breed Biotechnol 2014;2:195–212. doi:10.9787/PBB.2014.2.3.195.

[22] Semagn K, Babu R, Hearne S, Olsen M. Single nucleotide polymorphism genotyping using Kompetitive Allele Specific PCR (KASP): overview of the technology and its application in crop improvement. Mol Breed 2014;33:1–14. doi:10.1007/s11032-013-9917-x.

[23] Yang H, Tao Y, Zheng Z, Li C, Sweetingham M, Howieson J. Application of next-generation sequencing for rapid marker development in molecular plant breeding: a

case study on anthracnose disease resistance in *Lupinus angustifolius* L. BMC Genomics 2012;13:318. doi:10.1186/1471-2164-13-318.

[24]   Devran Z, Kahveci E, Özkaynak E, Studholme DJ, Tör M. Development of molecular markers tightly linked to Pvr4 gene in pepper using next-generation sequencing. Mol Breed 2015;35:101. doi:10.1007/s11032-015-0294-5.

[25]   Rabbi IY, Hamblin MT, Kumar PLL, Gedil MA, Ikpan AS, Jannink JL, et al. High-resolution mapping of resistance to cassava mosaic geminiviruses in cassava using genotyping-by-sequencing and its implications for breeding. Virus Res 2014;186:87–96. doi:10.1016/j.virusres.2013.12.028.

[26]   Rabbi I, Hamblin M, Gedil M, Kulakow P, Ferguson M, Ikpan AS, et al. Genetic mapping using genotyping-by-sequencing in the clonally propagated cassava. Crop Sci 2014;54:1384–96. doi:10.2135/cropsci2013.07.0482.

[27]   Hart JP, Griffiths PD. Genotyping-by-sequencing enabled mapping and marker development for the potyvirus resistance allele in common bean. Plant Genome 2015;8:1-14. doi:10.3835/plantgenome2014.09.0058.

[28]   Sonah H, Bastien M, Iquira E, Tardivel A, Légaré G, Boyle B, et al. An improved genotyping by sequencing (GBS) approach offering increased versatility and efficiency of SNP discovery and genotyping. PLoS One 2013;8:1–9. doi:10.1371/journal.pone.0054603.

[29]   Egan AN, Schlueter J, Spooner DM. Applications of next-generation sequencing in plant biology. Am J Bot 2012;99:175–85. doi:10.3732/ajb.1200020.

[30]   Wang Z, Gerstein M, Snyder M. RNA-Seq: a revolutionary tool for transcriptomics. Nat Rev Genet 2009;10:57–63. doi:10.1038/nrg2484.

[31]   Lopez C, Jorge V, Piégu B, Mba C, Cortes D, Restrepo S, et al. A unigene catalogue of 5700 expressed genes in cassava. Plant Mol Biol 2004;56:541–54. doi:10.1007/s11103-004-0123-4.

[32]   Anderson JV, Delseny M, Fregene MA, Jorge V, Mba C, Lopez C, et al. An EST resource for cassava and other species of Euphorbiaceae. Plant MolBiol 2004;56:527–39. doi:10.1007/s11103-004-5046-6.

[33]   Reilly K, Bernal D, Cortés DF, Gómez-Vásquez R, Tohme J, Beeching JR. Towards identifying the full set of genes expressed during cassava post-harvest physiological deterioration. Plant Mol Biol 2007;64:187–203. doi:10.1007/s11103-007-9144-0.

[34]   Yang J, An D, Zhang P. Expression profiling of cassava storage roots reveals an active process of glycolysis/gluconeogenesis. J IntegrPlant Biol 2011;53:193–211.

[35]   Sakurai T, Plata G, Rodríguez-Zapata F, Seki M, Salcedo A, Toyoda A, et al. Sequencing analysis of 20,000 full-length cDNA clones from cassava reveals lineage specific

expansions in gene families related to stress response. BMC Plant Biol 2007;7:66. doi: 10.1186/1471-2229-7-66.

[36] Utsumi Y, Tanaka M, Morosawa T, Kurotani A, Yoshida T, Mochida K, et al. Transcriptome analysis using a high-density oligomicroarray under drought stress in various genotypes of cassava: an important tropical crop. DNA Res 2012;19:335–45. doi: 10.1093/dnares/dss016.

[37] Maruthi MN, Bouvaine S, Tufan HA, Mohammed IU, Hillocks RJ. Transcriptional response of virus-infected cassava and identification of putative sources of resistance for cassava brown streak disease. PLoS One 2014;9:e96642. doi:10.1371/journal.pone. 0096642.

[38] Allie F, Pierce EJ, Okoniewski MJ, Rey C. Transcriptional analysis of South African cassava mosaic virus-infected susceptible and tolerant landraces of cassava highlights differences in resistance, basal defense and cell wall associated genes during infection. BMC Genomics 2014;15:1–30.

[39] Chen X, Xia J, Xia Z, Zhang H, Zeng C, Lu C, et al. Potential functions of microRNAs in starch metabolism and development revealed by miRNA transcriptome profiling of cassava cultivars and their wild progenitor. BMC Plant Biol 2015;15:1–11. doi: 10.1186/s12870-014-0355-7.

[40] Zeng C, Wang W, Zheng Y, Chen X, Bo W, Song S, et al. Conservation and divergence of microRNAs and their functions in Euphorbiaceous plants. Nucleic Acids Res 2009;38:981–95. doi:10.1093/nar/gkp1035.

[41] Tamiru M, Natsume S, Takagi H, Babil PK, Yamanaka S, Lopez-Montes A, et al. Whole genome sequencing of Guinea yam (*Dioscorea rotundata*). First Glob. Conf. Yam, Accra, Ghana: International Institute of Tropical Agriculture; Ibadan, Nigeria. 2013. p.20

[42] Mutuku JM, Yoshida S, Shimizu T, Ichihashi Y, Wakatake T, Seo M, et al. The WRKY45-dependent signaling pathway is required for resistance against Striga parasitism. 2015;168: 1152-1163. doi:10.1104/pp.114.256404.

[43] Chapman MA. Transcriptome sequencing and marker development for four underutilized legumes. Appl Plant Sci 2015;3:1400111. doi:10.3732/apps.1400111.

[44] Liu S, Yeh C-T, Tang HM, Nettleton D, Schnable PS. Gene mapping via bulked segregant RNA-Seq (BSR-Seq). PLoS One 2012;7:e36406.

[45] Goyer A, Hamlin L, Crosslin JM, Buchanan A, Chang JH. RNA-seq analysis of resistant and susceptible potato varieties during the early stages of potato virus Y infection. BMC Genomics 2015;16:472. doi:10.1186/s12864-015-1666-2.

[46] Humbert S, Subedi S, Cohn J, Zeng B, Bi Y-M, Chen X, et al. Genome-wide expression profiling of maize in response to individual and combined water and nitrogen stresses. BMC Genomics 2013;14:3. doi:10.1186/1471-2164-14-3.

[47] Mochida K, Yoshida T, Sakurai T, Yamaguchi-Shinozaki K, Shinozaki K, Tran LSP. In silico analysis of transcription factor repertoire and prediction of stress responsive transcription factors in soybean. DNA Res 2009;16:353–69. doi:10.1093/dnares/dsp023.

[48] Van Dijk EL, Auger H, Jaszczyszyn Y, Thermes C. Ten years of next-generation sequencing technology. Trends Genet 2014;30:418–26. doi:10.1016/j.tig.2014.07.001.

[49] Grover CE, Salmon A, Wendel JF. Targeted sequence capture as a powerful tool for evolutionary analysis. Am J Bot 2012;99:312–19. doi:10.3732/ajb.1100323.

[50] Reeves GA, Talavera D, Thornton JM. Genome and proteome annotation: organization, interpretation and integration. J R Soc Interface 2009;6:129–47. doi:10.1098/rsif.2008.0341.

[51] Hirsch CN, Foerster JM, Johnson JM, Sekhon RS, Muttoni G, Vaillancourt B, et al. Insights into the maize pan-genome and pan-transcriptome. Plant Cell 2014;26:121–35. doi:10.1105/tpc.113.119982.

[52] Varshney RK, Terauchi R, McCouch SR. Harvesting the promising fruits of genomics: applying genome sequencing technologies to crop breeding. PLoS Biol 2014;12:1–8. doi:10.1371/journal.pbio.1001883.

[53] Bzhalava D. Bioinformatics for viral metagenomics. J Data Mining Genomics Proteomics 2013;4:3–7. doi:10.4172/2153-0602.1000134.

[54] Lindner MS, Renard BY. Metagenomic abundance estimation and diagnostic testing on species level. Nucleic Acids Res 2013;41:1–8. doi:10.1093/nar/gks803.

[55] Sharpton TJ. An introduction to the analysis of shotgun metagenomic data. Front Plant Sci 2014;5:209. doi:10.3389/fpls.2014.00209.

[56] Schatz MC, Witkowski J, McCombie WR. Current challenges in de novo plant genome sequencing and assembly. Genome Biol 2012;13:243. doi:10.1186/gb4015.

[57] Fonseca NA, Rung J, Brazma A, Marioni JC. Tools for mapping high-throughput sequencing data. Bioinformatics 2012;28:3169–77. doi:10.1093/bioinformatics/bts605.

[58] Engström PG, Steijger T, Sipos B, Grant GR, Kahles A, Rätsch G, et al. Systematic evaluation of spliced alignment programs for RNA-seq data. Nat Methods 2013;10:1185–91. doi:10.1038/nmeth.2722.

[59] Cech TR, Steitz JA. The noncoding RNA revolution-trashing old rules to forge new ones. Cell 2014;157:77–94. doi:10.1016/j.cell.2014.03.008.

[60] Bond DM, Baulcombe DC. Small RNAs and heritable epigenetic variation in plants. Trends Cell Biol 2014;24:100–07. doi:10.1016/j.tcb.2013.08.001.

[61] Bock C. Analysing and interpreting DNA methylation data. Nat Rev Genet 2012;13:705–19. doi:10.1038/nrg3273.

[62] Meaburn E, Schulz R. Next generation sequencing in epigenetics: insights and challenges. Semin Cell Dev Biol 2012;23:192–99. doi:10.1016/j.semcdb.2011.10.010.

[63] Teeling H, Glöckner FO. Current opportunities and challenges in microbial metagenome analysis – a bioinformatic perspective. Brief Bioinform 2012;13:728–42. doi:10.1093/bib/bbs039.

[64] Bradbury PJ, Zhang Z, Kroon DE, Casstevens TM, Ramdoss Y, Buckler ES. Tassel: software for association mapping of complex traits in diverse samples. Bioinformatics 2007;23:2633–55.

[65] DePristo MA, Banks E, Poplin R, Garimella KV, Maguire JR, Hartl C, et al. A framework for variation discovery and genotyping using next-generation DNA sequencing data. Nat Genet 2011;43:491–98. doi:10.1038/ng.806.

[66] Danecek P, Auton A, Abecasis G, Albers CA, Banks E, DePristo MA, et al. The variant call format and VCFtools. Bioinformatics 2011;27:2156–58. doi:10.1093/bioinformatics/btr330.

[67] Li Y, Tollefsbol TO. DNA methylation detection: bisulfite genomic sequencing analysis. Methods Mol Biol 2011;791:11–21. doi:10.1007/978-1-61779-316-5_2.

[68] Krueger F, Kreck B, Franke A, Andrews SR. DNA methylome analysis using short bisulfite sequencing data. Nat Methods 2012;9:145–51. doi:10.1038/nmeth.1828.

[69] Hagen C, Frizzi A, Kao J, Jia L, Huang M, Zhang Y, et al. Using small RNA sequences to diagnose, sequence, and investigate the infectivity characteristics of vegetable-infecting viruses. Arch Virol 2011;156:1209–16. doi:10.1007/s00705-011-0979-y.

[70] Araki M, Ishii T. Towards social acceptance of plant breeding by genome editing. Trends Plant Sci 2015;20:1–5. doi:10.1016/j.tplants.2015.01.010.

[71] Andersen MM, Landes X, Xiang W, Anyshchenko A, Falhof J, Østerberg JT, et al. Feasibility of new breeding techniques for organic farming. Trends Plant Sci 2015;20:426–34. doi:10.1016/j.tplants.2015.04.011.

[72] Carroll D. Genome engineering with zinc-finger nucleases. Genetics 2011;188:773–82. doi:10.1534/genetics.111.131433.

[73] Carroll D. A CRISPR approach to gene targeting. Mol Ther 2012;20:1658–60. doi:10.1038/mt.2012.171.

[74] Joung JK, Sander JD. TALENs: a widely applicable technology for targeted genome editing. Nat Rev Mol Cell Biol 2013;14:49–55. doi:10.1038/nrm3486.

[75] Osakabe Y, Osakabe K. Genome editing with engineered nucleases in plants. Plant Cell Physiol 2015;56:389–400. doi:10.1093/pcp/pcu170.

[76] Fichtner F, Urrea Castellanos R, Ülker B. Precision genetic modifications: a new era in molecular biology and crop improvement. Planta 2014;239:921–39. doi:10.1007/s00425-014-2029-y.

[77] Kumar V, Jain M. The CRISPR-Cas system for plant genome editing: advances and opportunities. J Exp Bot 2015;66:47–57. doi:10.1093/jxb/eru429.

[78] Zhang Y, Zhang F, Li X, Baller JA, Qi Y, Starker CG, et al. Transcription activator-like effector nucleases enable efficient plant genome engineering. Plant Physiol 2012;161:20–27. doi:10.1104/pp.112.205179.

[79] Zhang F, Maeder ML, Unger-Wallace E, Hoshaw JP, Reyon D, Christian M, et al. High frequency targeted mutagenesis in *Arabidopsis thaliana* using zinc finger nucleases. Proc Natl Acad Sci U S A 2010;107:12028–33. doi:10.1073/pnas.0914991107.

[80] Jiang W, Zhou H, Bi H, Fromm M, Yang B, Weeks DP. Demonstration of CRISPR/Cas9/sgRNA-mediated targeted gene modification in *Arabidopsis*, tobacco, sorghum and rice. Nucleic Acids Res 2013;41:e188. doi:10.1093/nar/gkt780.

[81] Shukla VK, Doyon Y, Miller JC, DeKelver RC, Moehle EA, Worden SE, et al. Precise genome modification in the crop species *Zea mays* using zinc-finger nucleases. Nature 2009;459:437–41. doi:10.1038/nature07992.

[82] Marton I, Zuker A, Shklarman E, Zeevi V, Tovkach A, Roffe S, et al. Nontransgenic genome modification in plant cells. Plant Physiol 2010;154:1079–87. doi:10.1104/pp.110.164806.

[83] Palmgren MG, Edenbrandt AK, Vedel SE, Andersen MM, Landes X, Østerberg JT, et al. Are we ready for back-to-nature crop breeding? Trends Plant Sci 2015;20:155–64.

[84] Xing H-L, Dong L, Wang Z-P, Zhang H-Y, Han C-Y, Liu B, et al. A CRISPR/Cas9 toolkit for multiplex genome editing in plants. BMC Plant Biol 2014;14:327. doi:10.1186/s12870-014-0327-y.

[85] Comai L, Henikoff S. TILLING: practical single-nucleotide mutation discovery. Plant J 2006;45:684–94. doi:10.1111/j.1365-313X.2006.02670.x.

[86] McCallum CM, Comai L, Greene EA, Henikoff S. Targeting induced local lesions IN genomes (TILLING) for plant functional genomics. Plant Physiol 2000;123:439–42. doi:10.1104/pp.123.2.439.

[87] Waugh R, Leader DJ, McCallum N, Caldwell D. Harvesting the potential of induced biological diversity. Trends Plant Sci 2006;11:71–79. doi:10.1016/j.tplants.2005.12.007.

[88] Mba C, Afza R, Jankowicz-Cieslak J, Bado S, Matijevic M, Huynh O, et al. Enhancing genetic diversity through induced mutagenesis in vegetatively propagated plants. In: Shu Q, editor. Induc. Plant Mutat. Genomics Era, Food and Agriculture Organization of the United Nations, Rome: 2009, p. 262–65.

[89] Tadele Z, Mba C, Till BJ. TILLING for mutations in model plants and crops. In: Jain S, Brar S, editors. Mol. Tech. Crop Improv. 2nd ed., Rome, Springer Netherlands; 2010, p. 307–32.

[90] Gilchrist E, Haughn G. Reverse genetics techniques: engineering loss and gain of gene function in plants. Briefings Funct Genomics Proteomics 2010;9:103–10. doi: 10.1093/bfgp/elp059.

[91] Till BJ, Zerr T, Comai L, Henikoff S. A protocol for TILLING and Ecotilling in plants and animals. NatProtoc 2006;1:2465–77. doi:10.1038/nprot.2006.329.

[92] Tsai H, Howell T, Nitcher R, Missirian V, Watson B, Ngo KJ, et al. Discovery of rare mutations in populations: TILLING by sequencing. Plant Physiol 2011;156:1257–68. doi:10.1104/pp.110.169748.

[93] Zhu Q, Smith SM, Ayele M, Yang L, Jogi A, Chaluvadi SR, et al. High-throughput discovery of mutations in tef semi-dwarfing genes by next-generation sequencing analysis. Genetics 2012;192:819–29. doi:10.1534/genetics.112.144436.

[94] Pan L, Shah AN, Phelps IG, Doherty D, Johnson EA, Moens CB. Rapid identification and recovery of ENU-induced mutations with next-generation sequencing and paired-end low-error analysis. BMC Genomics 2015;16:1–13. doi:10.1186/s12864-015-1263-4.

[95] Marroni F, Pinosio S, Morgante M. The quest for rare variants: pooled multiplexed next generation sequencing in plants. Front Plant Sci 2012;3:1–9. doi:10.3389/fpls.2012.00133.

[96] Abe A, Kosugi S, Yoshida K, Natsume S, Takagi H, Kanzaki H, et al. Genome sequencing reveals agronomically important loci in rice using MutMap. Nat Biotechnol 2012;30:174–78.

[97] Bernardo R. Molecular markers and selection for complex traits in plants: learning from the last 20 years. Crop Sci 2008;48:1649–64. doi:10.2135/cropsci2008.03.0131.

[98] Salvi S, Tuberosa R. The crop QTLome comes of age. Curr Opin Biotechnol 2015;32:179–85. doi:10.1016/j.copbio.2015.01.001.

[99] Xu F, Sun X, Chen Y, Huang Y, Tong C, Bao J. Rapid Identification of major QTLs associated with rice grain weight and their utilization. PLoS One 2015;10:e0122206. doi:10.1371/journal.pone.0122206.

[100] Takagi H, Abe A, Yoshida K, Kosugi S, Natsume S, Mitsuoka C, et al. QTL-seq: rapid mapping of quantitative trait loci in rice by whole genome resequencing of DNA from two bulked populations. Plant J 2013;74:174–83. doi:10.1111/tpj.12105.

[101] Lu H, Lin T, Klein J, Wang S, Qi J, Zhou Q, et al. QTL-seq identifies an early flowering QTL located near Flowering Locus T in cucumber. Theor Appl Genet 2014; 127:1491–99. doi:10.1007/s00122-014-2313-z.

[102] Das S, Upadhyaya HD, Bajaj D, Kujur A, Badoni S, Laxmi, et al. Deploying QTL-seq for rapid delineation of a potential candidate gene underlying major trait-associated QTL in chickpea. DNA Res 2015:1–11. doi:10.1093/dnares/dsv004.

[103] Han Y, Lv P, Hou S, Li S, Ji G, Ma X, et al. Combining next generation sequencing with bulked segregant analysis to fine map a Stem Moisture Locus in Sorghum (*Sorghum bicolor* L. Moench). PLoS One 2015;10:e0127065. doi:10.1371/journal.pone. 0127065.

[104] Thomas T, Gilbert J, Meyer F. Metagenomics – a guide from sampling to data analysis. Microb Inform Exp 2012;2:3. doi:10.1186/2042-5783-2-3.

[105] Lebeis SL. Greater than the sum of their parts: characterizing plant microbiomes at the community-level. Curr Opin Plant Biol 2015;24C:82–86. doi:10.1016/j.pbi. 2015.02.004.

[106] Schloss PD, Handelsman J. Metagenomics for studying unculturable microorganisms: cutting the Gordian knot. Genome Biol 2005;6:229. doi:10.1186/gb-2005-6-8-229.

[107] Kellner H, Luis P, Portetelle D, Vandenbol M. Screening of a soil metatranscriptomic library by functional complementation of *Saccharomyces cerevisiae* mutants. Microbiol Res 2011;166:360–68. doi:10.1016/j.micres.2010.07.006.

[108] Luo C, Rodriguez-R LM, Johnston ER, Wu L, Cheng L, Xue K, et al. Soil microbial community responses to a decade of warming as revealed by comparative metagenomics. Appl Environ Microbiol 2014;80:1777–86. doi:10.1128/AEM.03712-13.

[109] Liu S, Vijayendran D, Bonning BC. Next generation sequencing technologies for insect virus discovery. Viruses 2011;3:1849–69. doi:10.3390/v3101849.

[110] Legg JP, Lava Kumar P, Makeshkumar T, Tripathi L, Ferguson M, Kanju E, et al. Cassava virus diseases: biology, epidemiology, and management. Adv Virus Res 2015;91:85–142. doi:10.1016/bs.aivir.2014.10.001.

[111] Geering ADW, Olszewski NE, Harper G, Lockhart BEL, Hull R, Thomas JE. Banana contains a diverse array of endogenous badnaviruses. J Gen Virol 2005;86:511–20. doi:10.1099/vir.0.80261-0.

[112] Filloux D, Murrell S, Koohapitagtam M, Golden M, Julian C, Galzi S, et al. The genomes of many yam species contain transcriptionally active endogenous geminiviral sequences that may be functionally expressed. Virus Evol 2015;1:vev002–vev002. doi: 10.1093/ve/vev002.

[113] Heslot N, Sorrels ME, Jannink J. Perspectives for genomic selection applications and research in plants. Crop Sci 2015;55:1–30. doi:10.2135/cropsci2014.03.0249.

[114] Poland J. Breeding-assisted genomics. Curr Opin Plant Biol 2015;24:119–24. doi: 10.1016/j.pbi.2015.02.009.

[115] Rivers J, Warthmann N, Pogson BJ, Borevitz JO. Genomic breeding for food, environment and livelihoods. Food Secur 2015;7:375–82. doi:10.1007/s12571-015-0431-3.

[116] Cooper M, Messina CD, Podlich D, Totir LR, Baumgarten A, Hausmann NJ, et al. Predicting the future of plant breeding: complementing empirical evaluation with genetic prediction. Crop Pasture Sci 2014;65:311–36. doi:10.1071/CP14007.

[117] Ceballos H, Kawuki RS, Gracen VE, Yencho GC, Hershey CH. Conventional breeding, marker-assisted selection, genomic selection and inbreeding in clonally propagated crops: a case study for cassava. Theor Appl Genet 2015. 128:1647-1667. doi: 10.1007/s00122-015-2555-4.

[118] De Oliveira EJ, de Resende MDV, da Silva Santos V, Ferreira CF, Oliveira GAF, da Silva MS, et al. Genome-wide selection in cassava. Euphytica 2012;187:263–76. doi: 10.1007/s10681-012-0722-0.

[119] Ray S, Satya P. Next generation sequencing technologies for next generation plant breeding. Front Plant Sci 2014;5:1–4. doi:10.3389/fpls.2014.00367.

[120] Ly D, Hamblin M, Rabbi I, Melaku G, Bakare M, Gauch HG, et al. Relatedness and genotype environment interaction affect prediction accuracies in genomic selection: a study in Cassava. Crop Sci 2013;53:1312–25.

[121] Crossa J, Pérez P, Hickey J, Burgueño J, Ornella L, Cerón-Rojas J, et al. Genomic prediction in CIMMYT maize and wheat breeding programs. Heredity (Edinb) 2014;112:48–60. doi:10.1038/hdy.2013.16.

[122] Crossa J, Pérez P, de los Campos G, Mahuku G, Dreisigacker S, Magorokosho C. Genomic selection and prediction in plant breeding. J Crop Improv 2011;25:239–61. doi: 10.1080/15427528.2011.558767.

[123] Hickey JM, Dreisigacker S, Crossa J, Hearne S, Babu R, Prasanna BM, et al. Evaluation of genomic selection training population designs and genotyping strategies in plant breeding programs using simulation. Crop Sci 2014;54:1476-1488. doi:10.2135/cropsci2013.03.0195.

[124] Anacleto R, Cuevas RP, Jimenez R, Llorente C, Nissila E, Henry R, et al. Prospects of breeding high-quality rice using post-genomic tools. Theor Appl Genet 2015;128:1449–66. doi:10.1007/s00122-015-2537-6.

[125] Huynh B-L, Ehlers JD, Ndeve A, Wanamaker S, Lucas MR, Close TJ, et al. Genetic mapping and legume synteny of aphid resistance in African cowpea (*Vigna unguiculata* L. Walp.) grown in California. Mol Breed 2015;35:36. doi:10.1007/s11032-015-0254-0.

[126] Kumar S, Rajendran K, Kumar J, Hamwieh A, Baum M. Current knowledge in lentil genomics and its application for crop improvement. Front Plant Sci 2015;6:1–13. doi: 10.3389/fpls.2015.00078.

[127] Jarquín D, Kocak K, Posadas L, Hyma K, Jedlicka J, Graef G, et al. Genotyping by se‐
quencing for genomic prediction in a soybean breeding population. BMC Genomics
2014;15:740. doi:10.1186/1471-2164-15-740.

[128] Bao Y, Kurle JE, Anderson G, Young ND. Association mapping and genomic predic‐
tion for resistance to sudden death syndrome in early maturing soybean germplasm.
Mol Breed 2015;35:128. doi:10.1007/s11032-015-0324-3.

[129] Pazhamala L, Saxena RK, Singh VK, Sameerkumar CV, Kumar V, Sinha P, et al. Ge‐
nomics-assisted breeding for boosting crop improvement in pigeonpea (*Cajanus ca‐
jan*). Front Plant Sci 2015;6:1–12. doi:10.3389/fpls.2015.00050.

[130] Fernandez-Pozo N, Menda N, Edwards JD, Saha S, Tecle IY, Strickler SR, et al. The
Sol Genomics Network (SGN) – from genotype to phenotype to breeding. Nucleic
Acids Res 2014;43:D1036–41. doi:10.1093/nar/gku1195.

[131] Cobb JN, DeClerck G, Greenberg A, Clark R, McCouch S. Next-generation phenotyp‐
ing: requirements and strategies for enhancing our understanding of genotype-phe‐
notype relationships and its relevance to crop improvement. Theor Appl Genet
2013;126:867–87. doi:10.1007/s00122-013-2066-0.

[132] Rousseau D, Chéné Y, Belin E, Semaan G, Trigui G, Boudehri K, et al. Multiscale
imaging of plants: current approaches and challenges. Plant Methods 2015;11:1–9.
doi:10.1186/s13007-015-0050-1.

[133] Bergsträsser S, Fanourakis D, Schmittgen S, Cendrero-Mateo MP, Jansen M, Scharr
H, et al. HyperART: non-invasive quantification of leaf traits using hyperspectral ab‐
sorption-reflectance-transmittance imaging. Plant Methods 2015;11:1–17. doi:10.1186/
s13007-015-0043-0.

[134] Araus L, Elazab A, Vergara O, Cabrera-Bosquet L, Serret MD, Zaman-Allah M, et al.
New technologies for phenotyping. In: Fritsche-Neto R, Borem A, editors. Phenom‐
ics, Springer International Publishing, Switzerland; 2015. p.1-14. doi:
10.1007/978-3-319-13677-6_1.

[135] Zaman-Allah M, Vergara O, Araus JL, Tarekegne A, Magorokosho C, Zarco-Tejada
PJ, et al. Unmanned aerial platform-based multi-spectral imaging for field phenotyp‐
ing of maize. Plant Methods 2015;11:35. doi:10.1186/s13007-015-0078-2.

[136] Bansal KC, Lenka SK, Mondal TK. Genomic resources for breeding crops with en‐
hanced abiotic stress tolerance. Plant Breed 2014;133:1–11. doi:10.1111/pbr.12117.

[137] Dwivedi SL, Upadhyaya HD, Stalker HT, Blair MW, Bertioli DJ, Nielen S, et al. En‐
hancing crop gene pools with beneficial traits using wild relatives. Plant Breed Rev
2008;30:179–230.

[138] Koo B, Pardey PG, Wright BD. The economic costs of conserving genetic resources at
the   CGIAR   centers.   Agric   Econ   2003;29:287–97.   doi:10.1111/j.
1574-0862.2003.tb00165.x.

[139] Lee S-H, Tuberosa R, Jackson SA, Varshney RK. Genomics of plant genetic resources: a gateway to a new era of global food security. Plant Genet Resour 2014;12:S2–5. doi: 10.1017/S1479262114000513.

[140] Romay MC, Millard MJ, Glaubitz JC, Peiffer JA, Swarts KL, Casstevens TM, et al. Comprehensive genotyping of the USA national maize inbred seed bank. Genome Biol 2013;14:R55. doi:10.1186/gb-2013-14-6-r55.

[141] Elhoumaizi MA, Saaidi M, Oihabi A, Cilas C. Phenotypic diversity of date-palm cultivars(*Phoenix dactylifera* L.) from Morocco. Genet Resour Crop Evol 2002;49:483–90. doi:10.1023/A:1020968513494.

[142] Duminil J, Di Michele M. Plant species delimitation: a comparison of morphological and molecular markers. Plant Biosyst – An Int J Deal with All Asp Plant Biol 2009;143:528–42. doi:10.1080/11263500902722964.

[143] Börner A, Khlestkina EK, Chebotar S, Nagel M, Arif MAR, Neumann K, et al. Molecular markers in management of ex situ PGR – A case study. J Biosci 2012;37:871–77. doi:10.1007/s12038-012-9250-2.

[144] Girma G, Hyma KE, Asiedu R, Mitchell SE, Gedil M, Spillane C. Next-generation sequencing based genotyping, cytometry and phenotyping for understanding diversity and evolution of guinea yams. Theor Appl Genet 2014;127:1783–94.

[145] Padi FK, Ofori A, Takrama J, Djan E, Opoku SY, Dadzie AM, et al. The impact of SNP fingerprinting and parentage analysis on the effectiveness of variety recommendations in cacao. Tree Genet Genomes 2015;11:44. doi:10.1007/s11295-015-0875-9.

[146] Wallace JG, Upadhyaya HD, Vetriventhan M, Buckler ES, Tom Hash C, Ramu P. The genetic makeup of a Global Barnyard Millet Germplasm Collection. Plant Genome 2015;8:1-7. doi:10.3835/plantgenome2014.10.0067.

[147] McCouch S, Baute GJ, Bradeen J, Bramel P, Bretting PK, Buckler E, et al. Agriculture: feeding the future. Nature 2013;499:23–24. doi:10.1038/499023a.

[148] Girma G, Korie S, Dumet D, Franco J. Improvement of accession distinctiveness as an added value to the global worth of the yam (*Dioscorea* spp) genebank. Int J Conserv Sci 2012;3:199–206.

[149] Galperin MY, Rigden DJ, Fernández-Suárez XM. The 2015 Nucleic Acids Research Database Issue and molecular biology database collection. Nucleic Acids Res 2015;43:D1–5. doi:10.1093/nar/gku1241.

[150] Shirasawa K, Isobe S, Tabata S, Hirakawa H. Kazusa Marker DataBase: a database for genomics, genetics, and molecular breeding in plants. Breed Sci 2014;64:264–71. doi: 10.1270/jsbbs.64.264.

[151] Grant D, Nelson RT, Cannon SB, Shoemaker RC. SoyBase, the USDA-ARS soybean genetics and genomics database. Nucleic Acids Res 2010;38:D843–46. doi:10.1093/nar/gkp798.

[152] Schaeffer ML, Harper LC, Gardiner JM, Andorf CM, Campbell DA, Cannon EKS, et al. MaizeGDB: curation and outreach go hand-in-hand. Database (Oxford) 2011;2011:bar022. doi:10.1093/database/bar022.

[153] Goodstein DM, Shu S, Howson R, Neupane R, Hayes RD, Fazo J, et al. Phytozome: a comparative platform for green plant genomics. Nucleic Acids Res 2012;40:D1178–86. doi:10.1093/nar/gkr944.

[154] Kehoe MA, Coutts BA, Buirchell BJ, Jones RAC. Plant virology and next generation sequencing: experiences with a Potyvirus. PLoS One 2014;9:e104580. doi:10.1371/journal.pone.0104580.

[155] Li R, Gao S, Hernandez AG, Wechter WP, Fei Z, Ling K-S. Deep sequencing of small RNAs in tomato for virus and viroid identification and strain differentiation. PLoS One 2012;7:e37127. doi:10.1371/journal.pone.0037127.

[156] Adams IP, Glover RH, Monger WA, Mumford R, Jackeviciene E, Navalinkiene M, et al. Next-generation sequencing and metagenomic analysis: a universal diagnostic tool in plant virology. Mol Plant Pathol 2009;10:537–45. doi:10.1111/J.1364-3703.2009.00545.X.

[157] Seguin J, Rajeswaran R, Malpica-López N, Martin RR, Kasschau K, Dolja V V, et al. De novo reconstruction of consensus master genomes of plant RNA and DNA viruses from siRNAs. PLoS One 2014;9:e88513. doi:10.1371/journal.pone.0088513.

[158] Dennis ES, Ellis J, Green A, Llewellyn D, Morell M, Tabe L, et al. Genetic contributions to agricultural sustainability. Philos Trans R Soc Lond B Biol Sci 2008;363:591–609. doi:10.1098/rstb.2007.2172.

[159] Fridman E, Zamir D. Next-generation education in crop genetics. Curr Opin Plant Biol 2012;15:218–23. doi:10.1016/j.pbi.2012.03.013.

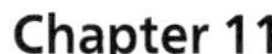

Chapter 11

Hop-variety Identification Using First- and Second-generation Sequencing

Hiromasa Yamauchi

Additional information is available at the end of the chapter

http://dx.doi.org/10.5772/61673

Abstract

Twenty-one hop varieties from Europe and the United States were successfully identified by DNA analysis, based on single nucleotide polymorphisms (SNPs; including insertion/deletion sequences) as identification markers. Several dozen megabases of transcriptome sequencing data were obtained by next-generation sequencing of samples from three hop varieties and compared to search for the regions containing SNPs. Consequently, four SNP-rich regions were selected as candidates for exploring identification markers in the hop varieties. Sequence data from these regions in all the tested varieties were obtained by the normal Sanger method and compared for the SNPs present. Combination of these SNPs could work well for identification of the 21 hop varieties. Moreover, the mixture of two varieties could be correctly evaluated by using this method. Hop pellet samples of two different varieties were mixed in various ratios and DNA sequencing was carried out. As a result, 5% contamination of a different variety could be detected by examining the electropherogram of the SNP positions. More quantitative methods for mixture evaluation could be expected using DNA techniques, such as quantitative real-time PCR. Because this SNP-based identification method utilizes the DNA sequence itself, it could be a reproducible tool for accurate identification of the hop varieties.

Keywords: hop, identification, NGS, SNP, transcriptome, variety

1. Introduction

Accurate identification and use of hop (*Humulus lupulus*) varieties is very important for the production of quality beer. Hop varieties are usually identified by sensory analysis (taste, appearance, and smell), detection of the differences in the cone structure, and content of different biochemical substances, including alpha acids and essential oils. However, these methods present certain limitations, as accurate identification of the pelletized hop is not

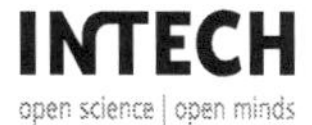

possible by observing its external appearance. Moreover, the content of biochemical substances in hop can vary depending on the cultivation conditions.

There are several reports on the use of DNA-based analytical techniques such as random amplified polymorphic DNAs (RAPDs) [1–5], restriction fragment length polymorphisms (RFLPs) [3,6], amplified fragment length polymorphisms (AFLPs) [3,4,7,8], and microsatellites (single sequence repeats, SSRs) [7, 9–14], besides other approaches like markers in the spacer or noncoding regions [15], sequence-tagged site (STS) markers [3, 13, 16], and diversity arrays technology (DArT) [17] for the assessment of the genetic diversity in hops. Since most of these methods are based on fingerprinting approach, the results obtained are sometimes unclear and prone to misjudgment, thereby limiting the detection of contaminating varieties.

Analysis of single nucleotide polymorphisms (SNPs; differences of single nucleotide in homologous DNA among different varieties) in genomic DNA might be a better and more reproducible tool for the identification of varieties. SNPs are widely distributed in the genome and could be used as markers for the assessment of genotypes. For example, variation in DNA sequence and expression of valerophenone synthase (VPS) gene, a key gene of the bitter acid biosynthesis pathway, has been investigated in hop, using SNPs [18]. However, a large amount of DNA sequence is needed to obtain sufficient SNPs in order to identify the different varieties. In this context, high throughput next-generation sequencing (NGS) generally provides several hundred thousand–times more sequence data in a single analysis compared to the conventional Sanger method, but the whole genome sequencing by either method is still very expensive and time-consuming. In fact, genome sizes of two representative hop varieties, lupulus and neomexicanus, are 2.74 and 2.97 Gb, respectively [19], which are comparable to that of the human genome [20].

To overcome these problems, transcriptome analysis has been employed for the identification of hop varieties. Transcriptome is the entire mRNA content, transcribed from the genome, and its size ranges from one hundredth- to two hundredth-parts of the genome. Nevertheless, even by a conservative estimate of an average of one SNP per 1000 bp, based on the frequency of SNPs observed in the human genome [20], 13.5K to 30K SNPs could be expected in a relatively short period. Such a high frequency of SNPs would be enough for the identification of hop varieties. The discovery of a large number of SNPs and their specific combinations in each variety could lead to the identification of many hop varieties and detection of contaminants in mixed varieties using these specific SNP-combination-based markers. In the present study, we developed an SNP-based identification method for the hop varieties [21].

2. Research protocols, methods, results, and discussion

2.1. Identification of SNP markers by second generation sequencing and transcriptome analysis

2.1.1. SNPs

In order to obtain intravariety DNA polymorphic regions required for developing a hop variety identification technique, we attempted searching for SNPs in a large amount of sequence data obtained using NGS. We focused on the transcriptome because transcriptome analysis requires about 100-times less data processing than whole-genome analysis, thereby reducing the lead time and cost. Besides, according to our calculation, there are already available data for as many as 15000 SNPs in the transcriptome analysis; the data size, however, is smaller than that for the whole-genome analysis. Thus, we performed an intravariety SNP analysis, using this technique, based on the assumption that SNPs required for the identification of many varieties could be obtained, thereby.

2.1.2. Sample collection and storage

The hop varieties to be identified were Saaz, Sládek, and Premiant, which originated in Czech Republic; Tradition, Spalter, Spalter Select, Perle, Tettnang, Brewer's Gold, Northern Brewer, Magnum, Herkules, German Nugget, and Taurus, which originated in Germany; and Cascade, Zeus, Summit, Galena, Super Galena, Nugget, and Columbus/Tomahawk, which originated in the United States (here, as is widely assumed, we considered that Columbus and Tomahawk were genetically identical). Pellets or dried samples of these varieties were obtained from appropriate suppliers. Three varieties (referred to as A, B, and C for convenience) were selected, and fresh leaves were collected from these varieties. The leaves were sampled and stored according to the procedure described below:

Tissue: Leaves as young (small, yellow-green, and soft) as possible were collected. Those with white foreign matter on the surface were excluded.

Methodology: To prevent RNase contamination, leaves were collected with gloved hands and were soaked in a reagent (RNA Save; Biological Industries Israel Beit Haemek Ltd., Israel) for preventing RNA degradation.

Storage: Although RNA was stable for at least 1 week even at room temperature, the leaves were stored under refrigeration for as much time as possible until being used for RNA isolation and transcriptome and SNP sequence analysis.

2.1.3. Transcriptome analysis

The collected samples were used for transcriptome analysis. The procedure was subcontracted to Eurofins Genomics (Ebersberg, Germany). Briefly, the total RNA was extracted from the samples using RNeasy Plant Mini Kit (Qiagen Inc., Valencia, CA, USA) according to manufacturer's procedure. The quality of total RNA was evaluated in terms of the degree of degradation of rRNAs with Bioanalyzer (Agilent Technologies, Santa Clara, CA, USA). Normalized cDNA library for use in Roche GS FLX Titanium sequencing was prepared as follows: poly (A) + RNA was isolated from the total RNA, and the first-strand cDNA synthesis was primed with an N6 randomized primer. Normalization was carried out by one cycle of denaturation and reassociation of the cDNA. Reassociated double-stranded (ds) cDNA was separated from the remaining single-stranded (ss) cDNA by passing the mixture through a hydroxylapatite column. The ss-cDNA was amplified by 9 PCR cycles. The cDNA library in the size range 500–700 bp was eluted from a preparative agarose gel. Emulsion PCR and sequencing were conducted according to standard protocols of Roche and the normalized cDNA library was sequenced in 1/2-plate run of GS FLX Titanium. Library preparations and their sequencing were carried out by Eurofins Genomics.

2.1.4. Preparation and assembly of contigs for SNP searches

Using the transcriptome sequence data obtained as described above, contigs were prepared under a subcontract to Eurofins Genomics. Briefly, the procedure comprised of sequence clustering and assembly for each of the varieties, based on the nucleotide sequences of the DNA fragments. De novo assembling from the unique single-read data was performed by MIRA Assembler Version 2.9.45 x 1 (for sequence assembly; Rheinfelden, Germany). To search for SNPs, contig and singlet data obtained in one of the hop varieties served as a reference for the single-read data obtained from the other two varieties. Specifically, with the nucleotide sequences of the contigs and singlets of variety C being used as reference sequences, single reads of varieties A and B were each applied and mapped to the reference sequences according to whether they shared a common portion. Further, contigs constituted by the mapped single reads were identified from the assembling information deployed on the analysis software. The reference sequences as well as the contigs and/or singlets of the other varieties were aligned to search for SNPs using bioinformatics analysis. Average reads per contig were 7 and 6 in variety A and B, respectively. The detected SNPs were reproducibly present in each variety and were therefore not the artifacts of error. Further, the nucleotide sequences of the contigs and singlets of variety B were used as reference sequences, and single reads of varieties A and C were compared and mapped to the reference sequences to search for SNPs in the same way, as mentioned above. A similar exercise was performed with the nucleotide sequences of the contigs and singlets of variety A being used as reference sequences, and the single reads of varieties B and C were applied and mapped to the reference sequences to search for SNPs.

The NGS performed in the 3 varieties generated a total of 589K to 638K reads with the total number of bases without keys, tags, and bad-quality bases being 191 to 227 Mb and the average read length without keys, tags, and bad-quality bases being 299 to 367. These values were comparable to the equipment spec (Table 1). Numbers of contigs (part of cDNAs) assembled in each variety were 42K to 45K. Among these contigs, there were about 4500–6700 contigs with a length of 1000 bp or more (Table 2).

2.1.5. Evaluation of SNP detection by NGS RNA method

SNPs were searched in the contigs by comparing among the 3 varieties. As a result, 10.4K to 19.3K SNPs were obtained, as shown in Table 2. The numbers of SNPs were almost compatible with the expected numbers, 13.5K to 30K.

2.1.6. Results for SNP analytical regions

To call variants, mapping analysis was performed among the three hop varieties, which were combined with the contigs (as reference sequences) and single reads of each other. They were mapped and called by GS Mapper Software (Roche Applied Science, Penzberg, Germany).

Large run results	Variety A	Variety B	Variety C	Equipment spec
Total number of reads	618207	588711	638443	450–650 K
Total number of bases without keys, tags, and bad-quality bases	227199992	210506914	191071744	180–280 Mb
Average read length without keys, tags, and bad-quality bases (bp)	367	357	299	350–450

Table 1. NGS run results for 3 hop varieties.

		Variety A	Variety B	Variety C
Assembly results	Number assembled	546411	516494	549226
	Number too short	14436	16175	25343
Sum of large contigs[a]	Total number of reads	290726	274772	232407
	Number of large contigs	6725	6157	4563
	Total number of bases	10096155	9165669	6562275
Sum of all contigs	Total number of reads	546411	516494	549226
	Number of all contigs	43638	42395	45432
	Total number of bases	29918028	28215799	26612919
Total number of SNPs		10472	14408	19330

[a]Contigs ≥1000 bp.

Table 2. NGS results of assembly, contigs, and SNPs.

Numbers and types of SNPs per contig or singlet were obtained. For example, if 16 single reads were selected as candidate DNA fragments containing SNPs, in some cases, all of them had the same nucleotide and were different from the reference, whereas in other cases, some of them had same nucleotide and the others had a nucleotide same as that of the reference. We called the former case "HOMO," in which identification was thought to be done more easily than in the latter case, designated as "HETERO."

We selected the contigs that had more "HOMO" SNPs per single contig. For example, a contig (A1 c1675) containing 6 different SNPs was selected when the mapping was performed in the A1 region contig as a reference with single reads of variety B. This contig (A1 c1675) had 4 SNPs when single reads of variety C were used. In the same way, the other SNP-rich regions were selected. Thus, 4 SNP-rich regions, A1, B1, C1, and A1-2, were obtained.

The results are shown in the Table 3.

Reference/ variety supplied	Total number of contigs	Total number of SNPs detected	Number of SNPs homozygous in 2 varieties other than reference (per contig)	Contig size (bp)	Analysis region
Variety A	43638	10472	6	1.4k	A1
				719	A1-2
Variety B	42395	14408	9	1.0k	B1
Variety C	45432	19330	24	2.8k	C1

Table 3. Results for SNP analytical regions.

Primers were designed for each region using DNASIS Pro software (Hitachi Software Engineering Co., Ltd.; Tokyo, Japan), and PCR amplifications of the four regions were performed for further confirmation of the analysis regions.

2.2. Application of NGS-SNP genotypes to identify hop varieties by Sanger sequencing

2.2.1. DNA extraction from hop varieties

DNA was extracted from the pellets or dried cones of the three hop varieties (A, B, and C), used in the transcriptome analysis described above. DNA extraction by the cetyltrimethylammonium bromide (CTAB; Sigma-Aldrich Co. LLC., St. Louis, USA) method was carried out as follows. The CTAB solution comprised of 2% (w/v) CTAB, 100 mM Tris–HCl (pH 8.0), 20 mM EDTA (pH 8.0), 1.4 M NaCl, and 1% (w/v) polyvinylpyrrolidone (PVP). About 10–50 g of hop pellets or 1 g of dried cones were ground in a mortar with or without liquid nitrogen. Next, 650 µL of the CTAB solution and 2 µL 1 mg/mL RNaseA solution were added to the ground material in a 1.5 mL microtube and stirred well. This microtube containing the sample and the CTAB solution was submerged in a constant temperature water bath held at 65°C such that the content of the tube was completely underwater; the mixture was incubated for 1 h to disrupt hop cells. An equal volume (650 µL) of chloroform/isoamyl alcohol (24:1; Sigma-Aldrich Co. LLC.) was subsequently added, and the mixture was manually mixed by inversion for 3 min. The mixture was centrifuged in a Beckman's Allegra 21R centrifuge (with F2402H rotor) at 15,000 rpm (ca. 15,000×g) for 1–5 min and thereby fractionated into an organic solvent layer (lower) and an aqueous layer (upper). The aqueous layer (ca. 400 µL) was removed to a new tube. After the addition of an equal volume of isopropyl alcohol (Wako Pure Chemical Industries, Ltd.), the mixture was mixed by inversion and then centrifuged in the same way as described above. The supernatant was discarded and the remaining sediment was rinsed with about 500 µL of 70% ethanol (Wako Pure Chemical Industries, Ltd.) and dried in an MV-100 MicroVac Mini Vacuum-Centrifugal Evaporator (TOMY Seiko Co., Ltd.) for about 5 min. The residue was dissolved in 20–50 µL of TE buffer (pH 8.0, Nippon Gene Co., Ltd.) to obtain the DNA sample.

The extracted DNAs were subjected to amplification of the respective regions A1, B1, C1, and A1-2 using the primer sets shown in Table 4. The primers were designed using the DNASIS Pro software (Hitachi Software Engineering Co., Ltd.).

Primer	Nucleotide sequence	Length of amplified product (bp)
A1_3L	TAAGGTGTTGGGAGGGTTGA	651
A1_3R	CCACCAATAACAGGCTCCAC	
B1_1L	CAGACTTGTGGCTGTCAAAAA	729
B1_1R	CTTCTCCTTCGAACCTGTCG	
C1_1L	CGGCGTTTTTCAATTTTCAT	646
C1_1R	GTGATGACTCGGGCTTCAGT	
A1_2_1L	GAAATCTGCTTKGAGAAACCTGG	ca 1500
A1_2_1R	GCAGGTATCTTTGTAGGTACATC	
A1-2-M_F	ATTTTTGCTATGCCTGGCA	507
A1-2-M_R	ATTAGACCAGCACCAGTATG	

Table 4. PCR primers used in the study.

PCR was performed in a Veriti 96 Well Thermal Cycler (Life Technologies Japan Ltd.) with PerfectShot Ex Taq (Loading dye mix, Takara Bio Inc.), as described in its manual. The temperature during the 30 PCR cycles was 98°C for 10 s, 60°C or 50°C for 30 s, and 72°C for 60 s.

2.2.2. Confirmation of PCR amplification

Five microliters each of the PCR product obtained, as described above, was subjected to agarose gel electrophoresis, performed using a mini gel electrophoresis system, Mupid (gel: 3% NuSieve 3:1 Agarose; FMC BioProducts or Cambrex Bio Science Rockland). The electrophoresis was carried out at 100 V for 30 min, and the amplification products were visualized under ultraviolet light illumination (Printgraph, Atto Corp.) after staining with ethidium bromide (2 µg/mL) for about 40 min. The presence of the amplified DNA fragment of the intended size was ascertained for each DNA sample. The sizes of DNA fragments amplified using the respective primer sets are described in Table 4.

The purification of the resulting PCR products was performed using the QIAquick PCR Purification Kit (Qiagen Inc., Valencia, CA, USA) according to the protocol recommended by the manufacturer, as described below. Five volumes of PBI buffer (225 µL) was added to the PCR product (45 µL) and mixed. The resulting solution was placed in the QIA quickspin column and centrifuged at 13,000 rpm (ca. 11,000xg) for 1 min. The supernatant was discarded, 750 µL of PE buffer was added, and the mixture was centrifuged at 13,000 rpm for 1 min. The supernatant was again discarded and the remaining solution was centrifuged at 14,000 rpm (ca. 13,000×g) for 1 min. The supernatant was discarded, the column was transferred to a new 1.5 mL Eppendorf tube, and 30 µL of EB buffer was added. After being left to stand for 1 min, the solution was centrifuged at 13,000 rpm for 2 min to elute the purified PCR product.

2.2.3. Confirmation of SNP markers by Sanger DNA sequencing

Cycle sequencing was performed using the BigDye terminator v1.1 cycle sequencing kit (Life Technologies Japan Ltd.), according to the protocol prescribed by the vendor. The purification of the product as the template DNA for sequencing was performed by the Centri-Sep Spin Column (Life Technologies Japan Ltd.) according to the manufacturer's protocol. DNA sequencing was performed on an ABI PRISM 310 genetic analyzer (Life Technologies Japan Ltd.). Sequence data obtained from the 5' and 3' ends were checked, and the correct base sequence was determined. The nucleotide sequences determined from the tested varieties were aligned in each analysis region by using ClustalW (DDBJ; DNA Data Bank of Japan), which is a popular multiple sequence alignment program for DNA.

Thus, the amplified regions were confirmed. Comparison was also made with the data obtained using the next-generation sequencer, to confirm that the identification of the three varieties A, B, and C was possible. The size of the amplified products from the regions, A1, B1, C1, and A1-2, were 651, 729, 640/646, and ca. 1500 bp, respectively.

The PCR product from the B1 region was bigger in size than expected, and on close scrutiny, it was found that this DNA region included a 111-bp insertion sequence, which might be that of an intron.

For reference, the two different sizes of the amplicons obtained from the C1 region represented the size with or without the 6-nucleotide insertion in this region.

Since the fragment of region A1-2 had a length of about 1,500 bp, the sequencing data obtained for this region consisted of sequences from two regions: an analytical region, A1-2-L of 538 bp from the 5' end (primer L), and an analytical region A1-2-R of 516 bp from the 3' end (primer R).

It was determined that the analysis of regions A1, B1, C1, and A1-2 (and the SNPs contained, therein) was also applicable to the identification of other varieties in addition to the three mentioned above. Thus, analysis of a number of varieties was carried out.

Name	No. of SNPs[a]	Size (bp)
A1	24	541
B1	14	645
C1	43	559[a]
A1-2-L	21	538
A1-2-R	67	516
A1-2-R-2	59	542

[a]Including indel (insertion/deletion) sequence.

Table 5. Properties of SNP-rich analytical regions.

2.2.4. Identification markers for 21 hop varieties

Twenty-one varieties of hops were selected for identification based on the nucleotide sequence in region A1.

Nucleotide sequences were aligned to determine the consensus sequence in region A1. The nucleotide sequences determined in the varieties were evaluated for 24 SNPs in region A1 corresponding to the nucleotide positions 74, 77, 87, 103, 116, 118, 121, 125, 134, 135, 148, 192, 195, 197, 199, 203, 204, 226, 230, 235, 306, 316, 330, and 532. These 21 hop varieties showed 12 types (types 1 to 12) of combinations of 24 SNPs in region A1. The SNP positions are depicted in red in Figure 1.

```
A1 REGION

TGGTGGTGCA GAAAAGTCAG GATTTTGATG GTGGGGAGTC AGAGTTTAGG GCCAGTGAGG   60
AGGTAGAAGT AGAWGAYGGT AAAATTKTGG ATGGTGGGAA TGRTAAAGAT AACTCWGYCA  120
DTTTWGAAGA GAAKRATGAG AAGTTGGYCG AAGAAGATGG GGTGAGTCTT GGCGGAGATG  180
AGTCAGTGGT GRAAKCWGYG CARSTTAATG TCCCAGCTTC AAGAGWAGCY GATGYTGGAG  240
TTTCAGAAGA ACTTGATGAA GCTGAAATTA GAGGTGTAGA GCCTCCAGGA GGCGGGAACC  300
TTGGCYCTGG TTCTGWAGAA TTTGTTGGCW CAAAGTTGAT GCCTACAGAT TCTGAATCTG  360
ATGGAAATGT TGTGGGGTCT GTTACTGGTG GTCCTGATGA AGTTGATACC AAGCACGTAT  420
CAGCAGGAGA AGATGGTGGG CTAAAAGCTA ATTCTGAAGT TCATCAGAGC GGCCCCGTGG  480
TCGAGAAAGG TGCTGATAAT GAAAAAGTTC TGTCAGGTGA TGGAGTTGGT CSAAAGTTGA  540
T                                                             541
```

Figure 1. Nucleotide sequence of region A1. Each nucleotide is shown as per the IUPAC definition. Gaps are inserted after every 10 letters to increase clarity. Number at the right in every line denotes the number of nucleotides up to that position. Red letters represent the SNP positions.

Nucleotide sequences determined in the 21 varieties were aligned to determine the consensus sequence in region B1. These sequences were evaluated for 14 SNPs in region B1, corresponding to the nucleotide positions 178, 204, 227, 234, 245, 246, 247, 248, 370, 426, 439, 547, 562, and 624. The 21 hop varieties to be identified showed 9 types (types a to i) of combinations of 14 SNPs in region B1. The SNP positions are depicted in red in Figure 2.

Similarly, 43 SNPs were found in region C1 (6 of these 43 SNPs, at positions 129–134, constituted an indel portion) corresponding to the nucleotide positions 3, 13, 17, 76, 77, 87, 88, 93, 129, 130, 131, 132, 133, 134, 136, 138, 163, 165, 245, 254, 313, 321, 331, 356, 373, 375, 376, 380, 396, 398, 399, 421, 435, 438, 460, 474, 475, 476, 477, 480, 481, 500, and 547. The 21 hop varieties to be identified showed 5 types (types i to v) of combinations of 43 SNPs or an indel portion in region C1. The SNP positions are depicted in red in Figure 3.

The analyses of 24 SNPs in region A1, 14 SNPs in region B1, and 43 SNPs or an indel portion in region C1 made it possible to classify 16 of the 21 varieties, excluding Perle, Northern Brewer, Premiant, Zeus, and Summit, into distinct types, respectively. For identifying Perle, Northern

```
B1 REGION
CATTCCTCAG GATCTAAAGC GAATTATTAA GAAATACATT CAAATGAGAT TGCAAGATGG    60
AAAAGATGTG GACATCGACC ATATTTTGCA TATTCTTCCT TTGTCACAGG GAATGCTAAT   120
TAAGAAACAC ATGTGTTTCC CTATGTTAAA AAAAGTAAGT TATCTTTTAT AGTATATRTA   180
TGTCATTATT AAGTTTGATC TTTAATTTGA GCTATAACAT AGTATTRTTA TTTRATTGAT   240
TGATTGATTA TATGATTAAT TATAGGTTCC ATTATTTCAA AACACGGATG AACATGTTTA   300
CGAAACAATA TGCAAATATC TGAAACCAGT CACATATTCA GAGAAAAGTT ATATCATTCG   360
AAAAGGAGAR CCACTTGATA TGATTCTCTT CATCACACAA GGTGTTGTGT GGGCATTTGG   420
AAATGNTACT ACTCCCATRA GTCGACTTCA AAAAGGTGAT TTCTATGGAA ATGAACTCAT   480
AGAATGGCAA TTAAAGTCAA CATCCATTGA TGAGTTTCCT ATTTCGGTTG CTAATCTTAA   540
ATCCCAYACC AATGTTGAAG CYCTTGCTCT TATGGCCAAT GACTTGGAAC ATGTAGTCTC   600
CAATTGCTGG TTCAAGTTCT CCCBCACCTG CTCATCTATG CCTGA                   645
```
  * Variety Galena shows 2 genotypes, one of which contains deletion
  sequences from 245th to 248th nucleotide.

Figure 2. Nucleotide sequence of region B1. Please consult the legend of Figure 1 for details.

```
C1 REGION
TTYGACGTGA TCSAGTKGAG TGGTGGTATA TACGTTCCAT ATTATAAAGA TTACATTGTT    60
TTAATGGATA TACCARRGAA GGAGAAWKTA AAMCTCTCCA TCGCACTGCA AGCCAACCCC   120
GATGATACSA TGACTYTSTA CACTGATGCC ATCTTGAATG GCRTSGAAAT CTTCAAATTA   180
AGCGACTCCA ACGGAAATCT CGCCGGTCTG AATCTTGACC TTGTTCCGCA TGCGAAGCCA   240
CCAARCCAAC CATYATGGAA GTTGAAAAAT CATCAATCAG AGATTATTGG CATTTCCATT   300
GGTGTAGTTT GCWGCGTTGT YTTGCTCTGC RTAATTGGAT TCCTATTTCT CCGGCRAGGT   360
AGAAAAGTCA AARGMWCAAK GCTCATTTCC TTGTCHASWA CCAGGTCAAG CAAGACCGGA   420
RAATCATCAT TGCCRTTKGA TCGGTGTCGT TACTTTTCAY TGGCTGAGAT CATWRMYGCM   480
RCAAACAACT TCGAAGATAK TTTCATTATT GGGGTTGGAG GATTCGGAAA CGTGTATAAA   540
GGGCACRTCG ACAATGGGA                                                559
```
  * Underlined part contains deletion sequence.

Figure 3. Nucleotide sequence of region C1. Please consult the legend of Figure 1 for details.

Brewer, Premiant, Zeus, and Summit, the nucleotide sequences in region A1-2 of these varieties were further analyzed. These nucleotide sequences were aligned to determine the consensus sequence in region A1-2-L. The nucleotide sequences were evaluated for 21 SNPs in region A1-2-L (10 of these 21 SNPs constitute indel portions) corresponding to the nucleotide positions 34, 101, 118, 124, 164, 168, 171, 186, 187, 188, 189, 190, 191, 192, 193, 194, 393, 398, 399, 459, and 502 (positions 186–194 and position 399 each constituted an indel portion). The SNP positions are highlighted in red in Figure 4.

These nucleotide sequences were aligned to determine the consensus sequence in region A1-2-R. The nucleotide sequences determined in the varieties were evaluated for 67 SNPs in region A1-2-R (4 of these 67 SNPs, at positions 57–59 and 65, constituted an indel portion) corresponding to the nucleotide positions 1, 2, 3, 5, 8, 9, 10, 11, 12, 13, 14, 15, 16, 17, 20, 21, 25, 26, 27, 28, 29, 30, 31, 33, 35, 36, 37, 38, 41, 42, 43, 44, 46, 47, 48, 50, 51, 56, 57, 58, 59, 63, 65, 68, 72, 78, 79, 84, 86, 88, 90, 92, 118, 153, 154, 191, 205, 206, 226, 228, 233, 254, 289, 315, 350, 392, and 405. The SNP positions are highlighted in red in Figure 5.

Zeus, Summit, and Premiant were subjected to further analysis for region A1-2-R2. In region A1-2-R2 (34 of these 59 SNPs constituted an indel portion), the SNPs corresponded to the nucleotide positions 3, 8, 19, 20, 27, 28, 40, 41, 46, 47, 57, 64, 65, 66, 67, 68, 69, 70, 71, 72, 73, 74, 75, 76, 77, 78, 79, 80, 81, 82, 83, 84, 85, 90, 112, 116, 118, 120, 121, 122, 123, 124, 125, 126, 127, 128, 129, 130, 131, 140, 156, 178, 191, 192, 244, 266, 271, 377, and 430 (positions 64–85, and 120–131 constituted the indel portions). The SNP positions are depicted in red in Figure 6.

Using nucleotides at the SNP positions in the fragments of A1-2-L (sequenced from 5′ primer) and A1-2-R/R2 (sequenced from 3′ primer), Perle and Northern Brewer as well as Premiant, Zeus, and Summit were successfully identified, when 21 and 67 SNPs were found between Perle and Northern Brewer, and 59 SNPs were found among Premiant, Zeus, and Summit.

```
A1-2-L REGION  (PERLE AND NORTHERN BREWER)
CAGCTGAGCT TGAAAGTTAT GGCTATCGCC GCCRCCATTT CGGGTCCTCT GACAACTCCG    60
TCTCGGCGGC GCTCAGTCAC CTCCTTCAGC TCACTCTCCA WTTCTCATTC TCTTACGRGA   120
CAAYTGAGTT TTCTCAGAGC AAGTCGCCCC TGTATTGGCT TGTYAGCYAC WGCTTCTTCT   180
TCTTCTTCTT CTTCCATTTC CATGAGTCTC GAAGCCGCCG AGAAGGCCTC GCCGGTGTCG   240
TTCTTGGATC GCAGGGAGAC CGGTTTTCTT CATTTTGTCA AGTACCACGG CGTCGGCAAT   300
GACTTCATCT TGGTAAACTC GAAAATGGAG CTAGTTTTTC TCTATAGAGG AAAAGAAAGA   360
ATTTTTTTCT TCTAAATTTA TTGAGTAGTC TYTTTTTKTA TTGATGTAGG TTGATAATAG   420
GGATTCTTCA GAGCCTAGGA TTACTCCCGA GCAAGCGGYG AAGCTCTGTG ATCGGAACTT   480
TGGAATTGGA GCTGATGGGG TSATTTTTGC TATGCCTGGC ATCAATGGCA CTGACTAC     538
  * Underlined part contains deletion sequence.
```

Figure 4. Nucleotide sequence of region A1-2-L. Please consult the legend of Figure 1 for details.

2.2.5. Characterization of SNP-rich regions and identification of hop varieties

In every SNP-rich region, consensus sequence and SNP positions were detected by the alignment analysis. Nucleotide polymorphisms in each variety were evaluated at the SNPs positions in all the regions. Within the 21 studied hop varieties, 24 SNPs were identified in the A1 region and 14 SNPs (including indel) were observed in the B1 region. *H. lupulus*, with normally a diploid chromosome, had heterozygous or homozygous SNPs in each DNA region. For example, in the A1 region, European varieties had homozygous SNPs at 77th (C/T) and

```
A1-2-R REGION (PERLE AND NORTHERN BREWER)
RSWASGAWRS YYYRSSYGAY WTATYKWYRW RCYTRWRMAT KSSWAKRWAW RCACASGTAA    60
CAYATCAYAC AYACACAYRC ACAYAYAYAY AYATATACAT ATAATGTAAA TGTTGATWCT   120
CTATTGTGAT GATTTGCTTC TGAAACATGA TAWWAGAAAC AATAAAAAGA ACAAAGAAGT   180
ATTGGTTATT RGGAAGACCT CTTTYRGATT TCTTTGACAA TGCCTRTRTG TTYTATTGAT   240
GTAGCTTTAC TGTRCATACT GGTGCTGGTC TAATTATTCC AGAAATACWA GATGATGGTC   300
AGGTATAAAC TTCTWTACTT GCAAATTACC TAAATCTATT GGGTTCATAK GCTTCAAAAG   360
CAACATTCAT AAATGATTGC ATTTTGCTAC ARTTATGGCA GTTTKGCTTC TAATCTGGAT   420
TTGTTGAAGT TGCCAAACTA CTGGATAGCG ATTTTTGAGT ATTCAATTTA GCAGGGGTGC   480
TGTTTTGATT TCAGGTCAAA GTTGATATGG GTGAAA                            516
  * Underlined part contains deletion sequence.
```

Figure 5. Nucleotide sequence of region A1-2-R. Please consult the legend of Figure 1 for details.

```
A1-2-R2 REGION (PREMIANT, ZEUS, AND SUMMIT)
AGYACGAKGC TTTGCCCGWK TTATTGYYGA GCTTGAGAAW WTGCAWRGAA AGCACASGTA    60
ACAYATMTAT AGACMTATAC ATGCATATAY ACACACACAC ACACACACAC AYACAYAYAC   120
ACACACACAC ATATACATAK AATGTAAATG TTGATWCTCT ATTGTGATGA TTTGCTTYTG   180
AAACATGATA WWAGAAACAA TAAAAAGAAC AAAGAAGTAT TGGTTATTAG GAAGACCTCT   240
TTTRGATTTC TTTGACAATG CCTATRTGTT YTATTGATGT AGCTTTACTG TGCATACTGG   300
TGCTGGTCTA ATTATTCCAG AAATACAAGA TGATGGTCAG GTATAAACTT CTATACTTGC   360
AAATTACCTA AATCTAWTGG GTTCATAGGC TTCAAAAGCA ACATTCATAA ATGATTGCAT   420
TTTGCTACAR TTATGGCAGT TTGGCTTCTA ATCTGGATTT GTTGAAGTTG CCAAACTACT   480
GGATAGCGAT TTTTGAGTAT TCAATTTAGC AGGGGTGCTG TTTTGATTTC AGGTCAAAGT   540
GA                                                                 542
  * Underlined part contains deletion sequence.
```

Figure 6. Nucleotide sequence of region A1-2-R2. Please consult the legend of Figure 1 for details.

103th (A/G) positions. Such homozygous SNPs can be analyzed more easily than the heterozygous SNPs when mixed with another variety, having different nucleotides at the SNP positions. In a case, where the variety Saaz was mixed with the variety Sládek, position 77 SNPs were T and C, respectively, in the A1 region (data not shown), and these nucleotides could be easily distinguished on their electropherograms. On the other hand, position 74 SNPs were W (A and T) and A, respectively, in the same region. In this case, it was difficult to recognize whether the variety Saaz was mixed with the variety Sládek or not. Each variety had a specific combination of SNPs as markers, and 12 and 9 DNA types in the A1 and B1 regions, respectively, were identified among the 21 varieties. Indel was also found in the C1 region. Nucleotides at the SNP positions including indel were observed. Forty-four SNPs were found in this region, and 5 DNA types were identified among the 21 varieties. It was revealed that Galena had 2 DNA types in the B1 region and Cascade and Super Galena had 2 DNA types in the C1 region.

Additionally, the A1-2 region was searched because there was no difference in the combination of the SNPs in A1, B1, and C1 regions between Perle and Northern Brewer, among Premiant, Zeus, and Summit. Nucleotides at the SNP positions in the fragments of A1-2-L (sequenced from 5′ primer) and A1-2-R/R2 (sequenced from 3′ primer) were shown, when 21 and 67 SNPs were found between Perle and Northern Brewer, and 59 SNPs were found among Premiant, Zeus, and Summit. Perle and Northern Brewer as well as Premiant, Zeus, and Summit were successfully identified.

For confirmation, we tried to distinguish between Columbus and Tomahawk, considered genetically identical [22–24], by analyzing the 4 regions and, additionally, the middle area of the A1-2 region, with newly designed primers, A1-2-M_F and A1-2-M_R (Table 4). No differences in the nucleotide sequences were detected between them. Therefore, we confirmed that these 2 varieties are indeed identical and could be considered a single variety.

Consequently, 21 hop varieties were successfully identified by a combination of these genotypes of SNPs, with differences in the 4 SNP-rich regions. The summary results are shown in Table 6.

Origin	Variety	Diplotype				
		A1	B1	C1	A1-2	A1+B1+C1+ (A1-2)
Czech Republic	Saaz	1	a	i		A
	Sládek	2	b	i		B
	Premiant	2	c	i	β1	C
Germany	Tradition	3	d	ii		D
	Spalter	4	e	i		E
	Spalter Select	2	f	ii		F
	Perle	2	d	i	α1	G
	Tettnang	5	g	i		H
	Brewer's Gold	7	c	i		I
	Northern Brewer	2	d	i	α2	J
	Magnum	2	d	iii		K
	Herkules	6	d	ii		L
	German Nugget	9	c	i		M
	Taurus	8	d	i		N
USA	Cascade	2	d	iv		O1

Origin	Variety	Diplotype				
		A1	B1	C1	A1-2	A1+B1+C1+ (A1-2)
				i		O2
	Zeus	2	c	i	β2	P
	Summit	2	c	i	β3	Q
	Galena	2	h	i		R1
			i			R2
	Super Galena	11	c	i		S1
				v		S2
	Nugget	10	c	i		T
	Columbus/Tomahawk	12	c	i	γ	U

Table 6. Successful identification of 21 hop varieties

2.2.6. Comparison of DNA samples prepared from hop pellets and cones

Comparison was made between the results obtained in the two cases where DNA samples were extracted from either the hop pellets or the dried hop cones, as described in Section 2.2. It was confirmed that DNA extraction and sequencing were possible with both types of DNA samples. Also, analyses using DNA samples of both types yielded the same results. This result further demonstrates that inspection at a processing step (e.g., inspection for contamination at a pelletization step) is technically possible.

2.2.7. Comparison between three Saaz clones

About 1 g each of dried cones of three Saaz clones (Osvald's clones 31, 72, and 114) was ground in a mortar in the presence of liquid nitrogen, and the DNA was extracted from about 50 mg each of the ground materials by the CTAB method described in Section 2.2. Each of the extracted DNA sample was subjected to amplification of the DNA fragments from regions A1, B1, and C1 and followed by sequencing of the amplified fragments, according to the procedures as described above. For each region, the nucleotide sequences of the three clones were aligned for comparison with each other.

The results obtained confirmed that there was no difference among the three Saaz clones in terms of the nucleotide sequences in the analyzed regions. In other words, it was found that any of Saaz clones could be identified through the above-described analysis using the inventive variety identification regions. These results demonstrated that the analysis using regions A1, B1, and C1 as the variety identification regions required no determination by clone.

2.2.8. Identification of variety mixtures using the newly identified SNP markers

Because it is important to detect contamination of other varieties, we developed a method for detecting such contamination by using the SNPs markers. The mixed samples of Saaz and

Premiant hops were analyzed (for region A1). To prepare different samples, pellets of these varieties were ground as described above followed by mixing of the ground materials in the relative proportions by weight as mentioned in Table 7.

A representative electropherogram, containing the SNP position 77 in the A1 region (A1_#77), is shown in Figure 7. Peaks in the electropherogram represent fluorescence intensity of 4 different nucleotides at each DNA positions, which are depicted in different colors; A, C, G, and T, are shown in green, blue, black, and red, respectively. Variety I is homozygous (TT) at position 77, and variety II is homozygous (CC) at the same position. In the case of mixing of varieties in 50% proportion, overlap of 2 peaks of T and C was observed at this position, reflecting contamination. Figure 7 also shows peaks in the same region when variety II was mixed at 5 and 10%. Peaks in blue at this position, derived from variety II, were detected even at 5% contamination. It was the same for A1_#199 and A1_#204, in which variety I was heterozygous (GC) and variety II was homozygous (CC), so it was not easy to recognize the contamination by peak height of electropherogram.

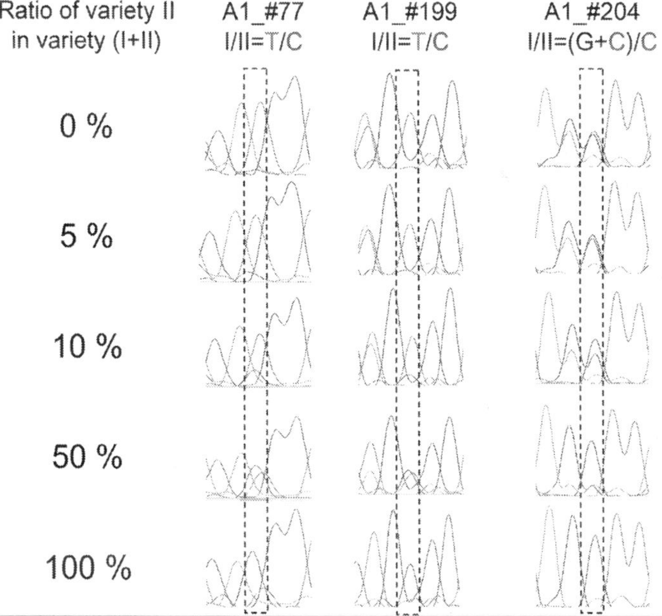

Figure 7. Representative electropherogram containing the SNP positions 77, 199, and 204 in the A1 region (A1_#77, A1_#199, and A1_#204): "T" is represented in red color, and "C" is in blue color.

We estimated more SNPs, with a focus on homozygous SNPs, and calculated an average of the mixing rate in variety II. As a result, we obtained a closer estimate of the mixing rate. We postulate that contamination at levels lower than 5% could be estimated; however, the acceptable contamination level for us might be 5% with reference to the genetically modified organism contamination in Japanese food. Thus, the values below 5% have a slight importance.

Proportion of Premiant as a contaminant	1	2	3	4	5
	0%	5%	10%	50%	100%
Saaz	30 mg	28.5 mg	27 mg	15 mg	0 mg
Premiant	0 mg	1.5 mg	3 mg	15 mg	30 mg
Detection of Premiant	–	○	○	○	○

Table 7. Preparation of the 2-variety mixtures and results obtained for each sample.

Each sample was prepared by mixing pellets of two varieties in specified proportions by weight.

3. Conclusions and future directions

The results obtained in the present study suggest that the SNP-combination method has high reliability as it utilizes the sequence data. Computational handling of SNP data can be easily carried out so that analysis among many varieties could be easily performed with digital information. Other SNPs identified in the future could be used as additional identification markers. Therefore, using this method, enhancement of accuracy and repeatability in the variety identification could be accomplished in a relatively simple manner.

As SNP-rich DNA regions are only 0.6–1.5 kb in size, they are much less likely to be damaged during the processing of hop products. However, upon degradation and fragmentation of the SNP-rich regions, newly designed primers for the shorter fragments generated might be useful for the amplification of the fragments and may contain several useful SNPs which can be used as identification markers.

The SNP-based information could be also used for quantitative determination of the ratio of variety mixture. In the future, more accurate results will be obtained by using quantitative real-time PCR and/or NGS, which may provide a huge amount of sequence data and increase reliability.

Acknowledgements

I appreciate the technical support and advice offered by Dr. Toshiya Yamamoto (National Institute of Fruit Tree Science, Tsukuba, Japan), Dr. Jun Onodera (Operon Biotechnologies, K.K., Eurofins Genomics, Japan), Dr. Eiichiro Ono (Research Institute, Suntory Global Innovation Center Limited, Japan), and my collaborators.

Author details

Hiromasa Yamauchi*

Address all correspondence to: Hiromasa_Yamauchi@suntory.co.jp

Suntory Business Expert Ltd, Kawasaki, Japan

References

[1] Araki S, Tsuchiya Y, Masachika T, Tamaki T, Shinotsuka K. Identification of hop cultivars by DNA marker analysis. J. Am. Soc. Brew. Chem. 1998;56:93–98. DOI: 10.1094/asbcj-56-0093.

[2] Murakami A. The practical application of PCR for the verification of hop variety. MBAA Technical Quarterly. 1998;35:185–188.

[3] Patzak J. Assessment of somaclonal variability in hop (*Humulus lupulus* L.) *in vitro* meristem cultures and clones by molecular methods. Euphytica. 2003;131:343–350. DOI: 10.1023/A:1024096401424.

[4] Patzak J, Nesvadba V, Henychova A, et al. Assessment of the genetic diversity of wild hops (*Humulus lupulus* L.) in Europe using chemical and molecular analyses. Biochem. Syst. Ecol. 2010;38:136–145. DOI: 10.1016/j.bse.2009.12.023.

[5] Sustar-Vozlic J, Javornik B. Genetic relationships in cultivars of hop, *Humulus lupulus* L., determined by RAPD analysis. Plant Breed. 1999;118:175–181. DOI: 10.1046/j.1439-0523.1999.118002175.x.

[6] Pillay M, Kenny S. T. Structure and inheritance of ribosomal DNA variants in cultivated and wild hop, *Humulus lupulus* L. Theor. Appl. Genet. 1996;93:333–340. DOI: 10.1007/BF00223173.

[7] Jakse J, Kindlhofer K, Javornik B. Assessment of genetic variation and differentiation of hop genotypes by microsatellite and AFLP markers. Genome. 2001;44:773–782. DOI: 10.1139/g01-071.

[8] Seefelder S, Ehrmaier H, Schweizer G, et al. Genetic diversity and phylogenetic relationships among accessions of hop, *Humulus lupulus*, as determined by amplified fragment length polymorphism fingerprinting compared with pedigree data. Plant Breed. 2000;119:257–263. DOI: 10.1046/j.1439-0523.2000.00500.x.

[9] Andreja Č, Jernej J, Branka J. Identification and differentiation of Hop varieties using simple sequence repeat markers. J. Am. Soc. Brew. Chem. 2004;62:1–7. DOI: 10.1094/ASBCJ-62-0001.

[10] Jakse J, Satovic Z, Javornik B. Microsatellite variability among wild and cultivated hops (*Humulus lupulus* L.). Genome. 2004;47:889–899. DOI: 10.1139/g04-054.

[11] Kanai D, Kirita M, Sakamoto K. Method for judging kind of hop using microsatellite DNA. JP Patent Publication number 2006-34142, 2006-2-9.

[12] Patzak J. Comparison of RAPD, STS, ISSR and AFLP molecular methods used for assessment of genetic diversity in hop (*Humulus lupulus* L.). Euphytica. 2001;121:9–18: DOI: 10.1023/A:1012099123877.

[13] Patzak J, Nesvadba V, Krofta K, Henychova A, Marzoev A. I, Richards K. Evaluation of genetic variability of wild hops (*Humulus lupulus* L.) in Canada and the Caucasus region by chemical and molecular methods. Genome. 2010;53:545–557. DOI: 10.1139/g10-024.

[14] Syvolap IuM, Zakharova O. O, Kozhukhova N. E, Ihnatova S. O, Prystavs'kyĭ M. S, Zelenina H. A. Modern biotechnologies in estimation of genetic diversity of Ukrainian varieties of hop (*Humulus lupulus* L.). Tsitol Genet. 2010;44:3–12. Cf. DOI: 10.3103/S0095452710050014.

[15] Murakami A, Darby P, Javornik B, Pais MSS, Seigner E, Lutz A, Svoboda P. Molecular phylogeny of wild Hops, *Humulus lupulus* L. Heredity. 2006;97:66–74. DOI: 10.1038/sj.hdy.6800839.

[16] Vrba L, Matoušek J, Patzak J. New STS molecular markers for assessment of genetic diversity and DNA fingerprinting in hop (*Humulus lupulus* L.). Genome. 2007;50:15–25. DOI: 10.1139/g06-128.

[17] Howard EL, Whittock SP, Jakše J, Carling J, Matthews PD, Probasco G, Henning JA, Darby P, Cerenak A, Javornik B, Kilian A, Koutoulis A. High-throughput genotyping of hop (*Humulus lupulus* L.) utilising diversity arrays technology (DArT). Theor. Appl. Genet. 2011;122:1265–1280. DOI: 10.1007/s00122-011-1529-4.

[18] Castro C. B, Whittock L. D, Whittock S. P, Leggett G, Koutoulis A. DNA sequence and expression variation of hop (*Humulus lupulus*) valerophenone synthase (VPS), a key gene in bitter acid biosynthesis. An Bot. 2008;102:265–273. DOI: 10.1093/aob/mcn089.

[19] Grabowska-Joachimiak A, Śliwińska E, Piguła M/, Skomra U, Joachimiak AJ. Genome size in *Humulus lupulus* L. and *H. japonicus* Siebold and Zucc. (*Cannabaceae*). Acta Societatis Botanicorum Poloniae. 2006;75:207–214. DOI: 10.5586/asbp.2006.024.

[20] Venter JC, Adams MD, Myers EW, Li PW, Mural RJ, et al. The sequence of the human genome. Science 2001;291:1304-1351. DOI: 10.1126/science.1058040.

[21] Yamauchi H, Mukouzaka Y, Taniguchi T, Nakashima K, Furukubo S, Harada M. Newly developed SNP-based identification method of hop varieties. J. Am. Soc. Brew. Chem. 2014;72:239–245. DOI: 10.1094/ASBCJ-2014-1006-01.

[22] Hatch L. Brewbase Encyclopedia. http://members.tripod.com/~Hatch_L/bbase-hops.html, (cf. 2013-08-20).

[23] Hopsteiner. Varieties - United States. http://www.hopsteiner.com/varieties/united-states.php, (cf. 2013-08-20).

[24] Lewis G. K, Zimmermann C. E, Hazenberg H. Hop variety named 'Columbus'. U. S. Patent 10,956. 1999-06-15.

Next Generation Sequencing in Humanomics

Chapter 12

Analysis of Haplotype Sequences

Sally S. Lloyd, Edward J. Steele and Roger L. Dawkins

Additional information is available at the end of the chapter

http://dx.doi.org/10.5772/61794

Abstract

In this era of whole-genome, next-generation sequencing, it is important to have a clear understanding of the concept of "haplotype". We show here that most of the important regions of the genome can be described in terms of polymorphic frozen blocks (PFB). At each PFB, there are numerous, even hundreds, of alternative ancestral haplotypes. Haplotypes, not genes, can be regarded as the principal unit of inheritance. We illustrate how sequence data can be analysed to reveal and define these ancestral haplotypes.

Keywords: Ancestral haplotypes, Polymorphic frozen blocks, Genomic evolution

1. Introduction

Comparative analyses of haplotype sequences allow many efficiencies. It is not surprising that there are many enthusiastic claims. Haplotypes, by any of many definitions, offer opportunities to understand the inheritance of polymorphic traits and their regulation. The most useful are markers of extensive complex polymorphic sequences of evolutionary significance even when the functional components, whether coding or noncoding, are yet to be elaborated.

Substantial advances became possible with the elucidation of genomic structure and function more than 20 years ago and long before recent advances in sequencing technology [1] and bioinformatics [2]. It became clear that haplotypes, *not genes*, can be regarded as the principal unit of inheritance.

This chapter evaluates some competing strategies and illustrates the power now available through NGS.

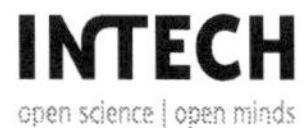

2. Haplotype terminology

A review of current literature reveals a staggering collection of terms synonymous with haplotypes, as listed in Table 1.

Ancestral haplotypes
Conserved extended haplotypes
Linkage groups
Linkage disequilibrium haplotypes
Hapmaps
Haplogroup
Haplobanks
Haploblocks
Haplotype block

Table 1. Terminology

Even if it were possible to define the various neologisms, it seems certain that confusion will remain until there is recognition of the conceptual background.

We introduced the term *ancestral haplotypes* to emphasise the persistence of the founding pool [3, 4]. Such haplotypes are conserved over thousands of generations; they allow identification of remote ancestors and their contributions to the creation of individual members of the species with their diseases. Unfortunately, others use the same term in different ways and even in the opposite sense, that is, to refer to *the single* original haplotype which is presumed to have mutated to give rise to all the so-called variants now present. Indeed, as just one example of the problem, the reader has to be able to interpret the following: "we identified all nonredundant haplotypes with a frequency of ≥10% and consisting of at least 10 SNPs, which are likely to represent the nonrecombinant descendants from a single ancestor" [5].

To yet further confound matters, increasingly, the term *haplotype* is being used to describe any combination of alleles or markers, such as SNPs, without regard to their reproducibility, inheritance, polymorphism or biological significance. Currently, there are conflicting methods of detection. The problems appear to be increasing as ephemeral concepts diverge and as claims for better approaches focus on just one or another competing technology or bioinformatic package.

Several other aspects are clear.

- Linkage groups relate to closely linked loci but do not define haplotypes.

- Linkage disequilibrium is affected by relative frequencies and therefore fails to detect rare haplotypes.

- Trios can be misleading since the coverage of the family is limited.

- Haplobanks. The Tokunaga group has established some important principles with the intention of establishing haplotype-matched pluripotential stem cell banks [6]. Unfortunately, and amazingly, there is now uncertainty as to how to define the haplotypes. For example, a recent paper urges international collaboration to avoid fragmentation [7]. It would be wise to avoid neologisms and such redefinitions without clarity of meaning.

3. Definitions and concepts

In the presequencing era, there was a clear understanding of what was meant by the term *haplotype*: Combinations of alleles at different loci segregating together in multigenerational family studies [8]. Some seem unaware of this long history and have had to rediscover the concept [2].

The implications were apparent at least 50 years ago: a specific allele A1 at locus A is inherited together with a specific allele B1 at an adjacent, "closely linked" locus B [9]. The fact that these two alleles segregated together through multiple generations was unexpected and lead to controversy but, in retrospect, clearly implied that

1.   The two alleles were encoded on the same chromosome, whether paternal or maternal.

2.   The two loci were closely linked.

3.   Recombination was rare.

4.   The two loci arose by duplication.

5.   Duplication is associated with polymorphism.

The repeated cosegregation of alleles came to be known as a haplotype: from ἁπλφούς = single [9].

It is worth emphasizing that it was the cosegregation as haplotypes through "phased" multigenerational families (rather than "unphased" populations) which foretold the later demonstration that there was a continuous haplospecific sequence. It is also pertinent, with the benefit of hindsight and in view of recent confusion, that the haplotypes, defined in one family, occurred in other families of similar remote ancestry raising the radical possibility of conservation beyond that expected from close linkage alone. In other words, recombination is patchy and does not necessarily disperse the components of duplications, even after thousands of meioses. The issue of linkage disequilibrium and the limits of LD mapping are considered below.

The implications of haplotypes, as listed above, became even clearer as the HLA A and HLA B locus alleles and then HLA DR alleles were defined during the 1970s. However, in this case, the loci were widely separated. Over time, it became clear that each of the A-B and B-DR haplotypes were some 800 kb in length. Patently, close linkage could not explain these haplotypes; either there was selection for *cis* interaction or there was suppression of recombination [3, 4].

Through their studies of diseases, the Alper–Yunis group discovered that the B-DR haplotypes contained specific alleles at duplicated loci which had no structural or functional relevance to HLA (i.e. complement and 21 hydroxylase loci) but which happen to be located within the major histocompatibility complex [10–16]. Thus, *cis* interaction alone could be rejected as the sole explanation.

The importance of discovery through disease was illustrated at a meeting held in 1982 [3, 4]. As shown in Table 2, it was disease associations which allowed the initial discovery of ancestral haplotypes; note, these three disease-associated haplotypes could have only been discovered through their associations. Two share DR3 and two share B18 but the frequencies differ. Thus, the three haplotypes cannot be detected by linkage disequilibrium.

Designation	A	Cw	B	Bf	C2	C4A	C4B	DR	Disease
8.1	1	7	8	S	C	Q0	1	3	MG, SLE, IDDM
18.2	–	–	18	F1	C	3	Q0	3	IDDM
18.1	25	–	18	S	Q0	4	2	2	C2 deficiency

MG = myasthenia gravis, SLE = systemic lupus erythematosus, IDDM = insulin-dependent (type 1) diabetes mellitus.

Adapted from ref. [4]

Table 2. MHC haplotypes and disease associations

Once the numerous other ancestral haplotypes were defined, multigenerational family studies identified cosegregating combinations of multiple alleles at separated loci, i.e. haplotypes stretching over nearly 2 Mb from HLA A to DR. A haplotype was defined by the alleles "inherited *en bloc* from one parent and implies the transmission of all of the chromosomal segment" from one generation to the next [4].

When haplotypes defined in one family were compared with those identified in apparently unrelated families, sharing was immediately apparent. There were specific combinations of alleles at all the numerous unrelated loci as these were defined and typed. However, and increasingly relevant today, as summarized in refs. [3, 4, 17, 18]:

1. The combinations observed are *not* a simple function of allele frequencies; only some of the components inherited *en bloc* are in linkage disequilibrium.

2. Many haplotypes are rare combinations of frequent alleles at some loci but rare alleles at other loci.

3. Very few alleles are entirely haplospecific.

4. Haplotype frequencies are often less than 1%.

5. The same haplotypes are found in multiple, apparently unrelated, families.

6. Many of these nonrandom combinations are associated with a disease (such as systemic lupus erythematosus) or function (such as TNF production).

7. With a few dramatic exceptions (such as 21 hydroxylase and C2 deficiency carried by what we now call the 47.1 and 18.1 ancestral haplotypes), the individual alleles do not explain the haplospecific effects on disease and function.

8. Penetrance is low. That is to say, the haplotypes are *sine qua non* in that they permit particular diseases and functions but only in the presence of other genetic, infectious, environmental, hormonal and age-related factors.

9. Recombination is rare and difficult to demonstrate even within multigenerational families with the potential to confirm a meiotic recombinant. Nevertheless, over the life of an ancestral haplotype — say 10, 000 meioses — there have been recombinations which have resulted in shuffling between ancestral haplotypes [18, 19].

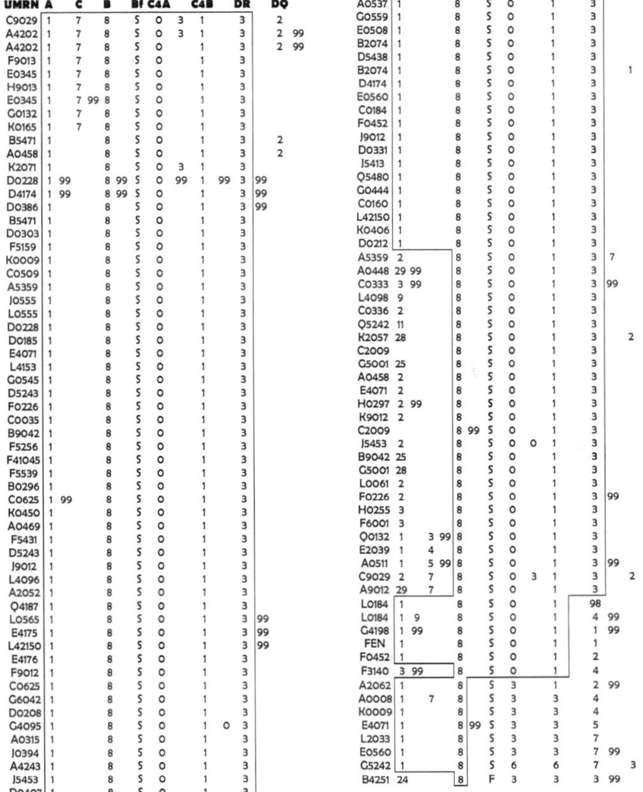

Adapted from ref. [18].

Figure 1. Historic recombinations of AH 8.1. The HLA-B8 allele is carried by one ancestral haplotype marked by A1, Cw7, B8, BfS, C4AQ0, C4B1, DR3. All the haplotypes in data set 1 carrying HLA-B8 are represented. These haplotypes have been sorted so that haplotypes that carry all alleles of 8.1 from HLA-A to DR are shown at the top of the figure, followed by haplotypes that extend from HLA-B to DR. Telomeric recombinants are shown at the bottom. The boxed areas represent those portions of the 8.1 ancestral haplotype that are carried by unrelated B8-containing haplotypes. Vertical lines approximately indicate the region where historical recombination has occurred.

Some of these points are illustrated in Figure 1. It can be seen that subjects with B8 can be listed to show conservation but also historic recombinations between HLA A and B, between C4B and DR, and between HLA B and Bf.

By the mid-1990s, and long before the rediscoveries of the 2000s [2], such analyses led to the conclusion that there are polymorphic frozen blocks (PFB), as illustrated in Figure 2.

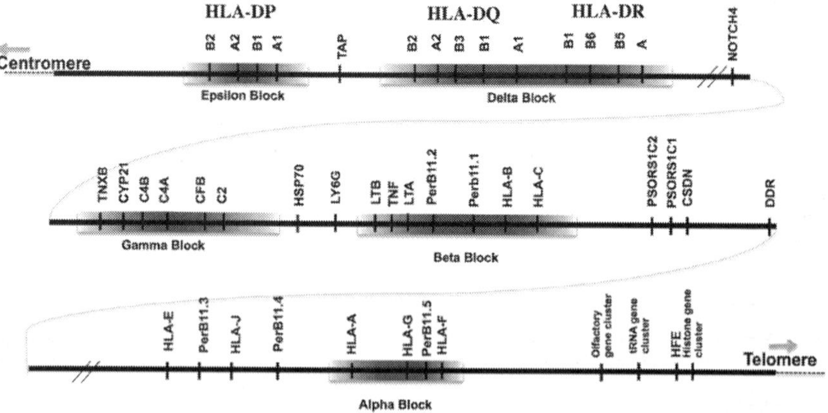

Figure 2. Ancestral haplotypes and polymorphic frozen blocks within the human major histocompatibility complex. Each ancestral haplotype has its own unique DNA sequence which includes single nucleotide polymorphisms (SNPs), copy number variations, segmental duplications, insertion and deletion events (indels) including retroviral and retroviral-like elements (RLEs). The full length is approximately 4 Mb. Higher degrees of diversity indicated by shading define polymorphic frozen blocks (PFB). Recombination occurs far more frequently between, rather than within, these blocks. Mutations within blocks are effectively suppressed. Adapted from refs. [17, 20] and [21]. Reproduced with permission from ref. [22].

PFB throughout the genome are the latter-day equivalents of loci. Sequences which define ancestral haplotypes are the equivalent of alleles. The diversity is multifactorial with contributions from reiterative speciation as follows [17]:

- Retroviral integration

- Duplication

- Indels

- Polymorphism

These elements all contribute to the haplospecificity of the sequence of ancestral haplotypes as shown in Figure 3. Similar distribution of diversity has been found by many others [5, 17, 19, 20, 23, 24]. The same patterns are also found in primates [25].

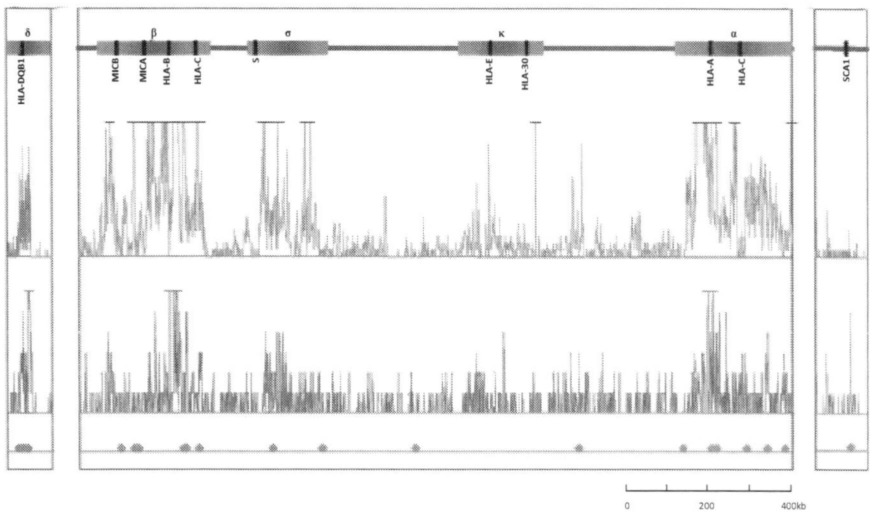

Adapted from ref. [26].

Figure 3. Sequence diversity is packaged as polymorphic frozen blocks (PFB). SNPs and indel occur in similar locations within PFB. (a) The SNP profile after removing indels. Peaks higher than 20 SNPs per 1000 nucleotides are truncated. (b) The location of indels. Peaks higher than six indels per 1000 nucleotides are truncated. (c) The position of indels greater than 100 nucleotides.

4. Use of ancestral haplotypes

Here, we illustrate the potential of sequence analysis, if designed to identify conserved, extended, ancestral haplotypes. The utility depends very largely on the concept behind the analysis. However, it also depends upon the genomic region actually sequenced and whether it is possible to interpret the patterns in the context of the heterogeneous architecture of the genome. Within PFB, there will be a multitude of alternative sequences to compare. In the genome between these blocks, there is much less diversity with long stretches of monomorphic sequence. Thus, the recent fashion for identifying homozygosity [27, 28], without regard to diversity, shifts the focus to less informative regions of the genome. Of course, by way of explanation for the fashion, homozygosity within PFB is much more difficult to find; the most common ancestral haplotypes with frequencies of 0.1 will be homozygous in only 1% of the general population. Until high-throughput NGS became available, it was necessary to examine disease panels or consanguineous families.

The conceptual background is summarised in the following figures which contrast two approaches. *Population genetics* teaches that free recombination effectively prevents the packaging of polymorphism. The reality, designated here as *quantal genomics*, emphasises clustering and conservation of polymorphism. Each haplotype is a specific sequence which regulates expressed genes by *cis, trans* or *epistatic* interaction. The whole sequence is conserved. Linkage disequilibrium, when it occurs, is simply a reflection of this conservation which includes haplotypes with alleles which are relatively common in one haplotype when compared with others. Each is ancestral, in the sense that they are shared by apparently unrelated families separated by hundreds or even thousands of generations. It follows that the polymorphisms are actively conserved and could not be a consequence of recent mutation.

Some of the implications are illustrated in Figures 4 and 5.

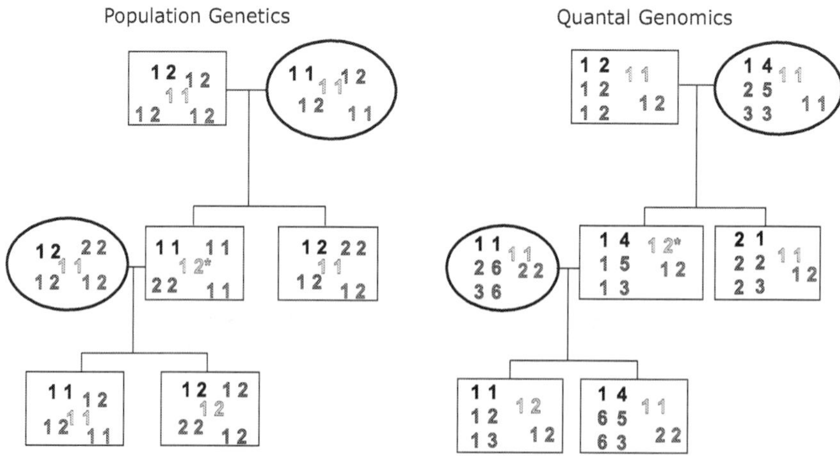

Figure 4. Importance of clustering functional genes. Colours represent loci and numbers represent alleles at those loci. On the left is the basis of the infinitesimal model used in population genetics. Loci are biallelic and can be homozygous or heterozygous. Free recombination occurs between loci and alleles segregate independently. On the right, loci are within polymorphic frozen blocks (PFB), shown by alignment of loci. Alleles within PFB segregate *en bloc*, forming haplotypes, which are inherited intact through many generations. Important genes are carried within PFB, conserving their *cis* interactions. Loci within PFB have multiple alleles, allowing for a greater degree of polymorphism clustered within the block. There can be hundreds of ancestral haplotypes for each PFB. *Trans* interactions between haplotypes increase the diversity expressed in the population. The loci shown in green and yellow are outside the PFB and follow a pattern of inheritance similar to population genetics. *De novo* mutations are indicated by asterisk—on the right the mutations occur at loci outside of conserved PFB and will have little if any consequence because truly important differences are encoded within PFB. Monogenic diseases or traits are the partial exceptions. On the left, mutations can occur at any loci but are generally assumed to occur at loci that were monoallelic. They may or may not be important, depending upon frequency, context, repair and heritability. Adapted with permission from ref. [22].

By 1987, it was clearly established that each ancestral haplotype has a specific content of genomic features such as duplications and indels. These too are actively conserved and can themselves be used as signatures for haplotypes of hundreds of kilobases and even megabases. These observations were very difficult to explain in terms of any form of neo-Darwinism, natural selection, random errors or population genetics as taught then and today. Rather, we realised, the genome is not actually homogeneous but partitioned into protected quanta or PFB [17, 22, 26, 29].

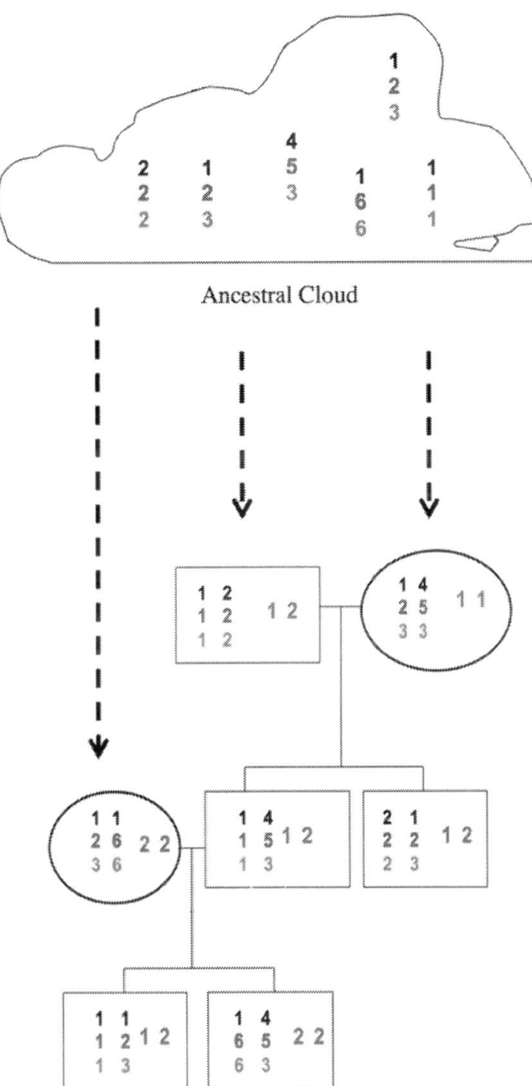

Figure 5. Modern haplotypes are derived from the deep past — they are ancestral haplotypes.

5. Sequencing of critical genomic regions

By 1992, there was sufficient sequencing to confirm the earlier prediction that each ancestral haplotype is actually a frozen sequence.

Haplotype	Geometric element at CL1	Length	Geometric element at CL2	Length
57.1	$(TC)^{12}(TG)^6(TC)^{14}(TG)^3(TC)^{12}$	94	TA $(TC)^{18}$ TT $(TC)^9$	58
18.2	$(TC)^{14}$	28	Deleted	
8.1	$(TC)^{28}$	56	$(TC)^{15}$ TG $(TC)^6$ TG $(TC)^8$ TG $(TC)^5$	96
7.1	$(TC)^{12}(TG)^6(TC)^{14}(TG)^3(TC)^{12}$	94	$(TC)^{14}$ TG $(TC)^6$ TG $(TC)^8$ TG $(TC)^5$	94

Adapted from ref. [30].

Table 3. Haplospecific geometric elements. Ancestral haplotypes have specific sequence signatures at each of the duplicons. Note in 18.2, the duplication did not occur or has been deleted.

We now know that examples of the 8.1 ancestral haplotype are almost identical over megabases [31, 32].

We illustrate the differences between different haplotype sequences in Figure 6. It can be seen that there are certain sites where haplotypes differ. Importantly, haplospecificity is conferred by the whole sequence rather than single nucleotide polymorphisms. For example, reading from left to right, 8.1 and 18.2 differ in T/G but not A/G, etc. Note also that some of the differences are due to indels. Of critical importance is accurate, unmolested sequencing over kilobases, as is now possible through NGS. It is clear, however, that assembly is hazardous especially in areas of duplication and polymorphism. Note also, that there is no justification for regarding *one* particular sequence as the reference. Rather, it is necessary to compare each output with a library of known sequences within each PFB.

The number of differences depends on which haplotypes are compared (see Table 4). Two of the most common Caucasian haplotypes, 8.1 and 7.1, differ by a hundred positions, representing approximately 1% nucleotide diversity. The most different haplotypes are 18.2 and 7.1, having 2.5% nucleotide diversity. Interestingly, these haplotypes are different functionally; 18.2 permits insulin-dependent diabetes mellitus whereas 7.1 is protective.

AH Haplotype	44.2	62.1	7.1	44.1*	8.1
44.2	0				
62.1	187	0			
7.1	249	221	0		
44.1*	73	154	227	0	
8.1	224	219	101	204	0
18.2*	184	130	250	137	245

Table 4. Pairwise differences between haplotypes. Total differences between each pair of haplotypes in the 9277 bp region at HLA-B.

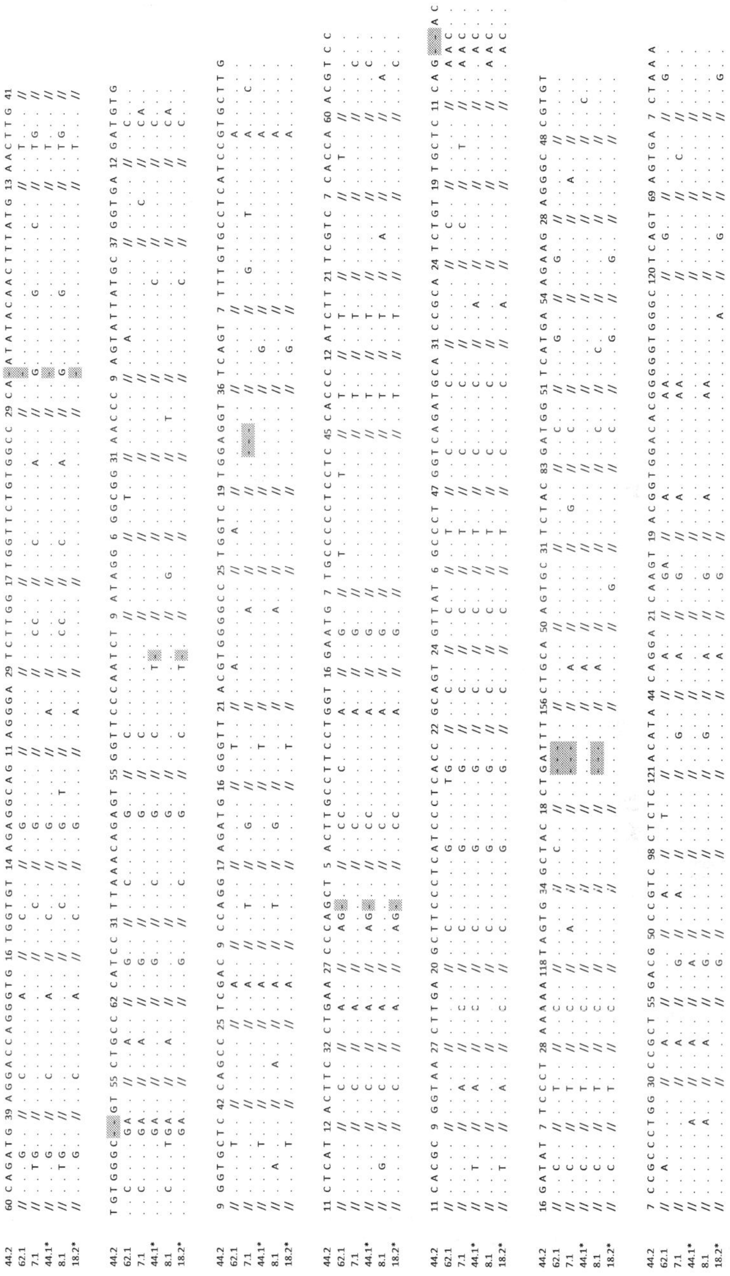

```
44.2    60 CAGATG 39 AGGACCAGGGTG 16 TGGTGT 14 AGAGGCAG 11 AGGGA 29 TCTTGG 17 TGGTTCTGTGGCC 29 CA▓ATATACAACTTTATG 13 AACTTG 41
62.1    // ...G.. // ..C....A.. // ..C... // ..G.... // ..... // ...... // ............. // ..G........C.. // ..T... //
7.1     // ..TG.. // .......... // ...C.. // ..G.... // ..CC.. // ...C...A.. // ..G.....G....... // ..TG.. //
44.1*   // ...G.. // ..C....A.. // ..C.. // ..G.... // ..A.. // ............. // ..G........... // ..T... //
8.1     // ..TG.. // .......... // ...C.. // ..G..T.. // ..... // ..CC.... // ..G.....G....... // ..TG.. //
18.2*   // ...G.. // ..C....A.. // ..C.. // ..G.... // ..A.. // ............. // ..G........... // ..T... //

44.2    TGTGGGC▓▓GT 55 CTGCC 62 CATCC 31 TTAAACAGAGT 55 GGTTCCAATCT 9 ATAGG 6 GGCGG 31 AACCC 9 AGTATTATGC 37 GGTGA 12 GATGTG
62.1    ..C....GA.. // ..A.. // ..G.. // ..C....G.. // ..C..... // ...... // ...... // ..T.. // ..... // ..A.... // ..... // ..C...
7.1     ..C....GA.. // ..A.. // ..G.. // ........G.. // ..C..... // ...... // ...... // ..... // ..... // ..C... // ..CA..
44.1*   .......GA.. // ......G.. // ..C....G.. // ..C....T▓ // ...... // ...... // ..... // ..... // ..C... // ..C..
8.1     ..C..TGA.. // ..A.. // ..G.. // ........G.. // ...G.. // ...... // ..... // ..T.. // ..... // ..... // ..CA..
18.2*   .......GA.. // ..G.. // ..C....G.. // ..C....T▓ // ...... // ...... // ..... // ..... // ..C... // ..C..

44.2    9 GGTGCTC 42 CAGCC 25 TCGAC 9 CCAGG 17 AGATG 16 GGGTT 21 ACGTGGGGCC 25 TGGTC 19 TGGAGGT 36 TCAGT 7 TTTGTGCCTCATCCGTGCTTG
62.1    // ...T.. // ..A.. // ..... // ..... // ..T.. // ..A.. // ...... // ..A.. // ...... // ...... // ..A.....
7.1     // ...... // ..A.C // ..T.. // ..G.. // ..... // ..... // ..A.. // ...... // ▓▓▓... // ..G.....T....A..C.
44.1*   // ...T.. // ..A.. // ..... // ..... // ..T.. // ..... // ..... // ...... // ...G.. // ..A.....
8.1     // ..A.. // ..A.. // ..T.. // ..G.. // ..... // ..... // ..A.. // ...... // ...... // ..A.....
18.2*   // ...T.. // ..A.. // ..T.. // ..... // ..... // ..... // ..G.. // ...... // ..A.....

44.2    11 CTCAT 12 ACTTC 32 CTGAA 27 CCCAGCT 5 ACTTGCCTTCCTGGT 16 GAATG 7 TGCCCCCTCCTC 45 CACCC 12 ATCTT 21 TCGTC 7 CACCA 60 ACGTCC
62.1    // ..... // ..C.. // ..A.. // ..AG▓. // ..CC..C..A.. // ..G.. // ..T..T.. // ..T.. // ..T.. // ..... // ..T.. // .....
7.1     // ..... // ..C.. // ..A.. // ..... // ..CC....A.. // ..G.. // ...... // ..T.. // ..T.. // ..... // ..... // ..C..
44.1*   // ..... // ..C.. // ..A.. // ..AG▓. // ..CC....A.. // ..G.. // ...... // ..T.. // ..T.. // ..... // ..... // ..C..
8.1     // ..G.. // ..C.. // ..A.. // ..... // ..C....A.. // ..G.. // ...... // ..T.. // ..T.. // ..A.. // ..... // ..A..
18.2*   // ..... // ..C.. // ..A.. // ..AG▓. // ..CC....A.. // ..G.. // ...... // ..T.. // ..T.. // ..... // ..... // ..C..

44.2    11 CACGC 9 GGTAA 27 CTTGA 20 GCTTCCCTCATCCCTCACC 22 GCAGT 24 GTTAT 6 GCCCT 47 GGTCAGATGCA 31 CCGCA 24 TCTGT 19 TGCTC 11 C▓AC
62.1    // ..... // ..... // ..... // ..C....G.....TG.. // ..C.. // ..C.. // ..T.. // ..C....C.. // ..... // ..C.. // ..... // .AAC..
7.1     // ..... // ..A.. // ..C.. // ..C....G.....G.. // ..C.. // ..C.. // ..T.. // ..C....C.. // ..... // ..C.. // ..T.. // .AAC..
44.1*   // ..T.. // ..A.. // ..C.. // ..C....G.....G.. // ..C.. // ..C.. // ..T.. // ..C....C.. // ..A.. // ..C.. // ..... // .AC..
8.1     // ..... // ..... // ..... // ..C....G.....G.. // ..C.. // ..C.. // ..T.. // ..C....C.. // ..... // ..... // ..... // .AAC..
18.2*   // ..T.. // ..A.. // ..C.. // ..C....G.....G.. // ..C.. // ..C.. // ..T.. // ..C....C.. // ..A.. // ..... // ..... // .AC..

44.2    16 GATAT 7 TCCCT 28 AAAAA 118 TAGTG 34 GCTAC 18 CTGATT 156 CTGCA 50 AGTGC 31 TCTAC 83 GATGG 51 TCATGA 54 AGAAG 28 AGGGC 48 CGTGT
62.1    // ..C.. // ..T.. // ..C.. // ..... // ..C.. // ..▓▓▓.. // ...... // ...... // ...... // ..C.. // ..G.. // ..G.. // ...... // .....
7.1     // ..C.. // ..T.. // ..C.. // ..A.. // ...... // ..▓▓▓.. // ..A.. // ...... // ..G.. // ..C.. // ...... // ...... // ..A.. // .....
44.1*   // ..C.. // ..T.. // ..C.. // ...... // ...... // ...... // ..A.. // ...... // ...... // ...... // ...... // ...... // ...... // ..C..
8.1     // ..C.. // ..T.. // ..C.. // ...... // ...... // ..▓▓▓.. // ..A.. // ...... // ...... // ...... // ..C.. // ...... // ...... // .....
18.2*   // ..C.. // ..T.. // ..C.. // ...... // ...... // ...... // ...... // ..G.. // ...... // ..C.. // ..G.. // ..G.. // ...... // .....

44.2    7 CCGCCCTGG 30 CCGCT 55 GACG 50 CCGTC 98 CTCTC 121 ACATA 44 CAGGA 21 CAAGT 19 ACGGTGGACACGGGGGTGGGC 120 TCAGT 69 AGTGA 7 CTAAA
62.1    // ..A.....G.. // ..A.. // ..... // ..A.. // ..T.. // ...... // ..A.. // ..GA.. // ..A.......AA.. // ..... // ..G.. // ..G..
7.1     // .......... // ..A.. // ..G.. // ..A.. // ...... // ..G.. // ..A.. // ..G.. // ..A.......AA.. // ...... // ...... // ..C.. //
44.1*   // .......A.. // ..A.. // ..A.. // ...... // ...... // ...... // ...... // ...... // ...... // ...... // ..... //
8.1     // .......A.. // ..A.. // ..G.. // ...... // ..G.. // ..A.. // ..G.. // ..A.......AA.. // ...... // ...... //
18.2*   // .......... // ..G.. // ...... // ...... // ...... // ..A.. // ..G.. // ..A.....G.. // ...... // ..G.. //
```

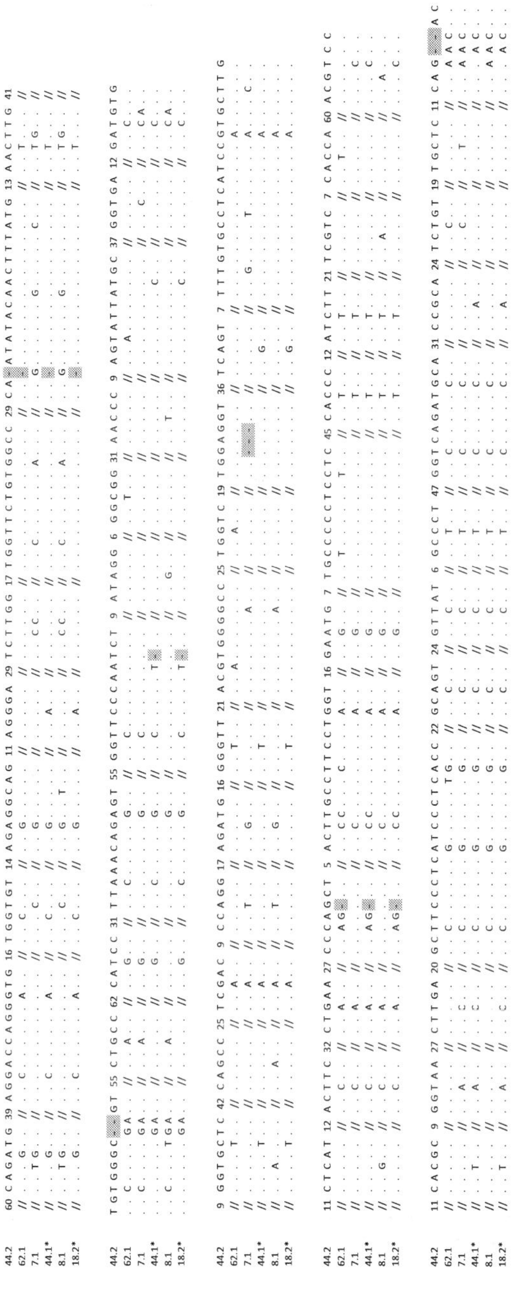

```
44.2    6 ACCAC 26 TCTCC 17 CCACTGCCCCACCCACCCCCAGACCTGCCACCCCACC 69 TGCCT 87 CCGCCCCCATCA 52 TGCCC 6 GGGAC 12 GGGCC 21 CTCGT
62.1    // . . G . . // . . . . . // . . . . . . . . . . . . . . . . . . C . . . . . . . . . . . . . . // . . G . . // . . A . . . . C . // . T . // . . . . . // . . A . . // . . . . .
7.1     // . . . . . // . . C . . // . . T . . . . . . . . . . . . . . . . . . . . . . . . . . . . . . // . . . . . // . . A . . . . C . // . T . // . . . . . // . . . . . // . . A . .
44.1*   // . . . . . // . . . . . // . . . . . . . . . . . . . . . . . . . . . . . . . . . . . . . . . // . . . . . // . . A . . . . . . // . . . // . . . . . // . . . . . // . . . . .
8.1     // . . . . . // . . . . . // . . . . . . . . . . . . . . . . . . . . . . . . . . . . . . . . C // . . . . . // . . . . . . . . . // . . . // . . . . . // . . . . . // . . . . .
18.2*   // . . . . . // . . . . . // . . T . . . . . . . . CT . . [----------] . C . . . C . . . G . . // . . G . . // . . A . . . . C . // . T . // . . . . . // . . . . . // . . . . .

44.2    4 GACCC 32 CAAGG 124 CACCAAGGTGA 4 TCCGTC 57 TGCGT 11 TGGATGCTGCTTC 93 GAGCT 18 AGCAG 64 GACGG 11 GACGG 11 GAAGG 28 GG[GCTCCA]
62.1    // . . A . . // . . G . . // . . T . . . . . C . . // . T . . . // . . . . . // . . . . . . . . . . . . . // . . . . . // . . T . . // . . T . . // . . T . . // . . G . . // . . GCTCCA
7.1     // . . . . . // . . G . . // . . T . . . . . . . . // . . A . . // . . . . . // . . . . . C . . . . . . . // . . A . . // . . . . . // . . . . . // . . . . . // . . G . . // . . [----]
44.1*   // . . . . . // . . . . . // . . . . . . . . . . . // . . . . . // . . . . . // . . . . . . . . . . . . . // . . . . . // . . . . . // . . . . . // . . . . . // . . . . . // . . [----]
8.1     // . . . . . // . . . . . // . . . . . . . . . . . // . . . . . // . . . . . // . . . . . . . . . A . . . // . . . . . // . . . . . // . . . . . // . . . . . // . . G . . // . . [----]
18.2*   // . . A . . // . . . . . // . . T . . . . . . . . // . . . . . // . . T . . // . . . . . . . . . . . . . // . . . . . // . . T . . // . . T . . // . . T . . // . . G . . // . . GCTCCA

44.2    [GAAGG]GC 16 AAGAG 163 TCGGT 58 AAGCC 20 TGACC 27 ACATG 51 CTCTCATGGGAC 80 GCCTGGACGC 15 TCTCCTA 34 AGGGA 105 CACGG 39 CAGTATTCT
62.1    GAAGG . . // . . C . . // . . . . . // . . . . . // . . G . . // . . . . . // . . . . . . . . . . . . // . . . . . . . . . . // . . . . . . . // . . . . . // . . . . . // . . C . . C . .
7.1     [----] . . // . . . . . // . . A . . // . . A . . // . . G . . // . . G . . // . . T . . . . . . . . . // . . . . . . . . . . // . . . . . . . // . . . . . // . . . . . // . . . . . . . .
44.1*   [----] . . // . . . . . // . . . . . // . . . . . // . . . . . // . . . . . // . . . . . . . . . . . . // . . . . . . . . . . // . . . . . . . // . . . . . // . . . . . // . . . . . . . .
8.1     [----] . . // . . . . . // . . A . . // . . . . . // . . G . . // . . G . . // . . . . . . . . . C . . // . . G[--]. . T . . // . . . . . . . // . . . . . // . . . . . // . . . . . . . .
18.2*   GAAGG . . // . . . . . // . . . . . // . . . . . // . . G . . // . . . . . // . . . . . . . . . . . . // . . . . . . . . . . // . . [---] . . // . . A . . // . . T . . // . . . . . . . .

44.2    36 ATCCC 6 GTCCT 57 AAGGG 102 CCCGCGCGCTGCAGCGTCTC 15 GTATC 6 GCGAC 7 ACAGGC 14 CTCAGCT 6 CCACA 36 GCGGT 4 GCCGC 9 GCTCA
62.1    // . . . . . // . . . . . // . . . . . // . . . . . . . . . . . . . . . . . . . . // . . . . . // . . C . . // . . . . . // . . CA . . // . . T . . // . . . . . // . . . . . // . . . . .
7.1     // . . T . . // . . [-] . . // . . C . . // . . A . . . . . . . . . C . . . T . G . . // . . . . . // . . C . . // . . TC . . // . . . . . // . . T . . // . . . . . // . . G . . // . . G . .
44.1*   // . . . . . // . . . . . // . . . . . // . . . . . . . . . . . . . . . . . . . . // . . . . . // . . . . . // . . . . . // . . . . . . GTC // . . . . . // . . . . . // . . . . . // . . . .
8.1     // . . . . . // . . . . . // . . . . . // . . . . . . . . . C . . . G . . . . . . // . . . . . // . . C . . // . . GT . . // . . . . . . GTC // . . . . . // . . . . . // . . . . . // . . G .
18.2*   // . . . . . // . . . . . // . . . . . // . . . . . . . . . . . . . . . . . . . . // . . G . . // . . C . . // . . GT . . // . . . . . . . . // . . . . . // . . . . . // . . . . . // . . . .

44.2    36 CGTCCTGGTCATACC 41 ATCCTCTGGATGATG 12 CCCGG 13 CCCGTCCCCC[-]GA 91 GTCTG 16 TCGGGG[--]GC 36 GTACG 28 CCGGG 36 GCGGAGCGCGG
62.1    // . . GA . . . . . . . . G . // . . G . . . . . . . G . G . // . . A . . // . . . . . . . . . . [-] . . // . . T . . // . . A . . . GG . // . . . . . // . . A . . // . . C . C . AG . T
7.1     // . . A . . . . . . . . G . . // . . G . . . . . . . G . G . // . . A . . // . . . . . . . . . . . . . // . . . . . // . . A . . . AG . // . . . . . // . . . . . // . . C . C . AG . T
44.1*   // . . . . . . . . . . . . . // . . . . . . . . . . . . . . // . . . . . // . . . . . . . . . . . . . // . . . . . // . . . . . . [--] . // . . . . . // . . . . . // . . . . . . . . . .
8.1     // . . A . . . . T . G . . // . . G . . . . . . . G . G . // . . . . . // . . C . . . . . . . . . . . // . . . . . // . . A . . . AG . // . . C . . // . . . . . // . . C . C . AG . T
18.2*   // . . GA . . . . . . . G . . // . . G . . . . . . . G . G . // . . . . . // . . C . . . . . . . . . . . // . . . . . // . . A . . . GG . // . . . . . // . . . . . // . . C . C . AG . T

44.2    TGCGCAGGTTCTCTCGGTAAGTCTGTGTGTTGGTCTTGGAG 6 GTCTCC 20 TCCTG 7 CATGG 4 CGCGGCTCCTTCCT 6 CGTGG 21 ACAGCGTGTCG 12
62.1    . C . . . . . C . . . . . . . . . . . . . . . . . . . . . . . . . . . . . . . . . // . . . . . . // . . . . . // . . . . . // . . G . . G . A . . . . // . . C . . // . . T . G . . . . . . //
7.1     . C . . . . . C . . . . . . . C . . . . . CC . G . C . . . T . . . G . T . . // . . . . . . // . . C . . // . . . . . // . . . . . . . . . . CT . // . . C . . // . . T . G . . . . . . //
44.1*   . . . . . . . . . . . . . . . . . . . . . . . . . . . . . . . . . . . . . . . . . // . . . . . . // . . . . . // . . . . . // . . . . . . . . . . . . // . . . . . // . . . . . . . . . . . //
8.1     . C . . . . . C . . . . . . . . . . . . . . . . . . . A . . // . . G . T . . // . . . . . // . . . . . // . . . . . . . . . . CT . // . . C . . // . . . T . . . . . . . //
18.2*   . C . . . . . C . . . . . . . . . . . . . . . . . . . . // . . G . T . . // . . T . . // . . . . . // . . G . . . . . . . G . . . // . . C . . // . . T . G . . C . . //

44.2    ACGGTGA 31 CATGGCGGTGTAGA 24 GGGGCGAG 40 CCCCGGG 25 TCTCTCCTCCCCACA 12 CTCCCGACCCCGCACTCACCGGC 18 CACTGCCCCCAG
62.1    . T . C . // . . . . . . . G . // . . . . . . . . // . . . . . . . // . . G . . . . . . . . . . . . // . . . . . G . . . . . . . . . . . . // . . GG . T . . G .
7.1     . T . A . // . . C . A . . . . . . G . . // . . T . . // . TA . . // . . G . . . . . . . . . GG . // . . . . . . . . . [--] . . . . . . // . . GG . . G . G .
44.1*   . . . . . // . . . . . . . . . . . . . // . . . . . // . . . . . // . . . . . . . . . . . . . . // . . . . . . . . . [--] . . . . . . // . . . . . . . . . .
8.1     . . T . A . // . . . . . . . C . // . . . . . . . . // . . . TA . . // . . G . . . . . . . . . GG . // . . . . . . . . . [--] . . . . . . // . . GG . . G . G .
18.2*   . . T . A . // . . C . A . . . . G . . // . . [--] . A . . // . . . . . . . // . . G . . . . . . . . . . . // . . . . . G . . . . . . . . . A . . // . . . . . . . . . .
```

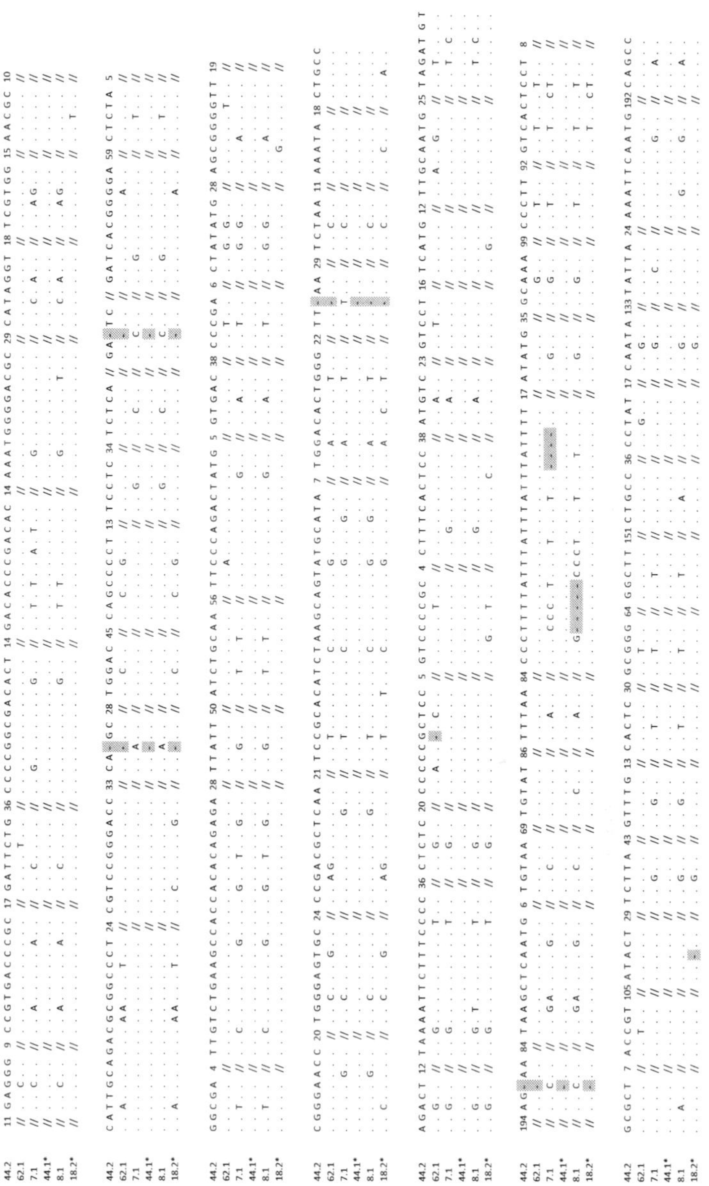

Figure 6. Alignment of 9 kb sequence at HLA-B. Sequences of 6 individuals with homozygous ancestral haplotypes were downloaded from UCSC browser [33] at HLA B and aligned using ClustalX2 [34]. For the purposes of illustration only, common sequences were removed and the interruption marked as //. The nucleotides of AH 44.2 are displayed in

the first row. Nucleotides of AH 62.1, 7.1, 44.1*, 8.1 and 18.2* are given only where they differ from AH44.2 and otherwise marked with a dot. Missing nucleotides are marked with a dash and shaded grey. The sequences are described by Horton et al. [24], whereas AH haplotypes have been assigned from the HLA allele types given by Horton, according to Cattley [35].

The degree of conservation of each ancestral haplotype is truly remarkable. For example, Smith et al. [32] found variation at only 11 of 3, 600, 000 positions between HLA-A and DR. Similar findings have been reported by others, including Aly et al. [31], see Figure 7. Mutation and recombination must be suppressed.

Figure 7 illustrates the importance of interpreting nucleotide diversity according to the block structure of the genome. Thus, conservation in the intervening, essentially monomorphic regions, is of minor interest, whereas differences within PFB allow the discovery of evolution, function and disease susceptibility.

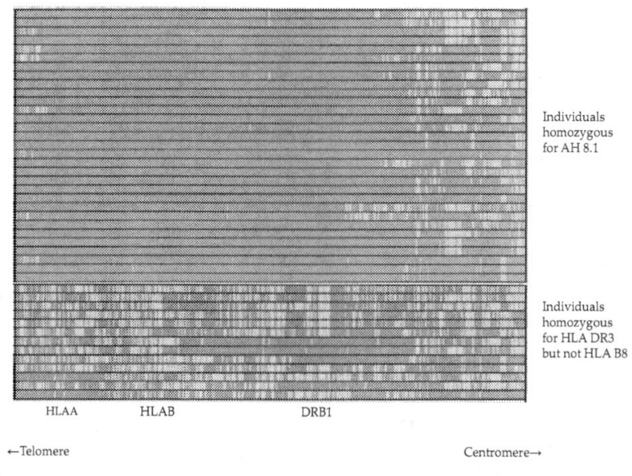

Adapted from ref. [31].

Figure 7. Remarkable conservation within 8.1 haplotypes. A total of 656 SNPs spanning 4.8 Mb in the MHC region are depicted. The lower frequency allele (row) for each SNP along each haplotype column is highlighted in yellow. The top group depicts SNP results from 8.1 AH haplotypes (n = 31), the lower group are HLA-DR3, non-B8 haplotypes (n = 13). The 29.9 Mb range between HLA and DRB1 was >99.9% conserved, with only 9 variant alleles of the 10, 768 alleles identified for the 384 SNPs in the 31 8.1 AHs.

The inescapable conclusion is that some parts of the genome have *not* two or three but hundreds of alternative ancestral sequences.

6. Sequence analysis of ancestral haplotypes

The challenge in terms of sequence analysis is to compile a sufficient matrix to be able to recognize each haplotype and its extent. Assume access to multigenerational families with accurate, truly phased but unmolested raw sequences of at least 100, 000 bases:

1. Clustering of these by independent criteria relating to as many as hundreds of distinct ancestral haplotypes.

2. Alignments which take account of haplospecific duplicons, indels and retroviral-like elements (RLE).

3. Functional information to address biological and disease significance.

Given NGS, this approach is now feasible, even if daunting.

Importantly, those regions which are complex because of duplications and indels should be included rather than "corrected" based on the assumption that there is a single reference or "wild" sequence. Some examples are shown in Figure 6.

In designing better algorithms [36], the strategy for comparative analysis will be crucial. In many polymorphic regions, the density of differences can be as high as 1 per 10 bases when different haplotypes are compared but as low as 0 if the haplotypes are the same. It follows that analysis without haplotype assignment will be misleading.

7. Finding polymorphic frozen blocks and their ancestral haplotypes

The best clue to the location of these blocks is segmental duplication [17, 37].

To characterize the PFB, it is helpful to amplify haplospecific geometric elements [30], see also Table 3. Essentially, this approach reveals duplications as seen in Figure 8. McLure developed the approach to find PFB throughout the genome [36]. Paralogous regions are also helpful as shown in Figure 9.

Once identified, we recommend tracking the polymorphism through panels of multigenerational families as illustrated in Figure 10. Although the region is over 10 megabases, recombination was not found. The different haplotypes in the three breeds must have been conserved for at least hundreds of generations and mark differences in function such as the melting point of fat [37].

8. Applications to NGS and the 1000 genomes project

8.1. Mapping PFB from 1000 genomes data

Since it is known that PFB can be mapped by plotting diversity measurements (see Figure 3), we asked whether it would be possible to use data from the 1000 Genomes Project [39] in the same way.

Earlier work was based on haplotypes defined in multigenerational families. Initially, sequences of haplotypes were determined from Sanger sequencing of homozygous cell lines. In contrast, variations in 1000 genomes are determined from NGS for heterozygous and unrelated

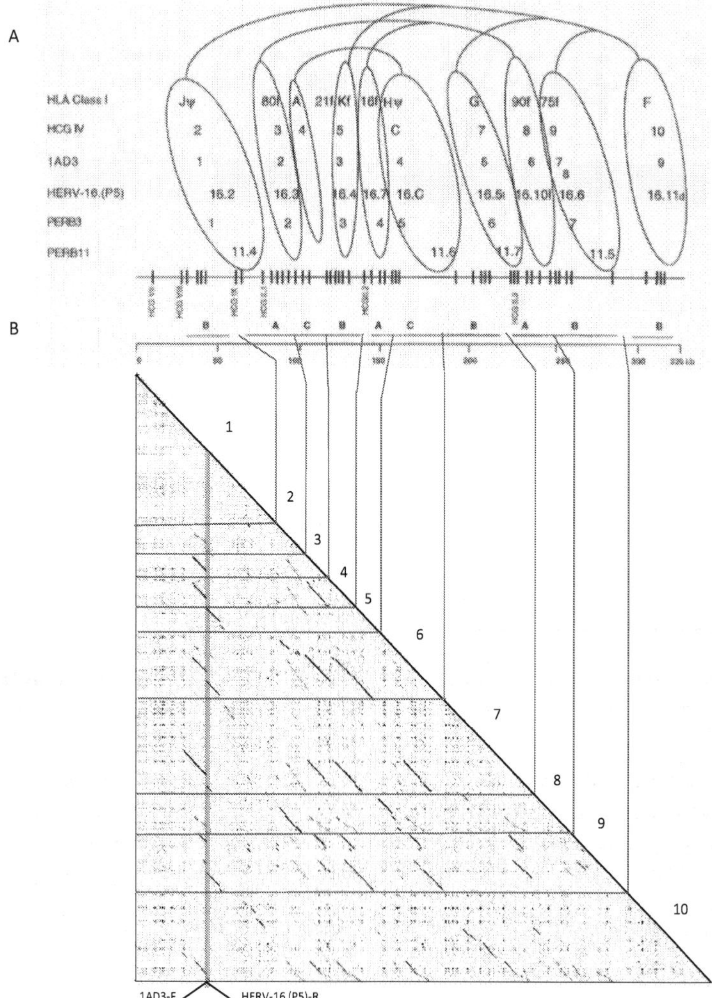

Figure 8. Segmental duplications in MHC alpha block. (a) Gene families and retroelements PERB 11, HLA, HCGIV, AD-3, HERV-16, PERB3 are duplicated to form an ordered pattern within the alpha block of the MHC, indicating that a segment containing multiple genes and retroelements has been duplicated to give 10 duplicons. Full-length duplicons consist of PERB11, HLA, HCGIV, 1AD3, HERV-16 (P5) and PERB3 genes. HLA-80, HLA-A, HIA-K, HLA-16, HLA-90 and HLA-F duplicons lack PERB11 gene. f = fragment, 1 = LTR only, d = discontinuous. ψ = pseudogene. A, B and C represent subgroups of duplicons with greater similarity. (b) A dot plot of the 319 kb genomic sequence encompassing the alpha block was compared against itself. The oblique lines in the plot represent duplications whereas the dots represent retroelements. Lines connect regions of the dotplot to the appropriate duplicons. The primers shown amplify products of different lengths in each duplication. Sequence from GenBank accession number AF055066. Adapted from ref. [17].

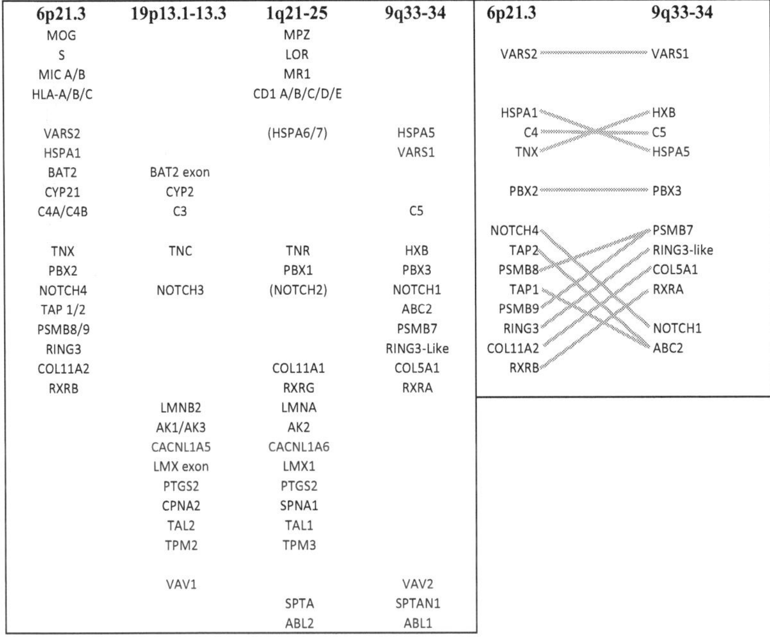

Figure 9. Paralogous locations of MHC genes. MHC genes are found on four chromosomes: 1, 9, 19 as well as chromosome 6. The arrangements of genes in each of the paralogous groups can be largely explained by duplication with and without inversion events. The genes common to chromosomes 6 and 9 are shown.

individuals. The phasing is an estimate based on ideas inherent in population genetics. It is known that the approach is a risky approximation. For example, artefactual "switch-overs" between haplotypes are misleading [40]. Since the reads tend to be short, such as just hundreds of bases, assembly can be fraught. There is a risk of missing complex polymorphisms and underestimating the number of ancestral haplotypes. Given these problems, we plotted several indices related to the 1000 genomes. The intention was to identify any similarities with the distribution as shown in Figure 3.

Unexpectedly, Figure 11 shows a remarkable correspondence between the classical measurements and our extraction from the 1000 Genomes database. The exception around 31.4 Mb was missed by the NGS reanalysis presumably because it is a region which is rich in complex iterative sequences, as shown in Figure 12.

These results are very encouraging in that the advantages of NGS can be coupled with identification of genomic architecture and therefore targeting of the most informative regions. The similarity, by simply counting the base differences per 10 kb, can be refined and applied to the whole genome. The plot of number of "haplotypes" is also promising, although clearly not indicative of the number of ancestral haplotypes.

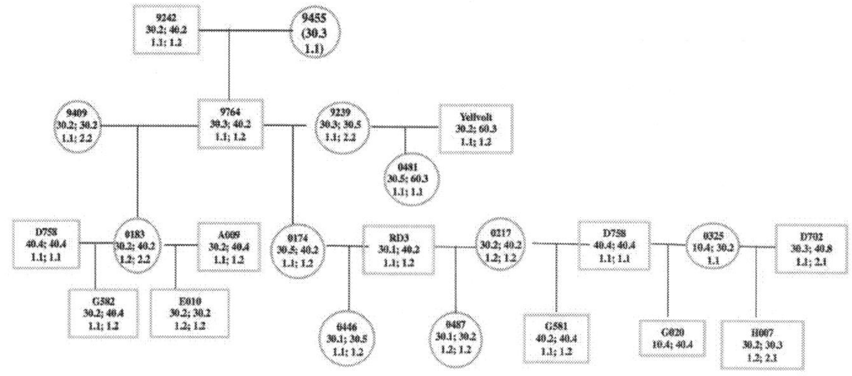

Reproduced with permission from ref. [22].

Figure 10. Tracing segregation through three generation families. The alleles at MRIP, now known as myosin phosphatase Rho-interacting protein, are used to designate haplotypes within the 5.5 Mb region of bovine chromosome 19 from SREBF1 to TCAP. Within this region, there are many genes involved in muscle development, growth and fatty acid synthesis. For further details, see Williamson et al. [38].

8.2. Comparing polymorphic sequences of well-characterised PFB

Since there are numerous ancestral haplotypes within a PFB, it is essential to compare as many sequences as possible. An example is shown in Figure 6.

It can be seen that

- Only a minority of sites are informative and these must be selected from the remainder.

- Kilobases need to be examined and reduced 10- to 100-fold, retaining the informative sites.

- Different haplotypes are defined by specific combinations of bases at those informative sites.

- Very few single nucleotide polymorphisms are specific for a particular ancestral haplotype. On the contrary, specific combinations may be best defined by comparison with a library of reference sequences.

- Indels are important: alignments can be misleading.

Thus, although the identification of each of the many haplotype remains challenging, the overall patterns of informative sites are helpful in screening for PFB and for localising haplospecific sequences.

9. Conclusion

In analysing NGS databases, we recommend:

1.   Screening for PFB.

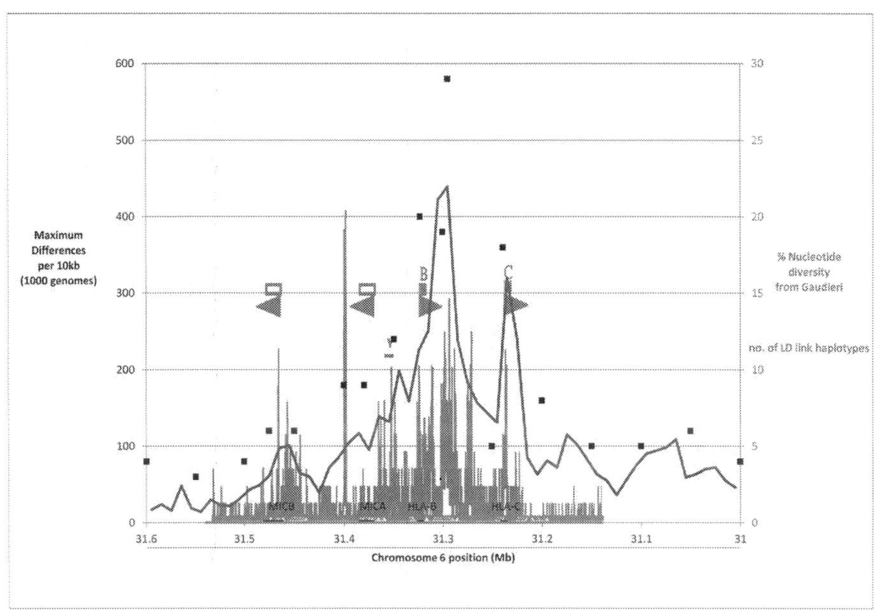

Figure 11. Regions of high sequence diversity within 1000 genomes are similar to previously identified PFB. Imputed haplotypes in the 600 kb region surrounding HLA-B from 553 individuals were downloaded from the 1000 Genomes browser [41]. The population groups chosen were of African, European and Asian origin (ACB, ASW, BEB, CEU, CHB and YRI). The majority of variations recorded in the 1000 Genomes vcf files are SNPs, but some indels up to 174 bp are recorded. For each imputed haplotype, we counted the number of differences from the reference sequence in 10 kb sections. Indels were counted as one difference, irrespective of length. The black curve represents the maximum difference at each 10 kb. The red lines, taken from ref. [42], show the amount of nucleotide diversity between two individual haplotypes, counted in 100 bp sections. Haplotypes compared for this section were 44.1 to 62.1, 44.1 to 8.1 and 8.1 to 14.1. Squares show the number of LD_link [41] "haplotypes", calculated from sets of adjacent variants in 500 bp intervals. LD link requires that variants be biallelic and only takes single nucleotide changes, not indels. Only variants with at least two examples in the CEU and YRI populations were included.

2. Alignment based on the ability to detect multiple, and even hundreds of ancestral haplotypes.

3. Analysis must recognise that haplospecificity is confirmed by many characteristics including RLE, indels, copy number and complex iterative sequences.

4. Analysis may be facilitated by examining paralogous regions which help to define interactions, including epistasis.

5. Validation of results by showing segregation in multigenerational family studies.

6. Confirming biological significance by demonstrating permissive or *sine qua non* associations.

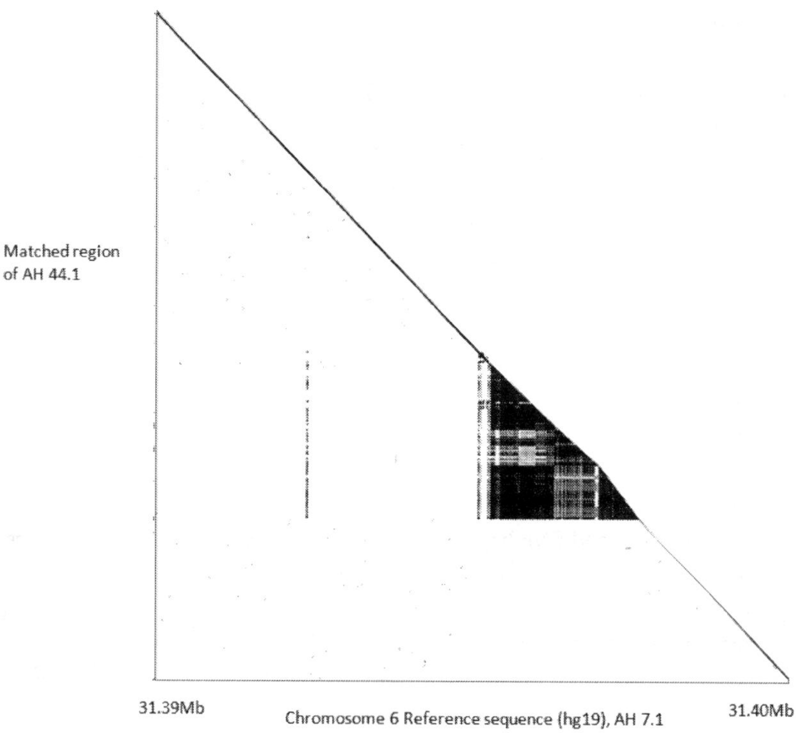

Figure 12. Complex iterative element. Dotplot of a 10 kb region in the MHC between MICA and MICB showing a complex iterative element. Gaudieri [42] shows high nucleotide diversity for this region which was not recorded within 1000 Genomes data. Example sequences for AH 7.1 and AH 44.1 downloaded from UCSC genome browser. Dotplot generated with Gepard [43] using word length 10.

Author details

Sally S. Lloyd[1], Edward J. Steele[1] and Roger L. Dawkins[1,2,3*]

*Address all correspondence to: rldawkins@cyo.edu.au

1 CY O'Connor ERADE Village Foundation, 24 Genomics Rise, Piara Waters, Western Australia, Australia

2 School of Veterinary and Biomedical Sciences, Division of Health Sciences, Murdoch University, Murdoch, Western Australia, Australia

3 Faculty of Medicine and Dentistry, University of Western Australia, Nedlands, Western Australia, Australia

References

[1] Kulski J, Suzuki S, Ozaki Y, Mitsunaga S. In Phase HLA Genotyping by Next Genera-tion Sequencing—A Comparison Between Two Massively Parallel Sequencing Bench-Top Systems, the Roche GS. In: Xi Y, editor. HLA Assoc. Important Dis., In-Tech; 2014, p. 141–81. doi:10.5772/57556.

[2] Lander ES. Initial impact of the sequencing of the human genome. Nature 2011;470:187–97. doi:10.1038/nature09792.

[3] Dawkins R, Christiansen F, Zilko P, editors. Immunogenetics in Rheumatology: Mus-culoskeletal Disease and D-Penicillamine. Excerpta Medica. Amsterdam-Oxford-Princeton; 1982.

[4] Dawkins RL, Christiansen FT, Kay PH, Garlepp M, McCluskey J, Hollingsworth PN, et al. Disease associations with complotypes, supratypes and haplotypes. Immunol Rev 1983;70:5–22.

[5] de Bakker PI, McVean G, Sabeti PC, Miretti MM, Green T, Marchini J, et al. A high-resolution HLA and SNP haplotype map for disease association studies in the ex-tended human MHC. Nat Genet 2006;38:1166–72. doi:10.1038/ng1885.

[6] Nakajima F, Tokunaga K, Nakatsuji N. Human leukocyte antigen matching estima-tions in a hypothetical bank of human embryonic stem cell lines in the Japanese pop-ulation for use in cell transplantation therapy. Stem Cells 2007;25:983–5. doi:10.1634/stemcells.2006-0566.

[7] Barry J, Hyllner J, Stacey G, Taylor CJ, Turner M. Setting Up a Haplobank: Issues and Solutions. Curr Stem Cell Reports 2015;1:110–7. doi:10.1007/s40778-015-0011-7.

[8] Bodmer WF, Trowsdale J, Young J, Bodmer J. Gene clusters and the evolution of the major histocompatibility system. Philos Trans R Soc Lond B Biol Sci 1986;312:303–15.

[9] Ceppellini R, Curtoni ES, Mattuiz PL, V.Miggiano, Scudeller G, Serra A. Genetics of Leukocyte Antigens: A Family Study of Segregation and Linkage. In: Curtoni ES, Mattiuz PL, Tosi RM, editors. Histocompat. Test. 1967, Munksgaard, Copenhagen: 1967, p. 149–87.

[10] Awdeh ZL, Raum D, Yunis EJ, Alper CA. Extended HLA/complement allele haplo-types: evidence for T/t-like complex in man. Proc Natl Acad Sci U S A 1983;80:259–63.

[11] O'Neill GJ, Pollack MS, Yang SY, Levine LS, New MI, Dupont B. Gene frequencies and genetic linkage disequilibrium for the HLA-linked genes Bf, C2, C4S, C4F, 21-hy-droxylase deficiency and glyoxalase I. Transplant Proc 1979;4:1713–5.

[12] O'Neill GJ, Yang SY, Dupont B. Two HLA-linked loci controlling the fourth component of human complement. Proc Natl Acad Sci U S A 1978;75:5165–9. doi:10.1073/pnas.75.10.5165.

[13] O'Neill GJ, Nerl CW, Kay PH, Christiansen FT, McCluskey J, Dawkins RL. Complement C4 is a Marker for Adult Rheumatoid Arthritis. Lancet 1982;320:214. doi:10.1016/S0140-6736(82)91057-1.

[14] Pollack MS, Levine LS, O'Neill GJ, Pang S, Lorenzen F, Kohn B, et al. HLA linkage and B14, DR1, BfS haplotype association with the genes for late onset and cryptic 21-hydroxylase deficiency. Am J Hum Genet 1981;33:540–50.

[15] Alper CA, Awdeh ZL, Raum DD, Yunis EJ. Extended major histocompatibility complex haplotypes in man: role of alleles analogous to murine t mutants. Clin Immunol Immunopathol 1982;24:276–85.

[16] Raum D, Awdeh Z, Yunis EJ, Alper CA, Gabbay KH. Extended Major Histocompatibility Complex Haplotypes in Type I Diabetes Mellitus. J Clin Invest 1984;74:449–54.

[17] Dawkins R, Leelayuwat C, Gaudieri S, Tay G, Hui J, Cattley S, et al. Genomics of the major histocompatibility complex: haplotypes, duplication, retroviruses and disease. Immunol Rev 1999;167:275–304. doi:10.1111/j.1600-065X.1999.tb01399.x.

[18] Degli-Esposti MA, Leaver AL, Christiansen FT, Witt CS, Abraham LJ, Dawkins RL. Ancestral Haplotypes: Conserved Population MHC Haplotypes. Hum Immunol 1992;34:242–52. doi:10.1016/0198-8859(92)90023-G.

[19] Gaudieri S, Leelayuwat C, Tay GK, Townend DC, Dawkins RL. The major histocompatibility complex (MHC) contains conserved polymorphic genomic sequences that are shuffled by recombination to form ethnic-specific haplotypes. J Mol Evol 1997;45:17–23.

[20] Trowsdale J, Knight JC. Major histocompatibility complex genomics and human disease. Annu Rev Genomics Hum Genet 2013;14:301–23. doi:10.1146/annurev-genom-091212-153455.

[21] Lloyd SS, Bayard D, Lester SA, Williamson JF, Dawkins RL. The Value of Haplotyping. INTERBULL Bull 2013;47:252–5.

[22] Dawkins RL. Adapting Genetics. Dallas, TX: Near Urban Publishing; 2015.

[23] Smith WP, Vu Q, Li SS, Hansen J a., Zhao LP, Geraghty DE. Toward understanding MHC disease associations: partial resequencing of 46 distinct HLA haplotypes. Genomics 2006;87:561–71. doi:10.1016/j.ygeno.2005.11.020.

[24] Horton R, Gibson R, Coggill P, Miretti M, Allcock RJ, Almeida J, et al. Variation analysis and gene annotation of eight MHC haplotypes: the MHC Haplotype Project. Immunogenetics 2008;60:1–18. doi:10.1007/s00251-007-0262-2.

[25] Shiina T, Ota M, Shimizu S, Katsuyama Y, Hashimoto N, Takasu M, et al. Rapid Evolution of Major Histocompatibility Complex Class I Genes in Primates Generates

New Disease Alleles in Humans via Hitchhiking Diversity. Genetics 2006;173:1555–70. doi:10.1534/genetics.106.057034.

[26] Longman-Jacobsen N, Williamson JF, Dawkins RL, Gaudieri S. In polymorphic genomic regions indels cluster with nucleotide polymorphism: Quantum Genomics. Gene 2003;312:257–61. doi:S0378111903006218 [pii].

[27] Curtis D, Vine AE, Knight J. Study of regions of extended homozygosity provides a powerful method to explore haplotype structure of human populations. Ann Hum Genet 2008;72:261–78. doi:10.1111/j.1469-1809.2007.00411.x.

[28] Clark AG. The size distribution of homozygous segments in the human genome. Am J Hum Genet 1999;65:1489–92. doi:10.1086/302668.

[29] Lloyd SS, Bayard D, Lester S, Williamson JF, Steele EJ, Dawkins RL. Ancestral Haplotypes, Quantal Genomics and Healthy Beef S. Proceedings, 10th World Congr. Genet. Appl. to Livest. Prod. Ancestral, 2014.

[30] Abraham LJ, Leelayuwat C, Grimsley G, Degli-Esposti M a, Mann A, Zhang WJ, et al. Sequence differences between HLA-B and TNF distinguish different MHC ancestral haplotypes. Tissue Antigens 1992;39:117–21.

[31] Aly T a., Eller E, Ide A, Gowan K, Babu SR, Erlich H a., et al. Multi-SNP analysis of MHC region: remarkable conservation of HLA-A1-B8-DR3 haplotype. Diabetes 2006;55:1265–9. doi:10.2337/db05-1276.

[32] Kent WJ, Sugnet CW, Furey TS, Roskin KM, Pringle TH, Zahler AM, et al. The Human Genome Browser at UCSC. Genome Res 2002;12:996–1006. doi:10.1101/gr.229102.

[33] Larkin MA, Blackshields G, Brown NP, Chenna R, Mcgettigan PA, McWilliam H, et al. Clustal W and Clustal X version 2.0. Bioinformatics 2007;23:2947–8. doi:10.1093/bioinformatics/btm404.

[34] Cattley SK, Williamson JF, Tay GK, Martinez OP, Gaudieri S, Dawkins RL. Further characterization of MHC haplotypes demonstrates conservation telomeric of HLA-A: Update of the 4AOH and 10 IHW cell panels. Eur J Immunogenet 2000;27:397–426. doi:eji226 [pii].

[35] Su SY, Balding DJ, Coin LJM. Disease association tests by inferring ancestral haplotypes using a hidden markov model. Bioinformatics 2008;24:972–8. doi:10.1093/bioinformatics/btn071.

[36] McLure CA, Hinchliffe P, Lester S, Williamson JF, Millman JA, Keating PJ, et al. Genomic Evolution and Polymorphism: Segmental Duplications and Haplotypes at 108 Regions on 21 Chromosomes. Genomics 2013;102:15–26. doi:10.1016/j.ygeno.2013.02.011.

[37] Lloyd SS, Valenzuela J, Bayard D, de Bruin S, Gilmour P, Steele EJ Dawkins RL. Heritability of fat melting temperature in beef cattle 2015. In preparation

[38] Williamson JF, Steele EJ, Lester S, Kalai O, Millman JA, Wolrige L, et al. Genomic evolution in domestic cattle: Ancestral haplotypes and healthy beef. Genomics 2011;97:304–12. doi:S0888-7543(11)00037-1 [pii] 10.1016/j.ygeno.2011.02.006.

[39] Abecasis GR, Altshuler DL, Auton A, Brooks LD, Durbin RM, Gibbs R A., et al. A map of human genome variation from population-scale sequencing. Nature 2010;467:1061–73. doi:10.1038/nature09534.

[40] Machiela MJ, Chanock SJ. LDlink®: A web-based application for exploring population-specific haplotype structure and linking correlated alleles of possible functional variants. Bioinformatics 2015.

[41] Pybus M, Dall'Olio GM, Luisi P, Uzkudun M, Carreño-Torres A, Pavlidis P, et al. 1000 Genomes Selection Browser 1.0: A genome browser dedicated to signatures of natural selection in modern humans. Nucleic Acids Res 2014;42:D903–9. doi: 10.1093/nar/gkt1188.

[42] Gaudieri S, Kulski JK, Dawkins RL, Gojobori T. Extensive nucleotide variability within a 370 kb sequence from the central region of the Major Histocompatibility Complex. Gene 1999;238:157–61.

[43] Krumsiek J, Arnold R, Rattei T. Gepard: A rapid and sensitive tool for creating dot-plots on genome scale. Bioinformatics 2007;23:1026–8. doi:10.1093/bioinformatics/btm039.

Chapter 13

On Genotyping Polymorphic HLA Genes — Ambiguities and Quality Measures Using NGS

Szilveszter Juhos, Krisztina Rigó and György Horváth

Additional information is available at the end of the chapter

http://dx.doi.org/10.5772/61592

Abstract

The major histocompatibility complex (MHC) region of the human genome is the most polymorphic sequence part on chromosome 6; this roughly 4 Mbase long stretch contains many genes involved in immune response and disease association. The HLA genes have a crucial role in transplantation; patients receiving organs or bone marrow from matching donors have significantly higher chance for survival. NGS-based HLA typing brings the hope of accurate genomic consensus sequences by relatively cheap and simple laboratory workflow. Using either targeted or whole-genome sequencing data, there are a lot of possibilities to get ambiguous results (combinations of several alleles as a result instead of a single pair). These can be sample- or reference-related, or the results of artifacts generated during the targeting and amplifying step. NGS technology itself has additional artifacts leading to ambiguity listed in our paper. The final bioinformatics step will not be able to resolve all the ambiguities; we are also proposing quality control metrics to assess the final ambiguity and typing failure.

Keywords: HLA, phasing, ambiguity, quality control, novel allele

1. Introduction

Every nucleated cell in our body expresses Class-I HLA genes (HLA-A, -B, and -C) and cells involved in immune function express some of the Class-II HLA genes (such as HLA-DRB1, -DQB1, etc.). These proteins on the cell membrane surface are the primary building blocks of antigen presentation and immunological memory mechanisms. Their role in transplantation became apparent about a hundred years ago [1], and for both solid organ and hematopoietic stem cell transplantation the general practice is to find donors with matching HLA genes for a patient. Besides transplantation, HLA loci (and MHC genes in general) have been found to

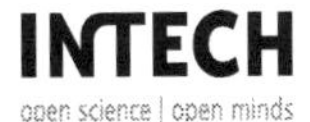

be associated with many traits and diseases [2]. Therefore, HLA genotyping from large datasets and finding further associations is an ever ongoing effort.

The HLA genes are codominant, both alleles in the two chromosomes are expressed, and are exceptionally polymorphic in their exons involved in antigen recognition (exon 2 and 3 for Class-I and exon 2 for Class-II loci). These peptide-binding highly variable regions are in the focus of HLA typing; there are 13,412 allele sequences in the IMGT/HLA reference database at the time of writing this article [3], compared to the 1250+ alleles known in 2002 [4]. This polymorphy, together with the high homology of these loci, makes the classical variant-call NGS pipelines impractical: it is not the individual SNPs or indels, but whole exon or whole gene sequences identifying alleles that have to be found by NGS-based HLA typing.

Sequence-based HLA typing (SBT) is relatively new, there are established methods to identify unique sequence patterns of HLA loci by sequence-specific oligonucleotides [5]. These methods are less precise though, it is not possible to obtain the whole sequence of an allele by using probes either. Furthermore, as SBT focuses primarily on the previously mentioned important exons, the phasing problem known from whole-genome assembly can be the main source of ambiguity. During phasing the individual base differences are assigned unambiguously to one of the chromosomes. Fortunately, phasing short reads is easier when the two alleles differ at many positions, making NGS-based HLA typing attractive. Unlike Sanger traces, the signal from the two chromosomes can be separated reassuringly as for each base there is only one signal, the base is treated unequivocally either A, C, G, or T.

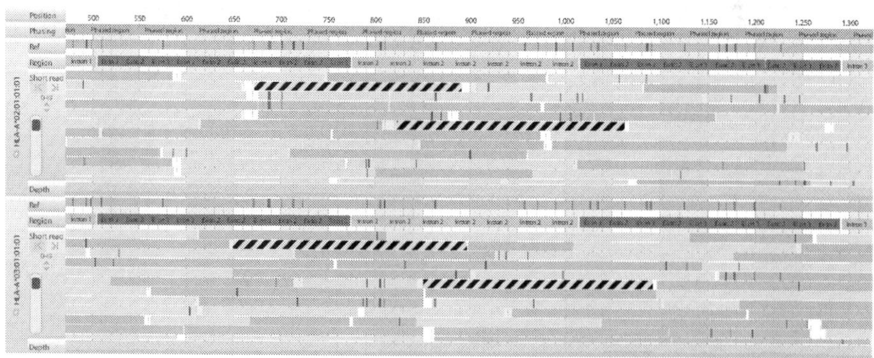

Figure 1. The figure illustrates how overlapping short reads can be used to phase exon 2 and exon 3 of HLA-A using the variants present in intron 2. Forward reads are colored pink/orange, reverse orientation is yellow. Colored bars in reads are depicting nucleotide differences from the reference, the reference track is gray at homozygous positions, only heterozygous bases are colored (A: red, C: blue, G: brown, T: green). Reads highlighted with black and yellow dashes show how step-by-step phasing can happen using the reads overlapping the consecutive heterozygous positions. Since all four marked reads overlap at the heterozygous position near the middle of intron 2, it is unambiguous which read belongs to which chromosome. Therefore, the phase between the heterozygous positions in exon 2 and exon 3 can be resolved too. Note that in practice phase resolution happens by considering large number of short reads for reliability. Alignment was created by the Omixon HLA Twin 1.1 software.

However, this cis/trans phase problem prevalent in HLA typing is not resolved in all cases, calculating the phase is hindered by sequencing artifacts, missing references, and other factors detailed below. Furthermore, these factors can introduce new typing issues different from phase ambiguity.

1.1. Short introduction into HLA nomenclature

The name of an HLA allele reflects the precision of the DNA sequence determining the actual allele. There are four fields separated by colons after the locus name and a star sign:

- The first field defines the general allele group: HLA-A*01 and HLA-A*02 belonging to different allele groups, their molecular structure at the binding site is very different from each other.

- The second field is related to a specific HLA protein: HLA-A*02:02:01 and HLA-A*02:02:02 differ only in their third fields, therefore, the sequence of their expressed proteins are the same.

- Differences in synonymous codons are expressed in the third field: the two alleles mentioned in the example above encode the same HLA proteins, but their coding DNA sequence differs.

- The fourth field denotes non-coding differences: HLA-C*07:01:01:01 and HLA-C*07:01:01:02 differs in two bases in intron 1: the importance of nucleotide diversity at splicing sites and regulatory locations (UTRs) is just emerging [6].

The ultimate source of HLA nomenclature is at [7] maintained by the Anthony Nolan Research Institute. The most up-to-date HLA reference database can be downloaded from [8].

1.2. The IMGT/HLA database

The IMGT/HLA database is part of the Immuno Polymorphism Database (IPD) system. Due to the high polymorphism of HLA alleles, allele information is stored in individual sequences, instead of a set of variants. Because of historical reasons (the first public release of IMGT/HLA was in 1998), the database is mainly populated with partial allele sequences. As it is now possible to obtain whole genomic sequences for many HLA loci, whole-gene (or near whole-gene) submission is now obligatory for the database and the raw sequencing data needs to be made public and available for independent analysis [3].

1.2.1. Undocumented regions and novel alleles

As the database is far from complete, finding novel sequences or known alleles with unknown intronic parts is pretty likely, even during a single sequencing run. According to our findings, most of the novelties are in introns/UTRs, since these regions were not investigated as thoroughly as exons. However, even for a small sample size, it is possible to find novelties in exons. In many cases, novelties have to be confirmed by an alternative method, and only high quality data should be accepted for confirmatory typing because algorithms frequently assign novel flags to low quality or failed samples.

1.3. NGS HLA typing

1.3.1. Pros and cons of switching to NGS HLA typing

One of the advantages of switching to NGS HLA typing is that inherent phasing ambiguities present in Sanger sequencing can be eliminated. As mentioned before, the two chromosomes produce separate reads, and an adequate bioinformatics workflow can separate these reads and assemble them into phased consensuses. Furthermore, using modern kits, it is not only possible to sequence the most polymorphic exons, but whole genes and many loci can be typed at once. This whole-gene sequencing approach provides an unprecedented precision, revealing novelties mainly in intronic and untranslated (UTR) regions. On the other hand, the high amount of data, the fundamentally different NGS workflow needs not only new laboratory equipments and reagents, but some bioinformatics and IT skills: sequence search, alignment, read filtering, database handling, etc. are among the daily routines of a HLA lab practitioner. The amount of generated data is more by magnitudes compared to the size of Sanger traces, and validating novelties by confirmatory typing can be cumbersome. In a low-throughput laboratory processing the samples in the wet lab have to be planned in advance; many kits accommodate more samples than the amount accumulating during a week/month.

Pros	Cons
Phasing problem inherent in Sanger traces is not present	There are still remaining ambiguities; some bioinformatics skills are desired
Multiple loci sequenced in one sample	Loads of data, needs serious IT infrastructure
Unprecedented precision: We do know that HLA expression is heavily affected by introns/UTRs, we are getting an insight into these sequences as well	Many novelties, mainly in introns
High-throughput lab workflow, more samples to process	In a low-throughput lab have to plane forward

Table 1. Main advantages and disadvantages of NGS HLA typing.

1.3.2. NGS HLA typing methods

Algorithms and kits for genotyping the HLA loci using NGS reads are in the focus of several publications in recent years [9]. Some of the authors use the straightforward read alignment followed by the variant call approach [10], and others developed designated genotyping algorithms for a wide variety of kits and sequencing approaches [11–14]. Since some of these authors are more interested in primer and sequencing workflow development, and others address the genotyping/bioinformatics problems concerning HLA typing, there is already a high diversity of available workflows.

The pioneering publications for NGS HLA typing were already considering targeted long-range PCR amplification and quality check measures [15–17] such as strand bias, though some cases managed to achieve high concordance for two fields only by using population frequency information. The ultimate goal is to have a primer set and a wet-lab and bioinformatics workflow to get phased, whole-gene consensus sequences with unambiguous four-fields typing [18, 19].

Other approaches are trying to extract HLA types from existing whole-exome (WES), whole-genome (WGS), or even RNA-Seq data. A short review of diverse methods addressing WES and WGS reads can be found in [20], exploring how to tackle problems regarding HLA gene homology (cross-mapping reads, see below) and missing intronic information.

It is expected that the number of both the kits and the typing algorithms will grow in the near future, and laboratories will use more than one strategy for confirmatory testing (for a comprehensive list of available HLA typing software see Table 2). Therefore, our goal was to give details about the possible source of ambiguity and mistyping.

Name	Availability	Web page
ATHLATES*	Academic non-commercial research purposes only	https://www.broadinstitute.org/scientific-community/science/projects/viral-genomics/athlates
Bwakit	Public	https://github.com/lh3/bwa/tree/master/bwakit
Conexio/Illumina TruSight HLA	Commercial	https://support.illumina.com/downloads/trusight-hla-analysis-software-conexio-assign.html
GenDx NGSengine	Commercial	http://www.gendx.com/products/ngsengine
HLA Caller*	Public	http://gatkforums.broadinstitute.org/discussion/65/hla-caller
HLAforest	Academic non-commercial research purposes only	http://code.google.com/p/hlaforest/
HLAminer	Public	http://www.bcgsc.ca/platform/bioinfo/software/hlaminer
HLAreporter	Public	http://paed.hku.hk/genome/software.html
hlaseq*	Public	http://sourceforge.net/projects/hlaseq/
HLAssign	Public	http://www.ikmb.uni-kiel.de/resources/download-tools/software/hlassign
NextGENe	Commercial	http://www.softgenetics.com/NextGENe_18.html
NXtype	Commercial	http://www.onelambda.com/en/about-us/news/recent-news/ngs-news.html
Omixon HLA Twin	Commercial	http://www.omixon.com/hla-twin/
OptiType	Public	https://github.com/FRED-2/OptiType
PHLAT	Academic non-commercial research purposes only	https://sites.google.com/site/phlatfortype/home
seq2hla	Public	https://bitbucket.org/sebastian_boegel/seq2hla
SOAP-HLA*	Public	http://soap.genomics.org.cn/SOAP-HLA.html

Table 2. Collection of available HLA typing software for NGS data. Entries with a star (*) are considered obsolete, their web pages have not been updated for more than two years.

2. Sources of ambiguity

While surveying donors can be done fast and relatively cheaply by methods other than sequence based HLA typing, finding the best match generally means that the nucleotide sequences of both recipients and provisional donors are determined either by Sanger capillary or by next-generation sequencing. Sanger sequencing can produce 1000 base-pairs long reads, but the signals from the two chromosomes are mixed. Therefore, there is an inherent phase ambiguity despite the long resulting reads. On the other hand, while reads from next-generation sequencers are from different chromosomes, their length are usually behind the stretch of Sanger traces, expected to be in the range of 4–500 basepairs that on average is 454 and 2 x 150 or 2 x 250 basepairs for Illumina sequencers. This again increases ambiguity: if the allele pair to be typed has a homozygous sequence region that is longer than the average read length and the insert between the pairs, the phase cannot be resolved. Instead of an allele pair, we get only a list of possible alleles having similar nucleotide sequences but possibly different expressed proteins.

Using the best sampling, targeting, and amplification technology combined with the latest HLA typing bioinformatics workflow can lead to ambiguity, when the two alleles of a heterozygous sample cannot be separated. The main causes for having multiple types instead of a single pair are discussed below.

2.1. Sample-related ambiguities

2.1.1. Long homozygous stretches

For NGS, we usually consider short reads, where the read length is less than 1000 base pairs. The longer the reads, the better the phase resolution, but there can be long homozygous stretches where even the best workflow fails to resolve the phase between the two chromosomes. Pacific Biosciences SMRT technology with thousands of base pairs length has the promise of covering a whole locus in a single read, but its clinical applicability has yet to come [21].

2.1.2. Novel alleles

For alignment-based algorithms where input data is processed read by read, the differentiation between mismatches imposed by the novel allele and mismatches related to random noise is not possible during the alignment. For assembly-based algorithms, when the final consensus is delivered including the novelty, then a name have to be proposed for the novel allele—or at least an allele to which the novel allele is the most similar. Consider the case when an exon 2 novelty is found to have impact on the protein sequence as well; this is not a situation where ambiguity of the naming and related closest alleles can be resolved automatically without human investigation or additional experiments.

2.2. Polymerase chain reaction related ambiguities

Polymerase chain reaction (PCR) is an essential part of most NGS workflows; in many cases it is a step of the library preparation process (it can be used for targeting and/or amplification) and in all major sequencing platforms PCR is part of the actual sequencing step (emulsion PCR in Ion Torrent and Roche 454 and bridge PCR in Illumina). Considering the major role that PCR plays in NGS, it is important to be aware of possible errors and artifacts that can originate from PCR, as these can greatly affect the outcome of HLA genotyping. PCR-related ambiguities are usually caused by two issues:

- signal loss caused by amplification imbalance or dropout can make consensus assembly difficult or can cause low coverage, both of which can increase ambiguity;

- mixed signals caused by PCR crossover artifacts or PCR stutter basically create a mix of artificial alleles in vitro that makes allele selection difficult.

2.2.1. Dropouts

From an HLA-typing perspective there are three main types of dropouts: both alleles drop out completely (locus dropout), one allele is amplified (and later successfully sequenced) but the signal for the other allele is missing completely (allele dropout), or one or both alleles are only partially amplified and/or sequenced (partial dropout). All three cases can be caused by issues in the pre-sequencing steps of the workflow. A locus dropout is very easy to detect at the end of the workflow, but the affected samples or loci need to be re-processed and re-sequenced in most cases, which can be very time consuming. This type of dropout can be caused by a long list of errors, ranging from input DNA issues, to primer design problems or even instrument malfunction or human error. An allele dropout is much harder to detect, as it can be basically indistinguishable from a homozygous result. Allele dropouts can be caused by technical errors (e.g., thermocycler malfunction or human error), protocol-related issues (e.g., primer design problems), or allele-related issues (e.g., novel variant in primer binding site). Although most cases of allele dropouts are likely PCR-related and generally can be considered extreme cases of allele imbalance, it needs to be noted that in some blood cancers (e.g., acute lymphocytic leukemia) and other cancer types, false homozygous HLA typing results due to chromosome 6 loss in cancer affected cells have also been reported [22].

2.2.2. Imbalance

Although some level of imbalance between amplicons within the same PCR reaction is expected even under ideal conditions, a high level of amplification imbalance can cause difficulties during HLA genotyping. When HLA alleles are amplified using a single pair of primers (either to amplify a partial gene sequence or the whole gene using, e.g., long range PCR), the main concern is imbalance between the two chromosomes. While most Sanger sequencing methods need a minimum of 5–20% minor signal strength for detecting the weaker signal, in some NGS-based HLA-typing methods, detectable imbalance as low as 2% have been reported [23]. Other studies put the safe level of allele imbalance between 20% and 25% [24, 25], so it needs to be noted that the level of acceptable imbalance for reliable detection of minor alleles might highly depend on the exact protocol (e.g., average coverage depth and targeting strategy), data characteristics (e.g., noise and artifact read percentage) and typing method used in the workflow. If multiplex PCR is used, amplification imbalance between amplicons derived from different chromosomes and between amplicons originating from the same chromosome can potentially be observed. Balance between amplicons is influenced by several factors. In a high number of cases, amplification imbalance is primer related. The high diversity of HLA alleles combined with the presence of homologous genes and pseudogenes make primer design for HLA loci difficult. Lack of sequence information for untranslated, non-coding, and even exonic regions in and near HLA alleles provides an additional challenge. Also, in many cases, multiple primer pairs are used for capturing multiple loci or simply all possible allele combinations and/or the whole gene sequence for a single locus that adds another layer of complexity to the primer selection and PCR optimization steps [19, 25]. Even if all available information is considered and the theoretically best primers have been designed for a specific workflow, it is always possible that previously unidentified novelties are present at or near the primer site in a specific sample that can significantly lower the efficiency of primer binding or even inhibit amplification altogether [26–29].

2.2.3. PCR crossover

PCR crossover artifacts can be generated by incomplete primer extension. After successful primer annealing, the extension step finishes prematurely. The resulting partial amplicon then re-anneals in the next cycle to a second amplicon and another extension cycle is started using this re-annealed partial amplicon as a starting point. The "target" of re-annealing can be either in a copy of the original contig or in the contig originating from the other chromosome (or even in contigs from other homologous amplified or co-amplified genes). As one of the possible causes behind incomplete extension is the annealing of already amplified complementary sequences and the concentration of these templates is the highest at the end of the PCR process, most PCR crossover artifacts are generated in the last few cycles of PCR. Reducing the number of amplification cycles can greatly reduce the amount of PCR crossover artifacts [30]. Both crossovers between homologous loci and between the two alleles within the same HLA loci [23] have been reported. Even crossover artifacts corresponding to HLA alleles found in the IMGT/HLA database have been described [30].

PCR crossover reads can be eliminated during the phasing process when the algorithms try to determine the correct base combination for each consecutive variant pair. For example, if a heterozygous position has bases A + C on the two chromosomes followed by another hetero-zygous position with bases T + G then based on the number of short reads (or read pairs) supporting the A $\rightarrow$ T + C $\rightarrow$ G combination compared to the read support of the A $\rightarrow$ G + C $\rightarrow$ T combination in most cases the correct phasing can be determined. If majority of the reads support one combination then the reads belonging to the other combination can be considered as crossover artifacts and can be ignored as a systematic noise.

If the crossover artifacts are strong and multiple artifact versions are present, it is not always possible to determine which reads can be ignored. In this case, unfiltered artifacts can cause phasing difficulties that can lead to increased ambiguity.

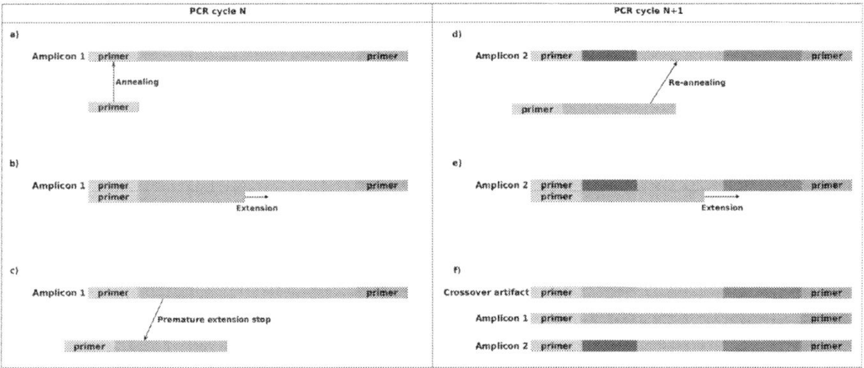

Figure 2. The formation of PCR crossover artifacts: a) a primer anneals to the primer binding site of amplicon 1; b) extension is started; c) the extension step is interrupted, a partial amplicon is created; d) the partial amplicon re-anneals to a complementary section of amplicon 2; e) the annealed partial amplicon is extended for the second time; f) the result of the second extension is an amplicon that contains sequence motifs from both amplicon 1 and amplicon 2.

2.2.4. PCR stutter

Short tandem repeats (STRs) are also present in HLA alleles, a well-known example is the low complexity region at the border of HLA-DRB1 exon 2 and intron 2. Amplification of these repeats can lead to PCR stutter [31] and ambiguity between alleles that differ only in the length of these very repeats. The consensus assembly of these low-complexity regions are itself difficult, and reads containing stutter artifacts are exacerbating this problem. For example, the HLA-DRB1*03:01:01:01 and HLA-DRB1*03:01:01:02 alleles differing only in an SNP in intron 1 and the length of GT repeats in intron 2. When the whole intron 1 of HLA-DRB1 is not sequenced (as for most of the available kits) these two alleles are hard to distinguish.

2.3. Next-gen sequencing technology artifacts leading to ambiguity

2.3.1. Missing coverage on important exons

While relatively deep coverage is desired in targeted gene experiments, coverage depth itself is actually not that important. Several publications report >90% concordance using reads from relatively shallow WGS sequencing with average ~ 20 reads depth [11, 12, 17, 32]. On the other hand, if important parts of the exons are not covered, there is no hope for acceptable typing for any sequencing depth. For targeted sequencing, it is expected that the most polymorphic exons are fully and evenly covered through the whole extent of the exons. Our experience is that even at parts where the coverage is low, at least eight reads are needed to support the reference, and it is the *extent of coverage* that really matters; if there are uncovered regions on the important exons the typing is unreliable and/or ambiguous.

2.3.2. Homopolymer errors

Homopolymer errors in reads of Roche 454 and Ion Torrent sequencers are common, but actually hardly effect the genotyping results. It is because aligner algorithms are dealing differently with flow-space and letter-space reads (Illumina reads are belonging to the latter category) and indels are tolerated by introducing a different error model into the aligner. Nevertheless, alleles differing in the length of the homopolymer can be displayed as ambiguities, such as HLA-A*03:21N where there is an insertion in the originally 7 bases-long C homopolymer in exon 4 of the allele compared to HLA-A*03:01:01:01. Similar to this null allele, pseudogenes, such as HLA-H, the pseudogene related to HLA-A can occur in typing results, particularly in typing from whole-genome data as these HLA-H alleles differ from the corresponding HLA-A alleles in the length of homopolymers.

Homopolymer errors occur for Illumina reads as well, though mainly arising not from the signal detection technology itself but due to polymerase slip on a homopolymer stretch [33]. A variation on polymerase slip is when it is not the length of the homopolymer that is changed, but a base surrounded by two homopolymers such as CCCCACCCC changing to CCCCCCCCC.

2.3.3. Low-quality reads

Apart from the cross-mapping ones, there are reads that can be generally considered as noise. The obvious ones are reads that are too short; excluding reads shorter than 90 bps will dramatically increase typing reliability [32]. With current sequencing technologies, it is possible to gain average read length much higher that 200 bps, but the low end of the read length distribution still should be excluded, especially when using enzymatic tagmentation [34].

2.3.4. Random artifact reads

Some reads do not map to our reference at all (off-target reads), or are not similar to any other reads in the data: if the ratio of these "orphan" reads is too high (the threshold can be set as a quality check metric), the resulting typing have to be treated with caution, particularly for homozygous cases in deep sequencing. If the typing/assembly algorithm is not prepared for random noise elimination, it can assemble bogus consensus sequences from noisy reads and present it as a candidate.

2.4. Reference-related ambiguities

2.4.1. Cross-mapping reads, either from pseudogenes or homologous sequences

The conserved exons of HLA genes coding cross-membrane and intracellular components are similar to each other. It is especially true for HLA-DRB1 and HLA-DQB1, where there is a strong homology between intronic parts of HLA-DRB1/3/4/5/7 and HLA-DQB1. Weaker cross-mapping can be seen among Class-I genes and between Class-I and Class-II sequences. Reads covering these exons bear little useful information, as they are the same for many alleles and should be marked as non-uniquely mapping. However, the concept of the "uniquely mapping read" is pretty murky; aligners use heuristics, the mapping quality is measured by the aligner itself. The actual reference database and introducing gaps can complicate the picture further. Repeats (e.g., few hundred bases long L2 and Alu stretches in intron 1 of DRB1) makes not only the primer design difficult, but when using whole genome data, reads from other parts of the genome can be mapped to these parts with little mismatch. Therefore, instead of using "mapping-uniqueness", a phred-scaled mapping probability is recommended [35, 36]. Using this metric, excluding/involving reads that are mapping to multiple genes can be assessed more objectively. Some algorithms simply discard these reads, risking coverage holes in homologous regions.

2.4.2. Allele ambiguity due to missing parts in IMGT/HLA

The IMGT/HLA reference database has many alleles with sequenced exons only; for most of the alleles, only the coding part is stored in the database, and for a number of the entries, only the important exons (exon 2 an 3 for Class-I and exon 2 only for Class-II) are presented, while some typing algorithms rely on the CDS sequences only [12, 17]. For example, the partially defined HLA-B*53:17:02 - HLA-B*78:02:01 allele pair can be resolved also as HLA-B*35:01:01 - HLA-B*52:01:01. If the phase information is available, these kinds of ambiguities can be resolved reassuringly. The list of ambiguous allele combinations can be found at the IPD IMGT/HLA webpage [37].

When selecting the most probable alleles identified in the sample data, comparisons are required between the alleles. Since most of the alleles are defined only partially, these comparisons cannot be always done properly. Regardless of the genotyping approach, deciding between two alleles defined on different regions when no perfect match is available cannot be done unambiguously. Consider the example if an allele has an SNP mismatch on exon 1 and the other has an SNP on exon 4 meanwhile the counterpart allele in each case has no sequence defined on the corresponding region, there is no clear decision between them. This applies even more to the coverage profile-based methods where the local mismatch information is not necessarily always available.

As an extremity, there are also situations where there are multiple alleles without any mismatch, even for whole gene targeting. In one of these situations the alleles of some exons are a subsequence of the other corresponding allelic regions that have no defining introns to let the algorithm distinguish between them. For example the frequent HLA-C*06:02:01:02 has a full genomic sequence, but the similar HLA-C*06:116N allele has only some exons sequenced, and exon 3 is five bases shorter than the same exon in HLA-C*06:02:01:02. Apart from this shorter exon, the two references are identical at every position; the latter is a subset of the former sequence. This means that it is possible to align the reads to both entries, and a consensus generated from raw data perfectly incorporates both sequences. Although the collection of null alleles [39] states that this allele is a result of a deletion: "615 > 619delCGCGG, in codon 181, causes a premature stop at codon 198", there is no further reference about the rest of the intron.

2.5. Ambiguities arising from typing workflow and bioinformatics

The process of determining genotypes based on the raw sequencing data contains multiple points where ambiguity might be introduced. Source of ambiguities in the software pipeline can be classified into the following categories:

- partial targeting of the gene(s)—by primer design—which results in lack of characterization for certain regions;

- the mechanism of the algorithm used for genotyping.

2.5.1. Targeting related ambiguities

Selecting the most appropriate target regions for PCR amplification within a gene or genomic region during primer design is necessary for reasons of technical and cost efficiency. As a result, some exons and introns have to be excluded for some loci, e.g., exon 1 and most of intron 1 of HLA-DRB1. The ambiguity introduced by partial targeting depends on the selection of the non-characterized regions. This is usually a compromise between precision and through-put. By analyzing the reference database, it is sometimes possible to omit exons/introns entirely without introducing ambiguity in the genotyping. However, note that consensus sequences will be still less specific by only covering parts of the gene.

Untranslated regions of Class-I loci are rarely targeted, although numerous alleles are differing from each other in a single base in the UTRs. Prime examples are HLA-A*02:01:01:01 and HLA-A*02:01:01:02L, the former having a significantly lower expression. The single T → C difference in the middle of the 5'UTR sequence has to be included into the whole gene consensus to precisely determine these alleles. Another example is HLA-B*35:01:01:01 and HLA-B*35:01:01:02 where the differentiating SNP is at the end of the 3'UTR: although both 5' and 3' UTR has influence to the gene expression after transcription, these parts are often left out from targeting.

Apart from UTRs, some Class-II loci, notably HLA-DRB1, have introns longer than 5 K base pairs incorporating repeats. For many DR loci the targeting primers are usually not in the UTR region, but skipping both exon 1 and the long intron 1 together with the rest of the gene after exon 4, where the remaining exons 5 and 6 are only 24 and 14 bases long, respectively. This makes space for ambiguities such as HLA-DRB1*12:01:01 vs. HLA-DRB1*12:10 that are differing in a single SNP on exon 1.

2.5.2. Algorithm-related ambiguities

Most genotyping algorithms incorporate reference alignment methods and/or assembly methods that reconstruct the sample DNA as a whole. Alignment methods investigate the raw sequencing data read by read (or read pair by read pair in case of paired data) and determine the genotypes by using some statistical approach at the end—alignment-based consensus generation and variant calling also fit into this category. Assembly methods consider multiple reads together to generate some consistently supported larger sequence set (a.k.a. consensus sequences) and infer genotypes by comparing the assumed sample DNA to the reference database.

Both alignment and assembly methods involve some statistical analysis that is inherently related to the nature of NGS; raw sequencing data contains partial measurements (reads) with significant error rate meanwhile providing high redundancy allowing the software pipelines to reduce the potential errors at the end to a really low value. These statistical parts always include some assumptions to avoid extremely high computation needs. When these assumptions fail this leads to ambiguity in the results.

Alignment methods have to tolerate certain levels of error otherwise random noise would prevent mapping significant proportion of the short reads. Since the alignment execution is essentially independent for each read/read pair aligners miss the capability of differentiating between random noise and systematic noise (e.g., artifacts). Meanwhile, random noise is not disturbing the statistical methods (variant calling, coverage profile analysis, etc.)—usually applied after the alignment step—systematic noise introduces significant error that might prevent unambiguous genotype resolution due to not enough reliable information available to decide between alleles.

Assembly methods have to consider only well-supported assembly paths to connect reads to each other to avoid the situation when artifacts mislead the assembly. Also they have to try keeping the whole targeted region continuous and not to be split into multiple separate contigs (continuous consensus sequence parts) even if there are regions where the amount of reads is relatively low (e.g., due to tandem repeats that are hard to sequence). When the assembly ends up with multiple separated contigs, this might lead to ambiguity since not only is phasing impossible between these separated parts but also in the in-between sequence when the distance separation is unknown.

3. Quality Control (QC)

Quality control consists of a set of metrics calculated independently from the core genotyping method to provide an additional control over the quality of the results. Here, independence is very important otherwise reliability would decrease. Each QC metric has reference values that behave as thresholds to map the actual values to QC result states (e.g., passed/failed).

Some metrics and methods routinely used in NGS quality control (e.g., read length, base quality, quality based trimming) can provide valuable information in NGS-based HLA genotyping as well. Other measures are more HLA typing-specific (e.g., number of result allele pairs, important exon coverage).

The QC metrics, based on their focus in the genotyping pipeline, can be classified into the following categories:

- Experiment qualification (e.g., fragment size, average read length, average read quality, read count): thresholds for these metrics should be established based on knowledge about the underlying technology and workflow. Failure for these QC tests generally indicates issues with the wet lab part of the genotyping workflow (e.g., over-fragmentation, unnoticed low input DNA concentration). These QC failures can usually be eliminated by repeating the experiment.

- Data qualification (e.g., cross-mapping read ratio, crossover PCR artifact ratio): the thresholds for these metrics are also experiment dependent, but a QC test failure is not necessarily a consequence of an error during the sequencing process, therefore, a repeated experiment won't necessarily resolve the issue. In most cases, these QC failures can be eliminated by further optimization of the workflow (e.g., PCR cycle number optimization).

- Result qualification (e.g., consensus continuity, consensus phasing, consensus coverage minimum depth, mismatch count): these metrics qualify the output, the result consensus and genotype, regardless of the input quality.

A special case of QC is the concordance calculation between two independent genotyping methods. In this case a complete alternative/secondary genotyping method is introduced to provide results comparable to the controlled primary genotyping method and the result is expressed as a concordance value that can be mapped to the standard QC result scheme (e.g., passed/failed).

4. Conclusion

As NGS-based HLA typing is getting more momentum, there is more and more accumulated knowledge and experience concerning ambiguities. At the present state of art, apparently the bioinformatics workflow and data management is the main hurdle that a HLA biologist has to face. Therefore, it is important to know the main sources of sequencing and data errors leading to ambiguities: when switching to NGS HLA typing, besides cost, consider its benefits and drawbacks to make sure you are ready to change the laboratory and informatics workflow. NGS-HLA is not a remedy for all the problems we have in Sanger SBT or in traditional non-sequence-based HLA typing methods: to have a whole-gene fully resolved phased consensus you have to use a kit that is designed to provide this sequence and a bioinformatics pipeline that is delivering this result. Sequence annotation is mostly unresolved; we get a flood of novel sequences, but assigning exon/intron/UTR boundaries is still a manual process. Sequencing and assembling consensuses with UTRs are problematic and missing UTRs can lead to ambiguities.

Introducing QC metrics can help find out the nature of ambiguities and failures; studying these metrics, it is possible to decide whether it is the whole experiment, the sequencing part, or the final bioinformatics workflow that needs to be repeated with altered input. Do not accept genotyping results blindly, reconsider the QC metrics, look at the actual alignments, and interpret the obtained ambiguities.

Author details

Szilveszter Juhos*, Krisztina Rigó and György Horváth

*Address all correspondence to: szilveszter.juhos@omixon.com

Omixon Ltd, H- Budapest, Hungary

References

[1] Marsh SGE, Parham P, Barber LD. The HLA FactsBook. 1st ed. London: Academic Press; 1999. 416 p.

[2] Trowsdale J: The MHC, disease and selection. Immunology Letters. 2011;137:1–8. DOI: 10.1016/j.imlet.2011.01.002.

[3] Robinson J, Halliwell J, Hayhurst J, Flicek P, Parham P, Marsh S: The IPD and IMGT/HLA database: allele variant databases. Nucleic Acids Research. 2014;43:D423–D431. DOI: 10.1093/nar/gku1161.

[4] Gerlach J: Human lymphocyte antigen molecular typing: How to identify the 1250+ alleles out there. Archives of Pathology & Laboratory Medicine. 2002;126:281–284.

[5] Bontadini A: HLA techniques: Typing and antibody detection in the laboratory of immunogenetics. Methods. 2012;56:471–476. DOI: 10.1016/j.ymeth.2012.03.025.

[6] Vandiedonck C, Taylor MS, Lockstone HE, Plant K, Taylor JM, Durrant C, Broxholme J, Fairfax BP, Knight JC: Pervasive haplotypic variation in the spliceo-transcriptome of the human major histocompatibility complex. Genome Res. 2011 Jul.; 21(7):1042–1054. DOI: 10.1101/g.116681.110.

[7] Nomenclature for Factors of the HLA System. 2015. Available from: http://hla.alleles.org/nomenclature/naming.html [Accessed: 2015–07–25].

[8] The IMGT/HLA Database. 2015. Available from: http://www.ebi.ac.uk/ipd/imgt/hla/download.html [Accessed: 2015–07–25].

[9] Erlich H: HLA typing using next-generation sequencing: An overview. Human Immunology. 2015. DOI: 10.1016/j.humimm.2015.03.001.

[10] Kazuyoshi H, Shigeki M, Hideki N, Ituro I: A Bead-based Normalization for Uniform Sequencing depth (BeNUS) protocol for multi-samples sequencing exemplified by HLA-B. BMC Genomics. 2014;15:645. DOI: 10.1186/1471-2164-15-645.

[11] Bai Y, Ni M, Cooper B, Wei Y, Fury W: Inference of high resolution HLA types using genome-wide RNA or DNA sequencing reads. BMC Genomics. 2014;15:325. DOI: 10.1186/1471-2164-15-325.

[12] Liu C, Yang X, Duffy B, Mohanakumar T, Mitra R, Zody M, Pfeifer J: ATHLATES: accurate typing of human leukocyte antigen through exome sequencing. Nucleic Acids Research. 2013;41:e142. DOI: 10.1093/nar/gkt481.

[13] Zhou M, Gao D, Chai X, Liu J, Lan Z, Liu Q, Yang F, Guo Y, Fang J, Yang L, Du D, Chen L, Yang X, Zhang M, Zeng H, Lu J, Chen H, Zhang X, Wu S, Han Y, Tan J, Cheng Z, Huang C, Wang W: Application of high-throughput, high-resolution and cost-effective next generation sequencing-based large-scale HLA typing in donor registry. Tissue Antigens. 2014;85:20–28. DOI: 10.1111/tan.12477.

[14] Warren R, Choe G, Freeman D, Castellarin M, Munro S, Moore R, Holt R: Derivation of HLA types from shotgun sequence datasets. Genome Medicine. 2012;4:95. DOI: 10.1186/gm396.

[15] Lank S, Wiseman R, Dudley D, O'Connor D: A novel single cDNA amplicon pyrosequencing method for high-throughput, cost-effective sequence-based HLA class I genotyping. Human Immunology. 2010;71:1011–1017.

[16] Erlich R, Jia X, Anderson S, Banks E, Gao X, Carrington M, Gupta N, DePristo M, Henn M, Lennon N, de Bakker P: Next-generation sequencing for HLA typing of class I loci. BMC Genomics. 2011;12:42. DOI: 10.1186/1471–2164–12–42

[17] Wang C, Krishnakumar S, Wilhelmy J, Babrzadeh F, Stepanyan L, Su LF, Levinson D, Fernandez-Viña MA, Davis RW, Davis MM, Mindrinos M: High-throughput, high-fidelity HLA genotyping with deep sequencing. PNAS. 2012;109(22):8676–8681. DOI: 10.1073/pnas.1206614109.

[18] Shiina T, Hosomichi K, Inoko H, Kulski J: The HLA genomic loci map: expression, interaction, diversity and disease. Journal of Human Genetics. 2009;54:15–39. DOI: 10.1038/jhg.2008.5.

[19] Ehrenberg P, Geretz A, Baldwin K, Apps R, Polonis V, Robb M, Kim J, Michael N, Thomas R: High-throughput multiplex HLA genotyping by next-generation sequencing using multi-locus individual tagging. BMC Genomics. 2014;15:864. DOI: 10.1186/1471–2164–15–864.

[20] Szolek A, Schubert B, Mohr C, Sturm M, Feldhahn M, Kohlbacher O: OptiType: precision HLA typing from next-generation sequencing data. Bioinformatics. 2014;30:3310–3316. DOI: 10.1093/bioinformatics/btu548.

[21] Mayor N, Robinson J, McWhinnie A, Ranade S, Eng K, Midwinter W, Bultitude W, Chin C, Bowman B, Braund MPH, Madrigal JA, Latham K, Marsh SGE: HLA Typing for the Next Generation. PLoS ONE. 2015;10:e0127153. DOI: 10.1371/journal.pone.0127153.

[22] Park H, Hyun J, Park S, Park M, Song E: False Homozygosity Results in HLA Genotyping due to Loss of Chromosome 6 in a Patient with Acute Lymphoblastic Leuke-

mia. The Korean Journal of Laboratory Medicine. 2011;31:302. DOI: 10.3343/kjlm. 2011.31.4.302.

[23] Lange V, Bohme I, Hofmann J, Lang K, Sauter J, Schone B, Paul P, Albrecht V, Andreas J, Baier D, Nething J, Ehninger U, Schwarzelt C, Pingel J, Ehninger G, Schmidt A: Cost-efficient high-throughput HLA typing by MiSeq amplicon sequencing. BMC Genomics. 2014;15:63. DOI: 10.1186/1471–2164–15–63.

[24] Nelson W, Pyo C, Vogan D, Wang R, Pyon Y, Hennessey C, Smith A, Pereira S, Ishitani A, Geraghty D: An integrated genotyping approach for HLA and other complex genetic systems. Human Immunology. 2015. DOI: 10.1016/j.humimm.2015.05.001.

[25] Ozaki Y, Suzuki S, Kashiwase K, Shigenari A, Okudaira Y, Ito S, Masuya A, Azuma F, Yabe T, Morishima S, Mitsunaga SS, Satake M, Ota M, Morishima Y, Kulski JK, Saito K, Inoko H, Shiina T: Cost-efficient multiplex PCR for routine genotyping of up to nine classical HLA loci in a single analytical run of multiple samples by next generation sequencing. BMC Genomics. 2015;16. DOI: 10.1186/s12864-015–1514–4.

[26] Cheng C, Kashi Z, Martin R, Woodruff G, Dinauer D, Agostini T: HLA-C locus allelic dropout in Sanger sequence-based typing due to intronic single nucleotide polymorphism. Human Immunology. 2014;75:1239–1243. DOI: 10.1016/j.humimm. 2014.09.016.

[27] Deng Z, Wang D, Xu Y, Gao S, Zhou H, Yu Q, Yang B: HLA-C polymorphisms and PCR dropout in exons 2 and 3 of the Cw*0706 allele in sequence-based typing for unrelated Chinese marrow donors. Human Immunology. 2010;71:577–581. DOI: 0.1016/j.humimm.2010.03.001.

[28] Lam C, Mak C: Allele dropout caused by a non-primer-site SNV affecting PCR amplification—a call for next-generation primer design algorithm. Clinical Chimica Acta. 2013;421:208–212. DOI: 0.1016/j.cca.2013.03.014.

[29] Bru D, Martin-Laurent F, Philippot L: Quantification of the detrimental effect of a single primer-template mismatch by real-time PCR using the 16S rRNA gene as an example. Applied and Environmental Microbiology. 2008;74:1660–1663.

[30] Holcomb C, Rastrou M, Williams T, Goodridge D, Lazaro A, Tilanus M, Erlich H: Next-generation sequencing can reveal in vitro-generated PCR crossover products: Some artifactual sequences correspond to HLA alleles in the IMGT/HLA database. Tissue Antigens. 2013;83:32–40. DOI: 10.1111/tan.12269.

[31] Walsh P, Fildes N, Reynolds R: Sequence analysis and characterization of stutter products at the tetranucleotide repeat locus vWA. Nucleic Acids Research. 1996;24:2807–2812.

[32] Major E, Rigó K, Hague T, Bérces A, Juhos S (2013) HLA Typing from 1000 Genomes Whole Genome and Whole Exome Illumina Data. PLoS ONE 8(11): e78410. DOI: 10.1371/journal.pone.0078410.

[33] Schlötterer C, Tautz D: Slippage synthesis of simple sequence DNA. Nucleic Acids Ressearch. 1992;20:211–215.

[34] Lan JH, Yin Y, Reed EF, Moua K, Thomas K, Zhang Q: Impact of three Illumina library construction methods on GC bias and HLA genotype calling. Hum Immunol. 2015 Mar.;76(2–3):166–175. DOI: 10.1016/j.humimm.2014.12.016.

[35] Li H: Mapping uniqueness [Internet]. 2009. Available from: http://lh3lh3.users.sourceforge.net/mapuniq.shtml [Accessed: 2015-07-24].

[36] Li H. and Durbin R: Fast and accurate short read alignment with Burrows-Wheeler Transform. Bioinformatics, 2009;25:1754–60.

[37] Ambiguous Allele Combinations. 2015. Available from: http://www.ebi.ac.uk/ipd/imgt/hla/ambig.html [Accessed: 2015-07-25].

[38] Null and Alternatively Expressed Alleles. 2015. Available from: http://hla.alleles.org/alleles/nulls.html [Accessed: 2015-07-25].

Chapter 14

DNA-based Diagnosis of Uncharacterized Inherited Macrothrombocytopenias Using Next-generation Sequencing Technology with a Candidate Gene Array

David J. Rabbolini, Marie-Christine Morel Kopp, Sara Gabrielli, Qiang Chen, William S. Stevenson and Christopher M. Ward

Additional information is available at the end of the chapter

http://dx.doi.org/10.5772/61777

Abstract

Inherited macrothrombocytopenias comprise a heterogeneous group of inherited platelet disorders that are characterized by large platelets, thrombocytopenia and bleeding tendencies in affected individuals. Diagnostic platforms have traditionally involved a battery of complex phenotypic tests that often fail to reach a diagnosis. Next-generation sequencing lacks the pre-analytical and analytical shortcoming of these tests and provides an attractive alternate diagnostic approach. Our group has developed a candidate gene array targeting genes known to affect platelet function and tested it in a large cohort of Australasian patients with presumed platelet function disorders, particularly macrothrombocytopenia. This array identified causative variants in a significant portion of patients with uncharacterized platelet disorders, including transcription factor mutations that cannot easily be diagnosed with standard platelet phenotyping procedures. We propose that targeted genotypic screening can identify the genetic basis of platelet function defects and has the potential to be developed into a powerful clinical platform to help clinicians diagnose these rare disorders.

Keywords: Inherited macrothrombocytopenia, next-generation sequencing, candidate gene array

1. Introduction

Platelets are essential for clot formation after tissue trauma. Initiation of the platelet plug occurs by adhesion of platelets to the damaged vascular endothelium mediated by interactions of glycoprotein Ib/IX/V complexes with von Willebrand factor (vWF), and GPVI and integrin

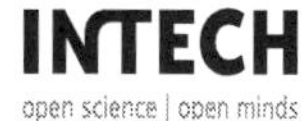

α2β1 with collagen [1]. Extension of the platelet plug requires activation of αIIbβ3 through an "inside-out" signaling cascade which enables receptor cross-linking with fibrinogen and vWF and activation of "outside-in" signaling events [1, 2].

Primary hemostasis relies on both adequate function and number of platelets. Abnormalities in platelet function and/ or number may be acquired (liver disease, chronic kidney disease) or inherited (inherited platelet function disorders, IPFDs or inherited platelet number disorders, IPNDs). The group of inherited macrothrombocytopenias is included in the heterogeneous IPNDs and are characterized by large platelets, thrombocytopenia and bleeding tendencies in affected individuals (Figure 1A, Figure 1B, Figure 1C and Figure 1D) [3].

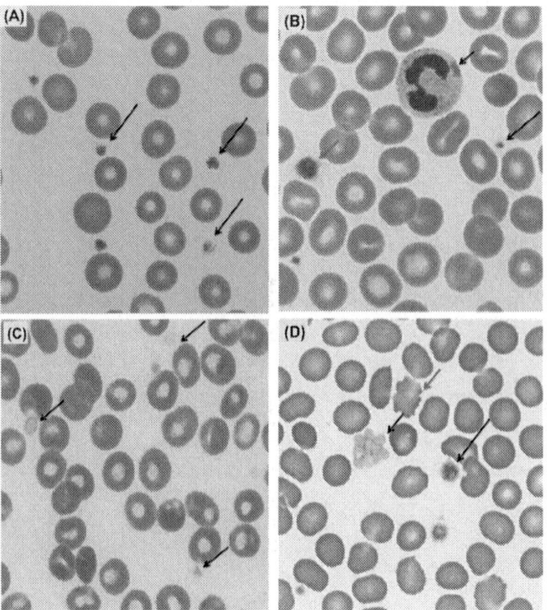

Figure 1. A normal blood film and three blood films demonstrating macrothrombocytopenia associated with mutations in different genes (*MYH9, NBEAL2* and *GFI1B,* respectively). (A) A blood film with platelets of normal appearance (black arrows). (B) *MYH9*-related disorder with characteristic inclusion bodies in the neutrophils (small black arrow) and large platelets (red arrow). Normal-sized platelets are also seen (long black arrow). (C) Gray platelet syndrome showing distinctive pale or gray platelets (black arrows). (D) *GFI1B*-related thrombocytopenia (c.880-881insC mutation) resulting in red cells with atypical shapes and sizes (red arrow) and thrombocytopenia with platelets that appear large with normal granulation (long black arrow) as well as hypogranular or gray (short black arrows).

Unfortunately, inherited macrothrombocytopenia is under-recognized with the presence of large platelets on blood film examination often leading to a misdiagnosis of immune thrombocytopenic purpura (ITP), resulting in subsequent inappropriate treatment with steroids or in some cases removal of the spleen [4]. Diagnostic algorithms have traditionally been based around biological laboratory tests examining functional properties and activation pathways in isolated platelets [3, 5–7]. This phenotypic approach is poorly standardized, technically difficult and not easily reproducible [6–11]. In addition, numerous pre-analytical variables may affect phenotypic test results. These variables include the effect of food (garlic), alcohol, drugs (herbal remedies, non-steroidal anti-inflammatory drugs, anti-platelet medications) and stimulants (smoking and caffeine) on platelet function, activation of platelet samples during venipuncture and transport necessitating careful sample handling as well as the relatively large volume of blood needed (which becomes a major problem when assessing pediatric samples) [12–14]. Despite these complex phenotypic tests, many cases remain without a definitive diagnosis.

Genetic technology may overcome many of the problems surrounding phenotypic testing for thrombocytopenia as DNA is stable, can easily be transported long distances and is not affected by diet or drugs. Moreover, genetic-based tests have provided opportunities to reduce redundancy and heterogeneity of diagnostic algorithms and have shifted our ability to describe inherited platelet disorders from a level of the defective platelet pathway involved, to a molecular level.

The Sanger sequencing method [15] has long been considered the "gold standard" technology to rapidly analyze small regions across a limited number of samples, but it is not suited to screening large numbers of genes in multiple patients [16]. The emergence of next-generation sequencing (NGS) technologies as a diagnostic approach has been able to generate more test sequence increasing the number of gene targets and decreasing the costs [17, 18]. Human whole genome sequencing (WGS) or whole exome sequencing (WES) [19, 20] have proven to be clinically appropriate and practical modalities in describing new genetic mutations in families and identifying known pathogenic mutations in individuals formerly without a diagnosis [17].

Testing approaches may vary depending on whether a novel genetic mutation is likely. WGS and WES are powerful platforms in discovering novel causal variants in individuals with rare penetrant monogenic disorders [21], whilst a candidate gene approach allows assessment of known mutations in genes causing clinical phenotypes.

Whole genome approaches incorporating NGS have recently reported novel mutations in an essential platelet transcription factor GFI1B [22, 23], and a WES approach followed by targeted Sanger sequencing was used successfully to describe mutations in *ACTN1* causing macro-thrombocytopenia [24, 25]. Acknowledging these advancements, we employed a targeted candidate gene approach to explore cases of suspected inherited macrothrombocytopenia that remained uncharacterized despite phenotypic testing and hypothesized this to be an effective approach to diagnose inherited macrothrombocytopenia.

2. Materials and methods

2.1. Patients

Diagnostic assessment of patients with uncharacterized thrombocytopenia was performed as part of a human research ethics committee approved study conducted in accordance with the Declaration of Helsinki.

Following informed written consent, 20 ml of blood was taken from an antecubital vein and collected into EDTA tubes. This blood was easily transported, in some cases, over 1,000 km between diagnostic sites in Australia.

A total of 95 patient DNA samples were analyzed. This included two internal controls for which DNA-based diagnosis had previously been established by Sanger sequencing.

32 male patients (mean age 37.4 years, range 18–92 years) and 44 female patients (mean age 38.7 years, range 18–79 years) were included in the NGS assay. The mean age of the cohort was 38.1 years (range 18–92 years). Sixteen de-identified DNA samples were received from referring institutions for which no additional laboratory data were available.

Phenotypic testing data were available for 59 (62.1%) individuals. This included platelet functional analysis (PFA) (n = 25, 26.0% of the cohort), light transmission aggregometry / whole blood impedance aggregometry (LTA/WBIA) (n = 39, 41.3% of the cohort), flow cytometry (n = 45, 47.8% of the cohort) and electron microscopy (n = 12, 13% of the cohort). These phenotypic test results suggested a diagnosis to a "pathway level", that is, a description to the level of the suspected defective biochemical pathway, in only 11 cases. Pathway orientated defects included, storage pool disorders (n = 3), platelet glycoprotein deficiency (n = 3), platelet signaling defects (n = 2), platelet secretion defects (n = 2) as well as α-granule disorder (n = 1).

2.2. DNA preparation

Genomic DNA (gDNA) was isolated from peripheral blood leukocytes using the Wizard® Genomic DNA purification kit (Promega, Alexandria, NSW, Australia). DNA quality and concentration were assessed using the Nanodrop™ 1000 spectrophotometer (Thermo Scientific, Scoresby, Vic, Australia) that measures the purity of DNA by the ratio of absorbance of molecules at 260 and 280 nm. Samples with ratios between 1.8 and 2.0 were accepted for analysis whilst ratios lower than this may represent the presence of contaminants and these samples were not processed further [26]. At least, 250 ng of input gDNA was prepared per sample.

2.3. Candidate gene identification and gene panel design

An extensive literature search using public databases was performed to assemble an initial candidate gene list of all genes reasonably hypothesized to have an impact on platelet number and size (n = 173). A final list of candidate genes (n = 19) was derived by including those genes in which mutations were known to be definitively associated with IPNDs (predominantly, macrothrombocytopenia) and by excluding genes, which although known to result in thrombocytopenia, could easily be identified by conventional and clinical methods characterized by distinct clinical phenotypes.

A TruSeq custom amplicon (TruSeq® Custom Amplicon Kit, Illumina Inc., Scoresby, Vic, Australia) specific for the target regions of the selected 19 genes (Table 1, *ACTN1, CD36, ETS1, F2R, FLI1, GATA1, GFI1B, GP1BA, GP1BB, GP6, GP9, ITGA2, ITGA2B, ITGB1, ITGB3, MYH9, NBEAL2, P2RY12, RUNX1, TUBB1*) was designed as an entire custom pool using the web-based software tool, Illumina Design Studio (Illumina Inc.). This generated 201 gene targets that were either exons or gene regions that were split into 632 amplicons, each of approximately

250 base pairs (bps). There were no undesignable targets and a total coverage of 91% was predicted for the panel.

Gene	Description (OMIM)	Inheritance	Disorder (abbreviation in this paper, OMIM entry)
ACTN1	Alpha-Actinin-1	AD	α actinin-related thrombocytopenia (α actinin-RT, 615193)
CD36 (GPIV)	Thrombospondin receptor (Glycoprotein IV)	AD	Familial thrombocytopenia with GPIV deficiency (nd, 608404)
ETS1	V-Ets avian erythroblastosis virus E26 oncogene homolog 1	nd	nd
F2R	Coagulation factor II (thrombin) receptor	nd	nd
FLI1	Friend leukaemia virus integration 1	AD	Paris-Trousseau syndrome / Jacobsen syndrome (TCPT/ JBS, 188025, 600588)
GATA1	GATA-binding protein 1	XL	GATA1-related disorders (GATA1-RD, 300367, 314050)
GFI1B	Growth factor-independent 1B	AD	GFI1B-related thrombocytopenia (GFI1B-RT, 187900)
GP1BA	Glycoprotein 1b-alpha polypeptide	AR	Bernard Soulier syndrome (BSS, 231200)
		AD	Platelet type-von Willebrand disease (PT-VWD, 177820)
		AD	Velocardiofacial syndrome (VCFS, 192430)
		AD	Mediterranean thrombocytopenia (nd, 153670)
GP1BB	Glycoprotein 1b-beta polypeptide	AR	Bernard Soulier syndrome (BSS, 231200)
GP6	Glycoprotein VI	AR*	Bleeding disorder, platelet type 11 (614201)
GP9	Glycoprotein IX	AR	Bernard Soulier syndrome (BSS, 231200)
ITGA2	Integrin, alpha-2	AR	GPIa/IIa deficiency (giant platelets and mitral valve insufficiency) (nd,nd)
ITGA2B	Integrin, alpha-2B	AD	Monoallelic ITGA2B/ITGB3-related thrombocytopenia (ITGA2B/ITGB3-RT, 187800)
ITGB1	Integrin, beta-1	AR	GPIa/IIa deficiency (giant platelets and mitral valve insufficiency) (nd,nd)
ITGB3	Integrin, beta-3	AD	Monoallelic ITGA2B/ITGB3-related thrombocytopenia (ITGA2B/ITGB3-RT, 187800)
MYH9	Myosin heavy-chain 9	AD	MYH9-related disease (MYH9-RD,155100)
NBEAL2	Neurobeachin-like 2	AR	Gray platelet syndrome (GPS, 139090)
P2RY12	Purinergic receptor P2Y, G protein-coupled 12	AR*	Bleeding disorder, platelet type 8 (609821)
RUNX1	Runt-related transcription factor 1	AD	Platelet disorder, familial, with associated myeloid malignancy (FDP/AML, 601399)
TUBB1	Tubulin, beta-1	AD	β1 Tubulin-related thrombocytopenia (β1 tubulin-RT, 613112)

Table 1. Candidate gene list. OMIM, online Mendelian inheritance in man; AR, autosomal recessive; AD, autosomal dominant; XL, X-linked; nd, not defined, *In progress (OMIM)

2.4. Next-generation sequencing

The Truseq custom amplicon library preparation kit and the MiSeq Illumina sequencer platform (Illumina Inc.) were used to create the sequencing library and perform resequencing respectively. All steps were performed in-house according to the manufacturer's instructions [27, 28].

Library preparation was performed by enrichment of the target regions using an amplicon-based multiplex polymerase chain reaction (PCR) method. Here, a custom amplicon tube (CAT) containing upstream and downstream oligonucleotides specific for the target regions was hybridized to the unfragmented gDNA samples in a 96-well plate. Unbound oligonucleotides were then removed by a series of wash steps using manufacturer supplied reagents. A proprietary extension–ligation mix containing DNA polymerase and ligase (Illumina Inc.) extended and ligated the upstream bound oligonucleotide through the targeted region to the 5′ end of the downstream oligonucleotide. The resulting extension–ligation products containing the targeted genomic region flanked by common sequences required for amplification were then amplified by standard PCR on a thermal cycler. The amplicon size (250 bps), the number of amplicons in the CAT (632 amplicons) and the type of input DNA (high quality) determined the number of PCR cycles ($n = 24$). The PCR reaction incorporated two unique, sample-specific, multiplexing index sequences (barcoding) that would later be used by the alignment software (MiSeq reporter) to identify individual samples following library pooling, and common adapters required for cluster generation. PCR products were purified by AMPure XP beads (Beckman Coulter, Lane Cove, NSW, Australia) and the quantity of each library was normalized by an integrated bead-based method. Equal volumes of the normalized libraries were then combined, diluted in hybridization buffer (Illumina Inc.) and heat denatured.

The MiSeq Illumina instrument was used to resequence the pooled library by paired-end sequencing. The DNA library was immobilized to the single-use glass-based MiSeq flow cell through the adapter sequences. Bridge PCR amplification then generated clusters of clonal copies of each DNA molecule. These templates were then sequenced using platform-specific reversible dye terminator sequencing-by-synthesis chemistry. Sequence alignment to the reference genome (GRCh37/hg19) was performed using on-instrument software (MiSeq reporter software, Illumina Inc.) that aligned the reads in BAM format and outputted variant calls in.vcf files. Variant calls were generated using ANNOVAR software (http://www.open-bioinformatics.org/annovar) [29] with an acceptance threshold Q-score of 30, corresponding to a 1:1000 error rate and genomic datasets were viewed using the Integrative Genomics viewer (IGV) (www.broadinstitute.org/igv/) [30]. Sanger sequencing was performed to provide data for bases with insufficient coverage and validate variants of clinical significance.

2.5. Data analysis

The University of California, Santa Cruz (UCSC), genome browser (http://genome.ucsc.edu) was used for variant analysis and variants were cross-checked against databases including the NHLBI-Extended Sequencing Project (ESP), 1000 Genomes Project Database [31] and the Database of Single-Nucleotide Polymorphisms (dbSNP, http://www.ncbi.nlm.nih.gov/SNP/). Bioinformatic tools, Sorting Intolerant From Tolerant (SIFT, http://sift.jcvi.org/) [32], Polymorphism Phenotyping-2 (PolyPhen-2, http://genetics.bwh.harvard.edu/pph2/) [33] and Mutation taster (http://www.mutationtaster.org/) [34] were used to predict variant effects on protein structure and function in the cases of variants lacking published literature.

2.6. Nomenclature and descriptions for variant reporting

All variants identified were annotated according to Human Genome Variation Society (HGVS) nomenclature for clinical reporting (http://www.hgvs.org). The variant elements included gene name, zygosity, cDNA nomenclature, protein nomenclature, exon number and clinical assertion.

Descriptions of sequence variations were adapted from the American College of Medical Genetics and Genomics (ACMG) recommendations for standards for interpretation and reporting of sequence variations and are listed below [35]:

Pathogenic: The sequence variation has been reported in the literature and is a recognized cause of the disorder.

Likely pathogenic: The sequence variation is previously unreported and is of the type that is expected to cause the disorder.

Variant of uncertain significance (VUS): The sequence variation is previously unreported and is of the type which may or may not be causative of the disorder.

Likely non-pathogenic: The sequence variation is previously unreported and is probably not causative of disease.

Non-pathogenic: The sequence variation is previously reported and is a recognized neutral variant.

3. Results

3.1. Next-generation sequencing platform performance

Next-generation sequencing on the Illumina platform produced 13 690 589 (96.74%) reads that passed initial filtering. This process removes any clusters demonstrating excessive intensity corresponding to bases other than the called base. Only reads that passed the quality filter were assigned a quality score. A quality score of Q30 was accepted in the run predictive of an error probability of ≤0.1%. One sample was excluded from analysis due to poor DNA quality that generated poor-quality scores across all genomic regions.

Overall coverage across all genomic targets was 92.3%. This was consistent with the initial software prediction.

3.2. Candidate gene panel results

A total of 703 non-synonymous variants were detected; 75 of these variants were novel and had not been reported in the dbSNP database. An average of eight non-synonymous variants was detected per patient.

Two individuals with known mutations in *GFI1B*, *GP1BA* and *GP9* by Sanger sequencing were included as controls. NGS successfully called the first, *GFI1B* c.880-881insC, but failed to detect the second, a patient with a phenotype consistent with the inherited macrothrombocytopenia Bernard-Soulier syndrome (BSS). This patient's genotype had previously been confirmed by Sanger sequencing and included mutations in both the *GPIBA* (*GPIBA* c.2217C>T) and the *GP9* genes (c.1829A>G and c.1859T>G). Failure to detect these mutations may have been caused by sequencing errors introduced by GC-rich motifs in these regions [36, 37].

Pathogenic mutations were detected in 16 individuals (17.4% of the cohort) whilst 36 individuals (39.1%) had VUS and 40 individuals (43.0%) were without identifiable pathogenic mutations (Table 2, Table 3).

Genes	Number of individuals with pathogenic mutations	Number of mutations detected of uncertain significance
ACTN1	0	8
GP1BA	1**	2
GP1BB	0	2
GP9	0	1
MYH9	6	3
TUBB1	0	3
NBEAL2	1	7
FLI1	0	1
GATA1	0	3
GFI1B	3	2
RUNX1	2**	0
CD36	0	13
F2R	0	0
GP6	0	5
ITGA2	0	4
ITGA2B	3*	6
ITGB1	0	0
ITGB3	0	0
P2RY12	0	0
Total Number	16	60 mutations in 36 individuals
Number of individuals without pathogenic mutations identified: 40		

*Parents heterozygous; child with homozygous mutation giving rise to a Glanzmann thrombasthaenia phenotype.

** These mutations are likely pathogenic. That is, the detected variation is unreported in the literature to date, however, based on the type of variation, it's deleterious effect predicted using bioinformatic tools (see data analysis) and the associated phenotypic data, is of the type to cause the disorder

Table 2. Mutations detected in the candidate genes. Genes affecting the platelet cytoskeleton (top, white shading), the platelet granules (light gray shading) and platelet-related transcription factors (dark gray shading).

Gene	Chromosome	Zygosity	Nucleotide change	Protein alteration	Exon
*GP1BA***	17	Heterozygous	c.1432delT	p.Phe478fs	2
MYH9	22	Heterozygous	c.283G>A	p.Ala95Thr	2
		Heterozygous	c.287C>T	p.Ser96Leu	2
		Heterozygous	c.2104C>T	Arg702Cys	17
		Heterozygous	c.4339G>C	p.Asp1447His	31
NBEAL2	3	Compound heterozygous	c.5935C>T	p.Arg1979Trp	37
			c.7103dupA	His2368fs	45
GFI1B	9	Heterozygous	c.503G>T	p.Cys168Phe	4
*RUNX1***	21	Heterozygous	c.503–504ins ACCACAGAGCCATCAAA AT	p.Ile168fs	3
		Heterozygous	Stop/gain c.766C>T	p.Gln256X	5
*ITGA2B**	17	Homozygous	c.138–139insT	p.Gly47fs	1

* Parents heterozygous. Child with homozygous mutation giving rise to a Glanzmann thrombasthaenia phenotype.

** Mutations are likely pathogenic.

Table 3. Pathogenic genetic variants detected: nucleotide cDNA changes and corresponding protein alterations.

The candidate array was successful in detecting mutations in genes commonly associated with macrothrombocytopenia and included a total of nine *MYH9* mutations (six of which had previously been reported in the literature as pathogenic and three of which are of uncertain significance) (Figure 2) and a compound heterozygous mutation of *NBEAL2* in keeping with Gray platelet syndrome.

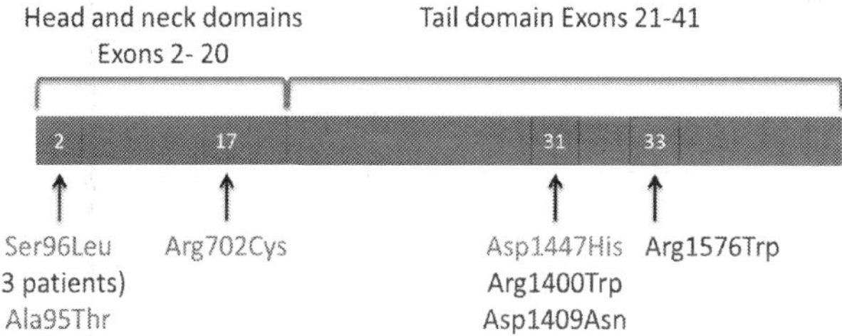

Figure 2. MYH9 variants detected in the candidate gene panel. Exons 2–20 encode the head and neck domains of NMMHC IIA (Blue block). Exons 21–41 encode the tail domains. Mutations were detected in exons 2, 17, 31 and 33. Six pathogenic mutations (red text) and three variants of uncertain significance (black text) were detected.

A homozygous mutation of *ITGA2B* was also detected and confirmed a suspected Glanzmann thrombasthenia phenotype. Several transcription factor variants were found, including a *FLI1* mutation of uncertain significance in one patient, three *GATA1* mutations of uncertain significance in three individuals from two families, three pathogenic *GFI1B* mutations in three individuals from two families and two of uncertain significance in two individuals in another two families. *RUNX1* mutations were identified in three individuals from three families; two of these were considered likely pathogenic, whilst the third was shown to represent a false positive result (*RUNX1*, heterozygous, stop/gain, c. 966T>G (p.Tyr322X), exon 6). False positivity was confirmed by Sanger sequencing that showed a wild-type sequence across that region.

Sanger sequencing was also performed in selected samples across regions of low coverage (Q < 30) from those genes in which the clinical significance is widely accepted and included, *GP9, GP1BA, GPIBB, FLI1* exon 3, *FLI1* exon 9, *MYH9* exon 20, *MYH9* exon 37 and *GFI1B* exon 5. This confirmatory step detected a novel mutation in *FLI1* [38], not identified by NGS.

4. Discussion

The diagnosis of IPFD and IPNDs using classic phenotypic methods poses a challenge to clinicians and laboratory scientists due to lack of consensus over classification and diagnostic criteria, poor standardization of tests and heterogeneity of traditional diagnostic approaches [6]. This diagnostic conundrum is evident in our cohort where only 11 patients received a suspected diagnosis to a pathway level following multiple previous phenotypic tests. In addition, only 62% of patients received any form of phenotypic test, reflecting the difficulty of accessing these specialized techniques in many centers.

Sanger sequencing is widely regarded as a reliable platform for routine diagnostic genetic testing and small-scale projects. However, effective analysis of numerous disease-associated genes by Sanger sequencing in a diagnostic setting is time-consuming, expensive and not always feasible [18]. A candidate gene array was selected as it has the potential to simultaneously analyze all of the selected coding regions of disease-targeted genes. Moreover, relative to WES and WGS, it provides good gene coverage and representation of exons, is relatively fast and cheap and minimizes the problems with unexpected findings and development of complex downstream bioinformatic pipelines for analysis [39].

We have demonstrated that high-quality sequence data can be generated from a candidate group of platelet genes using the Illumina MiSeq platform. Our candidate gene panel comprised 19 genes associated with IPNDs, predominantly inherited macrothrombocytopenia. Pathogenic mutations were detected in 17.4% of the cohort. The most number of mutations was detected in the *MYH9* gene. *MYH9*-related disorders are the most common forms of inherited thrombocytopenia and are frequently under-recognized or misdiagnosed as immune ITP [40–42]. Immunofluorescence staining of the peripheral blood film demonstrating abnormal clustering of non-muscle myosin heavy chain IIA (NMMHC IIA), seen as Döhle bodies on the blood film is regarded as a suitable diagnostic test [40], but is not available at all centers. A strong genotype–phenotype relationship is recognized in these disorders, with mutations affecting the motor (head and neck) region of NMMHC-IIA causing more severe thrombocytopenia and a higher risk for nephritis, cataracts and deafness, whilst those mutations affecting the tail region cause less severe thrombocytopenia and extra-hematological manifestations [43, 44]. Genetic confirmation of *MYH9*-related disorders, therefore, has prognostic significance. In our group of patients, three pathogenic mutations in five individuals were detected and were predicted to affect the motor region of NMMHC IIA. Knowledge of these mutations has provided an opportunity to offer advice regarding additional non-hematological surveillance tests such as audiograms, renal function assessments and ophthalmological screening for cataracts [40, 41, 45].

Transcription factors are the key regulators for the development of the hemostatic platelet from blood stem cells. Stem cells differentiate into a bipotent megakaryocyte-erythroid progenitor, then a committed megakaryocyte that undergoes endoreplication prior to extending proplatelet extensions from the cytoplasm into the bone marrow sinusoid forming platelets [46]. This complex differentiation pathway is orchestrated by the activation and repression of groups of genes important for blood cell development via transcription factors [46, 47]. The candidate gene panel contained four genes that encode hemopoietic transcription factors, FLI1, GATA1, GFI1B and RUNX1. Definitive diagnosis of platelet disorders caused by mutations in these genes solely by phenotypic testing is not possible. We detected a pathogenic mutation in one of these genes, *GFI1B*, and likely pathogenic mutations, in *RUNX1*. The *RUNX1* gene is responsible for the familial platelet disorder with a predisposition to acute myeloid leukemia (FPD/AML) [48]. The propensity to develop acute leukemia is determined by the action of the variant, with dominant negative and haploinsufficient mutations having different leukemogenic risk. The former has a higher risk (up to 40% in some reports) of progression to AML or myelodysplastic syndrome [49–51]. Other factors include the residual level of activity of wild-type RUNX1 [52], deregulation induced by dominant negative mutations on hamopoietic stem cell genes such as *NR4A3* [53] as well as effects on p53 genes-dependent genes that induce genomic instability of the granulomonocytic precursors [52]. The median age of onset of progression to myelodysplastic syndrome / acute leukemia is 33 years of age, and therefore, the detection of two, likely pathogenic, *RUNX1* mutations by our candidate gene panel is of obvious importance [49]. Despite their adverse risk, clinical guidelines regarding the best way to counsel, test and manage these patients and their family members are lacking and recommendations are largely based on expert opinion [54]. Initial referral to a specialist team comprising a physician as well as genetic counselor is recommended, as well as, full blood count analysis, bone marrow biopsy (to detect occult malignancy) and full human-leukocyte antigen (HLA) typing of patients and their first-degree relatives (in the event a bone marrow transplant is required in the future). A biannual follow-up schedule thereafter should be established to ensure close hematological surveillance [54]. GFI1B is another transcription factor that plays an essential role in hematopoiesis [46, 55]. Two recent publications [22, 23] described mutations in the DNA-binding zinc finger domain of *GFI1B* causing an autosomal dominant bleeding disorder in affected families. Our candidate gene array detected another mutation in a non-DNA-binding zinc finger domain of *GFI1B* (*GFI1B* c.503G>T). Further characterization of this c.503G>T mutation indicates a milder platelet phenotype with less clinical bleeding symptomatology than the DNA-binding mutants [56] (Figure 3). The detection of this non-DNA-binding mutation has afforded us an opportunity to propose a genotype–phenotype relationship associated with mutations in two different regions of GFI1B. This is important to enable classification, aid diagnosis and inform treatment strategies.

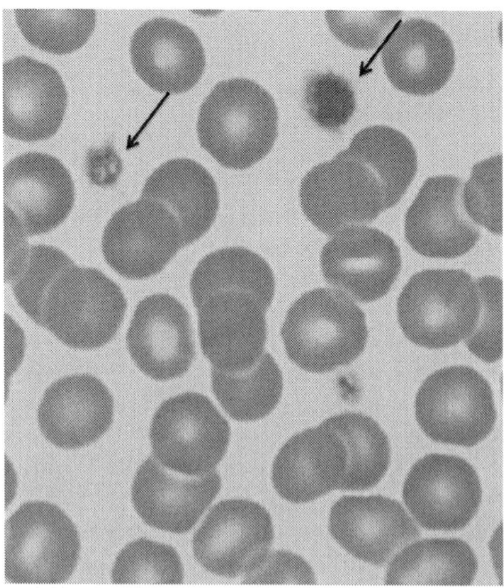

Figure 3. The blood film of an affected individual with the *GFI1B* c.503G>T mutation demonstrating macrothrombocytopenia. Platelets show normal granulation unlike the platelets seen in individuals with the *GFI1B* c.880-881insC mutation (Figure 1D) that have a heterogeneous appearance (some platelets appear hypogranular or gray whilst others have normal granulation).

The yield of pathogenic variants reported above may have been improved by more stringent patient selection criteria. In this study, all patients suspected of an inherited thrombocytopenia by treating hematologists were included regardless of the platelet phenotype. That is, not all patients demonstrated macrothrombocytopenia. In addition, in 16 cases only DNA was received and the platelet phenotype was not known. Noting that 15 of the 19 genes on the candidate panel are known to cause macrothrombocytopenia and that only 5 genes on the panel (*ETS1, P2RY12, F2R, GP6, RUNX1*) have an uncertain platelet phenotype or otherwise known to cause functional disorders with normal-sized platelets, the pre-test probability of detecting a pathogenic variant in samples where macrothrombocytopenia was not present was low. Furthermore, this candidate array was performed in a research laboratory and therefore included genes (*ETS1 and F2R*) where the association with inherited thrombocytopenia is not well delineated. Exclusive inclusion of genes with clear evidence of disease association may further improve the diagnostic yield.

Variants of uncertain significance (VUS) were detected in over a third of the cohort (39.1%). Thirteen samples contained more than one VUS. One sample contained five VUS in five different genes (*GFI1B, ITGA2, MYH9, NBEAL2 and TUBB1*). In many instances, these variants were novel. It is likely, as knowledge of the genes causing inherited platelet bleeding disorders increases, this percentage will decrease, the VUS either becoming recognized as pathogenic or definitely non-pathogenic. Our analytical pathway used three bioinformatics tools (SIFT, PolyPhen2, Mutation taster) in variants lacking published literature to assist variant annotation. Bioinformatic tools using sequence and/or structure to predict the effects of amino acid substitutions on protein function have been developed following observations that disease-causing mutations are more likely to occur at positions that show evolutionary conservation and/or common structural features which enable them to be distinguished from neutral substitutions [57–60]. These tools serve to guide future experiments and should not be used solely as a clinical predictor of pathogenicity. Consider the *ACTN1* missense mutation (*ACTN1*, heterozygous, c.580G>A [p.Gly194Arg], exon 6, rs145918825) detected in our candidate gene array. It is predicted to disturb the calponin homology domain (CHD) within the actin-binding domain (ABD) of α-actinin (an important platelet structural protein). All of the mutations described in the literature to date have identified *ACTN1* mutations within the functional domains (ABD and the C-terminal calmodulin-like domain [CaM]) but not within the spacer spectrin repeats [25, 61, 62]. Bioinformatic tools were applied to this variant. It is predicted to be deleterious by SIFT (sequence homology-based tool), whereas PolyPhen-2 (structure/sequence based tool) predicts the amino acid alteration to be benign. This highlights two points. Firstly, it is advisable that predictions are made by integrating the results from several tools as reliance on one tool may lead to incorrect annotation [63], and secondly, that bioinformatic tools provide predictions only. In this case, the functional consequences of the *ACTN1* DNA variant are yet to be described and thus the variant may or may not be significant. Further family studies and additional structural analyses of the protein may clarify the pathogenicity of the variant [35].

Coverage is a crucial metric for establishing accuracy as well as analytical sensitivity and specificity of a NGS testing platform [64]. Coverage requirements depend on the application of the NGS test. In general, sequencing more reads will increase the power of the assay. We determined the necessary coverage level based on recommendations forwarded by the Royal College of Pathologists of Australasia [65] whose guidance is in compliance with National Pathology Accreditation Advisory Council (NPAAC) standards for testing of human nucleic acids [66] and combined this advice with recommendations from published literature and other international bodies such as the ACMG [35]. Our accepted Q score (Q30) was met in 92.3% of all genomic targets and in 97% of exonic targets. The read coverage distribution curve displayed a classic Poisson-like distribution indicating uniformity of coverage, this data accompanied by the high quality of base calls suggested that the NGS platform is able to deliver reliable sequence data. However, there were also areas of lower coverage where the platform did not perform as well, and lacked sensitivity. These regions were identified at genomic targets in *FLI1, GP1BA, GP1BB, GP9, ITGB1* and *NBEAL2* and were predicted in the design studio report. Two false negative results were confirmed in regions where coverage was low. The first being the failed detection of *GPIBA* and *GP9* mutations in the second internal control sample and the second was a novel pathogenic mutation in *FLI1* that was confirmed by Sanger sequencing and additional laboratory investigations. To ensure coverage of the respective amplicons over the *GP9* region, parallel Sanger sequencing was performed. Targeted Sanger sequencing was also performed for *GP1BA* and *GP1BB* in cases in which phenotypic details had been provided by the referring clinician and where confident exclusion of a variant in those genes was necessary. Sanger sequencing performed over these regions did not detect additional mutations. Only a single false positive result was confirmed by Sanger sequencing (*RUNX1*, stop/gain, c.966T>G). This suggested good platform specificity. The question as to whether confirmatory Sanger sequencing need be performed is debated in the literature [39, 67]. Proponents argue that it is required to confirm a diagnosis as well as remove incorrect calls introduced by experimental errors. Whereas, opponents argue, in the setting where the NGS platform performance metrics have been established to be comparable to Sanger sequencing performance measures, a strategy dictated by the degree of coverage per nucleotide be adopted. Suggesting that parallel Sanger sequencing need not be performed as long as the coverage is >30 times per nucleotide at that genomic target, adding that confirmatory testing be performed where coverage is less than 20 times, and be determined by visual inspection with coverage between 20 and 30 times. Authors commented that the laboratory may also simply elect to exclude the target from the report if Sanger sequencing is not performed despite low coverage [39].

An important aspect of the post-analytical process is the timely provision of a genomic test report. In the setting of inherited platelet disorders, a false negative interpretation may lead to a falsely conservative bleeding prophylactic strategy at the time of surgery, in turn, placing the individual at a potentially increased risk of bleeding. A false positive result, on the other hand, may cause undue stress to the individual and their family. A genomic test report was therefore carefully and consistently structured taking into consideration recommendations from professional bodies such as the RCPA [65] and ACMG [68]. The report (Appendix 1) contained a summary of the genes analyzed and reflected the scope and limitation of the assay and indicated the context in which the test was performed. A clear, succinct, interpretative comment was made regarding the detected variant. This indicated whether or not the detected variant was associated with the clinical phenotype and highlighted variants of uncertain significance. The body of the report detailed, in a structured format (see materials and methods), any detected pathogenic or clinically relevant variants and whether these had been previously described. An interpretation on the significance of the detected variant was supported by relevant references where possible, and recommendations regarding additional validation tests and /or genetic counseling and clinical screening were provided. Following the main body of the report, DNA variants that were considered to be non-pathogenic were listed. The report was concluded by a description of the test method and limitations thereof.

In conclusion, our study has demonstrated the potential to successfully diagnose inherited macrothrombocytopenia in cases that remained uncharacterized by traditional phenotypic approaches. Optimization of this format will provide patients an opportunity for a "one stop, one step" testing platform that is cost-effective and not affected by the pre-analytical variables that hinder current testing methods based on functional analysis of platelets. However, the translation of NGS from a powerful research tool into the clinical laboratory will require co-operation from international groups to establish best practice, quality and reporting standards for these conditions, as well as to generate reliable databases that link platelet phenotypes to genotypes to provide best hemostasis clinician advice.

5. Appendix

Test performed: Candidate gene array of 19 genes (*ACTN1, CD36, F2R, FLI1, ETS1, GATA1, GFI1b, GP1BA, GP1BB, GP6, GP9, ITGA2, ITGA2B, ITGB1, ITGB3, MYH9, NBEAL2, P2RY12, RUNX1, TUBB1*) using the Illumina MiSeq next-generation sequencing platform.

Please Note:

This test has been performed for research purposes only and has not been NATA accredited in our laboratory.

Validation by Sanger sequencing has not been performed on clinically significant or novel detected variants and should be considered by the referring clinician.

Result: A mutation in a gene known or predicted to be associated with decreased platelet counts and/ or function has been identified. A second variant of uncertain significance has also been identified.

DNA variants: Variant 1: *MYH9*, Heterozygous, c.287C>T (p.Ser96Leu), Exon 2, rs121913657, **pathogenic.**

Variant 2: *NBEAL2*, Heterozygous, c.6178C>T (p.Arg2060Cys), exon37, **uncertain significance.**

Previously described: Variant 1: Yes (rs121913657)

Variant 2: No.

Interpretation: A heterozygous 287C-T transition in the MYH9 gene, resulting in a ser96-to-leu (S96L) substitution, has been predicted to disturb the helical region of the protein resulting in MYH9- related disorder (Epstein syndrome).

The pathogenicity of variant 2 is uncertain as information regarding this mutation is not available in the reported literature. Note that the classification of variants of uncertain/ unknown significance may change over time if additional information on these conditions becomes available in the reported literature.

References: Arrondel C, et al. Expression of the non-muscle myosin heavy chain IIA in the human kidney and screening for MYH9 mutations in Epstein and Fechtner syndromes. J Am Soc Nephrol 2002;13: 65–74.

Utsch B, et al. Bladder exstrophy and Epstein type congenital macrothrombocytopenia: evidence for a common cause? (Letter) Am J Med Genet 2006;140A:2251–3.

Kunishima S, et al. Immunofluorescence analysis of neutrophil non-muscle myosin heavy chain-A in MYH9 disorders: association of subcellular localization with MYH9 mutations. Lab Invest 2003;83:115–22.

Recommendations: The pathogenicity of detected candidate variants should be validated independently by Sanger sequencing. Where necessary, the functional significance of these variants should be confirmed independently by appropriate biological assays to replicate the phenotype of this patient.

MYH9-related disorders have an autosomal dominant inheritance. Genetic counselling is recommended for this individual and their family. Family screening may be appropriate after appropriate genetic counselling.

DNA variants detected of unlikely clinical significance:

NBEAL2, Heterozygous, c.1531C>G (p.Arg511Gly), Exon 13, rs11720139, likely **non-pathogenic**. *GP6*, Homozygous, c.691G>A (p.Ala231Thr), Exon 6, rs2304167, likely **non-pathogenic**. *MYH9*, Heterozygous, c.4876A>G (p.Ile1626Val), Exon 34, rs2269529, likely **non-pathogenic**.

Test method:

A TruSeq custom amplicon specific for the target regions of 19 genes, *ACTN1, CD36, F2R, FLI1, ETS1, GATA1, GFI1b, GP1BA, GP1BB, GP6, GP9, ITGA2, ITGA2B, ITGB1, ITGB3, MYH9, NBEAL2, P2RY12, RUNX1, TUBB1* was designed using Illumina design studio (Illumina, Inc, San Diego, CA, USA). Next-generation sequencing was performed using the MiSeq Illumina sequencer platform (Illumina, Inc.). Obtained sequences were aligned to the reference genome (GRCh37/hg19) using MiSeq reporter software (Illumina, Inc.) and the genomic datasets viewed using the Integrative Genomics viewer (IGV) (www.broadinstitute.org/igv/). Variant calls were generated using ANNOVAR software (http://www.openbioinformatics.org/annovar) with an acceptance threshold Q-score of 30, corresponding to a 1:1000 error rate. Sanger sequencing was performed to provide data for bases with insufficient coverage. The University of California, Santa Cruz (UCSC), genome browser (http://genome.ucsc.edu) was used for variant analysis and variants were cross-checked against databases including the NHLBI-extended sequencing project (ESP), 1000 genomes project database and the Database of Single-Nucleotide Polymorphisms (dbSNP). Bioinformatic tools (SIFT, PolyPhen-2 and Mutation taster) were used to predict variant effects on protein structure and function in the cases of variants lacking published literature.

Limitations: Overall gene coverage was 97% using this format. Therefore, it is possible that the genomic region where a disease causing mutation exists in the proband was not captured and therefore was not detected.

It is also possible that a particular genetic mutation was not recognised as the underlying cause of the genetic disorder due to incomplete scientific knowledge of the impact of all variants at this point in the literature.

Reported by:

An example of a NGS report.

Author details

David J. Rabbolini[1,2], Marie-Christine Morel Kopp[1,2], Sara Gabrielli[1,2], Qiang Chen[1,2], William S. Stevenson[1,2] and Christopher M. Ward[1,2*]

*Address all correspondence to: cward@med.usyd.edu.au

1 Northern Blood Research Centre, Kolling Institute of Medical Research, The University of Sydney, Sydney, Australia

2 Department of Haematology and Transfusion Medicine, Royal North Shore Hospital, Sydney, Australia

References

[1] Brass LF. Thrombin and platelet activation. Chest 2003;124(3 Suppl):18S–25S.

[2] Shattil SJ, Kashiwagi H, Pampori N. Integrin signaling: the platelet paradigm. Blood 1998;91(8):2645–57.

[3] Balduini CL, Cattaneo M, Fabris F, Gresele P, Iolascon A, Pulcinelli FM, et al. Inherited thrombocytopenias: a proposed diagnostic algorithm from the Italian Gruppo di Studio delle Piastrine. Haematologica 2003;88(5):582–92.

[4] Kunishima S, Saito H. Congenital macrothrombocytopenias. Blood Rev 2006;20(2): 111–21.

[5] Noris P, Pecci A, Di Bari F, Di Stazio MT, Di Pumpo M, Ceresa IF, et al. Application of a diagnostic algorithm for inherited thrombocytopenias to 46 consecutive patients. Haematologica 2004;89(10):1219–25.

[6] Gresele P, Harrison P, Bury L, Falcinelli E, Gachet C, Hayward CP, et al. Diagnosis of suspected inherited platelet function disorders: results of a worldwide survey. J Thromb Haemost 2014;12(9):1562–9.

[7] Gresele P. Diagnosis of inherited platelet function disorders: guidance from the SSC of the ISTH. J Thromb Haemost 2015;13(2):314–22.

[8] Israels SJ, El-Ekiaby M, Quiroga T, Mezzano D. Inherited disorders of platelet function and challenges to diagnosis of mucocutaneous bleeding. Haemophilia 2010;16(Suppl 5):152–9.

[9] Hayward CP, Eikelboom J. Platelet function testing: quality assurance. Semin Thromb Hemost 2007;33(3):273–82.

[10] Hayward CP, Rao AK, Cattaneo M. Congenital platelet disorders: overview of their mechanisms, diagnostic evaluation and treatment. Haemophilia 2006;12(Suppl 3): 128–36.

[11] Moffat KA, Ledford-Kraemer MR, Nichols WL, Hayward CP, North American Specialized Coagulation Laboratory A. Variability in clinical laboratory practice in testing for disorders of platelet function: results of two surveys of the North American Specialized Coagulation Laboratory Association. Thromb Haemost 2005;93(3):549–53.

[12] Favaloro EJ, Lippi G, Franchini M. Contemporary platelet function testing. Clin Chem Lab Med 2010;48(5):579–98.

[13] Harrison P, Mackie I, Mumford A, Briggs C, Liesner R, Winter M, et al. Guidelines for the laboratory investigation of heritable disorders of platelet function. Br J Haematol 2011;155(1):30–44.

[14] George JN, Shattil SJ. The clinical importance of acquired abnormalities of platelet function. N Engl J Med 1991;324(1):27–39.

[15] Sanger F, Nicklen S, Coulson AR. DNA sequencing with chain-terminating inhibitors. Proc Natl Acad Sci USA 1977;74(12):5463–7.

[16] Bonetta L. Genome sequencing in the fast lane. Nat Meth 2006;3(2):141–7.

[17] Johnsen JM, Nickerson DA, Reiner AP. Massively parallel sequencing: the new frontier of hematologic genomics. Blood 2013;122(19):3268–75.

[18] Shendure J, Ji H. Next-generation DNA sequencing. Nat biotechnol 2008;26(10):1135–45.

[19] Harismendy O, Ng PC, Strausberg RL, Wang X, Stockwell TB, Beeson KY, et al. Evaluation of next generation sequencing platforms for population targeted sequencing studies. Genome Biol 2009;10(3):R32.

[20] Smith ML, Wheeler KE. Weight-based heparin protocol using antifactor Xa monitoring. Am J Health-Syst Pharm 2010;67(5):371–4.

[21] Bamshad MJ, Ng SB, Bigham AW, Tabor HK, Emond MJ, Nickerson DA, et al. Exome sequencing as a tool for Mendelian disease gene discovery. Nat Rev Genet 2011;12(11):745–55.

[22] Monteferrario D, Bolar NA, Marneth AE, Hebeda KM, Bergevoet SM, Veenstra H, et al. A dominant-negative GFI1B mutation in the gray platelet syndrome. N Engl J Med 2014;370(3):245–53.

[23] Stevenson WS, Morel-Kopp MC, Chen Q, Liang HP, Bromhead CJ, Wright S, et al. GFI1B mutation causes a bleeding disorder with abnormal platelet function. J Thromb Haemost 2013;11(11):2039–47.

[24] Kunishima S, Okuno Y, Yoshida K, Shiraishi Y, Sanada M, Muramatsu H, et al. ACTN1 mutations cause congenital macrothrombocytopenia. Am J Hum Genet 2013;92(3):431–8.

[25] Bottega R, Marconi C, Faleschini M, Baj G, Cagioni C, Pecci A, et al. ACTN1-related thrombocytopenia: identification of novel families for phenotypic characterization. Blood 2015;125(5):869–72.

[26] Thermo Scientific technical bulletin: 260/280 and 260/230 ratios [Internet]. 2008. Available from: http://www.nanodrop.com/Library/T009-NanoDrop%201000-&-NanoDrop%208000-Nucleic-Acid-Purity-Ratios.pdf [Accessed: 2015-08-02].

[27] Illumina-Truseq Custom Amplicon Library Preparation Guide [Internet]. 2013. Available from: http://support.illumina.com/content/dam/illumina-support/documents/documentation/chemistry_documentation/samplepreps_truseq/truseqcustomamplicon/truseq-custom-amplicon-libraryprep-ug-15027983-c.pdf [Accessed: 2015-08-08].

[28] Illumina- MiSeq System user guide [Internet]. 2014. Available from: https://support.illumina.com/content/dam/illumina-support/documents/documentation/system_documentation/miseq/miseq-system-guide-15027617-o.pdf [Accessed: 2015-08-08].

[29] Wang K, Li M, Hakonarson H. ANNOVAR: functional annotation of genetic variants from high-throughput sequencing data. Nucleic Acids Res 2010;38(16):e164.

[30] Robinson JT, Thorvaldsdottir H, Winckler W, Guttman M, Lander ES, Getz G, et al. Integrative genomics viewer. Nat biotechnol 2011;29(1):24–6.

[31] Gunter C. Genomics: a picture worth 1000 genomes. Nat Rev Genet 2010;11(12):814.

[32] Kumar P, Henikoff S, Ng PC. Predicting the effects of coding non-synonymous variants on protein function using the SIFT algorithm. Nat Protocol 2009;4(7):1073–81.

[33] Adzhubei IA, Schmidt S, Peshkin L, Ramensky VE, Gerasimova A, Bork P, et al. A method and server for predicting damaging missense mutations. Nat Meth 2010;7(4): 248–9.

[34] Schwarz JM, Cooper DN, Schuelke M, Seelow D. MutationTaster2: mutation prediction for the deep-sequencing age. Nat Meth 2014;11(4):361–2.

[35] Richards CS, Bale S, Bellissimo DB, Das S, Grody WW, Hegde MR, et al. ACMG recommendations for standards for interpretation and reporting of sequence variations: revisions 2007. Genet Med 2008;10(4):294–300.

[36] Quail MA, Smith M, Coupland P, Otto TD, Harris SR, Connor TR, et al. A tale of three next generation sequencing platforms: comparison of Ion Torrent, Pacific Biosciences and Illumina MiSeq sequencers. BMC Genom 2012;13:341.

[37] Ross MG, Russ C, Costello M, Hollinger A, Lennon NJ, Hegarty R, et al. Characterizing and measuring bias in sequence data. Genome Biol 2013;14(5):R51.

[38] Stevenson WS, Rabbolini DJ, Beutler L, Chen Q, Gabrielli S, Mackay JP, et al. Paris-Trousseau thrombocytopenia is phenocopied by the autosomal recessive inheritance of a DNA-binding domain mutation in FLI1. Blood [Epub ahead of print]. 2015. Available from: http://dx.doi.org/10.1182/blood-2015-06-650887. [Accessed 2015-08-27]

[39] Sikkema-Raddatz B, Johansson LF, de Boer EN, Almomani R, Boven LG, van den Berg MP, et al. Targeted next-generation sequencing can replace Sanger sequencing in clinical diagnostics. Hum Mutat 2013;34(7):1035–42.

[40] Savoia A, De Rocco D, Panza E, Bozzi V, Scandellari R, Loffredo G, et al. Heavy chain myosin 9-related disease (MYH9 -RD): neutrophil inclusions of myosin-9 as a pathognomonic sign of the disorder. Thromb Haemost 2010;103(4):826–32.

[41] Balduini CL, Pecci A, Savoia A. Recent advances in the understanding and management of MYH9-related inherited thrombocytopenias. Br J Haematol 2011;154(2):161–74.

[42] Althaus K, Greinacher A. MYH9-related platelet disorders. Semin Thromb Hemost 2009;35(2):189–203.

[43] Althaus K, Greinacher A. MYH9-related platelet disorders. Semin Thromb Hemost 2009;35(2):189–203.

[44] Pecci A, Panza E, Pujol-Moix N, Klersy C, Di Bari F, Bozzi V, et al. Position of non-muscle myosin heavy chain IIA (NMMHC-IIA) mutations predicts the natural history of MYH9-related disease. Hum Mutat 2008;29(3):409–17.

[45] Althaus K, Greinacher A. MYH-9 related platelet disorders: strategies for management and diagnosis. Transfusion medicine and hemotherapy : offizielles Organ der Deutschen Gesellschaft fur Transfusionsmedizin und Immunhamatologie. 2010;37(5): 260–7.

[46] Doerks T, Copley RR, Schultz J, Ponting CP, Bork P. Systematic identification of novel protein domain families associated with nuclear functions. Genome Res 2002;12(1): 47–56.

[47] Tijssen MR, Ghevaert C. Transcription factors in late megakaryopoiesis and related platelet disorders. J Thromb Haemost 2013;11(4):593–604.

[48] Song WJ, Sullivan MG, Legare RD, Hutchings S, Tan X, Kufrin D, et al. Haploinsufficiency of CBFA2 causes familial thrombocytopenia with propensity to develop acute myelogenous leukaemia. Nat Genet. 1999;23(2):166–75.

[49] Liew E, Owen C. Familial myelodysplastic syndromes: a review of the literature. Haematologica 2011;96(10):1536–42.

[50] Beri-Dexheimer M, Latger-Cannard V, Philippe C, Bonnet C, Chambon P, Roth V, et al. Clinical phenotype of germline RUNX1 haploinsufficiency: from point mutations to large genomic deletions. Eur J Hum Genet 2008;16(8):1014–8.

[51] Matheny CJ, Speck ME, Cushing PR, Zhou Y, Corpora T, Regan M, et al. Disease mutations in RUNX1 and RUNX2 create nonfunctional, dominant-negative, or hypomorphic alleles. Embo J 2007;26(4):1163–75.

[52] Antony-Debre I, Manchev VT, Balayn N, Bluteau D, Tomowiak C, Legrand C, et al. Level of RUNX1 activity is critical for leukemic predisposition but not for thrombocytopenia. Blood 2015;125(6):930–40.

[53] Bluteau D, Gilles L, Hilpert M, Antony-Debre I, James C, Debili N, et al. Down-regulation of the RUNX1-target gene NR4A3 contributes to hematopoiesis deregulation in familial platelet disorder/acute myelogenous leukemia. Blood 2011;118(24):6310–20.

[54] Churpek JE, Lorenz R, Nedumgottil S, Onel K, Olopade OI, Sorrell A, et al. Proposal for the clinical detection and management of patients and their family members with familial myelodysplastic syndrome/acute leukemia predisposition syndromes. Leuk Lymphoma 2013;54(1):28–35.

[55] Vassen L, Okayama T, Moroy T. Gfi1b:green fluorescent protein knock-in mice reveal a dynamic expression pattern of Gfi1b during hematopoiesis that is largely complementary to Gfi1. Blood 2007;109(6):2356–64.

[56] Rabbolini DJ, Morel-Kopp MC, Chen Q, Gabrielli S, Dunlop L, Brighton T, et al. Abstracts. J Thromb Haemost 2015;13:1–997 (abstract PO421).

[57] Ng PC, Henikoff S. Predicting the effects of amino acid substitutions on protein function. Annu Rev Genomics Hum Genet 2006;7:61–80.

[58] Miller MP, Kumar S. Understanding human disease mutations through the use of interspecific genetic variation. Hum Mol Genet 2001;10(21):2319–28.

[59] Wang Z, Moult J. SNPs, protein structure, and disease. Hum Mutat 2001;17(4):263–70.

[60] Sunyaev S, Ramensky V, Bork P. Towards a structural basis of human non-synonymous single nucleotide polymorphisms. Trends Genet 2000;16(5):198–200.

[61] Kunishima S, Okuno Y, Yoshida K, Shiraishi Y, Sanada M, Muramatsu H, et al. ACTN1 mutations cause congenital macrothrombocytopenia. Am J Hum Genet 2013;92(3):431–8.

[62] Gueguen P, Rouault K, Chen JM, Raguenes O, Fichou Y, Hardy E, et al. A missense mutation in the alpha-actinin 1 gene (ACTN1) is the cause of autosomal dominant macrothrombocytopenia in a large French family. PloS one 2013;8(9):e74728.

[63] Gilissen C, Hoischen A, Brunner HG, Veltman JA. Disease gene identification strategies for exome sequencing. Eur J Hum Genet 2012;20(5):490–7.

[64] Gargis AS, Kalman L, Berry MW, Bick DP, Dimmock DP, Hambuch T, et al. Assuring the quality of next-generation sequencing in clinical laboratory practice. Nat biotechnol 2012;30(11):1033–6.

[65] The Royal College of Pathologists of Australasia: Massively Parallel Sequencing Implementation Guidelines [Internet]. 2014. Available from: https://www.rcpa.edu.au/getattachment/7d264a73-938f-45b5-912f-272872661aaa/Massively-Parallel-Sequencing-Implementation.aspx [Accessed: 2015-08-09]

[66] National Pathology Accreditation Advisory Council Requirements for medical testing of human nucleic acids. In: Health AGDo (Ed.) 2 edn [Internet]. 2013. Available from: https://www.health.gov.au/internet/main/publishing.nsf/Content/E688964F88F4FD20CA257BF0001B739D/$File/V0.25%20NAD%20Human%20Genetics.pdf [Accessed: 2015-08-09].

[67] Zhang W, Cui H, Wong LJ. Application of next generation sequencing to molecular diagnosis of inherited diseases. Top Curr Chem 2014;336:19–45.

[68] Rehm HL, Bale SJ, Bayrak-Toydemir P, Berg JS, Brown KK, Deignan JL, et al. ACMG clinical laboratory standards for next-generation sequencing. Genet Med 2013;15(9): 733–47.

Chapter 15

Clinical Implementation of Next-generation Sequencing in the Field of Prenatal Diagnostics

Gwendolin Manegold-Brauer and Olav Lapaire

Additional information is available at the end of the chapter

http://dx.doi.org/10.5772/61799

Abstract

The possibility to receive genetic information of the fetus from maternal blood during the course of pregnancy has been one of the main goals of research in prenatal medicine for decades. First, the detection of cell-free fetal DNA in maternal blood and finally, the development of the powerful technique of "next-generation sequencing" (NGS) were required to finally transfer this analysis into clinical practice. Since its introduction in 2011, the clinical demand for the technique of non-invasive prenatal testing (NIPT) has been enormous. NIPT initially was available for the most common aneuploidies (trisomy 21, 13, and 18), but the varieties of diseases that can be detected prenatally by NIPT are increasing rapidly.

In this chapter, we aim to describe the current basic concepts of NIPT, give an overview of the currently available NIPT tests and associated technical aspects. We will present our studies on the clinical uptake of NIPT into clinical care in two different European centers and its impact on prenatal diagnosis.

Keywords: Non-invasive prenatal testing, prenatal diagnosis, prenatal ultrasound, cell-free fetal DNA, fetal aneuploidies

1. Introduction

The analysis of the fetal genome by an indirect approach from maternal blood during pregnancy has been the focus of research in prenatal medicine for decades. The only option to investigate the genetic condition of the fetus so far had been an invasive procedure such as chorionic villous sampling and amniocentesis, which carries a 1% risk of miscarriage.

The basis of the current concepts to this non-invasive approach was the detection of cell-free fetal DNA (cffDNA) in maternal blood in 1997 [1]. It finally was the development of the

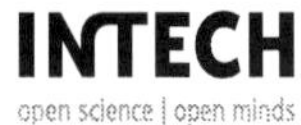

technique of next-generation sequencing (NGS) that lead to the transfer of this research into clinical practice. After the clinical availability and introduction of cell-free DNA analysis for the most common fetal aneuploidies (Trisomy 21, 13, and 18) in 2011, there has been an extremely high demand by pregnant women and to date approximately 1.4 million analyses have been performed worldwide assuming that there will be around 1 million/year in 2015 [2]. Most current tests count DNA fragments, map them to the chromosomes, and quantitatively compare the cell-free-DNA in maternal blood with a euploid reference genome. This new screening tool in prenatal diagnostics has marked the beginning of a new era in prenatal care and has significantly reduced the rate of invasive prenatal procedures such as chorionic villous sampling and amniocentesis.

With the broad availability of non-invasive prenatal genetic testing, a number of new issues have emerged concerning its reasonable clinical application, ethical concerns, integration into current public healthcare plans, counseling issues, and the role of prenatal ultrasound screening. In the following, we will discuss the current and future concepts of prenatal cell-free fetal DNA testing and show the current impact on clinical care among different risk groups taking into account medical, social, and ethical aspects.

2. Fetal cells and cell-free DNA

The idea that genetic information of the fetus can be discovered by investigating maternal blood during pregnancy stems from the historic concept of Georg Schmorl, who described cross-placental trafficking of fetal cells into the maternal circulation. Fetal trophoblast cells were first demonstrated in lung tissue in mothers who died from eclampsia [3]. The isolation of fetal cells has remained a challenge due to their very low quantity [4,5], the limited knowledge on the characteristics and suboptimal markers for identification [6]. The focus has moved to the analysis of fetal cell-free DNA fragments which were first described in 1997 [1]. Cell-free DNA in maternal blood is comprised of extracellular DNA fragments that can be found in the maternal plasma and serum. The majority of cell-free DNA in maternal circulation is of maternal origin and around 10% is of fetal origin. Cell-free fetal DNA is released into the maternal circulation from cells of the placenta. It can be detected very early in pregnancy and is cleared a few hours after birth [7].

Initially, it was only feasible to analyze sequences of paternal origin and de novo mutations that were different from the maternal genome due to the high percentage of maternal cell-free DNA. Therefore, early studies focused on fetal Rhesus-status and on the detection of autosomal-dominant disorders of paternal inheritance [8]. Real-time quantitative PCR technology proved to be suitable for the detection of fetal loci that are different from the maternal genome such as the Y chromosome. Fetal gender determination was applied in families with a high risk for X-chromosome-linked disorders in which only male fetuses are affected from the disease and for the detection of fetal Rhesus D in pregnancies at risk for hemolytic disease of the newborn [9–11]. Just recently, non-invasive prenatal testing for routine fetal Rhesus D genotyping in Rhesus-negative women has been proven to be highly accurate over a 2-year period after its implementation in Denmark and proved to have the ability to direct the use of Anti-D Rhesus prophylaxis in prenatal care [12].

With the technique of next-generation sequencing, it is now possible to also reliably quantify specific DNA sequences and therefore assess sequences that are not only present in the fetus but also present in the maternal genome. This is accomplished by comparing the measured quantity with a reference genome, hence offering the possibility for the widespread analysis for the detection of most common fetal aneuploidies [13].

3. Technical principles of the clinically available Non-Invasive Prenatal Tests (NIPT)

In the following passage, we will focus on the basic principles of the commercially available cell-free DNA test that offers analysis for the three most common aneuploidies today. Basically, there are three different types of approaches of prenatal cell-free DNA testing: whole genome sequencing, targeted genome sequencing, and single-nucleotide polymorphism (SNP)-based sequencing. Another fourth approach, epigenetic testing of fetal DNA methylation, which is not yet clinically available, has shown promising results. It detects fetal-specific epigenetic patterns and unique methylation profiles [14,15].

All techniques use massive parallel genomic sequencing (MPS) or NGS, which refers to the high-throughput DNA sequencing technology that can sequence millions of DNA molecules in parallel [13]. For prenatal testing, both cell-free DNA of maternal and fetal origin present in maternal peripheral blood are sequenced and these fragments are mapped to a reference chromosome. It is important to keep in mind that the majority of sequenced DNA is of maternal origin and that the difference between a normal fetus and fetus with an additional chromosome will only show a slight increase compared to a normal reference chromosome since the aneuploid part forms only about 10% of the sequenced DNA. Quantitative accuracy of the applied method, therefore, is crucial to exclude an aneuploidy. A minimum percentage of fetal DNA is required to reliably perform an analysis and is usually set at a minimum of 4%.

3.1. Whole genome sequencing

For this analysis, the entire cell-free DNA is sequenced in short reads and compared to a reference human genomic database and each sequence is matched to a specific chromosome. The counts observed in the individual probe are then compared to an euploid reference sample. If the fetus carries an additional chromosome (as in trisomy 21, 13, and 18), more fragments are expected for the additional chromosome compared with a normal fetus. However, it is necessary to sequence many millions of DNA fragments ($12\text{--}15 \times 10^6$ mapped sequences) to ensure that there are sufficient chromosome fragments (reads) from the specific chromosome to detect statistically significant differences between aneuploid and euploid fetuses. Also, there are several other aspects of sequencing and the fetal fraction as well as the guanine–cytosine content, etc. that need to be taken into account.

3.2. Targeted sequencing

Targeted sequencing sequences only the regions / chromosome of interest and thus can be more time- and cost-efficient compared to whole genome sequencing. The principle is to selectively amplify the regions from chromosome 21, 13, and 18 followed by NGS. This method is also referred to as digital analysis of selected regions (DANSR). The amount of sequencing for a reliable detection is significantly lower around 40,000 and 1 million mapped sequences / sample. Unique to this type, the analysis uses a fetal fraction optimized risk score (FORTE) and takes into account the a priori risk (maternal age and gestational age) and uses an odds ratio approach to calculate the risk for aneuploidy.

3.3. SNP-based sequencing

This third approach was the most recent method introduced to the variety of clinically available NIPT options. This technique involves targeted amplification and sequencing of single-nucleotide polymorphisms (SNPs). SNPs are single base pairs that occur approximately once / 300 base pairs on the human genome and can be used to distinguish individuals. In addition to the above mentioned applications, maternal and fetal DNA also can be distinguished by SNP analysis. For this analysis, both maternal DNA from white cells from the buffy coat and maternal plasma which includes fetal and maternal DNA are used. In the SNP-technology originally introduced by Zimmermann et al. [16], 19,488 SNPs on the chromosomes 21, 13, 18, X, and Y are analyzed simultaneously. Taking into account the parental genotype, the fetal fraction, and the fetal chromosome copy number, billions of possible genotypes at a specific locus are considered by a complex algorithm and the observed allele distributions are compared to the expected allele distributions. By this method, the most likely fetal genotype can be calculated and a specific risk score for the analyzed aneuploidies is reported [16–19].

4. Evidence on the quality of NIPT from published literature

The initial studies on test quality for the most common aneuploidies were performed in high-risk collectives and focused on the sensitivities and specificities of the different cell-free DNA tests [20–26]. After the rapid clinical application of NIPT including many women at low risk, there was a demand for information on the positive predictive value of each individual test. The positive predictive value then was found to vary widely depending on the investigated cohort and could be as low as 45.4% for trisomy 21 [27], meaning that when a NIPT-test was positive only 45.4% of the fetuses were affected. This underlines the fact that although cell-free DNA testing performs better than the previous screening algorithms for aneuploidy, a positive test result requires confirmation with an invasive procedure such as amniocentesis or chorionic villous sampling.

4.1. Trisomy 21, 13, and 18

The data for the three most common aneuploidies now stem from a number of large-scale studies from mainly high-risk collectives. The detection rate for trisomy 21 ranged from 97.5%

to 100%, with most of the studies showing sensitivities above 99%. For trisomy 18, the outcome is similar ranging from 92.8% to 100%. The sensitivities for trisomy 13 are slightly lower ranging from 78.6% to 100% [18–32]. All of the reported screening methods have significantly lower false positive rates below 1% compared to conventional first trimester screening, which typically is set at a 5% false positive rate.

4.2. Sex chromosome aneuploidies

While reporting of fetal gender is feasible with cell-free DNA testing with high sensitivities of more than 95%, the reporting of sex chromosomal aneuploidies is more challenging. The most common sex chromosomal aneuploidies are 45X0 (Turner syndrome), XXX (Triple X syndrome), XXY (Klinefelter syndrome), and XYY (Jacob syndrome).

While Turner syndrome can be detected on prenatal ultrasound, the others typically do not show sonographic signs but have been detected incidentally if an invasive procedure was performed for another reason. Compared to the most common aneuploidies, the detection rates of sex chromosomal aneuploidies have lower specificities leading to higher false positive rates [23,33]. This is most likely due to the guanine–cytosine content of the X chromosome, which affects the reliability and accuracy of the sequencing data, the small size of the Y chromosome, and the sequence similarity between the X and the Y chromosome. Furthermore, an unknown maternal or fetal mosaicism can interfere with the quantifications of the chromosomal representations. The reported numbers on detected sex chromosome aneuploidies other than Turner syndrome are very low with less than seven cases of each aneuploidy per study [23,34–36] so that reliable data are not present to date. The data on Turner syndrome need to be interpreted with caution since there may be a bias toward the non-viable cases and those detected with sonography. Furthermore, the follow-up data on test negative cases might be incomplete due to the fact that children with Turner syndrome might not show a noticeable phenotype at birth. Also, the rate of tests that do not receive a result due to difficulties with the interpretation of the sequencing data (non-reportables) seems to be higher compared to the autosomal aneuploidies. Taking into account some of these limitations, the detection rate for Turner syndrome ranges between 75% and 92% at a false positive rate of up to 0.3% [23,34–36].

4.3. Triploidy

The presence of a third additional copy of each chromosome is called triploidy. The third copy stems from either the mother (digynic triploidy) or the father (diandric triploidy) and is a challenge for NIPT. Since whole genome sequencing and targeted sequencing rely on the proportions of chromosomes in relation to each other, it is impossible to detect this condition. Only very few cases have been investigated in SNP-based arrays [37] and have shown that the detection of diandric triploidy is feasible but digynic triploidy is difficult, most likely due to the severe growth restriction and a very small placenta which is the typical phenotype associated with this condition that will lead to non-reporting of NIPT due to the low fetal fraction.

4.4. Mosaicism

In mosaic autosomal trisomies, the detection with NIPT is less effective compared to complete fetal trisomies. The major reason is that the representation of the fetal chromosome is only partial. The detection of a fetal mosaicism is dependent on the fetal fraction and on the percentage of abnormal cells in the mosaic. There have been two relevant studies investigating the ability of detecting mosaicisms showing far less sensitive results for mosaic aneuploidies with NGS. Since cell-free "fetal" DNA stems from the trophoblast, a confined placental mosaicism can be a reason for a false positive result. Also, maternal mosaicism can lead to false positive results. On the other hand, mosaicisms can be missed since it is more difficult to detect due to the lower percentage of abnormal cells [38]. However, mosaicism is found in approximately 0.25% of pregnancies in women undergoing amniocentesis and conventional karyotyping [39]. Finally, if NIPT is positive for a trisomy, the distinction of mosaic versus complete trisomy can only be made after karyotyping. This shows the importance of confirmation of the findings detected by NIPT through an invasive procedure as recommended by the professional societies.

4.5. Twins

Most of the approaches using whole genome NGS and targeted NGS offer an analysis for twin pregnancies. The analysis, however, is more complex since maternal blood then carries the cell-free DNA from three individuals. For monozygotic twins that usually carry the same genetic information, the analysis can be made analogue to singletons. In dizygotic twins it is likely that only one fetus is affected from an aneuploidy. NGS relies on a small increase of reads identified for the trisomic chromosome. The total cell-free fetal DNA fraction is larger compared to singleton pregnancies most likely due to a larger placental volume [40] and this would be an advantage for NGS compared to singletons. However, this advantage is reduced by the fact that in most cases only half of the fetal DNA fraction stems from the aneuploid fetus. Furthermore, it is possible that the cell-free-DNA, which is found in the maternal circulation, is not equally released half by half from each of the two fetuses. So the aneuploid fetal fraction could be lower compared to the euploid fetus [41]. To circumvent the mistakes of the total fetal fraction, the lower fetal fraction is used for the risk assessment. A consequence of this policy is that the rate of non-reporting will be higher for twin pregnancies.

The published data from twin pregnancies now count almost one thousand analyzed twin pregnancies [40,42–47]. The SNP-targeted approach does not yet offer twin analysis. The most recent analysis on 515 twin pregnancies showed a test failure rate of 5.6% compared to 1.7% in singletons. The median lower individual fetal fraction was lower than in singletons (8.7% versus 11.7%). Among the 351 pregnancies with complete follow-up and with a test result, there were no false positives among 334 euploid fetuses. All 5 cases of trisomy 18 were detected, but there was 1 false negative case of trisomy 21 among the 12 pregnancies discordant for trisomy 21 [43].

The analysis for twins, however, will not reach a diagnostic level with NGS from maternal blood since it will never be able to tell which one of the fetuses is affected until this information is acquired via separate analysis of each twin through an invasive procedure.

4.6. Factors explaining false positive and false negative results

Even though NIPT is the best available screening test for the detection of the three most common aneuploidies trisomy 21,13, and 18, the method of analyzing cell-free DNA in maternal blood by NGS, false negative, as well as false positive results are possible. To understand the technology, one has to keep in mind two essential things: first, cell-free "fetal" DNA stems from the trophoblast rather than from the fetus itself [7], and second, the cell-free DNA analysis of maternal and fetal cell-free DNA in NIPT uses maternal blood as the DNA source for the analysis. As known from chorionic villous sampling for many years, there is the phenomenon of feto-placental mosaicism in which only the cytotrophoblast but not the fetus is affected by the aneuploid cell line or vice versa [48]. If only the cytotrophoblast is affected, this would lead to a false positive result while a false negative NIPT result is expected if only the fetus but not the trophoblast is affected from the aneuploid cell line.

Another potential cause for a false positive result could stem from cell-free DNA from an unrecognized vanishing twin [42,49]. Fetal aneuploidy is a common reason for early fetal loss and has been described as a reason for a false positive NIPT result [42]. In fact, an additional fetal haplotype was identified in 0.42% of over 30,000 routine NIPT samples from a SNP-based assay [49].

If an abnormal karyotype is present in the mother, this might lead to a false positive result. False positive findings have been reported associated with maternal malignancies [50] or with maternal X-chromosome abnormalities in otherwise healthy women [51]. As mentioned before, the depth of sequencing and a low fetal fraction can be the causes of false negative results due to the counting technology.

5. Integration of NIPT into current prenatal care

Although NIPT has just reached clinical application, the broad use of NIPT in high-risk and low-risk pregnancies is remarkable. Most professional societies have given recommendations to limit the application to women at higher risk [52–54], but the number of studies emerging from low risk and general populations are increasing and models for integration into health care plans are emerging.

A growing number of trials have now shown that NIPT can also be used in women at low risk for aneuploidy [19,27,31,33,55,56]. Although the positive predictive value is assumed to be lower in low-risk patients, test performance is still superior to conventional first trimester screening [27]. With a broad acceptance among specialist societies that a positive NIPT result requires confirmation by invasive testing, there seems to be no reason to withhold NIPT from low-risk women.

Basically, there are two discussed options: one is to use NIPT as a primary screening test that is offered to every pregnant woman and the second is to use NIPT as a secondary (contingent) screening test used only in certain risk groups. This could be either women of increased maternal age or women that screen positive in conventional screening. All discussed options refer to NIPT for trisomy 21,13, and 18 in singleton pregnancies as in traditional first trimester screening. All the other available NIPT options are not considered in a form of general clinical screening at this point.

A primary screening would lead to the highest detection rates of aneuploidies by lowering the false positive rates and also the need for invasive procedures [32]. However, the benefit of the first trimester ultrasound screening apart from aneuploidy detection needs to be remembered carefully since correct pregnancy dating by measuring crown-rump length is crucial for lowering perinatal mortality. Furthermore, the determination of twin chorionicity and an evaluation of maternal adnexae are part of the routine workup in the first trimester. Also, the majority of major fetal malformations that are not necessarily associated with genetic changes can be assessed by ultrasound. Further, primary screening also would be an expensive option by neglecting other benefits of first trimester ultrasound.

Considering contingent screening makes more sense from a healthcare point of view.

Since first trimester screening is widely used in many countries, it would make sense to offer NIPT to a selected population which is screen positive after first trimester screening. Such an approach was modeled with a test positive cut-off of 1:2,500 by first trimester screening and showed an increase of the detection rate of Down Syndrome with a decrease of invasive testing [57] at considerably lower costs compared to first-line screening.

In cases of a positive result, there is consensus among the specialist societies such as the American College of Obstetricians and Gynecologists (ACOG), the Society of Maternal-Fetal Medicine (SMFM), the International Society of Prenatal Diagnosis and the National Society of Genetic counselors that they need to be confirmed with an invasive procedure and fetal karyotyping. This seems especially important when a termination of pregnancy is considered following a positive NIPT result. As discussed previously, this is mandatory due to the occasional false-positive results, especially in low-risk patients.

Switzerland is the first country in Europe to have introduced a national policy on obligatory health care coverage for NIPT for women with singleton pregnancies that have a risk of > 1:1,000 for trisomy 21, 13, or 18 after conventional first trimester screening.

6. Influence of NIPT on diagnostic procedures and changes in prenatal care

With the introduction of clinical available NIPT for the most common aneuploidies, a risk-free additional option of prenatal testing has become available. So far, most pregnant women in the western world had access to a detailed sonographic examination of the fetal anatomy (Figures 1 and 2), correct pregnancy dating based on Crown rump length at 11–14 weeks, and were offered the "combined first trimester test", which is a risk assessment for the trisomy 21, 13, and 18. The first trimester screening combines the statistical background risk of the mother incorporating her age, fetal anatomical markers, nuchal translucency measurements, and biochemical markers in maternal blood (pregnancy associated plasma–protein–A (PAPP-A) and free beta human chorionic gonadotropin (HCG). With this, aneuploidy screening for trisomy 21 can be achieved with a sensitivity of 90% at a false positive rate of 5% [58]. Women at increased risk would usually undergo an invasive procedure such as amniocentesis or chorionic villous sampling for karyotyping. Although this type of screening was better than any previous serum marker tests or using the maternal age-risk alone, it still lead to a large number of invasive tests and only few positive results. Putting mothers through an invasive procedure exposes them to a risk of fetal loss of 0.5–1% [59,60].

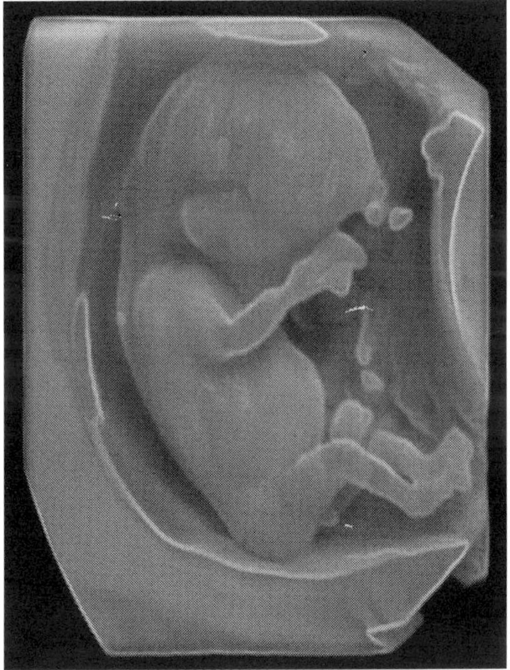

(Archive Dr. G. Manegold-Brauer, University of Basel, Department of Prenatal Medicine and Gynecologic Ultrasound)

Figure 1. 4D-ultrasound image of a fetus in the first trimester

With NIPT a new technology was introduced, which has lead to changes in algorithms previously used to guide patients. Since NIPT only requires a fetal blood sample, patients report that the greatest benefit is the decreased rate of miscarriage as compared to amniocentesis or chorionic villous sampling [61,62].

The medical profession rapidly had to face and solve many challenges on offering and counseling patients about NIPT. It is especially challenging to distinguish scientific information on the different NIPT tests from commercial announcements due to the many different laboratories that offer these tests and the flood of published studies that emerged in only a few years. Adequate counseling has become very complex and should incorporate all the options,

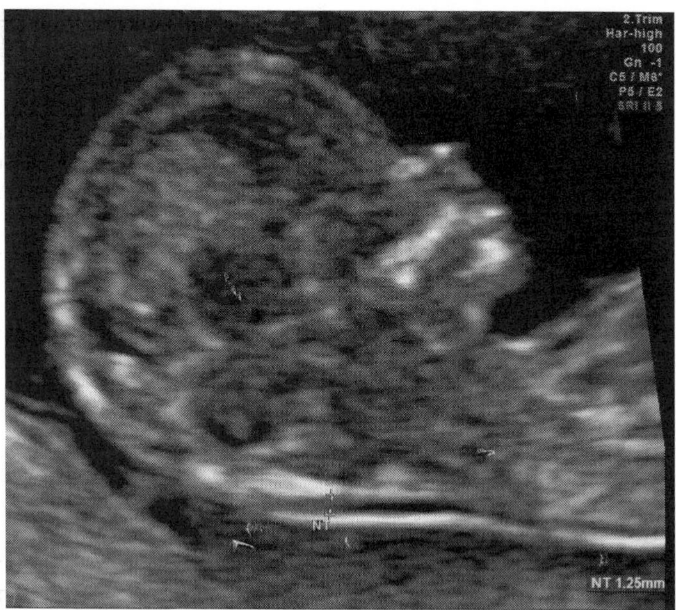

(Archive Dr. G. Manegold-Brauer, University of Basel, Department of Prenatal Medicine and Gynecologic Ultrasound)

Figure 2. 2D-ultrasound image of a fetal profile at 11–14 gestational weeks

limitations, and risks for each type of prenatal testing (ultrasound screening, biochemical screening, invasive procedures, NIPT, conventional karyotyping, and microarray analysis) in a non-directive manner and in the end should allow pregnant women to make an informed decision. For NIPT, it seems important to also counsel on non-reporting due to low fetal fraction in correlation to maternal weight and gestational age and fetal karyotype [63]. Further patients need to be informed on the need for an invasive procedure for confirmation in cases of positive findings.

However, in clinical practice the changes in prenatal care were incorporated differently in different health care systems and were highly dependent on the cohort that was investigated. The high costs associated with NIPT might also have played a role in the uptake in different societies. The introduction of NIPT has lead to an increased rate of prenatal testing in general. Many women that might have relied on first trimester screening in the past would now choose NIPT even if the results of first trimester screening were normal (Table 1). Not surprisingly, the increase of additional testing in the intermediate-risk group was most significant [64,65]. While the total number of invasive testing decreased by 70% in some studies [65], the reduction of invasive procedures was not significant in high-risk cohorts, especially when there is a high percentage of patients that present with anomalies seen on prenatal ultrasound. This management, however, is comprehensible since there is a high risk of chromosomal anomalies other than trisomy 21, 13, and 18 when ultrasound anomalies are present (about one third) that would not necessarily be picked up by NIPT but which can be detected by conventional karyotyping or microarray analysis.

Risk category after first trimester screening		n	No further tests (%)	IPT (%)	NIPT (%)	IPT special indication / termination (%)
Low risk	Group 1	431	95.36	2.09	0	2.55
	Group 2	391	92.58	1.02	5.88	0.51
	p		0.997	0.372	<0.001*	
Intermediate risk	Group 1	37	64.86	35.14	0	0
	Group 2	35	54.29	5.71	40.00	0
	p		0.835	0.018*	<0.001*	
High risk	Group 1	37	40.54	56.75	0	2.71
	Group 2	20	40.00	40.00	15.00	5.00
	p		0.333	0.054	0.103	

Table 1. Differences in prenatal testing according to risk category before and after the introduction of NIPT. Group 1: before the introduction of NIPT, group 2: after the introduction of NIPT (adapted from [63]) IPT: invasive prenatal testing; p: p-value comparison before and after the introduction of NIPT, significant differences are marked with *

	Structural abnormality (n = 69)	NT >95th percentile (n = 38)	Multiple softmarker (n = 43)	Normal scan (n = 32)
IPT	48 (69.6)	21 (55.3)	12 (27.9)	16 (50.0)
NIPT	0 (0.0)	1 (2.6)	3 (7.0)	8 (25.0)
No further tests	21 (30.4)	16 (42.1)	28 (65.1)	8 (25.0)

IPT: invasive prenatal testing; NIPT: non-invasive prenatal testing.

Data shows number (%).

Table 2. Management choices among high-risk patients after the introduction of NIPT. This table shows the presence or absence of sonographic findings (normal scan) in the high-risk group (n = 182) and management choices in the individual subgroups (adapted from [62]).

7. Ethical and social aspects

The introduction of NIPT by the technique of NGS used in prenatal diagnosis has raised some ethical and social concerns. NIPT can theoretically provide information on the entire genome of the mother and the fetus with relative ease. In fact, NIPT has already revealed a small number of occult malignancies [66]. The sequenced DNA, however, could also reveal a BRCA mutation or mutations on genes encoding for neurodegenerative diseases such as Chorea Huntington that would have major consequences for the mother and the unborn child [67]. It becomes obvious that the professional societies and national guidelines need to carefully regulate which data will be analyzed, stored, and reported. Clearly, the mother needs to give written informed consent to each specific analysis that is performed and needs to approve any individuals or institutions that receive this type of information. Although most of today's available NIPT tests directly report to the physician who indicated the test there remains a concern that NIPT could be offered directly to the pregnant woman without a medical request or indication. It seems of highest importance that the expectant mother is appropriately counseled by a trained health care professional who can offer and discuss all implications for testing, provide for and interpret all options, discuss prognosis and can assist with the management of the pregnancy and the subsequent prenatal care [68,69]. An important further aspect is that adequate educational material is offered to health care professionals and to the public, as it will assist in avoiding misunderstandings about the technology and possible misuse, thereby ease public anxieties [70].

8. Conclusion

With the technology of NGS, prenatal care has reached a new era. It has changed prenatal algorithms and has led to a reduction of invasive procedures which was one of the main goals of this technology [65,71]. At present, the main domain of NIPT is the detection of the three most common aneuploidies trisomy 21, 13, and 18, in singletons. However, further aneuploidies like sex chromosomal aneuploidies and some microdeletions are offered today in a clinical setting and research is aiming on sequencing the whole genome by a non-invasive approach with the ultimate dream of thereby opening an early "window of opportunity" for fetal therapy.

Acknowledgements

The authors thank Dr. Dr. Hans Ulrich Brauer for critical review of the manuscript.

Author details

Gwendolin Manegold-Brauer* and Olav Lapaire

*Address all correspondence to: gwendolin.manegold-brauer@usb.ch

University of Basel, Department of Prenatal Medicine and Gynecologic Ultrasound, Switzerland

References

[1] Lo YM, Corbetta N, Chamberlain PF, Rai V, Sargent IL, Redman CW, et al. Presence of fetal DNA in maternal plasma and serum. Lancet 1997;350:485–87.

[2] Bianchi DW. Pregnancy: prepare for unexpected prenatal test results. Nature 2015 Jun 4;522:29–30.

[3] Lapaire O, Holzgreve W, Oosterwijk JC, Brinkhaus R, Bianchi DW. Georg Schmorl on trophoblasts in the maternal circulation. Placenta 2007 Jan;28:1–5.

[4] Bianchi DW, Simpson JL, Jackson LG, Elias S, Holzgreve W, Evans MI, et al. Fetal gender and aneuploidy detection using fetal cells in maternal blood: analysis of NIF-TY I data. National Institute of Child Health and Development Fetal Cell Isolation Study. Prenat Diagn 2002 Jul;22:609–15.

[5] Hahn S, Jackson LG, Kolla V, Mahyuddin AP, Choolani M. Noninvasive prenatal diagnosis of fetal aneuploidies and Mendelian disorders: new innovative strategies. Expert Rev Mol Diagn 2009 Sep;9:613–21.

[6] Hatt L, Brinch M, Singh R, Møller K, Lauridsen RH, Uldbjerg N, et al. Characterization of fetal cells from the maternal circulation by microarray gene expression analysis–could the extravillous trophoblasts be a target for future cell-based non-invasive prenatal diagnosis? Fetal Diagn Ther 2014 Jan;35:218–27.

[7] Lo YM, Zhang J, Leung TN, Lau TK, Chang AM, Hjelm NM. Rapid clearance of fetal DNA from maternal plasma. Am J Hum Genet 1999 Jan;64:218–24.

[8] Daley R, Hill M, Chitty LS. Non-invasive prenatal diagnosis: progress and potential. Arch Dis Child Fetal Neonatal Ed 2014 Sep;99:F426–30.

[9] Zimmermann B, El-Sheikhah A, Nicolaides K, Holzgreve W, Hahn S. Optimized real-time quantitative PCR measurement of male fetal DNA in maternal plasma. Clin Chem 2005 Sep;51:1598–604.

[10] Lo YM, Tein MS, Lau TK, Haines CJ, Leung TN, Poon PM, et al. Quantitative analysis of fetal DNA in maternal plasma and serum: implications for noninvasive prenatal diagnosis. Am J Hum Genet 1998 Apr;62:768–75.

[11] Van der Schoot CE, Hahn S, Chitty LS. Non-invasive prenatal diagnosis and determination of fetal Rh status. Semin Fetal Neonatal Med 2008 Apr;13:63–8.

[12] Banch Clausen F, Steffensen R, Christiansen M, Rudby M, Jakobsen MA, Jakobsen TR, et al. Routine noninvasive prenatal screening for fetal RHD in plasma of RhD-negative pregnant women-2 years of screening experience from Denmark. Prenat Diagn 2014 Oct;34:1000–5.

[13] Manegold-Brauer G, Lapaire O, Hoesli IH. Pränatale Diagnostik-Molekularbiologische Methoden; in : Die Geburtshilfe. 2015, pp. 1–21.

[14] Lim JH, Kim SY, Park SY, Lee SY, Kim MJ, Han YJ, et al. Non-invasive epigenetic detection of fetal trisomy 21 in first trimester maternal plasma. PLoS One 2011 Nov 23;6:e27709.

[15] Lim JH, Lee DE, Park SY, Kim DJ, Ahn HK, Han YJ, et al. Disease specific characteristics of fetal epigenetic markers for non-invasive prenatal testing of trisomy 21. BMC Med Genomics 2014 Jan;7:1.

[16] Zimmermann B, Hill M, Gemelos G, Demko Z, Banjevic M, Baner J, et al. Noninvasive prenatal aneuploidy testing of chromosomes 13, 18, 21, X, and Y, using targeted sequencing of polymorphic loci. Prenat Diagn 2012 Dec;32:1233–41.

[17] Samango-Sprouse C, Banjevic M, Ryan A, Sigurjonsson S, Zimmermann B, Hill M, et al. SNP-based non-invasive prenatal testing detects sex chromosome aneuploidies with high accuracy. Prenat Diagn 2013 Jul;33:643–9.

[18] Nicolaides KH, Syngelaki A, Gil M, Atanasova V, Markova D. Validation of targeted sequencing of single-nucleotide polymorphisms for non-invasive prenatal detection of aneuploidy of chromosomes 13, 18, 21, X, and Y. Prenat Diagn 2013 Jun;33:575–9.

[19] Pergament E, Cuckle H, Zimmermann B, Banjevic M, Sigurjonsson S, Ryan A, et al. Single-nucleotide polymorphism-based noninvasive prenatal screening in a high-risk and low-risk cohort. Obstet Gynecol 2014 Aug;124:210–8.

[20] Ehrich M, Deciu C, Zwiefelhofer T, Tynan JA, Cagasan L, Tim R, et al. Noninvasive detection of fetal trisomy 21 by sequencing of DNA in maternal blood: a study in a clinical setting. Am J Obstet Gynecol 2011;204:205.e1–e11.

[21] Chiu R, Akolekar R, Zheng YWL, Leung T, Sun H, Chan K, et al. Non-invasive prenatal assessment of trisomy 21 by multiplexed maternal plasma DNA sequencing: large scale validity study. BMJ 2011;c7401.

[22] Palomaki GE, Kloza EM, Lambert-Messerlian GM, Haddow JE, Neveux LM, Ehrich M, et al. DNA sequencing of maternal plasma to detect Down syndrome: an international clinical validation study. Genet Med Off J Am Coll Med Genet 2011;13:913–920.

[23] Bianchi DW, Platt LD, Goldberg JD, Abuhamad AZ, Sehnert AJ, Rava RP. Genome-wide fetal aneuploidy detection by maternal plasma DNA sequencing. Obstet Gynecol 2012;119:1–13.

[24] Sparks AB, Struble CA, Wang ET, Song K, Oliphant A. Non-invasive prenatal detection and selective analysis of cell-free DNA obtained from maternal blood: evaluation for trisomy 21 and trisomy 18. Am J Obstet Gynecol 2012;206:322.e1–5.

[25] Ashoor G, Syngelaki A, Wagner M, Birdir C, Nicolaides KH. Chromosome-selective sequencing of maternal plasma cell-free DNA for first-trimester detection of trisomy 21 and trisomy 18. Am J Obstet Gynecol 2012 Apr;206:322.e1–5.

[26] Norton ME, Brar H, Weiss J, Karimi A, Laurent LC, Caughey AB, et al. Non-invasive chromosomal evaluation (NICE) study: results of a multicenter prospective cohort study for detection of fetal trisomy 21 and trisomy 18. Am J Obstet Gynecol 2012 Aug;207:137.e1–8.

[27] Bianchi DW, Parker RL, Wentworth J, Madankumar R, Saffer C, Das AF, et al. DNA sequencing versus standard prenatal aneuploidy screening. N Engl J Med 2014 Feb 27;370:799–808.

[28] Liang D, Lv W, Wang H, Xu L, Liu J, Li H, et al. Non-invasive prenatal testing of fetal whole chromosome aneuploidy by massively parallel sequencing. Prenat Diagn 2013 May;33:409–15.

[29] Song Y, Liu C, Qi H, Zhang Y, Bian X, Liu J. Noninvasive prenatal testing of fetal aneuploidies by massively parallel sequencing in a prospective Chinese population. Prenat Diagn 2013;33:700–706.

[30] Stumm M, Entezami M, Haug K, Blank C, Wüstemann M, Schulze B, et al. Diagnostic accuracy of random massively parallel sequencing for non-invasive prenatal detection of common autosomal aneuploidies: a collaborative study in Europe. Prenat Diagn 2014 Feb;34:185–91.

[31] Fairbrother G, Johnson S, Musci TJ, Song K. Clinical experience of noninvasive prenatal testing with cell-free DNA for fetal trisomies 21, 18, and 13, in a general screening population. Prenat Diagn 2013 Jun;33:580–3.

[32] Gil MM, Quezada MS, Bregant B, Ferraro M, Nicolaides KH. Implementation of maternal blood cell-free DNA testing in early screening for aneuploidies. Ultrasound Obstet Gynecol 2013 Jul;42:34–40.

[33] Song Y, Liu C, Qi H, Zhang Y, Bian X, Liu J. Noninvasive prenatal testing of fetal aneuploidies by massively parallel sequencing in a prospective Chinese population. Prenat Diagn 2013 Jul;33:700–6.

[34] Mazloom AR, Džakula Ž, Oeth P, Wang H, Jensen T, Tynan J, et al. Noninvasive prenatal detection of sex chromosomal aneuploidies by sequencing circulating cell-free DNA from maternal plasma. Prenat Diagn 2013 Jun;33:591–7.

[35] Nicolaides KH, Musci TJ, Struble CA, Syngelaki A, Gil MM. Assessment of fetal sex chromosome aneuploidy using directed cell-free DNA analysis. Fetal Diagn Ther 2014 Jan;35:1–6.

[36] Hooks J, Wolfberg AJ, Wang ET, Struble CA, Zahn J, Juneau K, et al. Non-invasive risk assessment of fetal sex chromosome aneuploidy through directed analysis and incorporation of fetal fraction. Prenat Diagn 2014 May;34:496–9.

[37] Nicolaides KH, Syngelaki A, Gil MDM, Quezada MS, Zinevich Y. Prenatal detection of fetal triploidy from cell-free DNA testing in maternal blood. Fetal Diagn Ther 2013 Oct 10; DOI: 10.1159/000355655

[38] Benn P, Cuckle H, Pergament E. Non-invasive prenatal testing for aneuploidy: current status and future prospects. Ultrasound Obstet Gynecol 2013 Jul;42:15–33.

[39] Wapner RJ, Martin CL, Levy B, Ballif BC, Eng CM, Zachary JM, et al. Chromosomal microarray versus karyotyping for prenatal diagnosis. N Engl J Med 2012 Dec 6;367:2175–84.

[40] Canick JA, Palomaki GE, Kloza EM, Lambert-Messerlian GM, Haddow JE. The impact of maternal plasma DNA fetal fraction on next generation sequencing tests for common fetal aneuploidies. Prenat Diagn 2013 Jul;33:667–74.

[41] Struble CA, Syngelaki A, Oliphant A, Song K, Nicolaides KH. Fetal fraction estimate in twin pregnancies using directed cell-free DNA analysis. Fetal Diagn Ther 2014 Jan; 35:199–203.

[42] Grömminger S, Yagmur E, Erkan S, Nagy S, Schöck U, Bonnet J, et al. Fetal aneuploidy detection by cell-free DNA sequencing for multiple pregnancies and quality issues with vanishing twins. J Clin Med 2014 Jun 25;3:679–692.

[43] Bevilacqua E, Gil MM, Nicolaides KH, Ordoñez E, Cirigliano V, Dierickx H, et al. Performance of screening for aneuploidies by cell-free DNA analysis of maternal blood in twin pregnancies. Ultrasound Obstet Gynecol 2015 Jan;45:61–6.

[44] Del Mar Gil M, Quezada MS, Bregant B, Syngelaki A, Nicolaides KH. Cell-free DNA analysis for trisomy risk assessment in first-trimester twin pregnancies. Fetal Diagn Ther 2014 Jan;35:204–11.

[45] Huang X, Zheng J, Chen M, Zhao Y, Zhang C, Liu L, et al. Noninvasive prenatal testing of trisomies 21 and 18 by massively parallel sequencing of maternal plasma DNA in twin pregnancies. Prenat Diagn 2014 Apr;34:335–40.

[46] Leung TY, Qu JZZ, Liao GJW, Jiang P, Cheng YKY, Chan KCA, et al. Noninvasive twin zygosity assessment and aneuploidy detection by maternal plasma DNA sequencing. Prenat Diagn 2013;33:675–681.

[47] Lau TK, Jiang F, Chan MK, Zhang H, Lo PSS, Wang W. Non-invasive prenatal screening of fetal Down syndrome by maternal plasma DNA sequencing in twin pregnancies. J Matern Fetal Neonatal Med 2013 Mar;26:434–7.

[48] Grati FR, Malvestiti F, Ferreira JCPB, Bajaj K, Gaetani E, Agrati C, et al. Fetoplacental mosaicism: potential implications for false-positive and false-negative noninvasive prenatal screening results. Genet Med 2014 Aug;16:620–4.

[49] Curnow KJ, Wilkins-Haug L, Ryan A, Kırkızlar E, Stosic M, Hall MP, et al. Detection of triploid, molar, and vanishing twin pregnancies by a single-nucleotide polymorphism-based noninvasive prenatal test. Am J Obstet Gynecol 2015 Jan;212:79.e1–9.

[50] Osborne CM, Hardisty E, Devers P, Kaiser-Rogers K, Hayden MA, Goodnight W, et al. Discordant noninvasive prenatal testing results in a patient subsequently diagnosed with metastatic disease. Prenat Diagn 2013 Jun;33:609–11.

[51] Wang Y, Chen Y, Tian F, Zhang J, Song Z, Wu Y, et al. Maternal mosaicism is a significant contributor to discordant sex chromosomal aneuploidies associated with noninvasive prenatal testing. Clin Chem 2014 Jan;60:251–9.

[52] Benn P, Borell A, Chiu R, Cuckle H, Dugoff L, Faas B, et al. Position statement from the Aneuploidy Screening Committee on behalf of the Board of the International Society for Prenatal Diagnosis. Prenat Diagn 2013 Jul;33:622–9.

[53] Devers P, Cronister A, Ormond K, Facio F, Brasington C, Flodman P. Noninvasive prenatal testing/noninvasive prenatal diagnosis:the position of the national society of genetic counselors. J Genet Couns 2013;22:291–295.

[54] Committee Opinion No. 545. Noninvasive prenatal testing for fetal aneuploidy. Obstet Gynecol 2012 Dec;120:1532–4.

[55] Dan S, Wang W, Ren J, Li Y, Hu H, Xu Z, et al. Clinical application of massively parallel sequencing-based prenatal noninvasive fetal trisomy test for trisomies 21 and 18 in 11,105 pregnancies with mixed risk factors. Prenat Diagn 2012 Dec;32:1225–32.

[56] Nicolaides KH, Syngelaki A, Ashoor G, Birdir C, Touzet G. Noninvasive prenatal testing for fetal trisomies in a routinely screened first-trimester population. Am J Obstet Gynecol 2012;207:374.e1–6.

[57] Nicolaides KH, Wright D, Poon LC, Syngelaki A, Gil MM. First-trimester contingent screening for trisomy 21 by biomarkers and maternal blood cell-free DNA testing. Ultrasound Obstet Gynecol 2013 Jul;42:41–50.

[58] Kagan KO, Wright D, Valencia C, Maiz N, Nicolaides KH. Screening for trisomies 21, 18 and 13 by maternal age, fetal nuchal translucency, fetal heart rate, free beta-hCG and pregnancy-associated plasma protein-A. Hum Reprod Oxford Engl 2008;23:1968–1975.

[59] Kollmann M, Haeusler M, Haas J, Csapo B, Lang U, Klaritsch P. Procedure-related complications after genetic amniocentesis and chorionic villus sampling. Ultraschall der Medizin 2013 Aug;34:345–8.

[60] Tabor A, Alfirevic Z. Update on procedure-related risks for prenatal diagnosis techniques. Fetal Diagn Ther 2010 Jan;27:1–7.

[61] Tischler R, Hudgins L, Blumenfeld YJ, Greely HT, Ormond KE. Noninvasive prenatal diagnosis: pregnant women's interest and expected uptake. Prenat Diagn 2011 Dec; 31:1292–9.

[62] Yi H, Hallowell N, Griffiths S, Yeung Leung T. Motivations for undertaking DNA sequencing-based non-invasive prenatal testing for fetal aneuploidy: a qualitative study with early adopter patients in Hong Kong. PLoS One 2013 Jan;8:e81794.

[63] Bianchi DW, Wilkins-Haug L. Integration of noninvasive DNA testing for aneuploidy into prenatal care: what has happened since the rubber met the road? Clin Chem 2013 Nov 19; DOI: 10.1373/clinchem.2013.202663

[64] Manegold-Brauer G, Berg C, Flöck A, Rüland A, Gembruch U, Geipel A. Uptake of non-invasive prenatal testing (NIPT) and impact on invasive procedures in a tertiary referral center. Arch Gynecol Obstet 2015 Feb 26; DOI: 10.1007/s00404-015-3674-5

[65] Manegold-Brauer G, Kang Bellin A, Hahn S, De Geyter C, Buechel J, Hoesli I, et al. A new era in prenatal care: non-invasive prenatal testing (NIPT) in Switzerland. Swiss Med Wkly 2013;143:w13915.

[66] Bianchi DW, Chudova D, Sehnert AJ, Bhatt S, Murray K, Prosen TL, et al. Noninvasive prenatal testing and incidental detection of occult maternal malignancies. JAMA 2015 Jul 13;314:162–9.

[67] Hahn S, Hoesli I, Lapaire O. Non-invasive prenatal diagnostics using next generation sequencing: technical, legal and social challenges. Expert Opin Med Diagn 2012;6:517–528.

[68] Skirton H, Goldsmith L, Jackson L, Lewis C, Chitty L. Offering prenatal diagnostic tests: European guidelines for clinical practice guidelines. Eur J Hum Genet 2013 Sep 11; DOI: 10.1038/ejhg.2013.205

[69] Sachs A, Blanchard L, Buchanan A, Bianchi DW. Recommended pre-test counseling points for noninvasive prenatal testing using cell-free DNA: a 2015 perspective. Prenat Diagn 2015 Aug 5; DOI: 10.1002/pd.4666

[70] Kelly SE, Farrimond HR. Non-invasive prenatal genetic testing: a study of public attitudes. Public Health Genomics 2012 Jan;15:73–81.

[71] Warsof SL, Larion S, Abuhamad AZ. Overview of the impact of noninvasive prenatal testing on diagnostic procedures. Prenat Diagn 2015 Apr 14; DOI: 10.1002/pd.4601

Chapter 16

Impact of Gene Annotation on RNA-seq Data Analysis

Shanrong Zhao and Baohong Zhang

Additional information is available at the end of the chapter

http://dx.doi.org/10.5772/61197

Abstract

RNA-seq has become increasingly popular in transcriptome profiling. One of the major challenges in RNA-seq data analysis is the accurate mapping of junction reads to their genomic origins. To detect splicing sites in short reads, many RNA-seq aligners use reference transcriptome to inform placement of junction reads. However, no systematic evaluation has been performed to assess or quantify the benefits of incorporating reference transcriptome in mapping RNA-seq reads. Meanwhile, there exist multiple human genome annotation databases, including RefGene (RefSeq Gene), Ensembl, and the UCSC annotation database. The impact of the choice of an annotation on estimating gene expression remains insufficiently investigated.

In this chapter, we systematically characterized the impact of genome annotation choice on read mapping and gene quantification by analyzing a RNA-seq dataset generated by Illumina's Human Body Map 2.0 Project. The impact of a gene model on mapping of non-junction reads is different from junction reads. We demonstrated that the choice of a gene model has a dramatic effect on both gene quantification and differential analysis. Our research will help RNA-seq data analysts to make an informed choice of gene model in practical RNA-seq data analysis.

Keywords: RNA-seq, gene quantification, gene model, RefSeq, UCSC, Ensembl

1. Introduction

In recent years, RNA-seq has become a powerful approach for transcriptome profiling [1–3]. RNA-seq not only has considerable advantages for examining transcriptome fine structure—

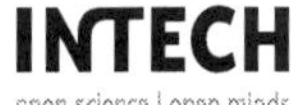

for example, in the detection of novel transcripts, allele-specific expression, and alternative splicing—but also provides a far more precise measurement of levels of transcripts than that of other methods such as microarray [4–7]. Previously, we had performed a side by side comparison of RNA-seq and microarray in investigating T cell activation, and demonstrated that RNA-seq is superior in detecting low abundance transcripts, differentiating biologically critical isoforms, and allowing the identification of genetic variants [7]. In addition, RNA-seq has a much broader dynamic range than microarray, which allows for the detection of more differentially expressed genes with higher fold-change. Furthermore, RNA-seq avoids technical issues in microarray related to probe performance such as cross-hybridization, limited detection range of individual probes, and nonspecific hybridization [5–7]. Thus, RNA-seq delivers unbiased and unparalleled information about the transcriptome and gene expression. By RNA-seq technology, the Genotype-Tissue Expression (GTEx) project generated large amount of RNA sequence data to investigate the patterns of transcriptome variation across individuals and tissues [8–9]. An analysis of RNA sequencing data in the GTEx project from 1,641 samples across 43 tissues from 175 individuals revealed the landscape of gene expression across tissues, and catalogued thousands of tissue-specific expressed genes. These findings provide a systematic understanding of the heterogeneity among a diverse set of human tissues.

Current RNA-seq approaches use shotgun sequencing technologies such as Illumina, in which millions or even billions of short reads are generated from a randomly fragmented cDNA library. The first step and a major challenge in RNA-seq data analysis is the accurate mapping of sequencing reads to their genomic origins including the identification of splicing events. Despite of the fact that a large number of mapping algorithms have been developed for read mapping [10–13] and RNA-seq differential analysis [14–15] in recent years, however, accurate alignment of RNA-seq reads is a challenging and yet unsolved problem because of exon-exon spanning junction reads, relatively short read lengths and the ambiguity of multiple-mapping reads. Nowadays, many RNA-seq alignment tools, including GSNAP [16], OSA [17], STAR [18], MapSplice [19], and TopHat [20], use reference transcriptomes to inform the alignments of junction reads. In fact, this has become a common practice in RNA-seq data analysis. However, no systematic evaluation has been performed to assess and/or quantify the benefits of incorporating reference transcriptome in mapping RNA-seq reads.

The second aspect of transcriptome research is to quantify expression levels of genes, transcripts, and exons. Acquiring the transcriptome expression profile requires genomic elements to be defined in the context of the genome. Gene models are hypotheses about the structure of transcripts produced by a gene. Like all models, they may be correct, partly correct, or entirely wrong. In addition to RefGene [21], there are several other public human genome annotations, including UCSC Known Genes [22], Ensembl [23], AceView [24], Vega [25], and GENCODE [26]. Characteristics of these annotations differ because of variations in annotation strategies and information sources. RefSeq human gene models are well supported and broadly used in various studies. The UCSC Known Genes dataset is based on protein data from Swiss-Prot/ TrEMBL (UniProt) and the associated mRNA data from GenBank, and serves as a foundation for the UCSC Genome Browser. Vega genes are manually curated transcripts produced by the

HAVANA group at the Welcome Trust Sanger Institute, and are merged into Ensembl. Ensembl genes contain both automated genome annotation and manual curation, while the gene set of GENCODE corresponds to Ensembl annotation since GENCODE version 3c (equivalent to Ensembl 56). AceView provides a comprehensive non-redundant curated representation of all available human cDNA sequences.

Although there are multiple genome annotations available, researchers need to choose a genome annotation (or gene model) while performing RNA-seq data analysis. However, the effect of genome annotation choice on downstream RNA-seq expression estimates is under-appreciated. Wu et al. [27] demonstrated that the selection of human genome annotation results in different gene expression estimates. Chen et al. [28] systematically compared the human annotations present in RefSeq, Ensembl, and AceView on diverse transcriptomic and genetic analyses. They found that the human gene annotations in the three databases are far from complete, although Ensembl and AceView annotate many more genes than RefSeq. In this paper, we performed a more comprehensive evaluation of different annotations on RNA-seq read mapping and gene quantification, including RefGene, UCSC, and Ensembl, and reported the main findings. More comprehensive reports were presented elsewhere [29–30].

2. Method

The Human Body Map 2.0 Project, using Illumina sequencing, generated RNA-seq data for 16 different human tissues (adipose, adrenal, brain, breast, colon, heart, kidney, leukocyte, liver, lung, lymph node, ovary, prostate, skeletal muscle, testis, and thyroid) and is accessible from ArrayExpress (accession number E-MTAB-513). We chose to analyze this public dataset because gene expression is tissue specific [9] and analyzing those 16 high-quality RNA-seq samples as a whole could result in less biased conclusions. The read length is 75 bp in all 16 samples, and there are 70 to 80 million reads for each sample (Supplementary Table 1 in [30]). To demonstrate the impact of read length on analysis results, we created a new dataset in which each original 75-bp long sequence read was trimmed to 50 bp. The same analysis protocol described below was applied to both datasets. In this chapter, we mainly presented the results for the read length of 75 bp, and for 50 bp reads, the detail reports could be found in [29–30]. We used the total number of reads mapped to each individual gene to represent expression level. For a given tissue sample, we analyzed the same RNA-seq dataset using the same aligner but with different gene models. The raw reads mapped to each gene across gene models can be compared directly.

The RefGene, Ensembl, and UCSC annotation files in GTF format were downloaded from the UCSC genome browser. Primary sequencing reads were first mapped to the reference transcriptome and the human reference genome GRCH37.3 using Omicsoft Sequence Aligner (OSA) [17]. Benchmarked with existing methods such as TopHat and others, OSA improves mapping speed 4–10 fold, with better sensitivity and fewer false positives.

As shown in Figure 1A, the mapping result of a sequence read is gene model dependent. For instance, read #2 can be uniquely mapped to gene #b if the gene model #A is chosen in the mapping step. However, this read became a multiple-mapped read when either gene model #B or #C is used instead, because it can be mapped to genes #b and #e equally well. For a junction read with short overlap with an exon, it can be aligned to genome with the help of a reference transcriptome. Otherwise, it might fail to map to a genomic loci without the usage of a gene model when mapping reads.

Note that none of the gene annotation is 100% complete. As a result, for those RNA-seq reads not covered by a gene annotation, whether to use the gene model in the mapping step has no impact on their mappings. Therefore, to fairly assess the impact of a gene model on RNA-seq read mapping, only those reads covered by a gene model were used. In this study, we devised a two-stage mapping protocol (Figure 1B) for our evaluation. In Stage #1, all RNA-seq reads were mapped to a reference transcriptome only, and then only mapped reads are saved into a new FASTQ file. In Stage #2, all remaining reads were re-mapped to the reference genome with and without the use of a gene model, respectively. The role of a gene model in the mapping step was then quantified and characterized by comparing the mapping results in Stage #2. The two-stage mapping protocol is crucial for a fair evaluation. Otherwise, the impact of a gene annotation on RNA-seq data analysis will be diluted or underestimated.

The effect of a gene model on RNA-seq read mapping could be characterized and quantified by comparing the read mapping results in different mapping modes. We focused on those uniquely mapped reads with a gene annotation and divided them into four categories (Figure 1C) with respect to their mapping results without a gene annotation in the mapping step: (1) "Identical", the same alignment results were obtained regardless of the use of a gene model; (2) "Alternative", the read was still mapped but mapped differently. It turns out that the majority of reads in this category were junction reads. A junction read could be either mapped as a non-junction read, or remain mapped as a junction read but with different start, end, and splicing positions; (3) "Multiple", a uniquely mapped read became a multiple-mapped one. When a read is mapped across the whole reference genome, it is more likely to be mapped to multiple locations; and (4) "Unmapped", i.e., a read could not be mapped to anywhere in the genome without the assistance of a gene model. Nearly all reads in this category were junction reads.

The impact of a reference transcriptome on read mapping is dependent upon whether a sequence is a junction read and how much it overlaps with an exon. Therefore, we split all mapped reads into junction and non-junction ones based upon the CIGAR string in the SAM files. Then we compared the mapping difference with and without a reference transcriptome in the mapping step, and summarized the difference in each category shown in Figure 1C. Additional analysis was performed on "Alternative" and "Unmapped" junction reads to characterize the splicing patterns in terms of their overlaps with exons.

3. Results

3.1. The coverage of different gene annotations

The RNA-seq read mapping summaries for all 16 samples are shown in Figure 2. There are two different mapping modes. In the "transcriptome only" mapping mode, all RNA-seq reads

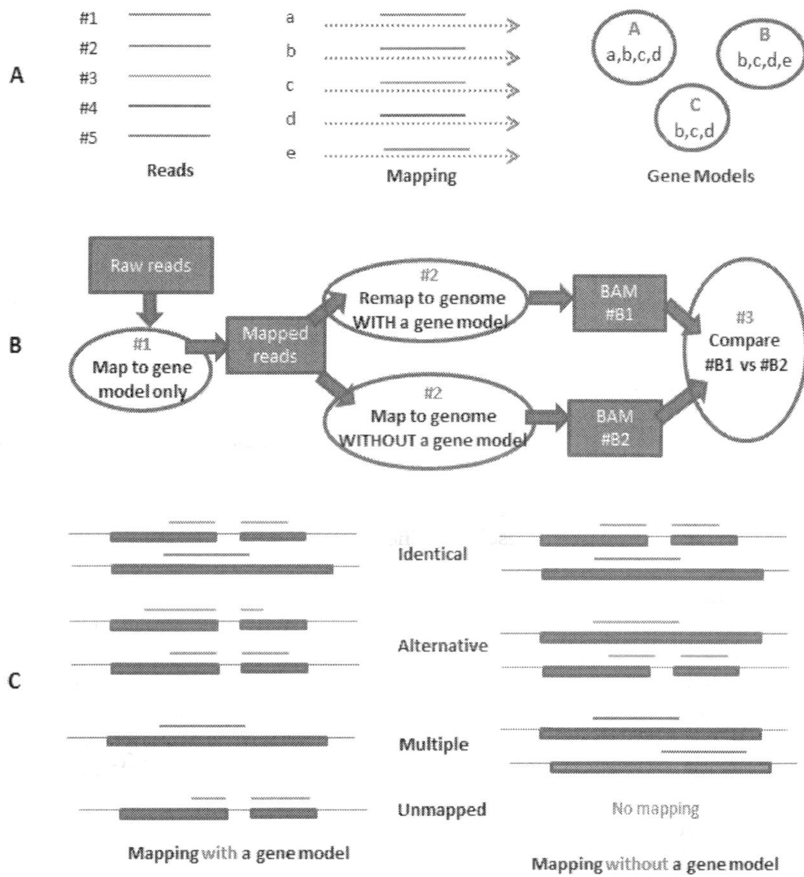

Figure 1. Analysis protocol. (A) The mapping result for a sequence read is gene model dependent; (B) "two-stage" mapping protocol: at Stage #1, all RNA-Seq reads are mapped to a reference transcriptome; at Stage #2, the mapped reads at Stage #1 are re-mapped to the genome with and without the use of a gene model, respectively; (C) the protocol for classifying uniquely mapped sequence reads into four categories, i.e., "Identical", "Alternative", "Multiple" and "Unmapped" (or Fail).

were mapped to a reference transcriptome only. If a read could not be mapped to a known gene region, it became unmapped, even though it could potentially be aligned to a genomic region without annotations. While in the "transcriptome + genome" mapping mode, reads were first mapped to a reference transcriptome, and then the unmapped ones were mapped to the reference genome. The impact of a reference transcriptome on the mapping of RNA-seq reads is attenuated in the "transcriptome + genome" mapping mode because every unmapped read has a second chance to be mapped to a genome.

In the "transcriptome only" mapping mode, more reads were mapped in Ensembl than in RefGene and/or UCSC. For each tissue type, the mapping rate was similar between RefGene and UCSC. The average read mapping rates across all 16 samples were 86%, 69%, and 70% for Ensembl, RefGene, and UCSC annotations, respectively. Short-read mapping is a basic step in RNA-seq data analyses, and to a certain extent, the percentage of reads mapped to a given transcriptome can roughly reflect the completeness or coverage of its annotated genes and transcripts. Thus, Ensembl annotation has much broader gene coverage than RefGene and UCSC. The patterns in "transcriptome + genome" mapping mode was different from those in "transcriptome only" mode (left panel on Figure 2). In the "transcriptome + genome" mapping mode, the average mapping rates for Ensembl, RefGene, and UCSC increased to 96.7%, 94.5%, and 94.6%, respectively, and the mapping rate difference among different gene models decreased. This large difference in the mapping rates between the two modes suggests the incompleteness of gene models: there are many reads that were mapped to the genomic regions without annotations.

Figure 2 shows that the read mapping percentage is also sample dependent, and this holds true for every gene model. For instance, only 52.5% of sequence reads in the heart were mapped to the RefGene model; while in leukocytes, 84.2% of reads could be mapped to RefGene. This mapping difference between heart and leukocyte results from, at least in part, the incompleteness of the RefGene annotation. As more expressed genes are annotated in a gene model, a higher percentage of reads will be mapped in the "transcriptome only" mapping mode.

In the "transcriptome only" mapping mode (the right panel in Figure 2), an average of 6.9%, 1.4%, and 1.8% of reads were multiple-mapped reads in Ensembl, RefGene, and UCSC gene models, respectively. The percentage of multiple-mapped reads in Ensembl is higher than in RefGene or UCSC. Usually, a more comprehensive annotation generally annotates more genes and isoforms, and thus, increases the possibility of ambiguous mappings. These ambiguous mappings directly translate to an increase in the percentage of non-uniquely mapped reads.

Different gene identifiers are used in different annotation databases; therefore, we mapped those database-specific identifiers into the unique HGNC gene symbols from the HUGO Gene Nomenclature Committee when comparing their gene quantification results across the different gene models originating from these databases. Considering that annotations are more or less incomplete in these databases, we only focused on common genes when comparing the results from different annotations. The Venn diagram in Figure 3 showed the overlap and intersection of RefGene, UCSC, and Ensembl annotations. Clearly RefGene has fewest unique genes, while more that 50% of genes in Ensembl are unique. In general, the different annotations have very high overlaps: 21,598 common genes are shared by all three gene annotations.

3.2. The impact of a gene model on RNA-seq read mapping

To evaluate the impact of a gene model on read mapping, the mapping summaries in Figure 2 were not sufficient. For instance, a read could be aligned differently with and without the assistance of a gene model in mapping, and in this scenario, the mapping summary could not tell such a difference. Thus, we compared the mapping details for every read, including start and end positions and splicing sites. For simplicity, in Stage #2, we focused on only uniquely

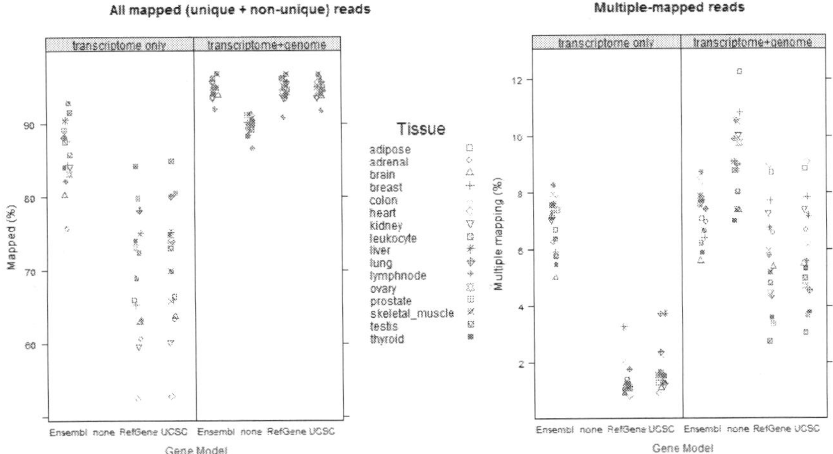

Figure 2. The read mapping summary for 16 tissue samples in the "transcriptome only" and "transcriptome+genome" mapping modes (note: read length = 75 bp). In the "transcriptome only" mode, more reads are mapped in Ensembl than in RefGene and UCSC (left panel), and more reads become multiple-mapped in Ensembl than in RefGene and UCSC (right panel). Note: the gene model "none" means the RNA-Seq reads are mapped to the reference genome directly without the use of a gene model.

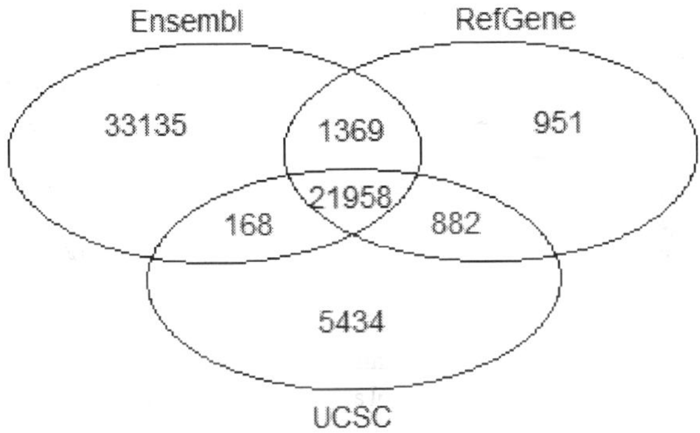

Figure 3. The overlap and intersection among RefGene, UCSC, and Ensembl annotations.

mapped reads in the "transcriptome only" mapping mode. A uniquely mapped read could be classified into four categories (Figure 1C) with respect to its corresponding mapping information without a gene model: (1) "Identical"—remaining mapped to the same genomic region; (2) "Alternative"—still uniquely mapped but differently; (3) "Multiple"—mapped to more locations; and (4) "Unmapped". The detailed evaluation results are summarized in Figure 4 (read length = 75 bp).

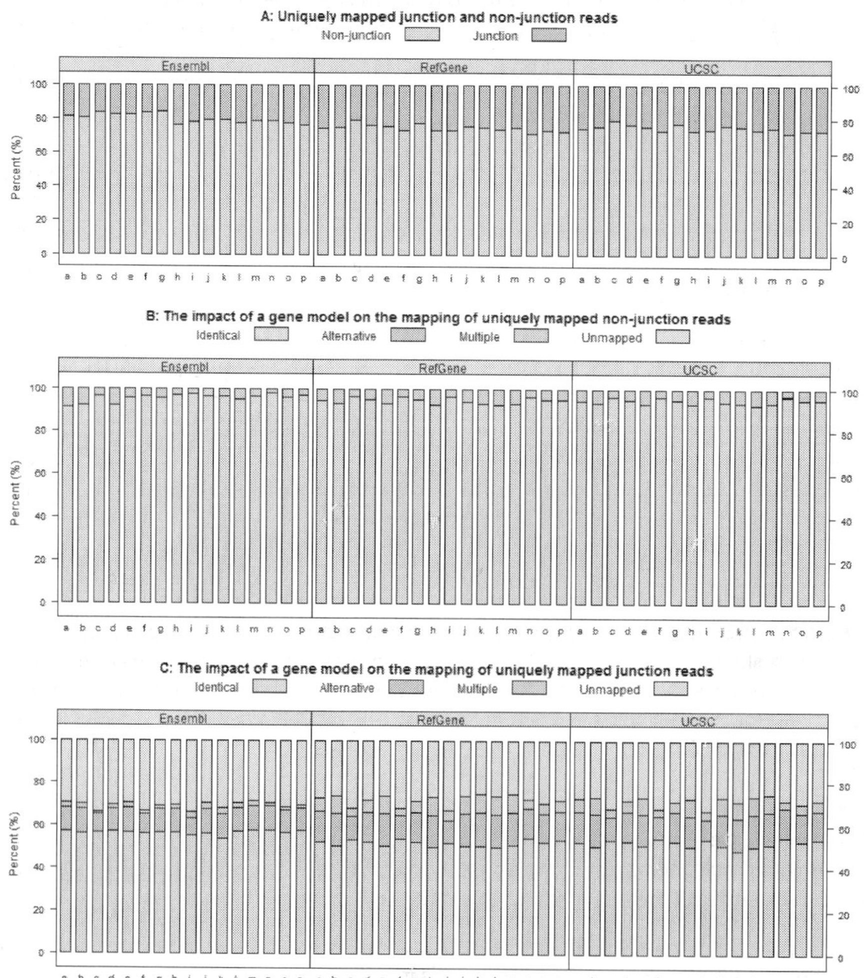

Figure 4. The impact of a gene model on RNA-Seq read mapping (read length = 75 bp). (A) Composition of mapped reads; (B) effect on mapping of non-junctions reads; (C) effect on mapping of junctions reads. (Note: The 16 tissue sample names are denoted as follows: a: adipose; b: adrenal, c: brain; d: breast; e: colon; f: heart; g: kidney; h: leukocyte; i: liver; j: lung; k: lymph node; l: ovary; m: prostate; n: skeletal muscle; o: testis; and p: thyroid.)

In Figure 4A, we divided uniquely mapped reads into two classes, i.e., non-junction reads and junction reads, and investigated the impact of a gene model on their mapping. Accordingly to Figure 4A, approximately 23% of mapped reads were junction reads, and the remaining 77% were non-junction reads. For non-junction reads (see Figure 4B), 95% remained mapped to exactly the same genomic location regardless of the use of a gene model. Without a gene model,

3% to 9% of non-junctions reads became multiple mapped reads. However, it is very rare for a non-junction read to become unmapped or alternatively mapped. In contrast, the mapping of junction reads was strongly impacted by the gene models (see Figure 4C). Without using a gene model, an average of 53% of junction reads remained mapped to the same genomic regions, 30% failed to map to any genomic region, and 10–15% of them mapped alternatively. Such alternative mappings are generally inferior compared to their corresponding mapping results using a gene model [29]. Similar to non-junction reads, an average of 5% of junction reads were mapped to more than one location without using a gene model. As shown in Figure 4C, more uniquely-mapped junction reads became multiple mapped reads in RefGene and/or UCSC than in Ensembl when the sequence reads were aligned to the reference genome without the use of gene models.

As we demonstrated, a gene model mainly affects the alignment of junction reads, but has little impact on non-junction reads. On average, 23% of reads in our samples were junction reads, and usually about one third of them failed to be mapped without the use of a gene model. Therefore, it is expected that when the read length is 75 bp, ~6% (23% * 0.33) of the mapped reads become unmapped without the use of a gene model. The percentage is expected to be higher when the read length is longer since a long read is more likely to span two or more exons.

3.3. The splicing patterns for "Identical", "Alternative", and "Unmapped" reads

As concluded above, a reference transcriptome mainly affects the mapping of junction reads. One interesting question is what kind of junction reads tend to be mapped identically, alternatively, or unmapped. In order to characterize the splicing patterns, we focus on only two-exon junction reads that are uniquely mapped when the RefGene annotation is used. For every junction read, we calculate the number of overlapping nucleotide bases with its left exon (OL) and right exons (OR), respectively. Then the minimum of OL and OR is chosen for histogram analysis (Figure 5). Only the results for lung, liver, kidney, and heart samples are shown in Figure 5, and for the rest of 12 samples, the patterns were very similar to those in Figure 5 (data not shown). Since the full read length is 75 bp long, the MOE (Minimum Overlap with an Exon, MOE = min(OL,OR)) ranges from 1 to 37 for any junction read.

For "Identical" junction reads, the typical MOE ranges from 15 to 37, and the frequency drops to nearly 0 when MOE is less than 10 (left panels in Figure 5). For "Alternative" junction reads, the most dominant MOE is 1 (middle panels in Figure 5), representing an average of one-third of cases. In general, those "Alternative" reads have very small MOE. For those junction reads with MOE of 1, 2, and 3, it is virtually impossible to map them 'correctly' without the prior knowledge on transcripts. The MOE for "Unmapped" reads has a much broader range with peaks from 4 to 12 (right panels in Figure 5). In order to map a junction read without a reference transcriptome, the read should have sufficient overlaps with exons at both ends. The majority of "Identical" reads meet this requirement (left panels in Figure 5). However, if the overlap with one end is too short, let's say 1 or 2 nucleotide bases, this read will be more likely mapped to only a single exon with the remaining couple of bases mapping to the intron region adjacent to that exon (middle panels in Figure 5). Otherwise, such junction reads become either unmapped or mapped to different genomic regions as non-junction reads if the overlap is something between (right panels in Figure 5).

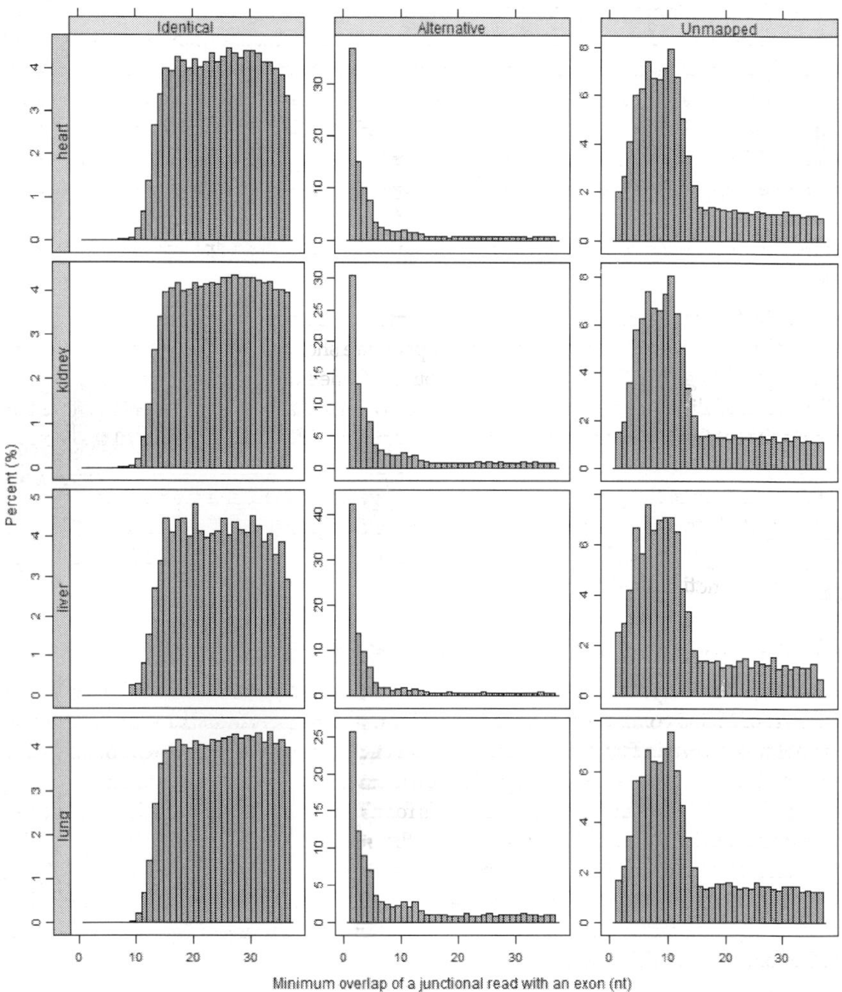

Figure 5. The splicing patterns and distribution of MOE (Minimum Overlap with an Exon) for junction reads. The typical MOE for "Identical" junction reads ranges from 15 to 37. For "Alternative" junction reads, the most dominant MOE is 1, representing an average of one-third of cases. In contrast, the MOE for "Unmapped" reads has a much broader range with peaks from 4 to 12. Note the scale for y-axis is not uniform.

3.4. Comparison of the mappings of "Alternative" reads

Since "Alternative" reads remain mapped but differently, we are more interested in the mapping difference in detail and the main reasons for alternative mapping. A typical example of "Alternative" reads is shown in Figure 6, in which 19 unique junction reads are nearly perfectly mapped to gene HSP90AB1 when RefGene is used in the mapping step. Without a reference transcriptome, four junction reads indicated by the red arrow remain mapped to the same gene HSP90AB1 but as non-junction reads with mismatches at one end. A few bases previously mapped to another exon are now mapped to the intron region. The remaining 15 junction reads are aligned to pseudogene gene HSP90AP3P as non-junction reads instead. The comparison reveals that the original mappings to HSP90AB1 for those 15 reads are nearly perfect, while they all have more mismatches when mapped to HSP90AP3P. Clearly, the alternative mapping for those junction reads in Figure 6 is getting worse without a reference transcriptome. In a sense, those 15 junction reads indicated by the blue arrow in Figure 6A are "forced" to be mapped to a different genomic region without the help of reference transcriptome.

"Alternative" junction reads are also likely to remain mapped to the same start and end positions but spliced differently. Two cases in point are shown in Figure 7. For those junction reads mapped to gene TCEA3 with and without RefGene model, both mappings are equally well in terms of alignment scores and gaps between exons. So there is no way to tell which one is right without the assistance of reference transcriptome. Likewise, the mappings of junction reads in gene FBXL3 are also equally well regardless of the usage of RefGene model. Despite the minor difference in splicing sites, the read mapped with RefGene model is considered as fully compatible to a known gene, and thus is counted in gene quantification. Collectively, the examples in Figure 6 and 7 illustrate the important role of a gene annotation in proper alignment of junction reads.

3.5. The impact of gene model choice on gene quantification

To investigate the impact of different gene models on gene quantification results, we focused on the set of 21,598 common genes (Figure 3). The overall correlation between RefGene and Ensembl was shown in Figure 8. Both x and y-axes represented log2(count+1). For all genes, 1 was added to the counts to avoid a logarithmic error for those genes with zero counts. Ideally, we should get identical counts of mapped reads for all common genes, regardless of the choice of a gene model; however, this was clearly not the case. Although the majority of genes had highly consistent or nearly identical expression levels, there were a significant number of genes whose quantification results were dramatically affected by the choice of a gene model. As shown in Figure 8, there were many genes for which the number of reads mapped to them was 0 in one gene model, but many in others.

To quantify the concordance between RefGene and Ensembl annotations, we first calculated the ratio of mapped read for each gene. For a given gene, we defined the raw read counts in RefGene and Ensembl annotations as #C1 and #C2, respectively. To prevent division by 0, 1 was added to all raw read counts before the ratios were calculated. The adjusted counts were denoted as #C1' (=#C1+1) and #C2' (=#C2+1), respectively. The ratio was calculated as

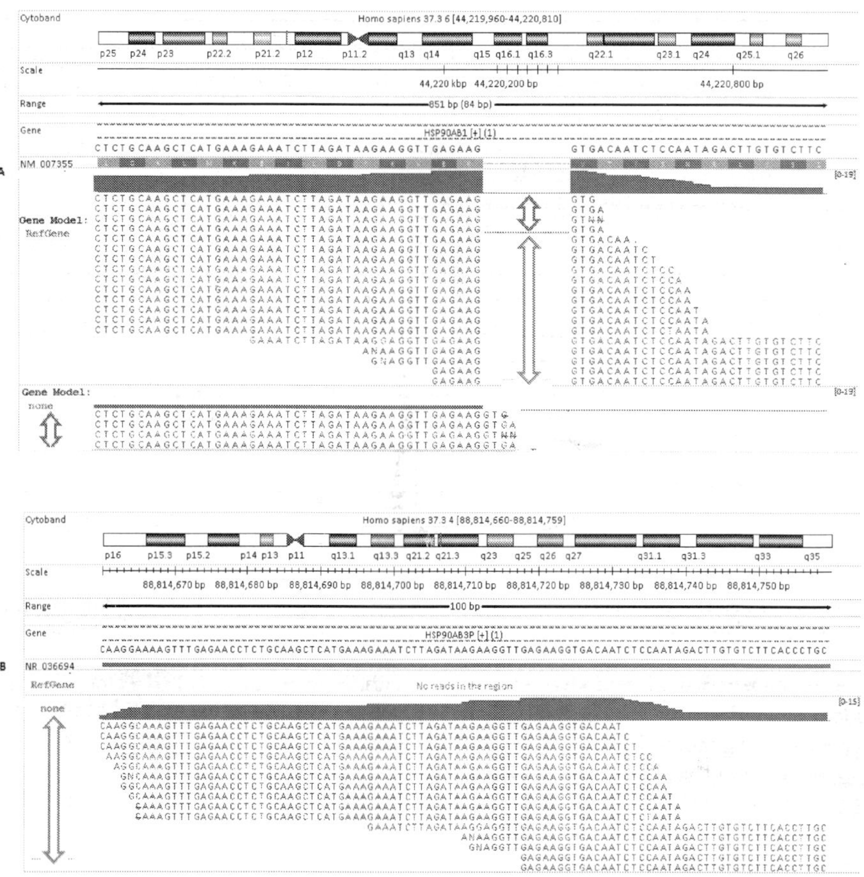

Figure 6. The impact of a reference transcripotome on the mapping of junction reads in gene HSP90AB1. (A) When RefGene is used, 19 unique junction reads are mapped to gene HSP90AB1 nearly perfectly. Four junction reads become non-junction ones with a few bases mapped to the intron region with mismatches without the usage of the RefGene model; (B) The remaining 15 reads (indicated by the blue arrow) are alternatively aligned to gene HSP90AP3P as non-junction reads without the assistance of RefGene annotation. Note the reads colored in blue are mapped to "+" strand, and colored in green when mapped to "-" strand. The mismatched nucleotide bases are colored in red.

Max(#C1′,#C2′)/Min(#C1′,#C2′). Therefore the calculated ratio was always equal or greater than 1. The distribution of ratios was summarized in Table 1 (read length = 75 bp). Among the 21,958 common genes, about 20% of genes had no expression at all in both annotations. Identical counts were obtained for only 16.3% of genes. Approximately 28.1% of genes' expression levels differed by 5% or higher, and among them, 9.3% of genes (equivalent to 2,038) differed by 50% or greater. As shown in Table 1 and Figure 8, the choice of a gene model had a large impact on gene quantification. Compared with Ensembl, UCSC had a much better

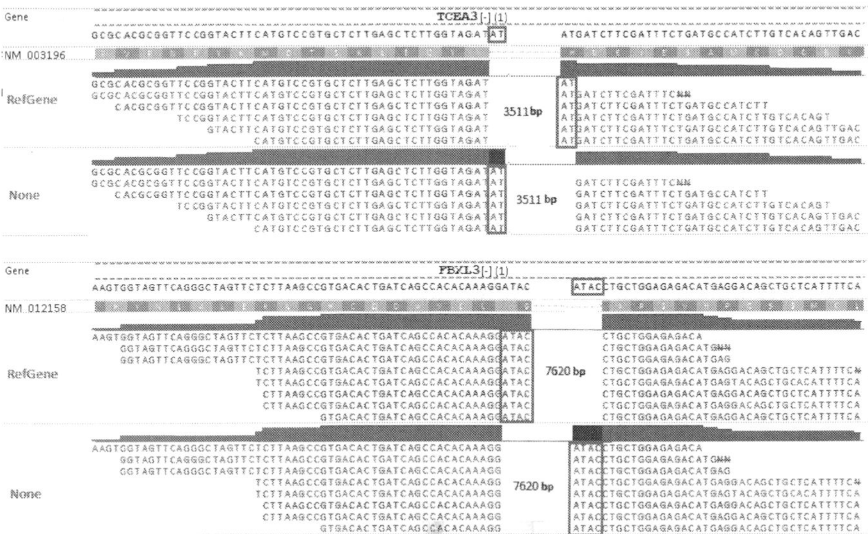

Figure 7. Alternative splicing with and without the use of RefGene annotation. All junction reads are still mapped to the same gene with the same start/end positions and intron size regardless of gene model, but are spliced differently.

concordance with RefGene, in terms of the gene quantification results [30]. 38.3% of genes had identical read counts, much higher than the 16.3% between Ensembl and RefGene. The percentage of genes with expression levels differing by 5% or more was only 11.3%, which was much less than the corresponding 28% between Ensembl and RefGene. Furthermore, only 3.24% of genes differed by 50% or greater, which was lower than the 9.3% between Ensembl and RefGene.

Why does the choice of a gene model have so dramatic an effect on gene quantification? If the gene definition is the same among different annotations, we expect the identical number of reads mapped to a given gene. Unfortunately, the gene definition varies from annotation to annotationm and can differ singnificantly for some genes. PIK3CA is a good example. The PIK3CA gene definition in both Ensembl and RefGene, and the mapping profile of RNA-seq reads were shown in Figure 9. In the liver sample, there were 1,094 reads mapped to PIK3CA in Ensembl annotation, while only 492 reads were mapped in RefGene. Clearly, the big difference in gene definition gives rise to the observed discrepancy in quantification. In Ensembl, there are three isoforms for PIK3CA, and the longest isoform is ENST00000263967. The total length of this transcript is 9,653 bp, comprising 21 exons, with a very long exon #21 (6,000 bp, chr3: 178,951,882-178,957,881). In RefGene, PIK3CA has only one transcript named NM_006218. This transcript is 3,909 bp long with a very short exon #21 (only 616 bp, located at chr 3:178,951,882-178,952,497). The definition of the PIK3CA gene in Ensembl seems more accurate than the one in RefGene, based upon the mapping profile of the sequence reads.

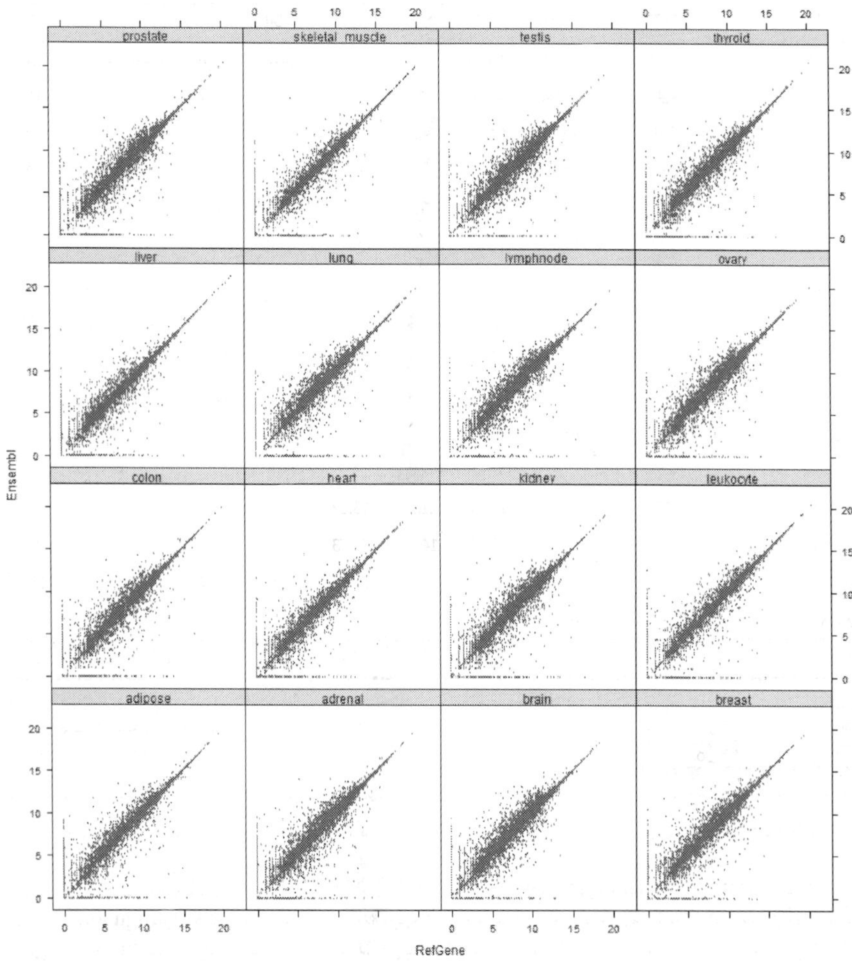

Figure 8. The correlation of gene quantification results between RefGene and Ensembl. Note both x and y-axes represent Log2(count + 1).

3.6. The effect of gene models on differential analysis

Generally, RNA-seq differential analysis requires biological replicates. However, we analyzed 16 different single tissue samples. To demonstrate the effect of gene models on differential analysis, the fold changes between heart and liver samples were calculated using RefGene and Ensembl annotations. The correlation of the calculated Log2Ratio (liver/heart) was depicted in Figure 10. The graph should show a perfect diagonal line if the choice of a gene model has no effect on differential analysis. Although the majority of genes have highly consistent or

Sample	No Expr	Same	1.05	1.10	1.20	1.50	2	5	10	100
adipose	19.97	16.53	26.16	19.64	14.51	8.81	5.65	1.96	0.94	0.16
adrenal	16.92	14.04	36.18	27.09	19.07	11.28	7.14	2.45	1.24	0.24
brain	16.79	15.22	32.94	24.91	17.95	10.78	6.73	2.29	1.08	0.20
breast	18.04	15.22	29.63	22.21	16.06	9.80	6.52	2.38	1.19	0.20
colon	20.50	17.41	25.85	19.43	14.30	8.95	6.10	2.30	1.17	0.19
heart	21.23	16.43	26.39	20.10	14.39	8.88	5.47	1.73	0.82	0.19
kidney	18.86	16.08	28.88	21.50	15.51	9.55	6.40	2.55	1.30	0.26
leukocyte	29.53	17.37	20.03	15.29	11.62	7.58	5.37	2.47	1.33	0.26
liver	24.60	19.16	23.20	17.43	12.84	8.24	5.42	2.00	1.02	0.15
lung	19.65	16.46	29.22	21.35	15.07	9.09	6.15	2.61	1.43	0.24
lymph node	20.94	16.79	31.74	24.16	17.21	10.26	6.65	2.69	1.44	0.24
ovary	16.90	13.42	31.46	23.30	16.72	10.23	6.63	2.31	1.13	0.20
prostate	18.21	16.29	28.33	21.14	15.17	9.43	6.51	2.49	1.27	0.23
skeletal muscle	29.60	23.48	18.65	14.40	10.73	6.88	4.81	2.34	1.39	0.21
testis	10.15	13.35	31.35	22.57	15.84	9.35	5.92	2.08	1.05	0.28
thyroid	17.41	14.25	30.08	22.23	15.88	9.39	5.88	1.97	1.03	0.24
Average	19.96	16.34	28.13	21.05	15.18	9.28	6.09	2.29	1.18	0.22

Note: Column "No Expr" represents the percentage of genes that do not express at all in both annotations. Column "Same" denotes the percentage of genes that have the same number of reads mapped to them in both gene models. The number in each cell after the column "Same" corresponds to the percentage of genes whose ratio is equal or greater than the threshold represented by the number.

Table 1. The distribution of the ratio of read counts between RefGene and Ensembl annotations (read length = 75 bp).

comparable expression changes, there are a number of genes whose ratios are dramatically affected by the choice of a gene model. Interestingly, some genes have a very high fold change in one gene model, but no change at all in another gene model. Evidently, the choice of a gene model has an effect on the downstream differential expression analysis, in addition to gene quantification.

4. Discussions

4.1. The effect of a gene model on read mapping is read length dependent

We performed the same analyses of the dataset with a 50-bp read length, and the results were detailed in [30]. Intuitively, the shorter a read, the more likely it is to map to multiple locations. As a result, the percentage of uniquely mapped reads decreases, and the percentage of

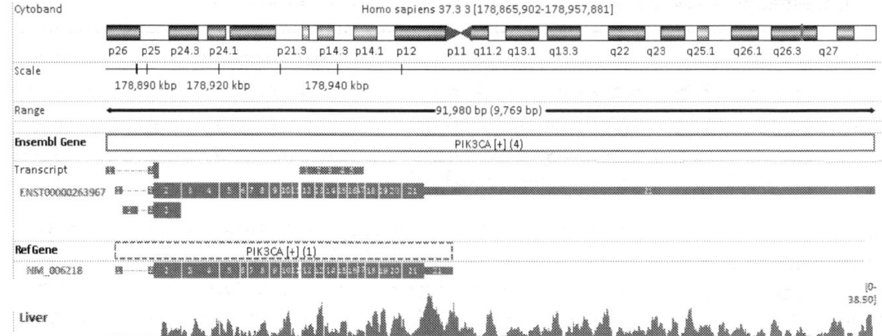

Figure 9. The different gene definitions for PIK3CA give rise to differences in gene quantification. PIK3CA in the Ensembl annotation is much longer than its definition in RefGene, explaining why there are 1,094 reads mapped to PIK3CA in Ensembl, while only 492 reads are mapped in RefGene.

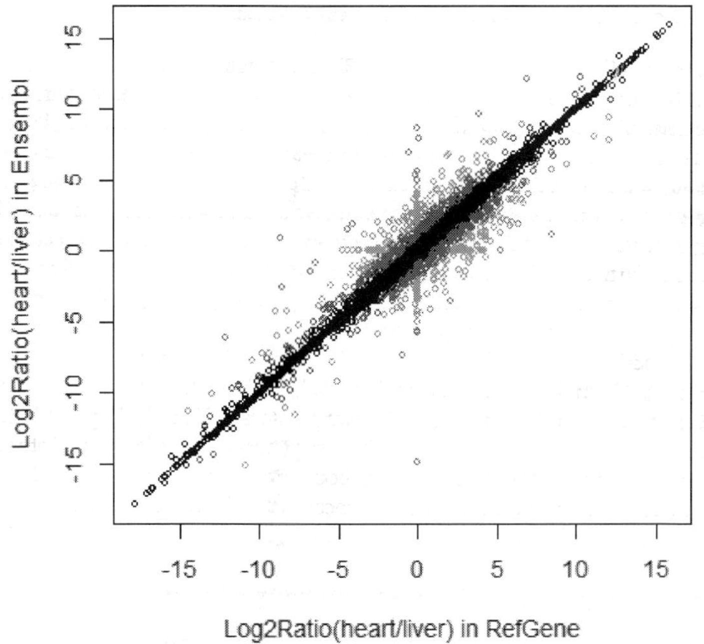

Figure 10. The correlation of the calculated Log2Ratio (heart/liver) between RefGene and Ensembl. The green, blue, and red points indicate corresponding absolute difference between the two Log2Ratios that were greater than 1, 2, or 5, respectively. Although the majority of genes have highly consistent expression changes, there are many genes that are remarkably affected by the choice of different gene models.

multiple-mapping reads increases. No matter which gene model was used in the mapping step, this observation held true. Thus, the mapping fidelity for a sequence read increases with its length, and this is especially true for junction reads. As demonstrated in Figure 4, when the read length was 75 bp, an average of 53% of junction reads remained mapped to the same genomic regions no matter whether a gene annotation was used. However, this percentage dropped to 42% when the read length was 50 bp long [30]. Thus, the effect of a gene model on the mapping of junction reads is significantly influenced by read length.

In the meantime, the relative abundance of junction reads is heavily determined by read length as well. According to Figure 4, on average, roughly 23% of sequence reads were junction reads when the read length was 75 bp. This percentage dropped to 16% when the read length was 50 bp [30]. This is explained by the fact that the longer the read, the more likely that it spans more than one exon. As sequencing technology evolves, the read length will become longer and longer. Consequently, more junction reads will be generated by short-gun sequencing technologies. Therefore, the need to incorporate genome annotation in the read mapping process will greatly increase.

4.2. The incompleteness and inaccuracy in gene annotation

Pyrkosz et al. [31] have explored the issue of "RNA-Seq mapping errors when using incomplete reference transcriptome" in detail. They used simulated reads generated from real transcriptomes to determine the accuracy of read mapping, and measured the error resulting from using an incomplete transcriptome. When 10% increments of the chicken reference transcriptome are missing, the true positive rate decreases by approximately 6–8%, while the false positive rate remains relatively constant until the reference is more than 50% incomplete. The number of false positives grows as the reference becomes increasingly incomplete. For model organisms such as human and mouse, their transcriptome models are relatively more complete compared to non-model organisms. Admittedly, RefGene, UCSC, and Ensembl are all not 100% complete and accurate, though the qualities in their annotations are constantly improving. For transcriptome-guided mapping of RNA-Seq reads, the more complete and accurate the transcriptome, the better. In addition, Seok et al. [32] have demonstrated that incorporating transcript annotations from reference transcriptome significantly improved the de novo reconstruction of novel transcripts from short sequencing reads for transcriptome research. The prior knowledge helped to define exon boundaries and fill in the transcript regions not covered by sequencing data. As a result, the reconstructed transcripts were much longer than those from de novo approaches that assume no prior knowledge.

4.3. The impact of gene annotation on variant effect prediction

The choice of a gene annotation has a big impact not only on RNA-seq data analysis, but also on variant effect prediction [33–34]. Variant annotation is a crucial step in the analysis of genome sequencing data. Functional annotation results can have a strong influence on the ultimate conclusions of disease studies. Incorrect or incomplete annotations can cause researchers both to overlook potentially disease-relevant DNA variants and to dilute interesting variants in a pool of false positives.

McCarthy et al. [33] recently used the software ANNOVAR [35] to quantify the extent of differences in annotation of 80 million variants from a whole-genome sequencing study with the RefSeq and Ensembl transcript sets as the basis for variant annotation. They demonstrated the large differences in prediction of loss-of-function (LoF) variation when RefSeq and Ensembl transcripts are used for annotation, highlighting the importance of the reference transcripts on which variant functional annotation is based. Choice of transcript set can have a large effect on the ultimate variant annotations obtained in a whole-genome sequencing study.

Frankish et al. [34] performed a detailed analysis of the similarities and differences between the gene and transcript annotation in the Gencode (v21) and RefSeq (Release 67) genesets in order to identify the similarities and differences between the transcripts, exons and the CDSs they encode. They demonstrated that the Gencode Comprehensive set is richer in alternative splicing, novel CDSs, and novel exons and has higher genomic coverage than RefSeq, while the Gencode Basic set is very similar to RefSeq. They presented evidence that the reference transcripts selected for variant functional annotation do have a large effect on variant annotation.

4.4. Which genome annotation to choose for gene quantification?

In practice, there is no simple answer to this question, and it depends on the purpose of the analysis. In this chapter, we compared the gene quantification results when RefGene and Ensembl annotations were used. Among 21,958 common genes, the expressions of 2,038 genes (i.e., 9.3%) differed by 50% or more when choosing one annotation over the other. Such a large difference frequently results from the gene definition differences in the annotations. Some genes with the same HUGO symbol in different gene models can be defined as completely different genomic regions. When choosing an annotation database, researchers should keep in mind that no annotation is perfect and some gene annotations might be inaccurate or entirely wrong.

Wu et al. [27] suggested that when conducting research that emphasizes reproducible and robust gene expression estimates, a less complex genome annotation, such as RefGene, might be preferred. When conducting more exploratory research, a more complex genome annotation, such as Ensembl, should be chosen. Based upon our experience of RNA-seq data analysis, we recommend using RefGene annotation if RNA-seq is used as a replacement for a microarray in transcriptome profiling. For human samples, Affymetrix GeneChip HT HG-U133+ PM arrays are one of the most popular microarray platforms for transcriptome profiling, and the genes covered by this chip overlap with RefGene very well, according to Zhao et al. [7]. Despite the fact that Ensembl R74 contains 63,677 annotated gene entries, only 22,810 entries (roughly one-third) correspond to protein coding genes. There are 17,057 entries representing various types of RNAs, including rRNA (566), snoRNA (1,549), snRNA (2,067), miRNA (3,361), misc_RNA (2,174), and lincRNA (7,340). There are 15,583 pseudogenes in Ensembl R74. For most RNA-seq sequencing projects, only mRNAs are presumably enriched and sequenced, and there is no point in mapping sequence reads to RNAs such as miRNAs or lincRNAs. Ensembl R74 contains 819 processed transcripts that were generated by reverse transcription of an mRNA transcript with subsequent reintegration of the cDNA into the genome, and are usually not actively expressed. In this scenario, a read truly originating from an active mRNA can be mapped to a processed transcript equally well or mapped to the processed transcript only, which is especially true for junction reads. Consequently, the true expression for the corresponding mRNA may be underestimated. Another downside of using a larger annotation database is calculation of adjusted P values, because the adjustment of the raw P value to allow for multiple testing is mainly determined by the number of genes in the model. If genes of interest are defined inconsistently across different annotations, it is recommended that an RNA-seq dataset is analyzed using different gene models.

5. Conclusions

RNA-seq has become increasingly popular in transcriptome profiling. Acquiring transcriptome expression profiles requires researchers to choose a genome annotation for RNA-seq data analysis. In this chapter, we assessed the impact of gene models on the mapping of junction and non-junction reads, characterized the splicing patterns for junction reads, and compared the impact of genome annotation choice on gene quantification and differential analysis. To fairly assess the impact of a gene model on RNA-seq read mapping, we devised a two-stage mapping protocol, in which sequence reads that could not be mapped to a reference transcriptome were filtered out, and the remaining reads were mapped to the reference genome with and without the use of a gene model in the mapping step. Our protocol ensured that only those reads compatible with a gene model were used to evaluate the role of a genome annotation in RNA-seq data analysis.

Ensembl annotates more genes than RefGene and UCSC. On average, 95% of non-junction reads were mapped to exactly the same genomic location without the use of a gene model. However, only an average of 53% junction reads remained mapped to the same genomic regions. About 30% of junction reads failed to be mapped without the assistance of a gene model, while 10–15% mapped alternatively. It is also demonstrated that the effect of a gene model on the mapping of sequence reads is significantly influenced by read length. The mapping fidelity for a sequence read increases with its length. When the read length was reduced from 75 bp to 50 bp, the percentage of junction reads that remained mapped to the same genomic regions dropped from 53% to 42% without the assistance of gene annotation.

There are 21,958 common genes among RefGene, Ensembl, and UCSC annotations. Using the dataset with the read length of 75 bp, we compared the gene quantification results in RefGene and Ensembl annotations, and obtained identical counts for an average of 16.3% (about one-sixth) of genes. Twenty percent of genes are not expressed, and thus have zero counts in both annotations. About 28.1% of genes showed expression levels that differed by 5% or higher; of these, the relative expression levels for 9.3% of genes (equivalent to 2,038) differed by 50% or greater. The case studies revealed that the difference in gene definitions caused the observed inconsistency in gene quantification.

In this chapter, we demonstrate that the choice of a gene model not only has a dramatic effect on both gene quantification and differential analysis, but also has a strong influence on variant effect prediction and functional annotation. Our research will help RNA-seq data analysts to make an informed choice of gene model in practical RNA-seq data analysis.

Author details

Shanrong Zhao* and Baohong Zhang

*Address all correspondence to: Shanrong.Zhao@pfizer.com

Clinical Genetics and Bioinformatics, Pfizer Worldwide Research & Development, Cambridge, MA, USA

References

[1] Mortazavi A, Williams BA, McCue K, Schaeffer L, Wold B. Mapping and quantifying mammalian transcriptomes by RNA-seq. Nat Methods. 2008;5(7):621-8.

[2] Wang Z, Gerstein M, Snyder M. RNA-seq: A revolutionary tool for transcriptomics. Nat Rev Genet. 2009; 10(1):57-63.

[3] Mutz KO, Heilkenbrinker A, Lönne M, Walter JG, Stahl F. Transcriptome analysis using next-generation sequencing. Curr Opin Biotechnol. 2013;24(1):22-30.

[4] McIntyre LM, Lopiano KK, Morse AM, Amin V, Oberg AL, et al. RNA-seq: technical variability and sampling. BMC Genomics. 2011;12:293.

[5] Hurd PJ, Nelson CJ. Advantages of next-generation sequencing versus the microarray in epigenetic research. Brief Funct Genomic Proteomic. 2009;8(3):174-83.

[6] Malone J, Oliver B. Microarrays, deep sequencing and the true measure of the transcriptome. BMC Biol. 2011;9:34.

[7] Zhao S, Fung-Leung W-P, Bittner A, Ngo K, Liu X. Comparison of RNA-seq and microarray in transcriptome profiling of activated T cells. PLoS One. 2014;9(1):e78644.

[8] GTEx Consortium. Human genomics. The Genotype-Tissue Expression (GTEx) pilot analysis: Multitissue gene regulation in humans. Science. 2015;348(6235):648-60.

[9] Melé M, Ferreira PG, Reverter F, DeLuca DS, Monlong J, Sammeth M, Young TR, et al. Human genomics. The human transcriptome across tissues and individuals. Science. 2015;348(6235):660-5.

[10] Garber M, Grabherr MG, Guttman M, Trapnell C. Computational methods for transcriptome annotation and quantification using RNA-seq. Nat Methods. 2011;8(6): 469-77.

[11] Engström PG, Steijger T, Sipos B, Grant GR, Kahles A, et al. Systematic evaluation of spliced alignment programs for RNA-seq data. Nat Methods. 2013;10(12):1185-91.

[12] Soneson C, Delorenzi M. A comparison of methods for differential expression analysis of RNA-seq data. BMC Bioinformatics. 2013;14:91.

[13] Borozan I, Watt SN, Ferretti V. Evaluation of alignment algorithms for discovery and identification of pathogens using RNA-seq. PLoS One. 2013;8(10):e76935.

[14] Anders S, Huber W. Differential expression analysis for sequence count data. Genome Biol. 2010;11(10):R106.

[15] Robinson MD, McCarthy DJ, Smyth GK. edgeR: A Bioconductor package for differential expression analysis of digital gene expression data. Bioinformatics. 2010;26(1): 139-40.

[16] Wu TD, Nacu S. Fast and SNP-tolerant detection of complex variants and splicing in short reads. Bioinformatics. 2010;26(7):873-81.

[17] Hu J, Ge H, Newman M, Liu K. OSA: A fast and accurate alignment tool for RNA-seq. Bioinformatics. 2012;28(14):1933-4.

[18] Dobin A, Davis CA, Schlesinger F, Drenkow J, Zaleski C, Jha S, et al. STAR: Ultrafast universal RNA-seq aligner. Bioinformatics. 2013;29(1):15-21.

[19] Wang K, Singh D, Zeng Z, Coleman SJ, Huang Y, Savich GL et al. MapSplice: Accurate mapping of RNA-seq reads for splice junction discovery. Nucleic Acids Res. 2010;38(18):e178.

[20] Kim D, Pertea G, Trapnell C, Pimentel H, Kelley R, Salzberg SL. TopHat2: Accurate alignment of transcriptomes in the presence of insertions, deletions and gene fusions. Genome Biol. 2013;14(4):R36.

[21] Pruitt KD, Tatusova T, Maglott DR. NCBI reference sequences (RefSeq): A curated non-redundant sequence database of genomes, transcripts and proteins. Nucleic Acids Res. 2007;35(Database):D61-5.

[22] Hsu F, Kent WJ, Clawson H, Kuhn RM, Diekhans M, Haussler D. The UCSC known genes. Bioinformatics. 2006;22(9):1036-46.

[23] Flicek P, Amode MR, Barrell D, Beal K, Billis K, Brent S, et al. Ensembl 2014. Nucleic Acids Res. 2014;42(Database issue):D749-55.

[24] Thierry-Mieg D, Thierry-Mieg J. AceView: A comprehensive cDNA-supported gene and transcripts annotation. Genome Biol. 2006;7 Suppl 1:1-14.

[25] Wilming LG, Gilbert JG, Howe K, Trevanion S, Hubbard T, Harrow JL. The vertebrate genome annotation (Vega) database. Nucleic Acids Res. 2008;36(Database):D753-60.

[26] Harrow J, Frankish A, Gonzalez JM, Tapanari E, Diekhans M, Kokocinski F, et al. GENCODE: The reference human genome annotation for the ENCODE project. Genome Res. 2012;22(9):1760-74.

[27] Wu P-Y, Phan JH, Wang MD. Assessing the impact of human genome annotation choice on RNA-seq expression estimates. BMC Bioinformatics. 2013;14 Suppl 11:S8.

[28] Chen G, Wang C, Shi L, Qu X, Chen J, Yang J, et al. Incorporating the human gene annotations in different databases significantly improved transcriptomic and genetic analyses. RNA. 2013;19(4):479-89.

[29] Zhao S. Assessment of the impact of using a reference transcriptome in mapping short RNA-seq reads. PLoS One. 2014;9(7):e101374.

[30] Zhao S, Zhang B. A comprehensive evaluation of ensembl, RefSeq, and UCSC annotations in the context of RNA-seq read mapping and gene quantification. BMC Genomics. 2015;16:97.

[31] Pyrkosz AB, Cheng H, Brown CT. RNA-Seq mapping errors when using incomplete reference transcriptomes of vertebrates. arXiv.org. 2013;arXiv:1303.2411v1.

[32] Seok J, Xu W, Jiang H, Davis RW, Xiao W. Knowledge-based reconstruction of mRNA transcripts with short sequencing reads for transcriptome research. PLoS ONE. 2012;7:e31440.

[33] McCarthy DJ, Humburg P, Kanapin A, Rivas MA, Gaulton K, Cazier JB, Donnelly P. Choice of transcripts and software has a large effect on variant annotation. Genome Med. 2014;6(3):26.

[34] Frankish A, Uszczynska B, Ritchie GR, Gonzalez JM, Pervouchine D, Petryszak R, et al. Comparison of GENCODE and RefSeq gene annotation and the impact of reference geneset on variant effect prediction. BMC Genomics. 2015;16 (Suppl 8):S2.

[35] Wang K, Li M, Hakonarson H. ANNOVAR: Functional annotation of genetic variants from high-throughput sequencing data. Nucleic Acids Res 2010;38:e164.

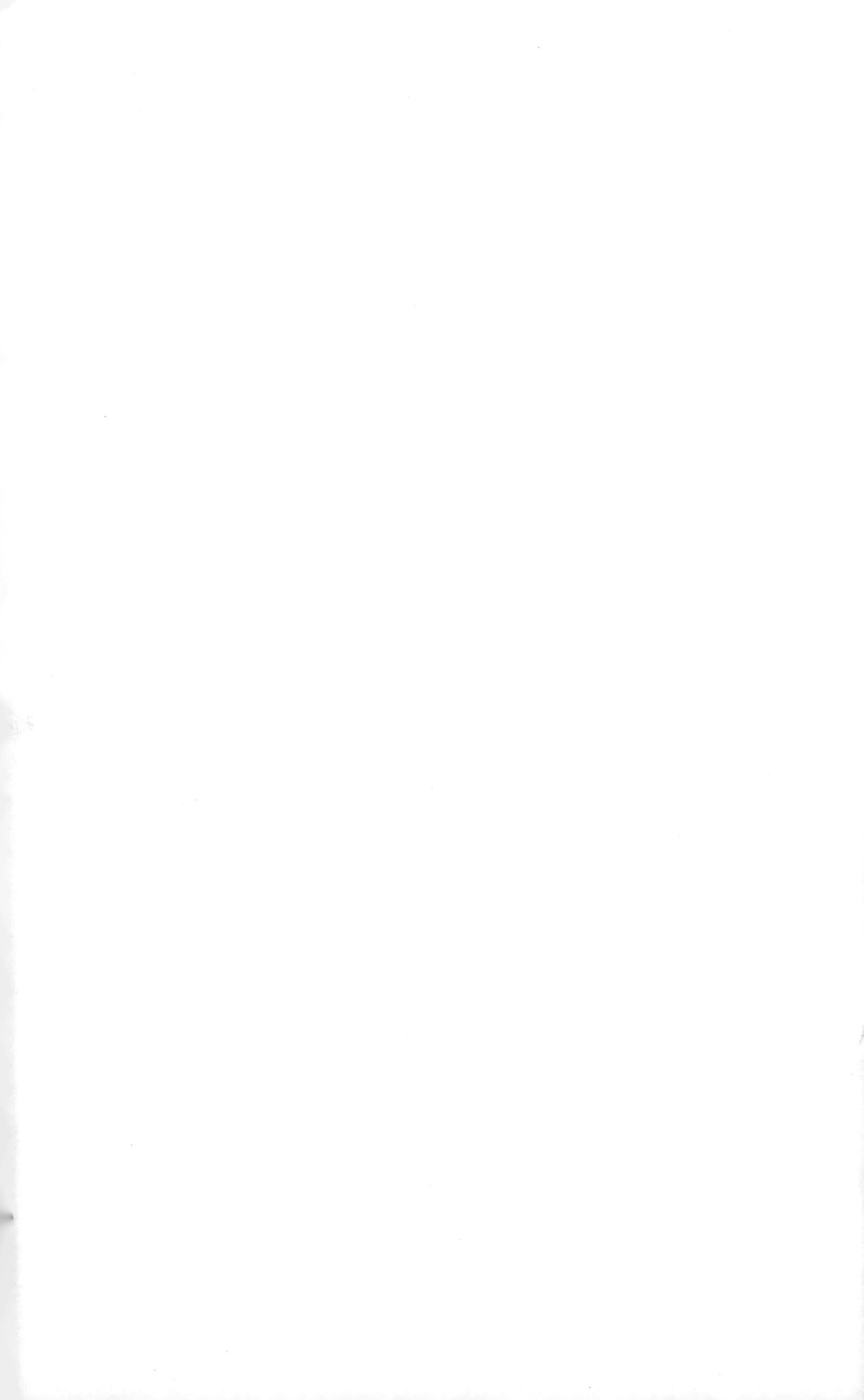